HEALTH AND HUMAN DEVELOPMENT

PUBLIC HEALTH YEARBOOK 2015

HEALTH AND HUMAN DEVELOPMENT
JOAV MERRICK - SERIES EDITOR –
NATIONAL INSTITUTE OF CHILD HEALTH AND HUMAN DEVELOPMENT, MINISTRY OF SOCIAL AFFAIRS, JERUSALEM, ISRAEL

Adolescent Behavior Research: International Perspectives
Joav Merrick and Hatim A Omar (Editors)
2007. ISBN: 1-60021-649-8

Complementary Medicine Systems: Comparison and Integration
Karl W Kratky
2008. ISBN: 978-1-60456-475-4

Pain in Children and Youth
P Schofield and J Merrick (Editors)
2008. ISBN: 978-1-60456-951-3

Alcohol-Related Cognitive Disorders: Research and Clinical Perspectives
Leo Sher, Isack Kandel and Joav Merrick (Editors)
2009. ISBN: 978-1-60741-730-9

Challenges in Adolescent Health: An Australian Perspective
David Bennett, Susan Towns and Elizabeth Elliott and Joav Merrick (Editors)
2009. ISBN: 978-1-60741-616-6

Children and Pain
P Schofield and J Merrick (Editors)
2009. ISBN: 978-1-60876-020-6

Living on the Edge: The Mythical, Spiritual, and Philosophical Roots of Social Marginality
Joseph Goodbread
2009. ISBN: 978-1-60741-162-8 (Hardcover)
2011. ISBN: 978-1-61470-192-7 (E-book)
2013. ISBN: 978-1-61122-986-8 (Softcover)

Obesity and Adolescence: A Public Health Concern
Hatim A Omar, Donald E Greydanus, Dilip R Patel and Joav Merrick (Editors)
2009. ISBN: 978-1-60692-821-9

Poverty and Children: A Public Health Concern
Alexis Lieberman and Joav Merrick (Editors)
2009. ISBN: 978-1-60741-140-6

Bone and Brain Metastases: Advances in Research and Treatment
Arjun Sahgal, Edward Chow and Joav Merrick (Editors)
2010. ISBN: 978-1-61668-365-8

Chance Action and Therapy: The Playful Way of Changing
Uri Wernik
2010. ISBN: 978-1-60876-393-1

International Aspects of Child Abuse and Neglect
Howard Dubowitz and Joav Merrick (Editors)
2010. ISBN: 978-1-61122-049-0

Advanced Cancer, Pain and Quality of Life
Edward Chow and Joav Merrick (Editors)
2011. ISBN: 978-1-61668-207-1

Advances in Environmental Health Effects of Toxigenic Mold and Mycotoxins
Ebere Cyril Anyanwu
2011. ISBN: 978-1-60741-953-2

**Alternative Medicine
Yearbook 2009**
Joav Merrick (Editor)
2011. ISBN: 978-1-61668-910-0

Behavioral Pediatrics, 3rd Edition
*Donald E Greydanus, Dilip R Patel,
Helen D Pratt and Joseph L Calles Jr.
(Editors)*
2011. ISBN: 978-1-60692-702-1

**Chance Action and Therapy:
The Playful Way of Changing**
Uri Wernik
2011. ISBN: 978-1-61122-987-5

**Child Health and Human Development
Yearbook 2009**
Joav Merrick (Editor)
2011. ISBN: 978-1-61668-912-4

Climate Change and Rural Child Health
*Erica Bell, Bastian M Seidel
and Joav Merrick (Editors)*
2011. ISBN: 978-1-61122-640-9

**Clinical Aspects of Psychopharmacology
in Childhood and Adolescence**
*DE Greydanus, JL Calles Jr.,
DP Patel, A Nazeer and J Merrick (Editors)*
2011. ISBN: 978-1-61122-135-0

**Drug Abuse in Hong Kong:
Development and Evaluation of
a Prevention Program**
*Daniel TL Shek, Rachel CF Sun
and Joav Merrick (Editors)*
2011. ISBN: 978-1-61324-491-3

**Environment, Mood Disorders
and Suicide**
*Teodor T Postolache
and Joav Merrick (Editors)*
2011. ISBN: 978-1-61668-505-8

**International Aspects of Child Abuse
and Neglect**
*Howard Dubowitz
and Joav Merrick (Editors)*
2011. ISBN: 978-1-60876-703-8

**Narratives and Meanings
of Migration**
Julia Mirsky
2011. ISBN: 978-1-61761-103-2

**Positive Youth Development:
Evaluation and Future Directions
in a Chinese Context**
*Daniel TL Shek, Hing Keung Ma
and Joav Merrick (Editors)*
2011. ISBN: 978-1-60876-830-1 (Hardcover)
2011. ISBN: 978-1-62100-175-1 (Softcover)

**Positive Youth Development:
Implementation of a Youth Program in
a Chinese Context**
*Daniel TL Shek, Hing Keung Ma
and Joav Merrick (Editors)*
2011. ISBN: 978-1-61668-230-9

**Principles of Holistic Psychiatry:
A Textbook on Holistic Medicine for
Mental Disorders**
Soren Ventegodt and Joav Merrick
2011. ISBN: 978-1-61761-940-3

Public Health Yearbook 2009
Joav Merrick (Editor)
2011. ISBN: 978-1-61668-911-7

**Randomized Clinical Trials and
Placebo: Can You Trust the Drugs Are
Working and Safe?**
Søren Ventegodt and Joav Merrick
2011. ISBN: 978-1-61470-151-4
(E-book)
2012. ISBN: 978-1-61470-067-8 (Hardcover)

Rural Child Health:
International Aspects
Erica Bell and Joav Merrick (Editors)
2011. ISBN: 978-1-60876-357-3

Rural Medical Education:
Practical Strategies
Erica Bell and Craig Zimitat
and Joav Merrick (Editors)
2011. ISBN: 978-1-61122-649-2

Self-Management and
the Health Care Consumer
Peter William Harvey
2011. ISBN: 978-1-61761-796-6

Sexology from a Holistic Point of View
Soren Ventegodt and Joav Merrick
2011. ISBN: 978-1-61761-859-8

Social and Cultural Psychiatry
Experience from the
Caribbean Region
Hari D Maharajh and Joav Merrick (Editors)
2011. ISBN: 978-1-61668-506-5

The Dance of Sleeping and Eating
among Adolescents: Normal and
Pathological Perspectives
Yael Latzer and Orna Tzischinsky (Editors)
2011. ISBN: 978-1-61209-710-7

Understanding Eating Disorders:
Integrating Culture,
Psychology and Biology
Yael Latzer, Joav Merrick
and Daniel Stein (Editors)
2011. ISBN: 978-1-61728-298-0 (Hardcover)
2011. ISBN: 978-1-61470-976-3 (Softcover)

Adolescence and Chronic Illness.
A Public Health Concern
Hatim Omar, Donald E Greydanus,
Dilip R Patel and Joav Merrick (Editors)
2012. ISBN: 978-1-60876-628-4

AIDS and Tuberculosis:
Public Health Aspects
Daniel Chemtob and Joav Merrick (Editors)
2012. ISBN: 978-1-62081-382-9

Alternative Medicine Yearbook 2010
Joav Merrick (Editor)
2012. ISBN: 978-1-62100-132-4

Alternative Medicine Research
Yearbook 2011
Joav Merrick (Editor)
2012. ISBN: 978-1-62081-476-5

Applied Public Health: Examining
Multifaceted Social or Ecological
Problems and Child Maltreatment
John R Lutzker and Joav Merrick (Editors)
2012. ISBN: 978-1-62081-356-0

Building Community Capacity:
Minority and Immigrant Populations
Rosemary M Caron and
Joav Merrick (Editors)
2012. ISBN: 978-1-62081-022-4

Building Community Capacity:
Skills and Principles
Rosemary M Caron and Joav Merrick
(Editors)
2012. ISBN 978-1-61209-331-4

Child and Adolescent
Health Yearbook 2009
Joav Merrick (Editor)
2012. ISBN: 978-1-61668-913-1

Child and Adolescent Health
Yearbook 2010
Joav Merrick (Editor)
2012. ISBN: 978-1-61209-788-6

Child Health and Human Development Yearbook 2010
Joav Merrick (Editor)
2012. ISBN: 8-1-61209-789-3

Conceptualizing Behavior in Health and Social Research: A Practical Guide to Data Analysis
Said Shahtahmasebi and Damon Berridge
2013. ISBN: 978-1-60876-383-2

Human Immunodeficiency Virus (HIV) Research: Social Science Aspects
Hugh Klein and Joav Merrick (Editors)
2012. ISBN: 978-1-62081-293-8

Our Search for Meaning in Life: Quality of Life Philosophy
Soren Ventegodt and Joav Merrick
2012. ISBN: 978-1-61470-494-2

Public Health Yearbook 2010
Joav Merrick (Editor)
2012. ISBN: 978-1-61209-971-2

Public Health Yearbook 2011
Joav Merrick (Editor)
2012. ISBN: 978-1-62081-433-8

Textbook on Evidence-Based Holistic Mind-Body Medicine: Basic Philosophy and Ethics of Traditional Hippocratic Medicine
Søren Ventegodt and Joav Merrick
ISBN: 978-1-62257-052-2

Textbook on Evidence-Based Holistic Mind-Body Medicine: Basic Principles of Healing in Traditional Hippocratic Medicine
Søren Ventegodt and Joav Merrick
2012. ISBN: 978-1-62257-094-2

Textbook on Evidence-Based Holistic Mind-Body Medicine: Healing the Mind in Traditional Hippocratic Medicine
Søren Ventegodt and Joav Merrick
2012. ISBN: 978-1-62257-112-3

Textbook on Evidence-Based Holistic Mind-Body Medicine: Holistic Practice of Traditional Hippocratic Medicine
Søren Ventegodt and Joav Merrick
2012. ISBN: 978-1-62257-105-5

Textbook on Evidence-Based Holistic Mind-Body Medicine: Research, Philosophy, Economy and Politics of Traditional Hippocratic Medicine
Søren Ventegodt and Joav Merrick
2012. ISBN: 978-1-62257-140-6

Textbook on Evidence-Based Holistic Mind-Body Medicine: Sexology and Traditional Hippocratic Medicine
Søren Ventegodt and Joav Merrick
2012. ISBN: 978-1-62257-130-7

The Astonishing Brain and Holistic Consciousness: Neuroscience and Vedanta Perspectives
Vinod D Deshmukh
2012. ISBN: 978-1-61324-295-7

Translational Research for Primary Healthcare
Erica Bell, Gert P Westert and Joav Merrick (Editors)
2012. ISBN: 978-1-61324-647-4

Treatment and Recovery of Eating Disorders
Daniel Stein and Yael Latzer (Editors)
2012. ISBN: 978-1-61470-259-7 (Hardcover)
2013. ISBN: 978-1-62808-248-7 (Softcover)

Adolescence and Sports
*Dilip R Patel, Donald E Greydanus,
Hatim Omar and Joav Merrick (Editors)*
2013. ISBN: 978-1-60876-702-1

**Advanced Cancer: Managing Symptoms
and Quality of Life**
*Natalie Pulenzas, Breanne Lechner,
Nemica Thavarajah, Edward Chow
and Joav Merrick (Editors)*
2013. ISBN: 978-1-62808-239-5

**Alternative Medicine Research
Yearbook 2012**
Søren Ventegodt and Joav Merrick (Editors)
2013. ISBN: 978-1-62808-080-3

**Building Community Capacity:
Case Examples from Around the World**
*Rosemary M Caron
and Joav Merrick (Editors)*
2013. ISBN: 978-1-62417-175-8

Bullying: A Public Health Concern
*Jorge C Srabstein
and Joav Merrick (Editors)*
2013. ISBN: 978-1-62618-564-7

Food, Nutrition and Eating Behavior
Joav Merrick and Sigal Israeli
2013. ISBN: 978-1-62948-233-0

**Health and Happiness from Meaningful
Work: Research in Quality of
Working Life**
*Soren Ventegodt and Joav Merrick
(Editors)*
2013. ISBN: 978-1-60692-820-2

**Health Promotion: Community Singing
as a Vehicle to Promote Health**
Joav Merrick (Editors)
2013. ISBN: 978-1-62618-908-9

**Health Promotion: Strengthening
Positive Health and Preventing Disease**
*Jing Sun, Nicholas Buys
and Joav Merrick (Editors)*
2013. ISBN: 978-1-62257-870-2

Health Risk Communication
Marijke Lemal and Joav Merrick (Editors)
2013. ISBN: 978-1-62257-544-2

**Human Development: Biology from a
Holistic Point of View**
*Søren Ventegodt, Tyge Dahl Hermansen and
Joav Merrick (Editors)*
2013. ISBN: 978-1-61470-441-6

Managed Care in a Public Setting
Richard Evan Steele
2013. ISBN: 978-1-62417-970-9

**Mental Health from an
International Perspective**
*Joav Merrick, Shoshana Aspler and
Mohammed Morad (Editors)*
2013. ISBN: 978-1-62948-519-5

Pain Management Yearbook 2011
Joav Merrick (Editor)
2013. ISBN: 978-1-62808-970-7

Pain Management Yearbook 2012
Joav Merrick (Editor)
2013. ISBN: 978-1-62808-973-8

**Pediatric and Adolescent Sexuality and
Gynecology: Principles for the Primary
Care Clinician**
*Hatim A Omar, Donald E Greydanus,
Artemis K Tsitsika, Dilip R Patel
and Joav Merrick (Editors)*
2013. ISBN: 978-1-60876-735-9

Public Health Concern: Smoking, Alcohol and Substance Use
Joav Merrick and Ariel Tenenbaum (Editors)
2013. ISBN: 978-1-62948-424-2

Public Health Yearbook 2012
Joav Merrick (Editor)
2013. ISBN: 978-1-62808-078-0

Alternative Medicine Research Yearbook 2013
Joav Merrick (Editor)
2014. ISBN: 978-1-63321-094-3

India: Health and Human Development Aspects
Joav Merrick (Editor)
2014. ISBN: 978-1-62948-784-7

Public Health: Improving Health via Inter-Professional Collaborations
Rosemary M. Caron
and Joav Merrick (Editors)
2014. ISBN: 978-1-63321-569-6

Public Health Yearbook 2013
Joav Merrick (Editor)
2014. ISBN: 978-1-63321-095-0

Suicide from a Public Health Perspective
Said Shahtahmasebi and Joav Merrick
2014. ISBN: 978-1-62948-536-2

Alternative Medicine Research Yearbook 2014
Joav Merrick (Editor)
2015. ISBN: 978-1-63482-161-2

Cancer: Bone Metastases, CNS Metastases and Pathological Fractures
Breanne Lechner, Ronald Chow, Natalie Pulenzas, Marko Popovic,
Na Zhang, Xiaojing Zhang,
Edward Chow and Joav Merrick (Editors)
2015. ISBN: 978-1-63483-949-5

Cancer: Pain and Symptom Management
Breanne Lechner, Ronald Chow,
Natalie Pulenzas, Marko Popovic,
Na Zhang, Xiaojing Zhang, Edward Chow
and Joav Merrick (Editors)
2015. ISBN: 978-1-63483-864-1

Cancer: Spinal Cord, Lung, Breast, Cervical, Prostate, Head and Neck Cancer
Breanne Lechner, Ronald Chow,
Natalie Pulenzas, Marko Popovic,
Na Zhang, Xiaojing Zhang, Edward Chow
and Joav Merrick (Editors)
2015. ISBN: 978-1-63483-904-4

Cancer: Survival, Quality of Life and Ethical Implications
Breanne Lechner, Ronald Chow,
Natalie Pulenzas, Marko Popovic,
Na Zhang, Xiaojing Zhang, Edward Chow
and Joav Merrick (Editors)
2015. ISBN: 978-1-63483-905-1

Forensic Psychiatry: A Public Health Perspective
Leo Sher and Joav Merrick (Editors)
2015. ISBN: 978-1-63483-339-4

Leadership and Service Learning Education: Holistic Development for Chinese University Students
Daniel TL Shek, Florence KY Wu
and Joav Merrick (Editors)
2015. ISBN: 978-1-63483-340-0

Mental and Holistic Health: Some International Perspectives
Joseph L. Calles Jr.,
Donald E Greydanus
and Joav Merrick (Editors)
2015. ISBN: 978-1-63483-589-3

Pain Management Yearbook 2014
Joav Merrick (Editor)
2015. ISBN: 978-1-63482-164-3

Public Health Yearbook 2014
Joav Merrick (Editor)
2015. ISBN: 978-1-63482-165-0

Cancer: Treatment, Decision Making and Quality of Life
Breanne Lechner, Ronald Chow, Natalie Pulenzas, Marko Popovic, Na Zhang, Xiaojing Zhang, Edward Chow and Joav Merrick (Editors)
2015. ISBN: 978-1-63483-863-4

Alternative Medicine Research Yearbook 2015
Joav Merrick (Editor)
2016. ISBN: 978-1-63484-511-3

Public Health Yearbook 2015
Joav Merrick (Editor)
2016. ISBN: 978-1-63484-514-4

HEALTH AND HUMAN DEVELOPMENT

PUBLIC HEALTH YEARBOOK 2015

JOAV MERRICK
EDITOR

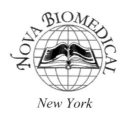

New York

Copyright © 2016 by Nova Science Publishers, Inc.

All rights reserved. No part of this book may be reproduced, stored in a retrieval system or transmitted in any form or by any means: electronic, electrostatic, magnetic, tape, mechanical photocopying, recording or otherwise without the written permission of the Publisher.

We have partnered with Copyright Clearance Center to make it easy for you to obtain permissions to reuse content from this publication. Simply navigate to this publication's page on Nova's website and locate the "Get Permission" button below the title description. This button is linked directly to the title's permission page on copyright.com. Alternatively, you can visit copyright.com and search by title, ISBN, or ISSN.

For further questions about using the service on copyright.com, please contact:
Copyright Clearance Center
Phone: +1-(978) 750-8400   Fax: +1-(978) 750-4470   E-mail: info@copyright.com.

NOTICE TO THE READER

The Publisher has taken reasonable care in the preparation of this book, but makes no expressed or implied warranty of any kind and assumes no responsibility for any errors or omissions. No liability is assumed for incidental or consequential damages in connection with or arising out of information contained in this book. The Publisher shall not be liable for any special, consequential, or exemplary damages resulting, in whole or in part, from the readers' use of, or reliance upon, this material. Any parts of this book based on government reports are so indicated and copyright is claimed for those parts to the extent applicable to compilations of such works.

Independent verification should be sought for any data, advice or recommendations contained in this book. In addition, no responsibility is assumed by the publisher for any injury and/or damage to persons or property arising from any methods, products, instructions, ideas or otherwise contained in this publication.

This publication is designed to provide accurate and authoritative information with regard to the subject matter covered herein. It is sold with the clear understanding that the Publisher is not engaged in rendering legal or any other professional services. If legal or any other expert assistance is required, the services of a competent person should be sought. FROM A DECLARATION OF PARTICIPANTS JOINTLY ADOPTED BY A COMMITTEE OF THE AMERICAN BAR ASSOCIATION AND A COMMITTEE OF PUBLISHERS.

Additional color graphics may be available in the e-book version of this book.

Library of Congress Cataloging-in-Publication Data

ISBN: 978-1-63484-514-4

Published by Nova Science Publishers, Inc. † New York

CONTENTS

Introduction   Ebola, public health and diverse cultures   xv
Cecilia S Obeng, Samuel Obeng and Joav Merrick

Section One - Inter-professional collaborations in improving health   1

Chapter 1   An inter-governmental approach to childhood obesity in Chicago, Illinois   3
Christine Bozlak, Adam Becker, Jennifer Herd, Andrew Teitelman, Judah Viola, Bradley Olson and Bechara Choucair

Chapter 2   Collaborative efforts towards an interdisciplinary and interprofessional dual degree program for public health training in a new rural medical school   15
Mark V White, Olapeju M Simoyan, Alberto JF Cardelle, Steven Godin, Elizabeth C Kuchinski, Erica L Townsend and Janet M Townsend

Chapter 3   Establishing partnerships between public health and academic partners to address infant mortality   27
Jennifer Mooney, Farrah Jacquez and William Scott

Chapter 4   Effect of a financial education program on the health of single, low-income women and their children   39
Kathleen A Packard, Julie C Kalkowski, Nicole D White, Ann M Ryan-Haddad, Lisa L Black, Kathleen A Flecky, Jennifer A Furze, Lorraine M Rusch and Yongyue Qi

Chapter 5   A novel financial education program for single women of low-income and their children   53
Nicole White, Kathleen Packard, Julie Kalkowski, Ann Ryan-Haddad, Kathy Flecky, Jennifer Furze, Lori Rusch and Lisa Black

Chapter 6	Utilization of peer teen advocates to increase awareness of human papillomavirus and vaccination among urban youth *Denise Uyar, Staci Young, Sarah Tyree-Francis and Mary Ann Kiepczynski*	63
Chapter 7	Innovations in continuing professional education: A model to impact interprofessional collaboration *Linda J Mast, Ateequr Rahman, Bard I Schatzman, Diane Bridges and Neil Horsley*	73
Chapter 8	*Community Wise*: A formative evaluation of a community-based health intervention *Liliane Cambraia Windsor, Lauren Jessell, Teri Lassiter, and Ellen Benoit*	89
Chapter 9	The promising potential role of sustainable development and conservation related bridging organizations in promoting health *Paivi Abernethy*	105
Chapter 10	The Lutiisi Academy Primary School: Using community-centered design as a catalyst for change *Peter J Ellery, Jane Ellery, John Motloch and Martha Hunt*	121
Chapter 11	Using concept mapping to mobilize a black faith community to address HIV *Magdalena Szaflarski, Lisa M Vaughn, Daniel McLinden, Yolanda Wess and Andrew Ruffner*	135
Chapter 12	Building interprofessional cultural competence: Reflections of faculty engaged in training students to care for the vulnerable *Joy Doll, Ann Ryan Haddad, Ann Laughlin, Martha Todd, Katie Packard, Jennifer Yee, Barbara Harris and Kimberly Begley*	153
Chapter 13	Building a co-created citizen science program with gardeners neighboring a superfund site: The gardenroots case study *Monica D Ramirez-Andreotta, Mark L Brusseau, Janick Artiola, Raina M Maier and A Jay Gandolfi*	163
Chapter 14	Community-engaged research and homeless adolescents: Capturing perceptions of health care and building lasting relationships with the community *Ricky T Munoz, Jeremy S Aragon and Mark D Fox*	181
Chapter 15	Bridge to care for refugee health: Lessons from an interprofessional collaboration in the Midwest *Ruth Margalit, Laura Vinson, Christine Ngaruiya, Kara Gehring, Pam Franks, Caci Schulte, Andrew Lemke, Joshua Blood, Tyler Irvine, Chelsea Souder, Deeko Hassan Andrea Langeveld, Carolyn Corn, Thu Hong Bui and Ann Marie Kudlacz*	191

Section Two - Substance abuse — 203

Chapter 16 Comorbidity and treatment in substance use disorders — 205
Brieana M Rowles, Aaron Ellington, Andrew R Tarr, John L Hertzer and Robert L Findling

Chapter 17 Substance abuse and adolescent girls — 221
Ruqiya Shama Tareen

Chapter 18 College students, prescription stimulant, and other substance abuse — 243
Brandon Johnson and Jeffrey H Newcorn

Chapter 19 Adolescent athletes and sports doping — 257
Dilip R Patel and Donald E Greydanus

Chapter 20 Teenage pregnancy: Prenatal drug exposure — 277
Colleen Dodich, Shalin Patel and Amanda Williams

Section Three - Public health issues — 293

Chapter 21 Measurements of social isolation and social support for rare lung disease patients: An integrative review — 295
Susan K Flavin

Chapter 22 Alcohol consumption in Russia during the past 50 years — 323
Sergei V Jargin

Chapter 23 Exercise culture among immigrants living in the Midwestern United States — 333
Goodwill Apiyo and Cecilia S Obeng

Chapter 24 Healthcare workers' breastfeeding practices and beliefs in Ghana — 343
Cecilia S Obeng and Donisha Reed

Chapter 25 Priapism in sickle cell disease: Need for imparting sex education in rural India — 349
Ranbir S Balgir

Chapter 26 Who do smokers feel ought to be responsible for informing people about the dangers associated with smoking and regulating smoking behaviors? — 359
Claire E Sterk, Hugh Klein and Kirk W Elifson

Chapter 27 Sero-prevalence of rubella-specific immunoglobulin G antibodies and its correlates among blood donors in Zambia — 381
Mazyanga L Mazaba-Liwewe, Mwaka Monze, Olusegun O Babaniyi, Seter Siziya, Dia Phiri, Joseph Mulenga and Charles Michelo

Chapter 28 Parents of children with autism: Issues surrounding childhood vaccination — 393
April M Young, Abigail Elliston and Lisa A Ruble

Section Four - Health and culture — 409

Chapter 29 — Immigrant college students' experiences with their American physicians — 411
Cecilia S Obeng, Roberta E Emetu and Sean Bowman

Chapter 30 — Food choices and eating patterns of international students in the United States: A phenomenological study — 419
Bobbie H Saccone and Cecilia S Obeng

Chapter 31 — Parents' strategies to increase physical activity among elementary-aged children in rural Indiana — 427
Sean M Bowman and Cecilia S Obeng

Chapter 32 — Oral health of immigrant African males in the United States — 433
Charity G Gichina and Cecilia S Obeng

Chapter 33 — The influence of religiosity on sexual behaviors: A qualitative study of young adults in the Midwest — 443
Jessica R Hauser and Cecilia S Obeng

Chapter 34 — Reflections of two-screen users: How people use information technology while watching sports — 453
Ryan P Vooris, Chase ML Smith and Cecilia S Obeng

Chapter 35 — Turkish immigrants' practices and perceptions of voluntary HIV testing and counseling in the United States — 461
Alper Kilic and Cecilia S Obeng

Chapter 36 — Significance of race in college athletics: Comparing mission statements across racial boundaries — 469
Chase ML Smith, Cecilia S Obeng and Gary A Sales

Chapter 37 — Encouraging Arab women to beat the cancer epidemic: An investigation into positive attributes that encourage Arab women to practice prevention methods for cancer — 487
Sara A Suhaibani and Cecilia S Obeng

Chapter 38 — Culture, health, and the use of household cleaning products by African women — 507
Nesrin Omer and Cecilia S Obeng

Section Five - Acknowledgments — 513

Chapter 39 — About the editor — 515

Chapter 40 — About the National Institute of Child Health and Human Development in Israel — 517

Section Six - Index — 521

Index — 523

Introduction
Ebola, public health and diverse cultures

Cecilia S Obeng[1,], PhD, Samuel Obeng[2], PhD, and Joav Merrick[3-7], MD, MMedSc, DMSc*

[1]School of Public Health
[2]African Studies Program and Linguistics Department, Indiana University, Bloomington, Indiana, United States of America
[3]National Institute of Child Health and Human Development, Jerusalem
[4]Office of the Medical Director, Health Services, Division for Intellectual and Developmental Disabilities, Ministry of Social Affairs and Social Services, Jerusalem
[5]Division of Pediatrics, Hadassah Hebrew University Medical Center, Mt Scopus Campus, Jerusalem, Israel
[6]Kentucky Children's Hospital, University of Kentucky College of Medicine, Lexington, Kentucky, United States of America
[7]Center for Healthy Development, School of Public Health, Georgia State University, Atlanta, United States of America

Introduction

In the 4th section of this Yearbook 2015, we have presented research on health issues in diverse cultures and especially at research around immigrants in the United States (US) from diverse backgrounds. Hispanic and Asian Americans make up the fastest growing sector of the US population and immigrants are often unable to access, seek, or receive health care due to barriers. Research and also clinical experience have found that recent immigrants who migrate to the US frequently experience a lack of access, high costs, and difficulty obtaining medical insurance along with barriers such as access to information, cultural or linguistic obstacles, and an inability to understand the healthcare system.

---

[*] Correspondence: Cecilia S Obeng, PhD, Associate Professor, Indiana University- School of Public Health, 1025 E 7th Street, SPH 116, Bloomington, IN 47405, United States. E-mail: cobeng@indiana.edu.

While we have worked on that research a new health concern emerged in West Africa, but it is slowly becoming a worldwide health issue of major proportions.

The Ebola virus, discovered in 1976, is one of the most lethal, contagious and poisonous pathogens, known to affect humans and such primate species as monkeys, gorillas, chimpanzees and macaques as well as fruit bats (1-5). It is a member of the filoviridae family of viruses and its morphology shows a typified long filamentous form making it unique in the world of viruses. Research indicates that the virus causes a raging disease that is characterized by severe fever that is accompanied by slow heart beats and hemorrhagic syndrome. The hemorrhagic fever occurs after an incubation period that varies between 2-21 days. Person-to-person transmission usually occurs after the incubation period. In its most severe form, the mortality rate associated with Ebola could reach up to 90% or even higher. Note that besides the hemorrhagic fever, patients may exhibit headache, chills, malaise (which may be extreme), and muscle pain of the torso and lower back (6).

On the African continent, there have been outbreaks of Ebola in the Democratic Republic of Congo, Uganda, and Gabon in the past. Current outbreak in West Africa has been in Nigeria and Senegal and more severely and on a larger scale in Guinea, Liberia, and Sierra Leone, where the toll on human life has been heavy and has led to panic in both West Africa, as well as in the United States and Western Europe due to international travel, but more especially due to the lack of understanding of the virus' biological morphology, the exact nature of how it functions in diseased individuals (especially the nature and type of changes it causes in patients), and its epidemiological status.

According to the World Health Organization (7), as reported by BBC African News, the current reported cases of Ebola infection and deaths reported by various Ministries of Health (and in the case of Guinea, by the French Embassy) in West Africa are:

Country	Source	Total Cases	Total Deaths
Liberia	WHO	4,249	2,458
Sierra Leone	MOH	3,412	1,200
Guinea	WHO	1,472	843
Nigeria	WHO	20	8
Senegal	WHO	1	0

Source: Ebola News Digest, October 14, 2014 (8).

The World Health Organization (7) notes further that Ebola is now entrenched in the capital cities (Monrovia, Conakry, and Free Town) of all three worst-affected countries Liberia, Guinea, and Sierra Leone respectively). The spread of the disease is said to be accelerating in almost all pockets of urban settlements (especially in slums), and in most domains of life. It is speculated that the spread could reach up to 10,000 per week in the worst affected areas if vaccines and other public health essentials are not put in place as a matter of urgency. So the numbers above is already outdated as we write.

EBOLA CAUSATION

An important aspect of Ebola causation has been linked to African food culture—that of depending, in some cases, on bush-meat for both nutritional sustenance and as an economic or financial resource via trading. In some rural areas in West Africa, the high cost of living has resulted in a situation where people depend solely on what they can get from their farms and from the forest. For such individuals, asking them not to depend on bush-meat is tantamount to forcing them to starve making such a suggestion unreasonable or inhumane. A way out of the crises could be through poverty reduction and gradual introduction to other sources of protein-rich nutrition that does not require dependence on bush-meat.

If it is indeed proven that humans get Ebola through our interaction with wildlife (either through living in close proximity to them, depending on them for nutrition and for financial sustenance, keeping them as pets without knowing what diseases they carry), then an obvious way to curtail the initiation and spread of such a deadly disease is to stop its pathogens' pathway or the 'viral traffic' from flowing either by limiting our interaction with such animals or co-existing with them without close co-habitation (9).

CO-HABITATION IN LARGE COMPOUND HOUSES

Another cultural practice that has led to the spread of Ebola in West Africa is the collectivist nature of West African societies which encourages compound housing with extended family members and tenants co-habiting and thus sharing rooms, eating from the same bowls or plates, sharing cups and other cooking utensils, as well as sharing toiletries, and clothing; a situation that easily leads to the transmission of bodily fluids. This cultural practice is exacerbated by abject poverty that reinforces and expands co-habitation and interdependence. With the possibility of up to 6 family members sharing a room, the extent of disease, especially infections and/or contagious diseases, spreading and getting out of hand becomes the norm rather than the exception.

DEATH AND BURIAL

In West African traditional religions, death does not mark the end of life; rather it is viewed as a transitional stage in life and requires lengthy rites of passage. The dead must be thoroughly washed (usually with bare hands using sponge and soap), dressed up in the deceased's best clothing, laid in state with hundreds of people coming close to it, and in most cases touching it, spending hours giving messages to the dead who are believed to be capable of transmitting such messages to other dead relatives of the living, among many other rituals. Given the 'power' of diseased individuals to act as links between people and their long dead relatives, corpses are literally venerated; to stay away from a corpse is to show disrespect toward the dead and people who do that are shunned and viewed as not properly socialized. In view of the close contact people come with the dead, it comes as no surprise, when infectious (especially deadly viral) diseases spread so quickly. In the current epidemic, even though corpses are cremated, some people feel it is a moral obligation to pay respects to the dead by observing proper funeral rites even if such practices may lead to some people contacting the disease. Thus, we see a clash between culture (the fear of a deceased coming back to haunt the living if not properly treated) and science (health) with each facet losing some of its crucial pathways.

BROKEN DOWN AND/OR LACK OF PUBLIC HEALTH INFRASTRUCTURE

The lack of adequate sanitation system, especially, the absence of sewerage infrastructure including running water, lack of disinfectants in public places of convenience, and its associated open defecation and urination in public places, creates fertile grounds for easy viral and bacterial transmission. The absence of simple and ordinary water to wash hands after using the toilet and the culture that encourages intensive socialization that is accompanied by handshakes, the holding of hands, and other forms of bodily contacts can all potentially worsen the Ebola outbreak. Associated with the above-mentioned factors is the irresponsible and sometimes ignorant ways in which refuse or garbage is disposed of and the ease with which women, children, and domestic animals come into contact with such refuse. Women are solely responsible for cleaning and transporting garbage to the dumpsite and it is common for children to play in such dumpsites making contact and contamination with virulent materials easy since no gloves or protective gears are worn by such individuals. The fact that some people search through dumped refuse for scraps also puts such people at risk of an infection. Poverty reduction, improved sewage system, proper hygiene, and cautions socialization can potentially mitigate or reduce the risk and spread of infection.

CREATING CULTURALLY CONGRUENT ISOLATION/QUARANTINE SYSTEM

In traditional African societies, people with infectious diseases self-isolated because of the support network that existed for isolated individuals. People with leprosy, for example, lived on the outskirts of the village and were provided with the most essential survival needs. Such camps were seen as necessary but temporary since there was the belief that recuperation was quicker and faster in such places. Also, public sympathy, empathy, and support for self-quarantined individuals were massive. In the current crises, especially in the urban areas, it is feared that people who are quarantined are stigmatized, even feared, and are therefore shunned and refused sufficient support. With such a situation it is not surprising that infected individuals are known to have left isolation places, mixed with the general population, and worsen the epidemic.

CONCLUSION

In sum, the fight against Ebola in West Africa can only be successful if attention is paid to the interconnectedness between the population's perception of the disease, their cultural practices relating to death, dying, and the treatment of corpses, their ecosystem (including their food culture, garbage disposal, and overall sanitation culture), their socialization methods, and their cultural practices and perceptions of isolation and human security.

It is essential for governments to provide essential information relating to the nature of the disease and the risks associated with it as well as create awareness through culturally congruent education and sensitization methods. West African governments must engage with community members and learn about their perceptions of the disease and of their own safety.

Public health providers must also learn about and utilize control and prevention strategies that are community-based. Any acts of prevention or curative methods that are perceived to be imposition may lead to failure and exacerbate the pandemic. The international community must know that panic and the imposition of cruel and drastic control measures and unreasonable international policy responses will only worsen the nature and extent of the pandemic. It is important for all to know that Ebola is not localized just in Africa; the fact that cases have been reported in the United States, Western Europe, and other parts of the world suggests the need for a global and international concerted effort in combating the disease.

REFERENCES

[1] Chua K, Bellini W, Rota P, Harcourt B, Tamin A, Lam S, et al. Nipah virus: A recently emergent deadly paramyxovirus. Science 2000;288:1432–35.

[2] Hahn BH, Shaw GM, De Cock KM, Sharp PM. Aids as a zoonosis: scientific and public health implications. Science 2000;287:607–14.

[3] Guan Y, Zheng BJ, He YQ, Liu XL, Zhuang ZX, Cheung CL, et al. Isolation and characterization of viruses related to the SARS coronavirus from animals in Southern China. Science 2003;302:276–8.

[4] Leroy EM, Kumulungui B, Pourrut X, Rouquet P, Hassanin A, Yaba P, et al. Fruit bats as reservoirs of Ebola virus. Nature 2005;438;575-6.

[5] Woolhouse MEJ, Gowtage-Sequeria S. Host range and emerging and reemerging pathogens. Emerg Infect Dis 2005;11:1842–7.

[6] Takada A, Robinson C, Goto H, Murti K, Gopal, Whitt MA, et al. A system for functional analysis of Ebola-virus-glycoprotein. Proceed Natl Acad Sci USA 1997;94(26):14764–9.

[7] World Health Organization online. Ebola is 'entrenched and accelerating' in West Africa. Accessed 2014 Oct 16. URL: http://www.bbc.com/news/world-africa-29563530.

[8] Ebola News Digest online. Accessed 2014 Oct 14. URL: http://star-tides.net/blog/2014/10/14/ebola-news-digest-october-14.

[9] Morse SS. Examining the origins of emerging viruses. In: Morse SS, ed. Emerging viruses. New York: Oxford University Press, 1993:10-28.

Section One - Inter-professional Collaborations in Improving Health

In: Public Health Yearbook 2015
Editor: Joav Merrick
ISBN: 978-1-63484-514-4
© 2016 Nova Science Publishers, Inc.

Chapter 1

AN INTER-GOVERNMENTAL APPROACH TO CHILDHOOD OBESITY IN CHICAGO, ILLINOIS

Christine Bozlak[1,*], PhD, MPH, Adam Becker[2,3], PhD, MPH, Jennifer Herd[4], MHLP, Andrew Teitelman[5], LCSW, Judah Viola[6], PhD, Bradley Olson[6], PhD, and Bechara Choucair[4], MD

[1]Department of Health Policy, Management, and Behavior, School of Public Health, University at Albany, Rensselaer, New York, United States of America
[2]Consortium to Lower Obesity in Chicago Children, Chicago, Illinois, United States of America
[3]Northwestern University, Evanston, Illinois, United States of America
[4]Chicago Department of Public Health, Chicago, Illinois, United States of America
[5]Chicago Housing Authority, Chicago, Illinois, United States of America
[6]National Louis University, Chicago, Illinois, United States of America

Childhood obesity continues to be a global epidemic. Prevention of this public health problem requires an inter-disciplinary and social ecological approach. This article describes the history, function, and structure of the City of Chicago's Inter-Departmental Task Force on Childhood Obesity (IDTF), a government coalition created in 2006 by four city agencies in Chicago with the support of staff from a multi-sectoral obesity prevention coalition, to confront the rising epidemic. Now with eleven member agencies, this award-winning task force offers lessons learned for other localities working to take a governmental approach to confront one of the greatest public health threats of our time. Recommendations are provided for governments of any size to consider as they address this global public health crisis.

Keywords: government collaboration, task force, childhood obesity, obesity prevention

---

[*] Corresponding author: Christine Bozlak, PhD, MPH, Assistant Professor, University at Albany, School of Public Health, Department of Health Policy, Management, and Behavior, One University Place, Room 173, Rensselaer, NY 12144, United States. E-mail: cbozlak@albany.edu.

INTRODUCTION

Over the last three decades, childhood obesity (1-3) has emerged as a significant public health crisis in the United States (4) and around the world (5). Almost 35 million of the 42 million children under the age of five who are overweight are located in developing countries (6). In the United States, childhood obesity is a major concern, with researchers there predicting that this generation of American children will be the first to have a shorter lifespan than the preceding generation (4, 7). Although some age groups (8) and localities, such as New York City and Los Angeles (9), are beginning to demonstrate decreases in childhood obesity rates, disparities still exist; especially for children in lower-income, African American, and Latino communities (10).

According to data analyzed by the Consortium to Lower Obesity in Chicago Children (CLOCC), in Chicago, Illinois, young children in this city have had considerably higher obesity rates than children in the rest of Illinois and across the US. However, there are signs of improvement. Data analyzed by CLOCC show a decrease in obesity prevalence among 3-7 year olds over a five year period. A recent report indicates declines in obesity exclusively among Chicago Public School students (11). These improvements cannot be attributed to one intervention but are, in part, the result of significant coordination of obesity efforts in Chicago since 2002 (3). One important aspect of this coordination is the City of Chicago's Inter-Departmental Task Force on Childhood Obesity (IDTF).

The purpose of this work is to align and coordinate Chicago governmental agency efforts to plan, implement, and evaluate policy, systems, and environmental change (PSE) strategies to address the childhood obesity epidemic in Chicago. The task force prioritizes children between the ages of 0-18. However, the IDTF acknowledges that early intervention is critical and thus interventions tailored for the early childhood years of 0-5 are emphasized.

BACKGROUND OF GOVERNMENT COLLABORATION ON CHILDHOOD OBESITY PREVENTION

Public health experts widely acknowledge that government has an essential role to play in protecting the public's health (12, 13). In the United States, state and local governments are authorized to protect the public's health, a concept known as "police power," and there is well-established precedent for government to exercise this power for childhood obesity prevention. For example, state and local governments have exercised this power to require the posting of nutritional information in restaurants, regulate the sale of junk food in schools, and impose zoning restrictions to limit the location of fast food establishments (14). Government is in a unique position to assess public health problems and coordinate implementation of policies, programs, and services to alleviate these issues (1, 13). Additionally, public health experts recognize the importance of an interdisciplinary approach with non-health governmental agencies' participation in the protection of the public's health (1).

Through Internet research and discussions with health departments across the US, the authors found that other obesity-focused government coalitions and task forces, such as those in the cities of New York, Boston, Baltimore, and Columbus, tend to convene for a delimited time to develop an agenda and work on specific topics on an as-needed basis. Some are created formally by legislation and others are developed based upon a call from a local government entity. Although other childhood obesity prevention task forces may exist, the authors believe that the City of Chicago's Inter-Departmental Task Force on Childhood Obesity is unique given the length of time it has been operational, its multi-pronged and multi-sector approach, and the city's ongoing commitment to its existence.

BACKGROUND OF CHICAGO'S INTERGOVERNMENTAL APPROACH TO CHILDHOOD OBESITY PREVENTION

The City of Chicago, situated in Northern Illinois, with a population of over 2.7 million (15) is a diverse urban area governed by a Mayor and City Council. In 2002, forty childhood obesity advocates convened to discuss a coordinated approach to the childhood obesity epidemic in Chicago (3, 16). This discussion resulted in the establishment of the Consortium to Lower Obesity in Chicago Children (CLOCC), housed at Ann and Robert H Lurie Children's Hospital of Chicago. This network connects hundreds of organizations to support, coordinate, and unite partners to promote healthy and active lifestyles for children and families. Consortium partners use data to guide their efforts and frame their priorities. For example, prevalence data collected from student health records and community-based surveys have helped to prioritize age groups and geographic locations within the City for intervention. Environmental audit data collected by researchers and community members (e.g., street and sidewalk conditions, merchandise in food retail establishments) have helped partners to prioritize strategies to improve access to healthy food and safe opportunities for physical activity. CLOCC's primary focus is on children aged zero to five, their caregivers, and their communities. CLOCC's work cuts across medical, government, corporate, academic, advocacy, and other sectors. Currently, more than 3,000 individuals representing over 1,300 organizations participate in the Consortium.

CLOCC initially engaged the government sector by creating a Governmental Policies and Programs working group. Co-chaired by representatives from two city agencies, the Chicago Department of Public Health and the Chicago Department of Family and Support Services, this working group was comprised of representatives from government agencies (including those who participated in the IDTF) and non-governmental organizations interested in policy (e.g., social service organizations, advocacy organizations dedicated to the prevention of obesity-related diseases, legal organizations that prioritize child health issues). Over time, CLOCC and city government leadership recognized the need for inter-governmental collaboration separate from efforts that included non-governmental partners.

In 2006, CLOCC's leadership approached the Chicago Department of Public Health (CDPH) with the idea of creating the Inter-Departmental Task Force on Childhood Obesity (IDTF). As the lead government agency, CDPH invited the Chicago Public Schools (CPS), the Chicago Department of Family and Support Services (DFSS), and the Chicago Park District (Parks) to join the effort. Since that time, seven other city agencies have joined (Table 1). In 2007, the IDTF hosted an event in a national series of "town-hall" meetings to gather input about childhood obesity. Six hundred Chicagoans attended the event, demonstrated support for the emerging IDTF, and helped develop its priorities.

Table 1. Inter-Departmental Task Force on Childhood Obesity Membership

IDTF Member Agency Name	Associated Acronym
Chicago Department of Public Health (lead agency)	CDPH
Chicago Department of Family and Support Services	DFSS
Chicago Department of Planning and Development	DPD
Chicago Department of Transportation	CDOT
Chicago Housing Authority	CHA
Chicago Park District	Parks
Chicago Police Department	CPD
Chicago Public Library	CPL
Chicago Public Schools	CPS
Chicago Transit Authority	CTA
Mayor's Office for People with Disabilities	MOPD
*Technical assistance provided by the Consortium to Lower Obesity in Chicago Children	CLOCC

METHODS

The IDTF was created to develop a coordinated governmental response to the childhood obesity epidemic in Chicago. This multi-agency approach was based on the premise that the complexity of childhood obesity requires inter-disciplinary solutions. City governments, because they are comprised of a range of agencies with diverse expertise, have an important opportunity to coordinate across disciplines (1). In 2006, the founding four IDTF agencies established the mission: "Chicago's city government will play a leading role in confronting childhood obesity through an unprecedented level of coordination, the strategic provision of services, and the advancement of evidence-based practices and policies to improve nutrition and physical activity in a wellness-enhancing environment." The IDTF follows a social ecological approach to childhood obesity prevention, meaning that its interventions are focused on the environments in which children are developing (2); not solely on the children themselves.

To accomplish its mission, the IDTF meets monthly. Each department's leader designates one or more staff members to represent their agency; most often those whose day-to-day work aligns most closely with IDTF objectives. The Commissioner of Health periodically convenes an IDTF leadership meeting to update the other agency executives on progress and future plans. Each year, the IDTF sets annual objectives, using a three-pronged strategic approach as a guiding framework.

Strategy #1: Primary prevention

The Task Force's primary prevention activities are intended to reach all children in Chicago. These activities include public education, data surveillance, environmental assessments, coordinated policymaking, and professional development for agency staff. The IDTF adopted CLOCC's 5-4-3-2-1 Go!® healthy lifestyle message which provides daily recommendations for children and families related to nutrition, physical activity, and screen-time (see www.clocc.net/partners/54321Go). Since 2008, the Task Force has disseminated 5-4-3-2-1 Go! by distributing materials throughout city facilities. In 2009, the IDTF contributed to a city-wide campaign to disseminate the message to 1.5 million Chicagoans with 8 million media impressions. Evaluation of the campaign suggests that those exposed to the message were more likely to adopt certain healthy behaviors than those who were not exposed (17).

A number of trainings delivered by IDTF member agencies were opened to staff from other IDTF agencies. The Department of Family and Support Services (DFSS) has invited partners to trainings on nutrition and physical activity in early childhood settings. The Park District has invited partners to physical activity trainings. These cross-training opportunities help to expand the capacity of city staff members who interact with young children.

In terms of surveillance, the Chicago Department of Public Health and Chicago Public Schools have a five-year inter-governmental agreement to share de-identified student health data collected through required health examinations at school entry, sixth grade, and ninth grade. CLOCC provided technical assistance on analysis methods that mirrored those implemented by the U.S. Centers for Disease Control and Prevention (CDC). The City published the first report on obesity prevalence among CPS students, which has helped guide the IDTF and the public health community to the areas in the city with the highest rates (11). A second report was released in late 2013 and showed a slight decline in childhood obesity rates among CPS kindergarten-aged students (18).

Strategy #2: Early childhood

The Task Force prioritizes activities that are focused on enhancing early childhood environments. Evidence increasingly points to the need to intervene early in order to curb the childhood obesity epidemic (19). In the US, infants and young children are increasingly cared for outside their home (20), thus, early childhood settings are a key context for childhood obesity intervention (21). As of 2011, there were almost 84,000 slots in licensed child care centers and homes in Chicago, demonstrating the potential reach of interventions when implemented in Chicago child care settings (22).

The IDTF's primary approach to early childhood is to strengthen the practices of childcare providers under the purview of city agencies. CDPH and DFSS led a policy change initiative to ensure that standards for nutrition, physical activity, and screen time in Chicago licensed childcare settings under CDPH's jurisdiction aligned with best practices. In 2009, CDPH and the Chicago Board of Health passed a joint resolution to this effect (23). CDPH then partnered with CLOCC and two other local non-profit organizations to provide training to childcare providers to support implementation of the standards.

Strategy #3: Geographic hubs

IDTF members developed a strategy that focuses on aligning partner resources in key geographic areas of Chicago where childhood obesity rates are expected or known to be highest. Known as Wellness Campuses, these areas of geographic concentration helped agencies to focus on priority neighborhoods and to align efforts for educational, programmatic, and clinical childhood obesity prevention services for children and their families. Early wellness campuses were anchored by Chicago Park District "Wellness Centers" – park district facilities equipped to provide enhanced fitness programming for youth. A 2009 CLOCC study found that when more resources and staff training were devoted to youth fitness through the Wellness Center structure, children engaged in more intensive physical activity for a longer period of time than those in parks without the centers. Other IDTF partners directed their activities to these geographic areas. For example, the Chicago Department of Transportation's (CDOT) Bike Ambassadors provide bicycle safety education at Wellness Centers.

Chicago Public Schools and the Chicago Park District identified ways to collaborate so that students in schools, including early childhood settings, with limited facilities for physical activity can use park resources. For example, through the Healthy Chicago Public Schools initiative, forty park sites have included thirty minutes of structured physical activity time in their existing early childhood programs. In addition, Chicago Park District staff members have been trained in the SPARK (www.sparkpe.org) early childhood program to promote physical activity in this population. The next step will be to connect nearby CPS schools who offer pre-kindergarten to the parks where the SPARK physical activity program will be implemented. The Chicago Park District staff trained in SPARK can also provide the training to CPS teachers.

More recently, other departmental strategies are anchoring geographically-defined settings around the city, and IDTF members are exploring opportunities to align their resources in these emerging locations. For example, CDOT is establishing "safety zones" where a variety of traffic-calming and enforcement approaches will be concentrated around schools and parks. CPS recently received funding from a U.S. Centers for Disease Control and Prevention's Community Transformation Grant to create "healthy school zones" that combine school wellness activities with efforts to improve the external food and activity environments. By focusing these collaborative efforts in the same geographic locations, the city has a coordinated approach in neighborhoods where obesity is a significant problem.

RESULTS

In addition to providing a foundation for collaborative alignment of existing resources, IDTF members have been able to leverage single opportunities into larger initiatives. The IDTF has been a foundation for new funding; expanding the capacity of city agencies to intervene to address childhood obesity in Chicago. In 2010, Chicago embarked on its largest federally-funded obesity prevention project to date, Healthy Places. This $5.8 million project was funded through a cooperative agreement from the Centers for Disease Control and Prevention (CDC) between CLOCC and the CDC under the U.S. Department of Health and Human Services' Communities Putting Prevention to Work initiative (CPPW). CLOCC served as the bona fide agent for the City of Chicago and led the effort in partnership with CDPH. The overall goal of Healthy Places was to implement sustainable policy, systems, and environmental changes that address obesity in Chicago by creating healthier environments where Chicagoans live, work, learn, and play. Several of the project's outcome objectives were integrated into "Healthy Chicago," the City of Chicago's official public health agenda (24).

Through the Healthy Places initiative, IDTF agencies worked together on projects, such as design guidelines for "complete streets," a framework that supports multi-modal use of streets with an emphasis on pedestrian and cyclist safety; a healthy food plan to guide government action to address access to healthy foods, and a safe park access plan, called "Make Way for Play." Although the federal funding period has ended, IDTF members are establishing mechanisms for ensuring the sustainability of Healthy Places efforts.

Evaluation of the IDTF

The Institute of Medicine (1) stresses the need to evaluate local obesity prevention efforts and encourage partnerships with local universities in this effort. In 2011, the IDTF commissioned an evaluation of its work and hired, with funding from CLOCC, two external researchers from a local university to work collaboratively with the Task Force to identify successes, challenges, and opportunities for improvement.

The evaluation identified outcomes in three main areas: 1) policy, 2) education, and 3) programs. Evaluation data pointed to a number of policy outcomes resulting from IDTF collaborations. The implementation of improved childcare standards, as well as policies for healthy vending across several member agencies, were found to be important policy outcomes. Programmatic outcomes included Safe Routes to School implementation, Open Streets (a day-long event that closes streets to vehicular traffic and opens them for recreational use), the Park District's fitness-related training, the dissemination of 5-4-3-2-1 Go!®, and the Healthy Places initiatives. The evaluation also found that the IDTF wellness campus initiative is a comprehensive concept in that it covers both physical activity and healthy eating promotion within the various community settings in which children interact.

IDTF members continue to integrate lessons learned from the evaluation into process improvements and intervention design. Evaluation results were shared with CDPH after transition to a new commissioner to keep the Department invested in the IDTF. In 2013, the IDTF began to explore options for an evaluation of the health impacts of the IDTF on Chicago children.

DISCUSSION

Establishing a coordinated, local governmental response to childhood obesity prevention is a critical strategy to address this epidemic (1). The experiences of the IDTF in Chicago can be helpful to other communities considering a similar, government-led, multi-disciplinary effort. The following recommendations are provided by IDTF members based on the IDTF evaluation findings.

1. Strong leadership: Identify one partner to lead with one or more dedicated staff members to coordinate the effort. Leadership from a government entity, ideally the health department, can help to keep city leadership informed and can provide access to city resources. In Chicago, CLOCC's expertise on childhood obesity enabled them to add technical and content support to CDPH's leadership. Communities with

similar non-governmental entities might consider their inclusion to provide similar support. On a regular basis, it is helpful for the task force to obtain an official endorsement of its work from local governmental leaders. With the IDTF, this is accomplished through an annual agency leadership meeting to keep high-level decision-makers informed. This meeting also provides the leadership a platform to discuss childhood obesity issues from their vantage point.

In Chicago, there is leadership from the top. Mayor Rahm Emanuel has made focusing on the child one of his main priorities of his administration for the past two years. In addition, the City's public health agenda, "Healthy Chicago" includes obesity as one of 12 priorities and articulates the critical role of public-private partnerships in meeting the goals set forth in the agenda. This top-level support is essential for the continuation of the IDTF and the engagement of its member agencies.

2. Task force membership: Think broadly and recruit diverse agencies. It will take every sector, even those not traditionally considered as health-focused (e.g., transportation, public safety, planning and land use) working together to address this complex epidemic. It is helpful to have budgetary support for this work across agencies. Inter-agency agreements may facilitate collaboration, solidify commitments, and ensure role clarity.

The IDTF operates under a multi-disciplinary model with mixed committee assignments to ensure that the City's member agencies, with differing missions and priorities, remain engaged in the process. IDTF member agencies also benefit from their participation in the IDTF because they know they can utilize the IDTF to leverage and support their own agency's objectives – a point emphasized in the next recommendation.

3. Maximize opportunities for collaboration: Maximize the potential for "synergy" with other efforts throughout the locality. Aligning objectives and activities with existing governmental priorities can increase the likelihood of successful implementation. Identifying ways that the collaborative work can support the individual priorities of member agencies helps to secure broad support. The work of a task force such as the IDTF could be integrated with other initiatives related to economic development, education, and public safety to accomplish other government goals.

4. Ensure effective communication: Government agency staffs are often pulled in multiple directions as leadership responds to well-established priorities and a constant stream of external pressures and demands. Organized and frequent communication among task force members can ensure that momentum is not lost even if members cannot attend every meeting. A centralized and cross-agency event calendar can help to increase awareness of member agency initiatives related to the task force and to identify opportunities for collaboration. Task force agencies can also help disseminate materials related to a partner agency's event. In addition, regularly update the local governmental leaders of the task force's work to increase support and buy-in from decision-makers. Establishing mechanisms to disseminate the task force's work and messaging to the local community and other public health professionals is also essential to increase support and participation from these entities.

Throughout the years, the IDTF has utilized various communication mechanisms and meeting schedules. The IDTF has functioned most efficiently when there was one staff-person dedicated to communicating with all the representatives of the member agencies via email and conference calls for scheduling and project coordination purposes. It is most effective to have one individual responsible for coordinating task force communication because this person can synthesize the communication within the task force and appropriately triage and follow-up on project-related responsibilities and other task force-related items. Throughout the existence of the IDTF, monthly in-person meetings helped to advance IDTF progress on its initiatives, and they also enabled the representatives from the member agencies to establish effective working relationships that would have otherwise not developed. Over time, this resulted in an unforeseen positive outcome from the IDTF in that there has been increased communication between member agencies on non-task force-related initiatives pertaining to the well-being of Chicago residents.

Staff turnover can be a challenge for any type of coalition. For the IDTF, individual representatives from the member agencies become internal champions for the work and are critical points of contact between task force staff and each participating agency. Encouraging members to identify more than one representative can help to ensure that the IDTF remains a priority for each of its member agencies and can help prevent disruptions in communications that might occur if a member's sole representative left his or her organization.

5. Prioritize task force projects: Utilize intervention research evidence and best practice guidelines to prioritize task force projects. It may be most efficient to charge one task force member or committee with the responsibility of staying current with the latest research on effective approaches to childhood obesity prevention and communicating this information to the group. In addition, the resources of a government task force may be used most effectively when directed towards agency practices and city policy, as opposed to programs delivered to citizens, because governments are uniquely situated to focus on the former. Such policy should include modifying the environment to make healthy choices practical and available to all community members. This approach is known as "Policy, Systems, and Environmental Change" (PSE), and is increasingly utilized by U.S. public health practitioners working in chronic disease prevention. By changing laws and shaping the landscape around us, a significant and sustainable impact can be made, often with fewer resources than one-time programmatic interventions with limited reach.

In addition to these recommendations, the challenges of creating and sustaining a task force of this nature must be recognized. It can be extremely helpful to measure the successes and challenges of the task force. Evidence of progress can help to keep city leaders engaged and identification of challenges can help the members to overcome them or prevent them in the future. Childhood obesity, because it is a chronic condition, may not be prioritized by governmental leadership amidst other, perhaps more visible issues (e.g., crime, academic achievement). Using data to illustrate the connections between childhood obesity and other priority health and/or social problems can help garner and maintain support. Finally, the current fiscal and structural challenges experienced by many local governments in the U.S., such as staff turnover, hiring freezes, and resource shortages, must also be considered when prioritizing work for the task force.

The City of Chicago's Inter-Departmental Task Force on Childhood Obesity is a unique entity that, since 2006, has grown to include eleven city agencies collaborating to effectively plan and implement childhood obesity prevention strategies. The work involves a broad cross-section of the governmental sector, including transit, housing, education, parks, health, urban planning, libraries, and public safety.

Since its creation, the IDTF has received national recognition for its innovative work. The IDTF strategy has also been presented at national conferences. In 2011, the Chicago Department of Public Health received a Model Practice Award from the National Association of County and City Health Officials for the IDTF. Most recently, the City of Chicago was recognized for its multi-sector obesity prevention efforts by the National League of Cities for its achievement in the Let's Move! Cities, Towns and Counties program. The City received this award in large part because of the accomplishments made possible by the IDTF collectively and its individual members.

Chicago's Inter-Departmental Task Force on Childhood Obesity illustrates the critical function of government agencies in tackling a complex public health problem. While not solely responsible for them, the IDTF has contributed to the steady declines in childhood obesity prevalence described earlier. Research evidence and national experts support the premise that the kinds of policy and environmental changes brought about by the IDTF do lead to improved nutritional and physical activity behaviors in children, which in turn result in improvements in population-level obesity rates. The experience of the IDTF can serve as a model for government leadership at the local level and demonstrates the important role that every government sector can and should play in reducing this epidemic among its most vulnerable and youngest citizens.

ACKNOWLEDGMENTS

The authors wish to thank the Otho SA Sprague Memorial Institute, the Michael and Susan Dell Foundation, and the Robert Wood Johnson Foundation for funding CLOCC's staff support of the IDTF, Dr Matt Longjohn for his advocacy that helped create the Task Force, and all the IDTF agencies and agency representatives who contributed to this work since 2006.

REFERENCES

[1] Institute of Medicine. Local government actions to prevent childhood obesity. Washington, DC: National Academies Press, 2009.
[2] Davison K, Birch, L. Childhood overweight: a contextual model and recommendations for future research. Obes Rev 2001; 2(3): 159-71.
[3] Becker A, Longjohn M, Christoffel K. Taking on childhood obesity in a big city: Consortium to Lower Obesity in Chicago Children (CLOCC). Prog Pediatr Cardiol 2008; 25(2): 199-206.
[4] US Department of Health and Human Services. The Surgeon General's call to action to prevent and decrease overweight and obesity. Washington, DC: US Government Printing Office, 2001.

[5] Prentice, A. The emerging epidemic of obesity in developing countries. Int J Epidemiol 2006; 35(1): 93-9.
[6] deOnis M, Blössner M, Borghi E. Global prevalence and trends of overweight and obesity among preschool children. Am J Clin Nutr 2010; 92(5): 1257-64.
[7] Olshansky J, Passaro D, Hershow R, Layden J, Carnes B, Brody J, et al. A potential decline in life expectancy in the United States in the 21st century. N Engl J Med 2005; 352(11): 1138-45.
[8] Ogden C, Carroll M, Curtin L, Lamb M, Flegal K. Prevalence of high body mass index in US children and adolescents, 2007-2008. JAMA 2010; 303(3): 242-49.
[9] US Department of Health and Human Services Centers for Disease Control and Prevention. Obesity prevalence among low income, preschool-aged children – New York City and Los Angeles County, 2003-2011. MMWR 2013; 62(2).
[10] Trust for America's Health. F as in Fat: How obesity threatens America's future 2012. 2013. Accessed 2012 November 20. URL: http://healthyamericans.org/report/100/.
[11] City of Chicago. Overweight and obesity among Chicago public schools students, 2010-2011. 2013. Accessed 20 November 2013. URL: http://www.cityofchicago.org/content/dam/city/depts/cdph/CDPH/OverweightObesityReportFeb272013.pdf.
[12] Jochelson K. Nanny or steward? The role of government in public health. Public Health 2006; 120(12): 1149-55.
[13] Turnock BJ. Public health: what it is and how it works, 4th ed. Burlington, MA: Jones and Bartlett, 2009.
[14] Mermin SE, Graff SK. A legal primer for the obesity prevention movement. Am J Health Behav 2009; 99(10): 1799-05.
[15] U.S. Census Bureau. State & County Quickfacts: Chicago, IL 2010. Accessed 2013 November 1. URL: http://quickfacts.census.gov/qfd/states/17/1714000.html
[16] Longjohn MM. Chicago project uses ecological approach to obesity prevention. Pediatr Ann 2004; 33(1): 55-7.
[17] Evans WD, Christoffel KK, Necheles K, Becker AB, Snider J. Outcomes of the 5-4-3-2-1 Go! childhood obesity community trial. Am J Health Behav 2011; 35(2): 189-98.
[18] City of Chicago. Healthy Chicago spotlight childhood obesity. Chicago, Illinois: City of Chicago, 2013. Accessed 20 November 2013. URL: http://www.cityofchicago.org/content/dam/city/depts/cdph/CDPH/HCObesityReport10302013.pdf.
[19] Nader P, Huang T, Gahagan S, Kumanyika S, Hammond R, Christoffel K. Next steps in obesity prevention: Altering early life system to support healthy parents, infants, and toddlers. Child Obes 2012; 8(3): 195-204.
[20] Baker M, Gruber J, Milligan K. Universal child care, maternal labor supply, and family well-being. J Polit Econ 2008; 116(4): 709-45.
[21] Kaphingst K, Story M. Child care as an untapped setting for obesity prevention: state child care licensing regulations related to nutrition, physical activity, and media use for preschool-aged children in the United States. Prev Chronic Dis 2009; 6(1): A11.
[22] Illinois Action for Children Research Department. Child care providers and capacity by Cook County Municipality. 2013. Accessed 2013 November 1. URL: http://www.actforchildren.org/site/DocServer/Commonly_Requested_Child_Care_Data_by_Cook_Municipality_.pdf?docID=2123.
[23] Bozlak C, Becker A. Using Evidence to Create Active Communities: Stories from the Field—Policy and Research with Chicago's Child Care Centers: a Commentary to Accompany the Active Living Research Supplement to Annals of Behavioral Medicine. Ann Behav Med 2013; 45 Suppl 1: s11-s13.
[24] Chicago Department of Public Health. Healthy Chicago Agenda. 2013. Accessed 2013 November 1. URL: http://www.cityofchicago.org/city/en/depts/cdph/provdrs/healthychicago.html.

In: Public Health Yearbook 2015
Editor: Joav Merrick

ISBN: 978-1-63484-514-4
© 2016 Nova Science Publishers, Inc.

Chapter 2

COLLABORATIVE EFFORTS TOWARDS AN INTERDISCIPLINARY AND INTERPROFESSIONAL DUAL DEGREE PROGRAM FOR PUBLIC HEALTH TRAINING IN A NEW RURAL MEDICAL SCHOOL

Mark V White[1],*, MD, MPH, Olapeju M Simoyan[1], MD, MPH, BDS, Alberto JF Cardelle[2], PhD, MPH, Steven Godin[2], PhD, MPH, Elizabeth C Kuchinski[1], MPH, Erica L Townsend[1], BS, and Janet M Townsend[1], MD

[1]Department of Family, Community, and Rural Health,
The Commonwealth Medical College (TCMC), Scranton,
Pennsylvania, United States of America

[2]The College of Health Sciences, Department of Health Studies,
East Stroudsburg University of Pennsylvania (ESU), Scranton,
Pennsylvania, United States of America

The purpose of developing the dual-degree MD/Master of Public Health program (MD/MPH) and the MD/Public Health Certificate (MD/PHC) program between The Commonwealth Medical College and East Stroudsburg University is to enrich the education of future primary care physicians, teachers, and researchers by developing and integrating a public health curriculum within traditional medical education. The partnership between TCMC, a new community-health and public-health focused allopathic (MD) medical school in rural northeastern Pennsylvania (NEPA) and ESU's public health programs will ultimately improve health outcomes and reduce health disparities in the regions our students serve. CEPH is an independent agency recognized by the US Department of Education to accredit public health programs. Educational training in public health is essential to better address the health inequities endemic experienced in our geographic region, which includes an aging population, a high rate of

---

* Corresponding author: Mark V White, MD, MPH, Department of Family, Community, and Rural Health, Associate Professor of Epidemiology, The Commonwealth Medical College, 525 Pine Street, Scranton, PA 18509, United States. E-mail: mwhite@tcmedc.org.

childhood poverty, and disproportionately high rates of cancer, cardiovascular disease and mental illness. Residents of NEPA are experiencing access to care issues, especially related to primary care, mental health, and dental care.

Keywords: public health, dual degree program, master of public health, interprofessional, medical education

INTRODUCTION

Practitioners, educators, and researchers working in the fields of public health and primary care strive for the common goal of improved health of individuals and their communities. Despite this mutual aim, the efforts of primary care physicians and public health practitioners are often disconnected from one another, to the detriment of their patients and communities. In a healthcare environment characterized by marked policy change, limited resources, and increasing need, the fields of primary care and public health will require more support from one another. A symbiotic relationship between these fields that involves interprofessional collaborations, community engagement, and collaborative evidence-based research endeavors will be essential to the achievement of the mutual goals of enhanced primary care and improved community health.

Medical schools provide natural opportunities to integrate public health training and primary care. To this end, The Commonwealth Medical College (TCMC) and East Stroudsburg University of Pennsylvania (ESU), both located in Northeastern Pennsylvania (NEPA), have collaborated to develop a curriculum that infuses public health training, community engagement, and interprofessional collaboration into traditional medical education. This collaboration has led to the development of two new programs: a Public Health Certificate (PHC) or a Master of Public Health (MPH) degree, available to TCMC medical students. These programs will prepare participants to make significant contributions to the healthcare environment in which they eventually practice, including increased access to quality health care and improved population health.

CURRENT STATE OF HEALTH CARE IN THE REGION

There is a shortage of primary care physicians in Pennsylvania, particularly in the northeast region. Presently, PA retains only 22% of its physician trainees and of these only: 16% practice primary care; 7% practice rural care; 4% practice rural primary care; and 0.5% practice rural underserved care.

Additionally, PA currently ranks 37th in the US in physicians per 10,000 elderly persons. The average age of physicians in Pennsylvania is 48.7, with those under 35 years of age consisting of only 8% of the physician workforce. Further, 21% of physicians currently practicing state that they will stop practicing within five years (1).

TCMC serves 16 counties, whose population ranges from 6,124 (Sullivan) to 311,983 (Luzerne). Only Lackawanna and Luzerne have significant "urban" centers- Scranton, population 72,233, and Wilkes-Barre, population 40,932; yet both counties have many rural communities. Williamsport, population 29,456, is the county seat for Pennsylvania's largest county, Lycoming County, which is rural.

The majority of 16 counties in TCMC's coverage region include federally designated shortage areas for primary care, dental, and/or mental health professionals. The residents of TCMC's region are disproportionately affected by mental health challenges and a lack of access, and experience high rates of obesity, heart disease, and other chronic diseases (2).

A Regional Health Needs Assessment conducted in 2009 by the Department of Family, Community and Rural Health (DFCRH) showed that mental health, transportation problems, lack of health insurance, lack of providers, lack of preventive care, drug and alcohol abuse, cultural and knowledge barriers to care and oral health care were areas of need. Interagency collaboration, the State Health Improvement Plan (SHIP) partnerships, volunteers, schools and churches as pillars of community were noted as strengths (3).

In 23 focus groups representative of 195 community agencies, participants reported mental health as a predominant concern in each county, and large gaps in mental health services: a lack of psychiatrists, scarce children's mental health services, long waiting lists and waits for appointments, lack of services for patients with concomitant substance abuse, and an enormous burden on primary care physicians and social service agencies trying to fill the gap. Isolation and depression, leading to poor physical health were identified as a major problem among seniors in the region. Lackawanna, Luzerne, and Schuylkill counties have very high youth suicide rate (3). The findings have been published (3, 4) and will continue to be used to guide development of the research, educational and clinical agendas of TCMC.

Public health education initiatives, such as this interprofessional dual degree program, encourage students to invest their time, energy, and efforts to approach patient care with a public health perspective. The theoretical framework for the programs is based on accountability to the public good, specifically in the NEPA region. The principles and practice of Community Based Participatory Research (CBPR), the World Health Organization's International Classification of Function, Disability, and Health(ICF) and social ecology models inform the curriculum and assessment strategies. Graduates of these programs will be equipped for positions in health departments, federally qualified health centers, and other organizations that require expertise in prevention strategies and healthcare policy.

GOALS AND OBJECTIVES

The main objective of the PHC and MPH programs is to provide training in environmental health, infectious disease control, disease prevention, health promotion, epidemiology, and injury control. TCMC is committed to the integration of community and public health in medical education, and these programs expand upon the standard curriculum, integrating population health skills, experiences, and core public health competencies that guide clinical practice and lead to improved access to quality care. Through ESU's MPH program, TCMC offers medical students a unique opportunity to receive a well-rounded curriculum in public health. The partnership between these two institutions will ultimately contribute to improving health outcomes and reduce health disparities in the regions the graduates ultimately serve.

METHODS

The Commonwealth Medical College (TCMC) is located in northeast and north central Pennsylvania and offers a community-based model of medical education with three regional campuses - North (Scranton), South (Wilkes-Barre), and West (Williamsport). The College was awarded degree granting authority by the Commonwealth of Pennsylvania in 2008, received preliminary LCME (Liaison Committee on Medical Education) accreditation in 2008; provisional accreditation in 2012, and accepted its first class of medical and master's students in 2009.

The four year MD Program features team and case-based learning, interprofessional education, early exposure to clinical care settings, medical simulation, standardized patients, and community health and research projects. TCMC is among the first United States medical schools to adopt the Longitudinal Integrated Clerkship (LIC) model as the standard clinical experience for the entire medical school class in the third year. As the core of the LIC, TCMC incorporates longitudinal ambulatory clerkships within each of the six core disciplines: medicine, surgery, pediatrics, psychiatry, obstetrics and gynecology, and family medicine. Students in these clerkships follow panels of patients longitudinally with their faculty. Interspersed with these longitudinal ambulatory half-days are group and case-based learning sessions and tutorials, inpatient rounds, emergency room experiences and self-directed learning.

The College attracts students from across the nation who are interested in studying evidence- and community-based medicine and who have a strong desire to serve their community. The students have early clinical experiences and are engaged with clinical mentors right from the start of their medical education. Each of the three campuses offers exposure to urban and rural settings and diverse clinical experiences. Medical students receive regional campus assignments following matriculation and are paired with community physicians who serve as continuity mentors throughout their education.

The Department of Family, Community, and Rural Health (DFCRH) played a major role in curriculum development for the medical school and faculty members conduct public health, epidemiologic and clinical research. Relationships with various community agencies became crucial when incorporating Community Health Research Projects (CHRPs) in the first year and the Family Centered Experience across the four years of the standard medical education curriculum. Advantages of being a newer institution include the opportunities for flexibility and innovation for faculty and students. There was a tremendous amount of institutional support for public health training at TCMC, a key factor in establishing these programs (5).

East Stroudsburg University of Pennsylvania

ESU is one of 14 state-supported institutions in the Pennsylvania State System of Higher Education (PASSHE), and is accredited by the Middle States Association of Colleges and Schools. The institution's MPH program, housed within ESU's Department of Health Studies, was approved by PASSHE in 1988 and has been continuously accredited by the Council on Education in Public Health (CEPH) since 1990. The MPH program at ESU consists of 45 credits aimed at preparing students in the core public health competencies (Epidemiology, Health Administration, Environmental Health, Social and Behavioral Sciences, and Biostatistics).

Requirements include a 300 hour internship requirement, a publishable paper and a comprehensive oral exam. An 18-credit Certificate of Public Health primarily for professionals working in the health and social services sectors is also available. This curriculum emphasizes population-based approaches, strengthening capacity for community-based prevention in order to promote healthy behaviors, and using environmental change strategies to enhance health and impact policy.

ESU public health programs aim to prepare the public health workforce to partner with communities while promoting collaboration and empowerment. The MPH and the public health certificate programs at ESU include training in cultural competency, addressing health disparities, use of technology in health care, and research methodology. Application of these skills to real-world scenarios during the required internship experience is an essential component of both programs.

FUNDING

Initial discussions and planning meetings involved key stakeholders from both institutions. A grant application was submitted to the Health Resources and Services Administration (HRSA) and TCMC were awarded funding in the amount of $1.5 million (T85HP24464) over a five-year period, with ESU and the NEPA Area Health Education Center (AHEC) as subcontractors. This grant provides partial tuition for students and also supports faculty time spent mentoring, preparing, advising, researching, and teaching public health students.

Program description

The ESU Master of Public Health program prepares students to enter the field of public health as researchers and practitioners working in the prevention of disease and improvement of the quality of life in communities. Through a well-integrated program of study, students receive instruction in the core public health disciplines of Biostatistics, Environmental Health, Epidemiology, Health Policy & Administration, and Social and Behavioral Sciences.

Students have opportunities to explore the intersection of the social behavioral sciences, information technology, human biology, and policy development. They have practical experiences in policy development, practice-based research, and program implementation. These internships are required to complete both the certificate and master's programs.

The challenge was to combine curricula from two separate institutions into one dual degree program. Please refer to Table 1 for a curriculum layout for all medical students pursuing either a MPH or PHC. It details the five year plan to infuse public health classes into the standard TCMC curriculum.

Both programs require internship experiences in a public health field to complete their certificate or degree requirements. TCMC and ESU have relationships with community leaders and healthcare providers dedicated to furthering public health in the communities which serve as internship sites for students.

How program addresses health needs

The establishment of TCMC, with its core mission of primary care training, has facilitated collaboration among research and health entities in NEPA to create an infrastructure that can effectively address the health disparities in the region. The collaboration with ESU allows TCMC to further integrate public health into primary care training. Previous collaborations with county-level State Health Improvement Plan Partners (SHIPs) and with community research areas have resulted in a "workforce" that is ready to address public health issues on a more systemic level.

For example, TCMC faculty and students have supported a community task force in Schuylkill County with their efforts at establishing a community health center (CHC). They have also assisted in creating the non-profit corporation that can evolve into a CHC, conducted surveys and are currently exploring the establishment of a medical reserve corps that can address public health needs in the county. It is anticipated that medical students in the public health training programs will be placed in meaningful internships in Schuylkill County to support these efforts. Other examples of community agencies that TCMC partners with include the Northeast Pennsylvania Cancer Research Institute, Wayne Memorial Hospital and the Children's Advocacy Center. These and numerous other partnerships will provide potential sites for student internships.

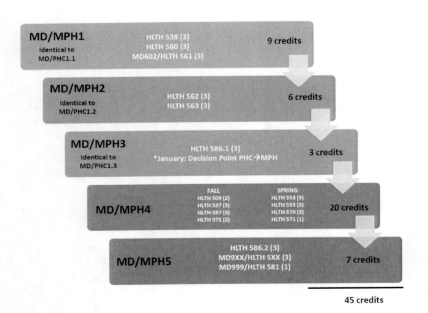

Figure 1. Curriculum Overview.

Strengthening existing community partnerships

A variety of community-based research, quality improvement, and summer research projects are essential components of TCMC's strategy to emphasize the value of community engagement and community partnerships within an allopathic medical curriculum.

First-year medical students at TCMC are required to complete a Community Health Research Project (CHRP) as a component of the "Physician and Society" course, where many core principles of public health are introduced. These projects involve a group of students working in collaboration with both an internal TCMC mentor and an external community agency or organization to contribute to improved health in the region by applying the concepts, strategies, and tools acquired in their studies (4).

Over the past five years, CHRPs have been conducted with a cadre of varied community agencies throughout NEPA, including the Northeast Regional Cancer Institute, the Lupus Foundation, the Lackawanna County Library System, Children's Advocacy Center, Volunteers in Medicine, the Care and Concern Clinic, and many more. The topics and scope of these projects change year to year depending upon the community partner agency and the type of research planned.

Each student group prepares and presents an academic poster documenting the rationale, research design, data analysis, and discussion of their project during an annual Research Symposium event, to which all of the current and past partnering community agencies are invited.

Multi-year CHRPs involving several stages/types of research on the same broad topic with the same community agencies are currently planned to further strengthen these existing community partnerships in an effort to maximize the impact on and benefit to the students and community partners involved.

Community engagement and interprofessional collaboration are again emphasized in the second year of TCMC's MD curriculum, when students are required to complete a Quality Improvement Community Collaborative (QuICC) project as a component of the "Art and Practice of Medicine" course. Working in groups, second-year medical students partner with a community-based team of health care professionals to measurably improve some aspect of patient care in a clinical setting. QuICC projects utilize the "Plan-Do-Study-Act" quality improvement cycle, and have focused on topics such as geriatric care, hand washing and vaccination rates, and guideline compliance for Pap smears, Constant Positive Airway Pressure (CPAP) use, and blood pressure monitoring. The settings for these projects range from small rural practices to busy hospital sites.

Often, the same community agencies and institutions that are collaborators for CHRPs are able to mentor QuICC projects as well; this internal consistency will augment alliances with community partners.

As with the first-year CHRPs, student groups prepare and present academic posters at TCMC's annual Research Symposium event. In addition to presentation to the TCMC community, many students involved in CHRP and QuICC projects have gone on to present their posters at national academic or professional conferences such as TCMC Annual Research Symposium, Pennsylvania Academy of Family Physicians (PAFP) conference, and American College of Physician's (ACP) annual meeting.

RESULTS

There are currently four TCMC medical students enrolled in the MD/public health program. They are the participants of the pilot program and have completed the first two semesters of the curriculum.

Recruitment

Recruitment is a crucial part of the success of any academic program. Recruitment strategies included partnering with student affairs and encouraging the enrolled students to serve as ambassadors for the programs. In the first year, recruitment was somewhat challenging as can be expected for any new program. The TCMC MD/MPH program coordinator was hired, whose responsibilities included student recruitment, assisting prospective students with the application process, and writing reports on all grant-related activities. In the future, prospective students applying to TCMC will receive information about the public health training programs, with the expectation that such opportunities will positively influence recruitment into the MD program. TCMC and ESU are exploring creative methods of marketing the program to current and prospective students.

The public health programs have been highlighted during admissions interviews, orientation and at other events, such as the TCMC revisit day, greatly increasing their exposure. Coordination of efforts between TCMC's Offices of Student Affairs, Academic Affairs, Marketing and Public Relations, and Curriculum has created a multi-tiered recruitment strategy with promising results.

Members of the newly-created Public Health Student Association will take an active role as recruitment ambassadors for the program, and create a mentorship program for those students newer to public health. Current MD/Public Health program students will also present a panel at a monthly Lunch and Learn seminar which is open to all students, faculty, and staff. Students will be encouraged to stay committed to the curriculum, create an internal support system and serve as ambassadors for public health within the institution.

DISCUSSION

Lack of lead time in recruitment during the first grant year limited the number of students enrolled in the program. When the HRSA grant was awarded, the team worked as quickly as possible to launch classes in July of 2013. The brief amount of time between the date of the grant award and the beginning of ESU coursework presented a barrier to acclimating students to the public health programs. All accepted students planned a visit to TCMC in the spring before their first year of medical school. The coordinators and faculty at that point reached out to the pre-matriculating students about the benefits of the programs. Due to limited exposure to the pre-matriculating students, enrollment for the pilot year of the programs was lower than anticipated.

A second challenge to recruitment is the time commitment needed for students pursuing an MD/MPH dual degree. Students must plan on a fifth year of study and are required to make significant personal, professional and financial commitments to the program early on in their medical training. Prospective students had concerns about graduating with their classmates and workload manageability during their first year of medical school. Two of the first group of enrollees dropped out shortly after enrolling.

Evaluation plans

The evaluation plan includes assessment of students' attainment of specific competencies in public health. Both quantitative and qualitative methodologies will be employed. TCMC's Department of Curriculum Development and Assessment will oversee program evaluation.

Student attitudes and perceptions will be assessed using data derived from questionnaires and focus groups; fund of knowledge from National Board of Medical Examiners (NBME) Subject Exams and NBME Comprehensive Clinical Science Self Assessments (CCSSA).

The Jefferson Scale of Physician Empathy (JSPE) will be completed at the beginning and the end of the academic year, which will allow 'empathy erosion' to be measured and compared over time. Students' career interests will be surveyed yearly to track changes over time using an internally administered survey, beginning with pre-matriculation to the MD Curriculum.

Students' attitudes to primary care will also be assessed prior to the beginning of the LIC and after completion of the LIC.

In addition, TCMC will survey graduates at 1 and every 5 years after completion of their medical education regarding career choice, primary care practice, and practice in HPSAs, MUAs or other underserved communities/populations as well as level of community engagement/public health activities. Residency directors will be surveyed during TCMC graduate's internship year to assess overall competence and qualities such as patient and community centeredness, team skills, and cultural competence.

Dissemination plans

It is anticipated that information about these collaborative programs will be disseminated at various national and international conferences, as well as through additional peer-reviewed publications.

FUTURE PLANS

Additional funding will be sought to ensure sustainability of the program beyond the five year funding period. It is anticipated that institutional funds from both partners will continue to be available to support the program. Potential modifications to the program include making more courses available online to facilitate scheduling and reduce costs. (Currently, a modest number of courses are offered online).

Additional partnerships with community agencies will be sought out in order to provide more practical opportunities for students while fulfilling the missions of both institutions.

Table 1. Acronyms Used

1.	TCMC	The Commonwealth Medical College
2.	ESU	East Stroudsburg University
3.	MPH	Master's of Public Health
4.	PHC	Public Health Certificate
5.	LIC	Longitudinal Integrated Curriculum
6.	CPAP	Constant Positive Airway Pressure
7.	NBME	National Board of Medical Examiners
8.	CHRP	Community Health Research Project
9.	QuICC	Quality Improvement Community Collaborative Project
10.	NEPA	Northeastern Pennsylvania
11.	CCSSA	Comprehensive Clinical Science Self Assessments
12.	JSPE	Jefferson Scale of Physician Empathy
13.	DFCRH	Department of Family, Community and Rural Health
14.	SHIP	State Health Improvement Plan
15.	CEPH	Council on Education for Public Health
16.	DFCRH	Department of Family, Community and Rural Health
17.	HPSAs	Health Professional Shortage Areas
18.	MUAs	Medically Underserved Areas
19.	HRSA	Health Resources and Services Association
20.	ICF	International Classification of Function, Disability, and Health
21.	PASSHE	Pennsylvania State System of Higher Education
22.	AHEC	Area Health Education Center
23.	PAFP	Pennsylvania Academy of Family Physicians
24.	LCME	Liaison Committee on Medical Education
25.	ACP	American College of Physicians

ACKNOWLEDGMENTS

Funding for this project was made possible in part by T85HP24464 from the Health Resources and Services Administration. The views expressed do not necessarily reflect the official policies of the Department of Health and Human Services nor does mention of trade names, commercial practices, or organizations imply endorsement by the US Government.

REFERENCES

[1] Quraishi SA, Orkin FK, Weitekamp MR, Khalid AN, Sassani JW. The health policy and legislative awareness initiative at the Pennsylvania State University college of medicine: theory meets practice. Acad Med 2005; 80(5): 443-7.

[2] Pennsylvania Department of Health. Pennsylvania: EpiQMS. Regional Health Statistics. Accessed 2012 April 14. URL: http://www.portal.state.pa.us/portal/server.pt?open=514&objID=596553&mode=2.

[3] Garrettson M, Walline V, Heisler J, Townsend J. New medical school engages rural communities to conduct regional health assessment. Fam Med 2010; 42(10): 693-701.

[4] Simoyan OM, Townsend JM, Tarafder MR, DeJoseph D, Stark RJ, White MV. Public and medical education: a natural alliance for a new regional medical school. Am J Prev Med 2011; 41(4S3): S220-7.

[5] Simoyan OM, Townsend JM. Improving the health of northeastern Pennsylvania through medical education and community engagement. Public Voices 2012; 12(2): 38-48.

In: Public Health Yearbook 2015
Editor: Joav Merrick

ISBN: 978-1-63484-514-4
© 2016 Nova Science Publishers, Inc.

Chapter 3

ESTABLISHING PARTNERSHIPS BETWEEN PUBLIC HEALTH AND ACADEMIC PARTNERS TO ADDRESS INFANT MORTALITY

Jennifer Mooney[1,*], *PhD, Farrah Jacquez*[2], *PhD, and William Scott*[1]

[1]Reproductive Health and Wellness Program, Maternal and Infant Health Division, Cincinnati Health Department, Cincinnati, Ohio, United States of America
[2]Department of Psychology, University of Cincinnati, Cincinnati, Ohio, United States of America

A partnership between a sociologist at a public health department and a psychologist at a university collaborated on a service learning project that addressed the high infant mortality rate in the region. By addressing unintended teen pregnancy and by examining factors contributing to fetal or infant loss, the partnership provided practicum students with opportunities to use the scientific method to examine infant mortality and disseminate findings to local stakeholders. The public health department benefited through additional workforce power in unbiased data analysis and reporting of results, which led to program enhancement. The students benefited by conducting translational research salient to our community. Strategies for building sustainable partnerships are discussed.

Keywords: partnership, infant mortality, public health, translational research

INTRODUCTION

Infant mortality, in a public health sense, serves as a gauge of overall community health and is defined as the death of an infant before his or her first birthday. The national infant mortality rate per one thousand births in the United States is 6.06 – a rate much higher than

---

[*] Corresponding author: Jennifer Mooney, PhD, Director, Reproductive Health and Wellness Program, Maternal and Infant Health Division, Cincinnati Health Department, 3101 Burnet Avenue, Cincinnati, Ohio 45229, United States. E-mail: jennifer.mooney@cincinnati-oh.gov.

that in other developed countries (1). Although infant mortality in the United States has declined in recent years (1), infant death in the Cincinnati-Hamilton County region of Ohio is nearly triple the Healthy People 2010 goal and double the national average (1, 2). Infant mortality has recently evolved to epidemic status in Cincinnati, although the issue has not affected all racial groups equally. At a rate of 17.8 deaths per 1000 births, African Americans have more than double the infant mortality rate of White residents (3-5). Considering the elevated overall infant mortality rate and the striking racial disparity in infant deaths, social and medical scientists are trying to untangle the web of factors that contribute to negative birth outcomes. Given the complexity of such disparities, interdisciplinary collaboration between public health and academic partners provides a unique way to dissect health concerns with greater rigor and objectivity.

Social determinants of infant mortality

The Cincinnati Health Department and its partnering social service agencies and community organizations have prioritized infant mortality as the key public health issue in our area and have started to investigate the unique social determinants of infant mortality in Cincinnati. Perhaps partially due to the fragmented landscape of health services for women in our area, understanding the perinatal risks for both women and their babies is multifaceted and therefore quite complicated. Unintended pregnancy, for instance, is documented as an indicator of poor birth outcomes (6). However, in a largely Catholic hospital delivery system, few post-partum women are discharged from the delivery hospital with contraception, thereby increasing the chances that these women might become pregnant before the recommended time of at least eighteen months post-delivery.

Pregnancy intention has been documented as a correlate of infant mortality, in that family planning can reduce infant mortality (7). Teen mothers are more likely to experience unintentional pregnancies, thereby increasing risks for adverse health outcomes. Proper prevention of unwanted pregnancy is also affected by the sociopolitical landscape. Research shows that young mothers with unwanted pregnancies are more likely to miss important prenatal visits (8), engage in risky behavior such as smoking or illicit drug use during pregnancy (9), and are more likely to suffer from postpartum depression than adult mothers who plan pregnancy (10). It has also been found that teen mothers often have poorer physical and mental health outcomes later in life than women who did not experience teen motherhood (11).

When attempting to promote optimal infant health and avoid mortality, social service agents and healthcare professionals tend to focus on those factors in which they have expertise. Primary care physicians may be more concerned with weight gain and hypertension as correlates of poor birth outcomes. Social workers may be more likely to contribute high infant mortality rates to domestic issues or access to social services. Obstetricians might focus on participation in prenatal healthcare as the primary target for intervention. In order to address the complex problem of infant mortality, collaboration among diverse stakeholders with varying skill sets and subjectivities is essential. Essentially, untangling the web of human behaviors that led to a pregnancy and ultimately a birth involves both social and medical perspectives.

University-public health department partnership

A truly successful partnership is considered to be a pooling of resources where each partner exercises power in decision-making (12). Research also suggests that successful collaboration be predicated on common interests and goals, mutual cooperation and shared responsibility, and expected mutual benefit (13). From a public health perspective, effective collaboration can be executed through evidence-based research that bridges the gaps between research, practice, and policy. Implementing a public health program through evidence-based research allows the data to inform the program policies and allows for replication of the program. Embracing a solid research foundation for government spending is vital for maximizing public health dollars; at the same time, the logistical barriers of conducting research in real-world programs must be understood by academic researchers (4). Prior examination of the relationship between research and policy has suggested that research must be rigorous, policy must be legitimate, acceptable, and socially relevant, and practice must have applicability (4). While seemingly fundamental, these guidelines for successful partnerships can prove quite challenging when the partnership demands energy and time above and beyond the scope of work for the collaborating partners.

Collaboration between academia and public health is not a new concept. Some partnerships are sustainable and others are time limited. For instance, when Connecticut experienced an increase of a vancomycin-resistant enterococci (VRE) incidence, registered nurses enrolled in a master's of science of nursing program collaborated with the physicians and epidemiologists of the Department of Public Health to address the issue (14). The emergency preparedness team found the resources necessary to address an epidemic and the nursing students were able to apply their skills to address an acute issue in the community. More sustainable academic-public health partnerships do not revolve around a single public health issue, have a longer developmental period, and tend to have less immediate results. For instance, Georgia's Fulton County Sickness Prevention Achieved through Regional Collaboration (SPARC) is a collaborative effort between public, nonprofit, and public health stakeholders to provide clinic-based preventive care to senior citizens. Over time, the dynamic collaboration has been flexible in changing strategies to meet its overall mission and has and scored high when evaluated for program effectiveness (12).

Like all partnerships, ideal university-public health partnerships are formed with the expectations of mutual benefits. Academic partnerships with public health departments can directly benefit students by guiding the career path of students toward public health; therefore, students gain education and experience while public health departments build their future workforce.

Previous literature has demonstrated that partnerships have been beneficial for student nurses who were naïve to nursing within the public health system until practicums opened for them to gain experience (15). Students gain access to resources offered by public health partnerships and can undertake training in order to shape their expertise and professional training (3). Based on their participation in public health activities as undergraduates, students are more likely to choose that path post-graduation (3).

The marriage of public health and academic research benefits public health departments by increasing scientific rigor of public health program efforts. For instance, partnerships with universities help protect against external bias because universities are less likely to have a conflict of interest. Financial incentives of outside parties, such as the pharmaceutical industry, play less into the direction of policy making when a non-biased academic institution is utilized instead as a partner (16). In addition, university-based partners (particularly students) have the benefit of naivety when collaborating in public health research. Unlike the hard-working public professionals who provide programming efforts and are highly invested in results, universities and students serve as an outside party with the goal of objectivity.

Barriers to healthy partnerships have been identified as the breakup of previously established networks and a risk of cost cutting on public health interventions that were previously shown to be effective (17). Partnerships should be manageable and when they are built on similar principles, values, and goals, the likelihood of sustainability increases (13).

Because public health is multidisciplinary, the opportunities for collaboration with academic partners are vast. However, the structure of the Cincinnati public health department employs methods that include surveillance, assessment, disease prevention, health education, and assuring access to public health services (18). With the many demands from the local public health system and the variety of skillsets of its employees, finding research minded individuals for academics to partner with could be challenging. The mission of academia, after all, is to provide unbiased guidance for tomorrow's leaders through education, peer review, and scientific rigor. The collaboration discussed in this paper holds that partnerships based on science and utilization of the naivety of research students is beneficial to public health epidemiology.

The goals of this project are to offer an effective strategy for building a sustainable university-public health partnership. The partnership we describe was established with careful planning, execution, and monitoring in part due to the sensitive nature of infant mortality as a subject matter. As a result of the collaboration, two successful public health projects targeting infant mortality were implemented. Each project provided benefits to both partners, generated useful knowledge for enhancing public health programs, and provided students with an active learning environment. We will discuss the partners, the process of establishing the partnership, the results of the collaboration, and the benefits and challenges of university-public health partnerships.

METHODS

We describe a university-public health department partnership to address infant mortality. The participants in the collaboration are the Cincinnati Health Department and the University of Cincinnati psychology capstone course.

Cincinnati Health Department

The first author, a sociologist at the CHD, serves as the public health partner in our university-health department collaboration. Within the division of Maternal and Infant Health at the CHD, Dr. Mooney oversees the data team of the Fetal and Infant Mortality Review (FIMR) program and is the director for the Cincinnati Hamilton County Reproductive Health and Wellness Program (RHWP), operating in CHD's six federally qualified health centers. FIMR and RHWP address infant mortality in two unique ways. The FIMR program examines fetal and infant death through a case review process while the RHWP prevents unintended pregnancy through family planning and contraception.

Fetal and Infant Mortality Review (FIMR)

FIMR serves women and families with a fetal or infant loss, is operated from the Cincinnati and Hamilton County Health Departments, and is intended to enhance the Greater Cincinnati community. Women and families are provided the opportunity to share the story of their baby's death with a trained interviewer, facilitating the grief process and providing opportunities for education and referrals. Traditionally, the FIMR process required the case review team to review individual level interview data and vital statistics to assess where system enhancements can be made. Prior to the current partnership, FIMR had never undergone any rigorous data analysis on the aggregate level. Suggestions to the community action team were usually made on a case-by-case basis. Trends were not mapped, nor were community level analyses conducted.

Reproductive Health and Wellness Program (RHWP)

The RHWP commenced in 2012 and serves the entire Hamilton County, although the majority of eligible patients live in Cincinnati proper. Federally funded through Title X, the RHWP is designed to improve the health and well-being of women, men, and children by improving their access to preventative and primary health care, promoting healthy behaviors and encouraging the establishment of a reproductive life plan. Patients are provided reproductive health care, including a wide variety of contraception, on a sliding scale. Rigorous program evaluation is ongoing for clinical visits although analysis on the existing RHWP outreach spinoffs is much needed. Outreach drives the mission of the clinical program and therefore, data analysis is critical.

University of Cincinnati Psychology Capstone Course

The academic partner in our university-health department partnership (second author) is a professor in the psychology department at the University of Cincinnati whose research focuses on community approaches to health disparities. Dr. Jacquez teaches the senior psychology capstone course, a class designed to provide advanced undergraduates with a culminating experience applying the knowledge and skills they acquired while progressing through the psychology major. Approximately 20 senior psychology students are enrolled in the capstone course each semester. Unlike other capstone options within the psychology department, students enrolled in this capstone participate in a service-learning experience designed to translate research skills into real-world settings. The goal of this course is for students to understand how psychological research can be used to address locally relevant questions about child health. By working with a community agency, students have the opportunity to see how research is crucial to solving real world problems. In addition, students provide a meaningful, much-needed contribution to our understanding of infant mortality in Cincinnati.

The capstone course is designed to provide advanced undergraduates with learning opportunities that make real community impact. Although service-learning projects each semester are unique, the goals of the course are fairly consistent. Students must demonstrate competency in a set of research skills, including reviewing academic literature, analyzing data, interpreting data in ways that will be meaningful to community partners, and writing research reports. Students collaborate directly with the public health partner throughout the semester, including off-site visits to the Cincinnati Health Department to learn more about programs and present results. Since the partnership between the CHD and the UC capstone course began approximately two years ago, three semesters of capstone students have had the opportunity to participate in service learning experiences directly or indirectly addressing infant mortality.

The current partnership

The purpose of collaboration is to pool the resources of academic partners (a clinical psychologist and advanced undergraduate psychology students) and public health partners (a sociologist and public health department staff) to address infant mortality in a way that progresses both (1) the program trajectory in public health, and (2) the pedagogy of psychology capstone students. Both supervising partners share similar interests and have backgrounds in research; particularly experimental design, human subjects protection, data integrity, and translation of findings to practice. In addition, both academic and community partners served on the Fetal and Infant Mortality Review (FIMR) case review team and are both interested in identifying and developing interventions to address the social determinants of infant mortality.

The current partnership was formed to address the often overlooked social determinants of health as contributors to the region's high infant mortality rate. We will present two examples of projects our partnership has completed: first, an in-depth analysis of FIMR interviews, and second, an evaluation of a program serving teens seeking reproductive health care in schools. Both semester long service-learning projects were designed to help 1) senior psychology students complete their capstones, 2) the CHD obtain quality data that informs program development, and 3) pave an avenue for further collaboration. Several logistical considerations have been made during each semester of collaboration. A "Not Human Subjects" exemption form was submitted to the Institutional Review Board (IRB) at the University as to exempt the project from being defined as "research." Project findings were to be used internally rather than shared with the public, and data was de-identified. Students were mandated to successfully complete a Collaborative Institutional Training Initiative (CITI) human subjects training course prior to beginning the project. Consent was received from the CHD and a Memorandum of Understanding (MOU) was on file prior to collaboration.

In each example project presented, the academic and community partner worked together closely when designing the course to plan activities that met both CHD and student needs. For instance, the syllabus was designed by both academic and community partners to ensure that outcomes of class activities could directly benefit CHD programs. The academic partner incorporated the community partner into elements of the classroom, added her name to the course syllabus as the Community Professor, and held class at the CHD on occasion so students might more easily translate their experience into real world practice. Finally, at the end of each project, students presented their written report in person to relevant stakeholders at the CHD.

RESULTS

Project #1: Fetal and Infant Mortality Review (FIMR)

The goal of the FIMR project was to utilize the research skills of capstone students to identify social determinants of health within existing FIMR data. Using qualitative methods and collaboratively taught by both academic and community partners, capstone students analyzed transcripts of FIMR interviews with mothers who had lost an infant. FIMR interviews contain a wealth of information about the life and healthcare experiences of women who experience a fetal/infant loss; however, until this partnership, the data had not undergone rigorous qualitative and quantitative analysis. The three objectives of the service learning project were 1) to identify themes common among mothers who experienced infant loss; 2) to describe how often mothers reported these themes; and 3) to identify significant relationships between demographic variables and themes. Themes derived from this project were to be used by FIMR to create recommendations for interventions.

The FIMR project had significant benefits for both the students and the health department. Students learned methods for conducting both qualitative and quantitative research, examined real incidences of fetal and infant death in the county, disseminated research findings through a formal report and presentation, and suggested four major implications for health professionals in Cincinnati. Unlike more traditional psychology capstone experiences in which student work does not leave the classroom environment, students in the CHD-partnered service learning capstone had the opportunity to translate research findings into meaningful deliverables that directly benefit public health in our area. The CHD also benefited from the FIMR project by gaining important insight into some of the driving mechanisms behind infant mortality.

Rigorous data analysis of rich content derived directly through structured interviews with women experiencing loss provided suggestions for policy based on evidence. Because public professionals are charged with huge responsibility in delivering programming, they often do not have the time or resources to delve into the mass of available data. Through the partnership, service-learning students fill that need by devoting time to analyzing existing data. Essentially, both academic and community partners benefited through this project, and since both partners were similarly aligned based on education, research interests, student investment, and community outcomes, the partnership continued.

Project #2: Reproductive Health and Wellness Program (RHWP)

Based on the success of the FIMR project and the mutual benefits for students and the CHD, both partners identified another issue to assess in the upcoming semester. In the second project, students worked with data from the RHWP to evaluate a school-based reproductive health program for adolescents. The CHD-funded program utilizes a Community Health Worker (CHW) to provide reproductive health education to adolescents and to help connect them to reproductive health services. The program is designed to increase the number of teens who seek reproductive health care as a means to prevent unintended pregnancy and lower STI incidence, thereby indirectly addressing the infant mortality issue in our area.

Capstone students analyzed data collected by the CHW. The teens visited the CHW in their school-based health clinic for education and consultation and when requested, the CHW connected them to a RHWP clinic to receive birth control and other reproductive services. To evaluate the program, capstone students identified three research objectives: 1) to describe adolescents utilizing the services of a Community Health Worker; 2) to explore how adolescents were connected to reproductive health education and services provided by the Community Health Worker; and 3) to explore the degree age was related to reproductive health knowledge, attitudes, and behaviors.

The RHWP project directly benefited both the public health department and the capstone student collaborators. The work completed by the capstone students was useful to the public health department because grant funding has limitations for data analysts. Until this partnership, the RHWP had no real obtainable way to measure the work the CHW was doing in the field. Findings from the students' analyses indicated that the CHW was successful in her role and more teens were accessing services, thereby preventing pregnancy and STIs. The RHWP project directly benefited students by providing them with the opportunity to experience the "real life" implications for research, statistics, and report writing. This project has continued with the next semester of college students to allow for an analysis of a larger sample size and more longitudinal data.

DISCUSSION

Over the course of eighteen months, the inter-professional collaboration between the University of Cincinnati and the Cincinnati Health Department has had three major impacts. First, academic partners integrated teaching, research, and service roles for community impact. Second, CHD has received much-needed assistance from outside researchers, uniquely able to apply scientific rigor to existing public health data. Third, the collaborative results have benefited infant vitality both directly and indirectly through addressing unintended pregnancy and other indicators of infant death. Each impact will be discussed and limitations and future directions of our long-term university-public health department partnership will be addressed.

The academic partners in our collaboration technically include both a research-track professor at a large urban university and the students enrolled in her capstone course over eighteen months. The academic partner continues to benefit significantly from the professional relationship formed with the public health partner. This academic-public health partnership provides a unique strategy to meet the research, teaching, and service requirements of academia while also making an impact in local communities. By focusing an undergraduate course on infant mortality, a topic relevant to personal research interests, the efforts of the academic professor fulfilled both research and teaching agendas. In addition, the results of the collaborative projects were directly translated to the local public health community in the form of presentations and reports, thereby contributing to community action efforts and fulfilling service requirements as well.

Students also served as academic partners in our interdisciplinary collaboration. By participating in service-learning at the health department, students had the opportunity to contribute to program enhancements through utilization of the scientific method to interpret meaningful results. Both in-class performance and feedback from students suggests that applying research methods to actual health problems in our local area enhances learning outcomes. Anecdotally, we have noticed that students become more engaged in even mundane research tasks when their purpose is important for the large goal. For example, students participating in the FIMR project carefully read countless pages of interview transcripts line-by-line to conduct qualitative analysis, staying after class and making additional time to ensure the analyses were thorough and complete. In end-of-semester course evaluations, students commonly describe the service-learning projects as highly beneficial and even transformative. Example student qualitative comments include, "I learned so much about the research process, more than any class I had taken before" and "having the opportunity to partake in research that yielded positive results for Cincinnati adolescents was the best and most rewarding thing I've ever done in any of my undergraduate classes."

The public health department in our partnership also experiences tangible benefits from the interdisciplinary collaboration. Public health departments by design are inviting to research dollars but often lack the infrastructure to manage research projects, interpret findings, and implement changes within the public health system. Service grants are sought instead since governmental positions can be posted, hired, and trained to implement the program with the grant dollars. With this, the pressure to implement a program, meet benchmarks, and apply for additional grants limits the capabilities of finding influential relationships in data. Therefore, much of the service provision grants cannot be rooted in real evidence because it has yet to be discovered. Public health departments are minefields for data but few have the skills and time to run analysis and interpret findings. Collaboration between both partners led to enhancing the FIMR and RHWP programs by increasing rigorous data analysis, and demonstrating efficacy in program expansion, respectively.

In addition to impact on academic and public health partners, the inter-professional collaboration also had direct and indirect impacts on infant vitality in our area. CHD's goal of eliminating health disparities and promoting health equity are better actualized with interdisciplinary collaboration since individual bias can be reduced, diversity is invited, and resources are pooled. By reducing unintended pregnancy in our region and by understanding the social forces behind infant loss, the two projects our partnership has completed will help promote the health and wellbeing of young women, infants, and families. Evidence-based programs promote our community by increasing opportunities to improve socioeconomic conditions and the career aptitude of the community. The care of undeserved women and men is an area of focus all its own and involves knowledge of the social determinants of health inequity and systematic approach to improving outcomes.

Prior to the academic-public health department collaboration there have been no scientific evaluations of the quality of these programs. Without evaluation, program development and improvement would be arbitrary. Data obtained from the two projects described is crucial for the improvement of programs aimed at reducing infant mortality. Consistent with the work of existing collaborations, this partnership utilized the principles of successful collaboration – common interests and goals, mutual cooperation and shared responsibility, and expected mutual benefit (13). In addition, this partnership found a way to be sustainable through replication. Each semester, the partnership renews and the principles are carefully reassessed prior to implementation.

In addition to the significant benefits experienced through our university-public health department partnership, we have dealt with challenges along the way. Many obstacles come in the form of logistical challenges that take some additional planning and compromise to overcome. For example, students enrolled in the capstone course often lack flexibility in their schedules, so activities with the health department are essentially limited to class time. Meetings at the health department are limited to no more than one hour to allow students to travel back to campus to attend classes immediately following ours. As principal collaborators, our project planning is limited to activities that do not require student attendance outside class time. Similarly, each project is limited to that which can be completed during the 10 weeks of an academic semester.

Some challenges also fell on the public health side of the partnership. For the RHWP project, we have overcome the semester challenge by designing the course to build on the results from the previous semester. Challenges from the public health side include issues with data cleaning and confidentiality. All data must be coded and cleaned prior to student analysis. This took additional time for the public health partner to complete so that informative results could be derived. In addition, data had to be de-identified according to the confidentiality standards set by the Department of Health and Human Services (HHA). Finally, as a former professor in the academic setting the public health partner was enthusiastic about teaching a few class sessions each semester, although lecture preparation took place outside the normal work day.

In conclusion, an academic-public health department collaboration that partners with psychology undergraduates to investigate locally relevant public health phenomena can be an effective strategy to meet both academic and public health department goals. By committing to a long-term partnership rather than single projects, the collaboration is better able to address the larger public health issue of infant mortality.

REFERENCES

[1] Jacquez F, Mooney J. Identifying themes in Fetal and Infant Mortality Review (FIMR) interviews. Cincinnati, OH: Department of Psychology, University of Cincinnati, 2012.
[2] James M Anderson Center for Health Systems Excellence. Preventing infant mortality. URL: http://www.cincinnatichildrens.org/service/j/anderson-center/community-population-health/infant-mortality/.
[3] Larkin M, Richardson E, Tabreman J. New partnerships in health and social care for an era of public spending cuts. Health Soc Care Commun 2011; 20(2): 199-207.
[4] Wehrens R, Bekker M, Bal R. Coordination of research, policy and practice: A case study of collaboration in the field of public health. Sci Public Policy 2011; 38 (10): 755-66.
[5] Pistella CY, Synkewecz CA. Community postpartum care needs assessment and systems development for low income families. J Health Soc Policy 1999; 11(1): 53-64.
[6] Gipson JD, Koenig MA, Hindin MJ. The effects of unintended pregnancy on infant, child, and parental health: A review of the literature. Stud Fam Plann 2008; 39(1): 18-38.
[7] The Guttmacher Institute. Family planning can reduce high infant mortality levels. New York, 2002. URL: http://www.guttmacher.org/pubs/ib_2-02.pdf.
[8] D'Angelo DV, Gilbert BC, Rochat RW, Santelli JS, Herold JM. Differences between mistimed and unwanted pregnancies among women who have live births. Perspect Sex Reprod H 2002; 36(5): 192-7.
[9] Orr ST, Reiter JP, James SA, Orr CA. Maternal health prior to pregnancy and preterm birth among urban, low income black women in Baltimore: The Baltimore preterm birth study. Ethn Dis 2011; 22(1): 85-9.

[10] Shanok AF, Miller L. Depression and treatment with inner city pregnant and parenting teens. Arch Womens Ment Health 2007; 10(5): 199-210.
[11] Patel PH, Sen B. Teen motherhood and long-term health consequences. Matern Child Health J 2012; 16: 1063-71.
[12] Sullivan BA. Inter-organizatonal relationships of health partnerships: Characteristics of the Fulton County Sparc Program. J Health Hum Serv Adm 2012; 35(1): 44-70.
[13] Staton-Tindall M, Rees JD, Oser CB, McNees B, Mooney Palmer J. Establishing partnerships between correctional agencies and university researchers to enhance substance abuse treatment initiatives. Corrections Today 2007: 42-45.
[14] Petroro R, Marola M, Ferreira T, Raboin K, Lewis KK. A win-win partnership between academia and public health practice. Public Health Nurs 2011; 28(6): 543-7.
[15] Landry L, Lee R, Greenwald J. The San Francisco collaborative: An evaluation of a partnership between three schools of nursing and a public health department. Public Health Nurs 2011; 26(6): 568-73.
[16] Johnston SC, Hauser SL, Desmond-Hellmann S. Enhancing ties between academia and industry to improve health. Nature Med 2011; 17(4): 434-6.
[17] Taylor-Robinson DC, Loyd-Williams F, Orton L, Moonan M, O'Flaherty M, Capewell S. Barriers to partnership working in public health: A qualitative study. PLoS ONE 2012; 7(1): 1-8.
[18] Maseru N. Cincinnati Health Department Mission Statement. Cincinnati Health Department, Cincinnati, OH, United States of America. URL: http://www.cincinnati-oh.gov/health/.

In: Public Health Yearbook 2015
Editor: Joav Merrick

ISBN: 978-1-63484-514-4
© 2016 Nova Science Publishers, Inc.

Chapter 4

EFFECT OF A FINANCIAL EDUCATION PROGRAM ON THE HEALTH OF SINGLE, LOW-INCOME WOMEN AND THEIR CHILDREN

Kathleen A Packard[2,*], PharmD, Julie C Kalkowski[1], MSW, Nicole D White[2], PharmD, Ann M Ryan-Haddad[2], PharmD, Lisa L Black[2], DPT, Kathleen A Flecky[2], OTD, Jennifer A Furze[1], DPT, Lorraine M Rusch[3], PhD, and Yongyue Qi[2], MS

[1]Financial Hope Collaborative,
Creighton University College of Business Administration, Omaha,
Nebraska, United States of America
[2]School of Pharmacy and Health Professions, Creighton University,
Omaha, Nebraska, United States of America
[3]School of Nursing, Creighton University, Omaha,
Nebraska, United States of America

Literature suggests an association between poverty, gender, and health. The Financial Success Program (FSP) provides financial education and support to low-income, single mothers. This study assessed the effect of the FSP on health and quality of life in participants and their children. From 2011-2012, 36 women and 28 children were enrolled. Indicators of health and quality of life were assessed pre-and post-year-long intervention. In addition to improvements in financial outcomes, participants demonstrated a significant reduction in fast food consumption and significant improvements in hopefulness and quality of life. Over 30% of mothers experienced weight loss, 52% a reduction in BMI, and 41% a reduction in body fat percentage. Many children experienced reductions in BMI and BMI percentile. This study is the first to report the health effect of financial education in low-income single mothers. When

---

[*] Corresponding author: Kathleen A. Packard, PharmD, MS, BCPS, Associate Professor of Pharmacy Practice, School of Pharmacy and Health Professions, Creighton University, 2500 California Plaza, Omaha, Nebraska, USA. Email: kpackard@creighton.edu.

designing multifaceted community-based cardiovascular risk reduction programs, financial stress should be addressed through education.

Keywords: financial, stress, women, education, cardiovascular disease

INTRODUCTION

In 2012, 40% of households reported living paycheck to paycheck, a trend more common in women than men, 36% versus 44% (1). The same survey demonstrated that 20% of workers were unable to make ends meet, which can lead to significant financial and socioeconomic stress. Increases in perceived life stress and impairments in well-being have been documented in individuals enduring financial strain (2-6).

Persons under stress can be more socially isolated and report elevated depressive and psychosomatic symptoms (7). They also engage in unhealthy behaviors such as smoking, alcohol consumption, overspending, and poor diet and exercise (8). This has been recently explained by the limited-resource model of self-control (8). Because the poor have less money, food, and expendable time, they are challenged to control behavior and resist urges more than others which exhaust self-control resources. Over time, people under stress are at a greater risk for chronic illness, particularly cardiovascular disease. Financial stress was shown to predict myocardial infarction and cardiac death in women in the Framingham Study and has been associated with coronary heart disease (9, 10).

While lifestyle factors can contribute to the development of chronic illness, lower socioeconomic status is also associated with biologic risk factors including hyperlipidemia, obesity, metabolic syndrome, diabetes, elevations in fibrinogen, cardiac rhythm abnormalities, and procoagulant blood profiles (11-13). Many researchers have postulated that the link between stress and poor health outcomes is sustained activation of autonomic and neuroendocrine responses (14). Increased activation of the hypothalamic-pituitary-adrenal axis leading to increased levels of cortisol is a major component of the stress pathway. Chronic cortisol elevations may contribute to insulin resistance, muscle atrophy, diabetes, abdominal fat, immune impairment, and hypertension (7, 15). Furthermore, increased sympathetic nervous system activity, specifically elevations in catecholamines, epinephrine and norepinephrine, has been shown in those of lower socioeconomic status (16). Poverty, low socioeconomic status, and financial stress can also affect health outcomes in children. Financial stress during childhood has been associated with increased childhood obesity and the development of diabetes and cardiovascular disease later in life (17-20).

The Financial Success Program (FSP), founded in 2010 at Creighton University, was developed to explore which financial education program components are most effective in creating behavior change for low-income single mothers. The FSP focuses on three core components: an outstanding trainer, one-on-one financial coaching, and an easy to use money management system. The program serves women in the Omaha, Nebraska metropolitan area who are predominantly African American. Participants have significantly more cardiovascular risk factors than other women in Nebraska including obesity, smoking, diminished exercise, hypertension, and diabetes (21).

During the FSP, participants meet weekly for nine weeks followed by monthly group meetings for one year. Participants are also assigned a coach for long-term financial advice.

Based on anecdotally-reported positive health changes in prior graduates of the FSP, this study was designed to evaluate the effect of the FSP on cardiovascular risk health indicators and financial outcomes in participants and their children. Figure 1 depicts a conceptual model to describe the relationship between financial education and health indicators. To date, there are no published studies assessing the effect of financial education interventions on health indicators.

METHODS

This study was approved by the Creighton University Institutional Review Board (#11-16171). All participants provided written informed consent/assent as applicable. The study was registered on clinicaltrials.gov as "Impact of a Financial Success Education Program in Women and Children," NCT01409291, on July 29, 2011.

All women enrolled in the FSP between September 2011 and May 2012 were approached for participation in the study. To qualify for the FSP, women were 19 years or older and currently employed. Women were excluded from the FSP if they were abusing alcohol or recreational drugs and were excluded from the study if they were pregnant or planning to become pregnant. Children between 3 and 18 years were also approached for participation in the study. A total of 36 women and 28 children chose to participate in the year-long study.

The FSP curriculum has been described in depth in another publication (22). Prior to the education intervention, baseline demographic, clinical, financial, and questionnaire data were obtained from participants and their children. The same data were collected at the one-year follow-up visit post-intervention. Demographic parameters collected in mothers included age, race, annual household income, education, smoking status, marital status, number of children, type of healthcare insurance, occupational status, frequency of exercise, consumption of fast food, medications, and chronic illnesses.

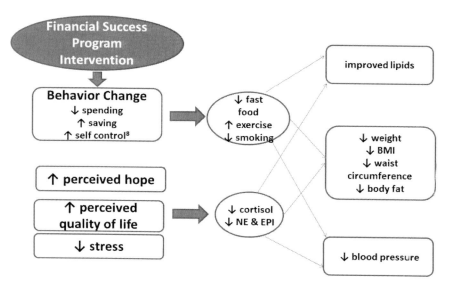

Figure 1. Conceptual Model of the Relationship between the FSP and Health Indicators.

Due to the outcome of cardiovascular risk reduction, the presence of certain chronic illnesses were defined as follows: hypertension as self-reported, a systolic blood pressure greater ≥140 mmHg, a diastolic blood pressure ≥90 mmHg, or use of an antihypertensive drug; diabetes as self-reported, a hemoglobin A1C ≥6.5%, or use of an anti-diabetic medication; and hyperlipidemia as either self-reported, a total cholesterol≥200 mg/dl, or use of a cholesterol-lowering medication. Demographic parameters collected in children included age, race, gender, smoking status, chronic illnesses, frequency of exercise, and consumption of fast food.

Clinical data collected in mothers included blood pressure, weight, body mass index (BMI), waist circumference, hemoglobin A1C, total cholesterol, low density lipoprotein cholesterol (LDL-C), high density lipoprotein cholesterol (HDL-C), triglycerides, and body fat percentage. Clinical data collected in children included blood pressure, weight, BMI, BMI percentile, and waist circumference. Blood pressure was measured in mothers and children three times using an Omron 10 Series digital sphygmomanometer (Omron Healthcare Co, Lake Forest, Illinois) on the dominant arm five minutes apart, at least 15 minutes after arrival. The average of three readings was recorded while the participant was seated. Weight was measured on a digital scale with shoes and coats off. BMI was calculated as weight in kg/(height in meters)^2. Waist circumference was measured by the same operator at both visits. A flexible tape measure was placed on the top of the iliac crest and recorded to the nearest half inch upon patient exhalation. A non-fasting lipid panel was obtained using the CholestechLDX^{TM} point of care device (Cholestech, Hayward, California) using reflectance photometry. Hands were cleaned with alcohol and the target finger was wiped with an alcohol pad. Enough blood to fill a capillary tube (approximately 5-10 drops) was obtained via fingerstick and was placed into the test cassette by depressing the plunger and inserted into the CholestechLDX^{TM} machine. Hemoglobin A1C was measured using a DCA Vantage™ Analyzer (Siemans, Deerfield, Illinois). The same fingerstick for the lipid panel was used to obtain the hemoglobin A1C sample. A bioelectrical impedance machine, Omron Model HBF-306C Fat Loss Monitor, (Omron Healthcare Inc., Bannockburn, Illinois) was used to measure body fat percentage.

Qualitative outcomes captured from the mothers at both visits included perceived hopefulness as measured by the Trait Hope Scale (23). Scores range from 8-64, with higher scores indicating more hopefulness. Quality of life was measured with the World Health Organization Quality of Life (WHOQOL)–BREF survey (24). Financial competency and financial health were measured with questions to capture objective and subjective data. For subjective questions, participants provided answers on a Likert Scale (1-5) coded as ordinal data for statistical analysis (1 = Never, 2 = Seldom, 3 = Sometimes, 4 = Frequently, 5 = Always).

Data analysis

Statistical analyses were performed using SPSS Statistics version 20 (IBM Corporation, Somers, New York). Descriptive statistics were used to describe most baseline demographics. Mean and standard deviations were calculated for continuous variables while a number and a percentage are reported for categorical variables. Comparisons of outcomes pre- and post-intervention were conducted. Dichotomous variables were compared using McNemar's test.

RESULTS

From September 2011 through May 2012, 36 women and 28 children were enrolled in the study. Follow-up continued through May 2013 with 29 women and 19 children returning for the final visit. Most women and children were African American (59% and 52%, respectively) with a mean annual income of $31,214 + $13,726 (Tables 1 and 2). The mean age was 35.8 + 6.1 years for mothers and 7.0 + 2.8 years for children. Interestingly, 95% of women were college educated and 66% were never married. Participants had contact with their financial coach an average of 6.9 times per month, either by phone, email, or face to face.

Financial outcomes

At the end of one year, participants experienced a significant reduction in the mean annual number of overdrawn bank accounts (pre-2.1 ±2.1, post-1.1 ±1.7, $p = .009$), annual shut off notices (pre-2.4 ±2.2, post-1.0 ± 1.2, $p = .003$), annual pay day lender utilization (pre-1.4 ± 2.3, post-0.3 ± 0.7, $p = .01$), and annual bills paid late (pre-3.7 ± 1.9, post-1.8 ± 1.8, $p < .0005$) (Figure 2). Participants also experienced significant improvements in mean annual medical care access and reductions in annual community agency use.

Table 1. Baseline Demographics in Mothers

Mean Age (years)	35.8 ± 6.1
Race	African American 17 (59%), White 11 (38%), Asian 1 (3%)
Mean Annual Household Income (dollars)	$31,214 ± $13,726
Education	College Graduate 14 (48%), Some College 13 (45%), Some High School 1 (3%), High School Graduate 1 (3%)
Marital Status	Never Married 19 (66%), Divorced 6 (21%), Separated 3 (10%), Married 1 (3%)
Mean Number of Children Living with Mother	1.83 ± 1.20

Table 2. Baseline Demographics in Children

Mean Age (years)	7.0 ± 2.8
Gender	Female 11 (58%), Male 8 (42%)
Race	African American 10 (52%), Mixed Race 6 (31%), White 3 (17%)

Survey data also indicated that the participants significantly reduced their financial stress including lost sleep over money, fighting with their partner about money, and allowing financial stress to affect health, relationships, and their ability to work (Figure 3).

Health indicators

There were no significant changes in the rate of chronic illness after the year-long intervention in women (Table 3).

At baseline, 41% of women had hypertension, 24% were smokers, 14% had diabetes, 17% had hyperlipidemia, and 17% reported depression. Though not significant, the rate of hypertension was reduced from 41% to 34% post-intervention. There were also no significant changes in the use of medications in women (Table 4). There were significant reductions in weekly fast food consumption in both women and children; 2.4 ± 1.7 weekly meals reduced to 1.5 ± 1.1, p = .010 and 1.9 ± 1.4 weekly meals reduced to 1.4 ± 1.3, p = .03 for women and children, respectively (Tables 5 and 6). There were also trends towards increased exercise in mothers, 120.0 ± 237.0 weekly minutes pre-intervention and 184.2 ± 404.2 minutes post-intervention, p = .35.

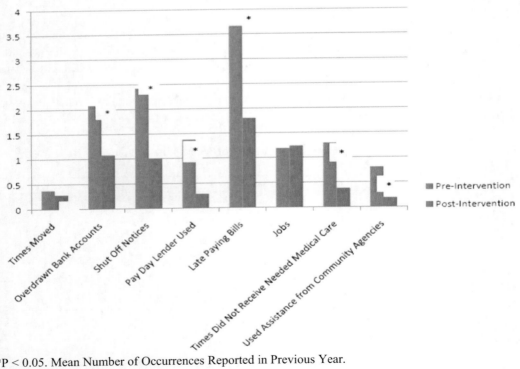

*P < 0.05. Mean Number of Occurrences Reported in Previous Year.

Figure 2. Objective Financial Health Data Pre- and Post-Intervention (n = 21).

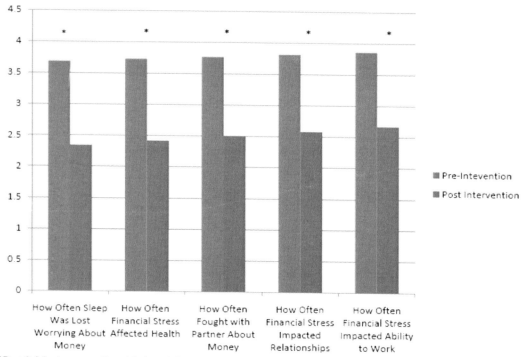

*P < 0.05. Answers Provided on Likert Scale on Occurrence in Previous Year (1 = Never, 2 = Seldom, 3 = Sometimes, 4 = Frequently, 5 = Always).

Figure 3. Subjective Financial Health Data Pre- and Post-Intervention (n = 21).

Table 3. Chronic Illness in Mothers Pre- and Post-Intervention

	Pre-Intervention	Post-Intervention	P Value
Allergies n(%)	2 (7%)	1 (3%)	1.00
Angina n(%)	0	1 (3%)	NA
Anxiety n(%)	4 (14%)	4 (14%)	1.00
Asthma n(%)	3 (10%)	2 (7%)	1.00
Attention Deficit Hyperactivity Disorder n(%)	1 (3%)	1 (3%)	1.00
Bipolar Disorder n(%)	2 (7%)	2 (7%)	1.00
Chrohn's Disease/Irritable Bowel Disease n(%)	1 (3%)	2 (7%)	1.00
Depression n(%)	5 (17%)	4 (14%)	1.00
Type II Diabetes n(%)	4 (14%)	4 (14%)	1.00
Gastroesophageal Reflux Disease n(%)	5 (17%)	5 (17%)	1.00
Headaches/Migraines n(%)	5 (17%)	4 (14%)	1.00
Hyperlipidemia n(%)	5 (17%)	6 (21%)	1.00
Hypertension n(%)	12 (41%)	10 (34%)	0.73
Insomnia n(%)	1 (3%)	0	NA
Narcolepsy n(%)	1 (3%)	1 (3%)	1.00
Obstructive Sleep Apnea n(%)	2 (7%)	2 (7%)	1.00
Osteoarthritis/Musculoskeletal Pain n(%)	2 (7%)	0	NA
Polycystic Ovarian Syndrome n(%)	1 (3%)	1 (3%)	1.00
Smokers n(%)	7 (24%)	6 (21%)	1.00

Table 4. Medications in Mothers Pre- and Post-Intervention

	Pre-Intervention	Post-Intervention	P Value
Allergy Medication: Antihistamine/Decongestant/Nasal Steroid n(%)	7 (24%)	7 (24%)	1.00
Antianxiety Medication n(%)	2 (7%)	3 (10%)	1.00
Antibiotic n(%)	1 (3%)	1 (3%)	1.00
Antidepressant n(%)	3 (10%)	3 (10%)	1.00
Antihypertensive n(%)	4 (14%)	5 (17%)	1.00
Antiviral n(%)	1 (3%)	0	NA
Asthma Medication n(%)	1 (3%)	1 (3%)	1.00
Diabetes Medication n(%)	3 (10%)	3 (10%)	1.00
Gastroesophageal Reflux Disease Medication n(%)	3 (10%)	4 (14%)	1.00
Headache/Migraine Medication n(%)	1 (3%)	1 (3%)	1.00
Multivitamin n(%)	7 (24%)	5 (17%)	0.73
Non-Steroidal Anti-Inflammatory or Acetaminophen n(%)	7 (24%)	6 (21%)	1.00
Opioid Analgesic n(%)	1 (3%)	0	NA
Oral Contraceptive n(%)	5 (17%)	4 (14%)	1.00
Psychostimulant n(%)	1 (3%)	2 (7%)	1.00
Sleep Aid n(%)	0	1 (3%)	NA

Table 5. Lifestyle Modifications in Mothers Pre- and Post-Intervention

	Pre-Intervention	Post-Intervention	P Value
Mean Minutes of Exercise per Week	120.0 ± 237.0	184.2 ± 404.2	0.35
Mean Weekly Fast Food Consumption	2.4 ± 1.7	1.5 ± 1.1	0.010*

*P < 0.05.

Table 6. Lifestyle Modifications in Children Pre- and Post-Intervention

	Pre-Intervention	Post–Intervention	P Value
Mean Minutes of Exercise per Week	404.5 ± 319.6	350.3 ± 246.8	0.38
Mean Weekly Fast Food Consumption	1.9 ± 1.4	1.4 ± 1.3	0.03*

Table 7. Cardiovascular Risk Factors in Mothers Pre- and Post-Intervention

	Pre-Intervention	Post-Intervention	P Value
Mean Systolic Blood Pressure (mmHg)	117.0 ± 15.5	118.4 ± 15.5	0.47
Mean Diastolic Blood Pressure (mmHg)	81.5 ± 13.1	82.3 ± 12.0	0.72
Mean Weight (pounds)	198.2 ± 58.5	197.3 ± 56.8	0.71
Mean Body Mass Index	33.4 ± 9.6	33.3 ± 8.6	0.81
Mean Waist Circumference (inches)	39.5 ± 7.2	40.0 ± 6.7	0.44
Mean Body Fat %	36.0 ± 8.8	37.2 ± 7.2	0.17
Mean Hemoglobin A1C %	5.7 ± 0.37	5.8 ± 0.80	0.25
Mean Total Cholesterol mg/dl	179.8 ± 29.3	173.4 ± 31.5	0.39
Mean Low-Density Lipoprotein Cholesterol mg/dl	93.0 ± 26.0	96.3 ± 30.4	0.58
Mean High-Density Lipoprotein Cholesterol mg/dl	53.1 ± 15.1	49.4 ± 12.8	0.11
Mean Triglycerides mg/dl	147.0 ± 75.0	147.2 ± 110.7	0.08

Table 8. Cardiovascular Risk Factors in Children Pre- and Post-Intervention

	Pre-Intervention	Post-Intervention	P Value
Mean Body Mass Index	18.4 ± 4.6	19.3 ± 5.6	0.05
Mean Body Mass Index Percentile	63.2% ± 30.1%	61.0% ± 33.1%	0.57
Mean Waist Circumference (inches)	25.1 ± 5.2	26.4 ± 5.2	0.001*
Mean Height (inches)	50.6 ± 6.5	53.2 ± 6.3	<0.0001*
Mean Weight (pounds)	71.1 ± 34.7	82.6 ± 41.6	<0.0001*
Mean Systolic Blood Pressure (mmHg)	95.8 ± 9.1	93.0 ± 9.1	0.30
Mean Diastolic Blood Pressure (mmHg)	62.7 ± 11.0	59.1 ± 8.0	0.20

*P < 0.05.

Table 9. World Health Organization Quality of Life-BREF Raw Score and Trait Hope Scale Score in Women Pre- and Post-Intervention

	Pre-Intervention	Post-Intervention	P Value
Mean Domain 1 Physical Health	21.2 ± 3.0	23.3 ± 3.0	0.001*
Mean Domain 2 Psychological	19.8 ± 3.2	20.8 ± 3.2	0.10
Mean Domain 3 Social Relationships	10.0 ± 2.5	10.8 ± 2.9	0.20
Mean Domain 4 Environment	26.6 ± 4.8	30.1 ± 5.6	<0.001*
Mean Trait Hope Scale Score	48.7 ± 7.9	52.7 ± 8.5	0.01*

*P < 0.05.

There were no significant changes in any of the mean cardiovascular risk factor or biometric data (Table 7) for mothers. While there was no difference in the mean change in weight, nine of the women (31%) lost weight, between 6 and 28 pounds. Fifteen women (52%) experienced a BMI reduction, ten (34%) experienced a waist circumference reduction, and 12 (41%) experienced a body fat percentage reduction.

Other than expected increases in normal growth, there were no significant changes in cardiovascular risk data for children (Table 8). While there were no significant differences in the mean change in BMI, eight children (42%) experienced a BMI reduction and six (32%) experienced a BMI percentile reduction. Quality of life in mothers improved for all domains assessed (Table 9). This was statistically significant for domain 1, physical health (pre-21.2 ±3.0 and post-23.3 ±3.0, p = .001) and domain 4, environment (pre-26.6 ±4.8 and post-30.1 ±5.6, p < .001).

Likewise, Trait Hope Scale scores significantly improved for mothers (pre-48.7 ±7.9 and post-52.7 ±8.5, p = .01)

DISCUSSION

Financial education through the FSP led to significant improvements in measurements of financial outcomes including reductions in overdrawn bank accounts, reductions in shut off notices, reductions in pay day lender use, reductions in late bill payments, improvements in health care access, and reductions in community agency use. These behavior changes also improved social and physical well-being including significant reductions in lost sleep over money, reductions in fighting with their partner about money, and less effect of financial stress on health, relationships, and ability to work.

This is the first study to demonstrate that a financial education program can affect physical health. Both women and children significantly reduced their consumption of fast food. This was probably due to the FSP emphasis of the negative effect of eating out not only on physical health but on finances. There were also trends towards increased weekly exercise in mothers, but not the children. Self-reporting of exercise in children was highly variable and anecdotally, mothers reported difficulty in estimating exercise, especially in their younger, more active children. Mothers were uncertain of physical activities their children engaged in during school-based physical education classes, recess, or after-school programs.

While there were no significant changes in any of the mean cardiovascular risk or biometric data for mothers, many of the women experienced weight loss and reductions in BMI, waist circumference, and body fat percentage. This is important as it has been shown in cohorts from the Nurses' Health Studies I and II that women gain, on average, approximately 3.35 pounds every four years (25). Data from the Behavioral Risk Factor Surveillance System similarly showed that women gain 0.3 kg or 0.7 pounds per year (26). The fact that so many women in this study lost weight needs to be further explored. Similarly, for children, while there were no significant differences in the mean change in BMI, many experienced a reduction in BMI and BMI percentile.

There are reasons why participants may not have experienced significant changes in blood pressure, lipid panels, hemoglobin A1C, and biometric parameters. First, the primary objective of the FSP is to improve immediate financial outcomes. There are only limited direct health interventions embedded within the program. Those that are implemented such as reduction of fast food or changing medications to generic or "$4 list" have a direct effect on finances and were significantly improved. Therefore, expansion of the program to integrate direct health interventions is planned for the future.

Second, a one year follow-up duration may not have been adequate for all participants to implement lifestyle changes necessary to reduce cardiovascular risk. While many of the women experienced weight loss and positive changes in their BMI, body fat percentage, and waist circumference, others remained the same or gained weight. Anecdotally, some women reported that one year was just enough time to become financially secure and now they could begin to focus on reducing cardiovascular risk. Therefore, investigators intend to follow participants for one more year to assess for further changes and determine sustainability of change.

A recent study in socially disadvantaged women assessing a two-year community-based primary prevention program to reduce cardiovascular risk supports this timeline to some degree (27). While the program was multi-faceted in that it encompassed exercise, nutrition, psychological and relaxation, it did not reportedly provide financial education. The findings indicated a significant decrease in metabolic syndrome at year one (64.7% versus 34.9%, $p = .01$) and even more at year two (28.2%, $p < .001$), driven by significant reductions in blood pressure and increases in HDL-C. Hemoglobin A1C was also further improved after two years of follow-up (6% at year one, 5.85% at year two ($p = .87$) and 5.8% at year three ($p < .01$)). Unlike the FSP, this study did not achieve significant reductions in fast food consumption, perhaps because it was not linked to a financial benefit. Similar to the FSP, this study did not achieve significant reductions in waist circumference or triglycerides.

FSP participants experienced statistically significant improvements in perceived hope and also quality of life for the domains of physical health and environment, with the most pronounced increase in environment. In the WHO QOL-BREF, the environment domain includes financial resources, information and skills, recreation and leisure, home environment, access to health and social care, physical safety and security, physical environment, and transport. Improvements in these domains are therefore consistent with other study results demonstrating improvement in financial and health indicators. In a recent study, perceived well-being was shown to be a strong predictor of health care outcomes including hospital admissions, emergency room visits, and health care costs (28). Each point increase in well-being was associated with a 1% reduction in health care costs and those with low scores had a 2.7 times increase in annual expenditures compared with those having high scores. Therefore, future research should be conducted to ascertain whether the FSP also reduces health care costs.

Limitations

Several important limitations of this study should be mentioned. Recruitment for the FSP is predominantly through word of mouth and there is an ongoing waiting list to enter the program. Therefore, these women may have been more motivated to change than other women in the general population. There is no control group that did not receive the financial intervention. While this is an important limitation, due to the wait list to enter the program, investigators did not feel it would be ethical to randomize a control group from this sample. Likewise, although these women are low-income, their mean income was $31,214±$13,726 and 95% of them had some college education or were college graduates. In 2012, the poverty threshold for a family of four was $23,050 (29). Only 34% of the women in this study fell below the poverty line. Therefore, it may be inappropriate to extrapolate these data to women living below the poverty line or those with less education. Also, because the study visits occurred in the evening after work, most were in a non-fasting state. This could have affected the lipid panel results. Likewise, fluid intake was not assessed and this can affect body fat percentage readings from the bioelectrical impedance machine. However, because the visits occurred at the same time both pre- and post-intervention, it is expected that these variables were equally distributed between both visits. Finally, the FSP also limits its enrollment in order to optimize group interactions. The small sample size restricts the generalizability of the results.

CONCLUSION

This study is the first to report the positive effect of a financial education program in low-income single women on health indicators. In this high risk population, it was found that a year-long financial education intervention led to significant reductions in fast food consumption, improvements in perceived hope and quality of life. While there were no significant changes in any of the mean cardiovascular risk factor or biometric data for mothers, many of the women experienced weight loss and reductions in BMI, waist circumference, and body fat percentage. Similarly, for children, while there were no significant differences in the mean change in BMI, many experienced a reduction in BMI and BMI percentile.

Multifaceted community-based cardiovascular risk reduction programs are important. When designing such interventions, financial stress, which is often a major barrier for single low-income women to adopt a healthy lifestyle, should be addressed through education. Further research needs to be conducted to determine the critical components of such programs and optimal follow-up.

ACKNOWLEDGMENTS

This work was supported by funding from the Creighton University Dr. George F. Haddix President's Faculty Research Fund, the Ruth and William Scott Family Foundation, Sherwood Foundation, Weitz Funds, and United Way of the Midlands. The authors would like to thank Kate Martens Stricklett and Ronna Sears-Fritz for their assistance and support throughout the investigation. None of the authors have any current or past commercial associations that may pose a conflict of interest. No financial disclosures were reported by the authors of this paper.

REFERENCES

[1] Careerbuilder.com. Percentage of U.S. workers living paycheck to paycheck reaches recession-era low, finds careerbuilder survey. Accessed 2013 July 09. URL: http://www.careerbuilder.com/share/aboutus/pressreleasesdetail.aspx?sd=8%2F15%2F2012&id=pr711&ed=12%2F31%2F2012.
[2] Kessler RC, Cleary PD. Social class and psychological distress. Am Social Rev 1980; 45: 463-78.
[3] Seeman TE, Crimmins E. Social environment effects on health and aging: integrating epidemiologic and demographic approaches and perspectives. Ann NY Acad Sci 2001; 954: 88-117.
[4] Turner RJ, Wheaton B, Lloyd DA. The epidemiology of social stress. Am Social Rev 1995; 60: 104-25.
[5] Garcia MC, de Souza A, Bella GP et al. Salivary cortisol levels in Brazilian citizens of distinct socioeconomic and cultural levels. Ann NY Acad Sci 2008; 1148: 504-8.
[6] Dettenborn L, Tietze A, Bruckner F, et al. Higher cortisol content in hair among long-term unemployed individuals compared to controls. Psychoneuroendocrinology 2010; 35(9): 1404-9.
[7] Grossi G, Perski A, Lundberg U, et al. Associations between financial strain and the diurnal salivary cortisol secretion of long-term unemployed individuals. Integr Physiol Behav Sci 2001; 36: 205-19.
[8] Vohs KD. Psychology. The poor's poor mental power. Science 2013; 341: 969-70.
[9] Eaker ED, Pinsky J, Castelli WP. Myocardial infarction and coronary death among women: psychosocial predictors from a 20-year follow-up of women in the Framingham Study. Am J Epidemiol 1992; 135: 854-64.
[10] Rosengren A, Hawken S, Ounpuu S, et al. Association of psychosocial risk factors with risk of acute myocardial infarction in 11,119 cases and 13,648 controls from 52 countries (the INTERHEART study): case-control study. Lancet 2004; 364: 953-62.
[11] Kunz-Ebrecht SR, Kirschbaum C, Steptoe A. Work stress, socioeconomic status and neuroendocrine activation over the working day. Soc Sci Med 2004; 58: 1523-30.
[12] Steptoe A, Phil D, Brydon L, et al. Changes in financial strain over three years, ambulatory blood pressure, and cortisol response to awakening. Psychosomatic Med 2005; 67: 281-7.

[13] Ogden CL, Lamb MM, Carroll MD, et al. Obesity and socioeconomic status in adults: United States. 2005-2008. 2010. NCHS Data Brief No. 50; 1-8.
[14] Dowd JB, Goldman N. Do biomarkers of stress mediate the relation between socioeconomic status and health. J Epidemiol Community Health 2006; 60: 633-39.
[15] Bjorntorp P, Rosemond R. The metabolic syndrome – a neuroendocrine disorder? Br J Nutr 2000; 83: 49-57.
[16] Janicki-Deverts D, Cohen S, Adler NE, et al. Socioeconomic status is related to urinary catecholamines in the Coronary Artery Risk Development in Young Adults (CARDIA) study. Psychosom Med 2007; 69: 514-20.
[17] Gundersen C, Mahatmya D, Garasky S, et al. Linking psychosocial stressors and childhood obesity. Obes Rev 2011; 12: e54-63.
[18] Chichlowska KL, Rose KM, Diez-Roux AV, et al. Life course socioeconomic conditions and metabolic syndrome in adults: the Atherosclerosis Risk in Communities (ARIC) Study. Ann Epidemiol 2009; 19: 875-83.
[19] Lidfeldt J, Li TY, Hu FB, et al. A prospective study of childhood and adult socioeconomic status and incidence of type 2 diabetes in women. Am J Epidemiol 2007; 165: 882-9.
[20] Galobardes B, Smith GD, Lynch JW. Systematic review of the influence of childhood socioeconomic circumstances on risk for cardiovascular disease in adulthood. Ann Epidemiol 2006; 16: 91-104.
[21] Gillespie N, Packard KA, Kalkowski J, et al. Cardiovascular risk factors of women and children in an urban financial education program. Presented at: Preventive Medicine Annual Meeting. Orlando, (FL), February 2012.
[22] White N, Packard K, Kalkowski J, et al. A novel financial education program in single women of low-income and their children. Int Pub Health J 2013, in Press.
[23] Snyder CR, Harris C, Anderson JR, et al. The will and the ways: development and validation of an individual-differences measure of hope. J Person Soc Psychol 1991; 60: 570-85.
[24] The WHOQOL Group. Development of the World Health Organization WHOQOL-BREF quality of life assessment. Psychol Med 1998; 28: 551–8.
[25] Mozaffarian D, Hao T, Rimm EB, et al. Changes in diet and lifestyle and long-term weight gain in women and men. N Engl J Med 2011; 363: 2392-2404.
[26] Wetmore CM, Mokdad AH. In denial: misperceptions of weight change among adults in the United States. Prev Med 2012; 55: 93-100.
[27] Gilstrap LG, Malhotra R, Peltier-Saxe D et al. Community-based primary prevention programs decrease the rate of metabolic syndrome among socioeconomically disadvantaged women. J Wom Health 2013; 22(4): 322-8.
[28] Harrison PL, Pope JE, Coberley CR, et al. Evaluation of the relationship between individual well-being and future health care utilization and cost. Pop Health Manag 2012; 15: 325-30.
[29] US Department of Health and Human Services. 2012 poverty guidelines. Accessed 2013 July 14. URL: http://aspe.hhs.gov/poverty/12poverty.shtml#thresholds.

Chapter 5

A NOVEL FINANCIAL EDUCATION PROGRAM FOR SINGLE WOMEN OF LOW-INCOME AND THEIR CHILDREN

Nicole White[1,], PharmD, Kathleen Packard[1], PharmD, MS, BCPS, Julie Kalkowski[2], MSW, Ann Ryan-Haddad[1], PharmD, Kathy Flecky[1], OTD, OTR/L, Jennifer Furze[1], PT, DPT, Lori Rusch[3], PhD, RN, CNE, and Lisa Black[1], PT, DPT*

[1]Creighton University School of Pharmacy and Health Professions, Omaha, Nebraska, United States of America
[2]Creighton University College of Business, Financial Hope Collaborative, Omaha, Nebraska, United States of America
[3]Creighton University School of Nursing, Omaha, Nebraska, United States of America

Financial stress is a condition that occurs commonly in the United States, especially in single-mothers and their children. This stress can be a barrier to optimal health and wellness. In an effort to reduce financial stress and improve money management skills in low income, single mother families, the Financial Success Program (FSP) was created. This novel program provides education and support to an underserved population and may also improve the health and well-being of the women and children enrolled. Through a unique interprofessional collaboration, a study was initiated to assess the effect of financial education on health indicators in single-mother families. A thorough discussion of the FSP and interprofessional model will be discussed as a framework for addressing public health needs in a financially stressed population.

Keywords: public health, cardiovascular risk, financial stress, interprofessional collaboration

---

[*] Corresponding author: Nicole White, PharmD, Assistant Professor, Pharmacy Practice, Creighton University, School of Pharmacy and Health Professions, 2500 California Plaza, Omaha, NE 68178, United States. E-mail: nicolewhite@creighton.edu.

INTRODUCTION

Traditional risk factors for heart disease include hypertension, hypercholesterolemia, diabetes, obesity, sedentary behavior, smoking and family history (1). Financial stress, however, has also been implicated in cardiovascular disease risk. In the Framingham heart study, financial stress was associated with coronary heart disease and was shown to predict myocardial infarction and cardiac death in women (2, 3). Additionally, lower socioeconomic status is associated with impaired well-being and biologic risk factors for heart disease including hyperlipidemia, metabolic syndrome and diabetes (4-6). Low socioeconomic status and financial stress also have deleterious effects on the health of children, including a greater rate of childhood obesity and subsequent development of diabetes and cardiovascular disease (7-10).

Financial stress is not uncommon. Up to 40% of American households report living paycheck to paycheck (11). Single-mother families may be especially affected by financial strain. A report from 2012 found that 63% of single mother families met the poverty rate in the United States versus a 17% rate of poverty in two-parent families (poverty rate based on the 50% of median income poverty standard) (12). Due to its prevalence and association with poor health outcomes, financial stress presents a novel target for public health interventions, especially in the single-mother family population.

PROGRAM HISTORY

In an effort to reduce financial stress and improve money management skills in low income, single mother families, the Financial Success Program (FSP) was created. The FSP was initially funded by a grant from the Financial Industry Regulatory Authority (FINRA) Investor Education Foundation in 2010 to explore what financial education program components are most effective in creating behavior change for low income single mothers. The FSP focuses on three core components: an outstanding trainer, financial coaching, and an easy to use money management system.

To be eligible for participation in the FSP, women must be earning a minimum of $12,000 annually, cannot be involved in a domestic violence situation or have an active addiction to alcohol or illicit drugs. They must also be willing to participate in both nine weeks of training and one year of financial coaching. The initial nine-week curriculum was created to address the immediate financial issues in a group of employed women who are struggling financially. The curriculum includes tracking expenses, saving for emergencies, and repairing credit reports. Information on taxes, insurance, predatory lending, legal issues, and the psychology of money are also provided. The nine-week curricular outline is described below (see Table 1). The classes are offered once a week for two-three hours in a local community meeting space. Program participants receive free dinner and daycare with each weekly class. Participants are also paired with a financial coach, with whom they work with for a year following the initial classes. Financial coaches review and assess saved receipts, expense tracking forms, pay stubs and credit reports with the women.

Table 1. Financial Education Curriculum

Session 1	Introduction to financial support team and program orientation. Active Learning: Intake form and baseline survey completion (assessing financial state, spending habits and hopefulness), family financial snapshot, financial journaling, asset bingo and receipt saving assignment
Session 2	Family financial snapshot and psychology of money Active Learning: Expense tracking
Session 3	Understanding predatory lending Active Learning: Expense tracking
Session 4	Banking and savings, guest speaker Active learning: expense tracking and assignment to collect paystub for next session
Session 5	Understanding credit and credit reports and how to increase income without a second job, guest speaker Active Learning: Learning how to read a credit report, what a credit score means and how your credit score affects your life, and how to fix and/or build credit, introduction to financial coach and expense tracking
Session 6	Level payment plan, guest speakers from local utility providers Active Learning: expense tracking and enrolling in the level payment plans for utilities
Session 7	Legal issues, guest speaker from Legal Aid Active Learning: Expense tracking, how to read your pay stub and meeting with financial coach
Session 8	Understanding insurance/retirement, guest speaker
Session 9	Graduation ceremony Active Learning: Follow-up survey completion (assessing financial state, spending habits and hopefulness)

From this evaluation, spending habits are discussed and women participants make plans for change. Frequency of interaction with the coach is agreed upon by the participant and coach and may vary throughout the year depending on needs. This may include face to face meetings, phone calls, or email interaction. To date 196 women have completed the FSP.

PROGRAM METHODOLOGY

The FSP is a two-phase program. Phase One involves the nine-week didactic curriculum in which women and their children receive a healthy dinner and live interactive educational sessions with an experienced trainer. Free childcare is available during these meetings. Phase Two occurs after graduation from the educational classes and involves one-on-one financial coaching from an assigned FSP representative, as well as monthly graduate follow-up meetings. Coaching is available for one year following the last didactic session and frequency of interaction is determined by the needs of the individual woman. Phase One curriculum is described below (see Table 1).

INTERPROFESSIONAL COLLABORATION

The FSP was developed and is currently directed by individuals affiliated with the Creighton University College of Business Administration in Omaha, Nebraska. Following the first year of program enrollment, the directors noted that cardiovascular risk indicators such as weight and overall well-being were improving in graduates as their financial health improved. Many graduates had either completely given up fast food or had significantly reduced the number of times they ate fast food per week. Based on these preliminary, anecdotal reports, the program directors sought out a partnership with health science colleagues to determine if better finances meant better health for the women and children enrolled in the FSP.

The FSP program directors reached out to the Creighton University School of Pharmacy and Health Professions Office of Interprofessional Scholarship, Service and Education (OISSE). The OISSE office is an established structure within Creighton University, designed to organize and promote interprofessional partnerships that offer teaching, scholarship and service opportunities for faculty and students in the health sciences. The OISSE office coordinated the recruitment of health science faculty, students, and residents to collaborate on this project.

This particular interprofessional collaboration is unique in that it bridges social sciences (business administration) with various health care disciplines. Members of the team include a social worker from the college of business administration, three pharmacists, an occupational therapist, a nurse, and three physical therapists.

Based on the hypothesis that decreased financial stress would also lead to cardiovascular risk reduction, an interprofessional study was initiated. The program directors continued to provide the financial education and support within the original structure of the FSP, while the health professional team measured pre and post-intervention biometric and quality of life data to assess for changes in cardiovascular risk and overall well-being. To date, there are no published studies assessing the impact of a financial education intervention on health.

Cardiovascular risk assessment

At the second FSP session, following consent, women are enrolled in the cardiovascular risk assessment study. At this time, baseline demographic, biometric and quality of life data are collected by the team of health care professionals. This data is comprehensive but includes among other measures: age, height, weight, body mass index (BMI), smoking status, cholesterol, hemoglobin A1c (HbA1c), blood pressure, body fat percentage, insurance coverage, income, and quality of life as measured by the World Health Organization (WHO) Quality of Life (QOL) survey (abbreviated version).

During the assessment visit, point of care blood pressure, cholesterol and A1c results are interpreted for each participant and referrals are made when urgent or emergent values are obtained. Additionally, short counseling sessions are completed regarding abnormal lab values and lifestyle behaviors that can be modified to improve biometric data. The risk assessment process is then repeated on the same set of women and children after approximately one year of participation in the FSP.

Not surprisingly, the women enrolled in the FSP were found to have great need for cardiovascular risk reduction. In addition to poor financial status, the women enrolled in FSP also present with significantly more risk factors for cardiovascular disease than other women in Nebraska including greater rates of obesity, tobacco use, diminished exercise, hypertension, and diabetes (see Table 2) (13-17). The children of single-mothers enrolled in the FSP were also at increased risk of chronic disease. Compared to 31.5% of children (aged 10-17) in Nebraska, 42.1% of the children assessed in the FSP were overweight or obese (as measured by a BMI > 85th percentile for age) (24).

Table 2. Comparison of FSP Participants to Average Women in Nebraska

	Women Enrolled in FSP	Women in Nebraska
Race		
Caucasian	38%	89.2%[16]
African American	59%	3.3%[16]
No health insurance	6.9%	12.6%[16]
Overweight or Obese BMI (≥25.0)	79.3%	57.3%[14]
Obese BMI (≥30)	58.6%	26.3%[14]
Current Smoker	20.7%	15.1%[13]
Physically Inactive (0 min/week reported)	24.1%	11.6%[15]
Diabetes	13.8%	7.2%[16]
Elevated Cholesterol	34.5%	35.3%[17]
Hypertension	34.5%	25.3%[17]

Table 3. Healthy People 2020 Goals Addressed by the FSP and Interprofessional Cardiovascular Risk Assessment

Goal	2020 Target
HDS 4 – Increase the proportion of adults who have had their blood pressure measured within the preceding 2 years and can state whether their blood pressure was normal or high	92.6%
HDS 5.1 – Reduce the proportion of adults in the population with hypertension	26.9%
HDS 5.2 – Reduce the proportion of children and adolescents in the population with hypertension	3.2%
HDS 6 - Increase the proportion of adults who have had their blood cholesterol checked within the preceding 5 years	82.1%
HDS 7 - Reduce the proportion of adults with high total blood cholesterol levels	13.5%
HDS 8 - Reduce the mean total blood cholesterol levels among adults	177.9 mg/dl
HDS 11 - Increase the proportion of adults with hypertension who are taking the prescribed medications to lower blood pressure	69.5%
HDS 12 – Increase the proportion of adults with hypertension whose blood pressure is under control	61.2%

HDS: Heart Disease and Stroke.

PUBLIC HEALTH IMPLICATIONS

Due to its prevalence and negative implications on health and well-being, financial stress is a novel target for public health interventions. On a broad level, the FSP, in conjunction with the interprofessional cardiovascular risk assessment, aligns well with several of the Healthy People 2020 goals (see Table 3) (18).

Additionally, the FSP and interprofessional cardiovascular risk assessment fulfill several of the ten Essential Services of Public Health, as defined by the National Public Health Performance Standards Program (NPHPSP) (19). Specifically, eight Essential Services are demonstrated in the FSP. These include:

1. Monitor health status to identify and solve community health problems
2. Diagnose and investigate health problems and health hazards in the community
3. Inform, educate, and empower people about health issues
4. Mobilize community partnerships and action to identify and solve health problems
5. Link people to needed personal health services and assure the provision of health care when otherwise unavailable
6. Assure competent public and personal health care workforce
7. Evaluate effectiveness, accessibility, and quality of personal and population-based health services
8. Research for new insights and innovative solutions to health problems

The pre/post cardiovascular risk assessments allow the team to monitor the health status and identify health problems affecting single mothers and their children with financial stress (Essential Service 1). The study team has identified that women in the FSP have a higher incidence of obesity, smoking, physical inactivity, diabetes, and hypertension compared to women in Nebraska (Essential Service 2). The FSP program and faculty team members provided health education to empower study participants to implement lifestyle modifications and to seek healthcare to address specific health issues identified in the health assessments (Essential Service 3). The campus-community partnership was successfully developed (with the university infrastructure in place) to recruit health science faculty team members interested in participating with colleagues in business administration to develop a research project assessing the impact of the FSP on women's cardiovascular health (Essential Service 4). On many occasions, team members were able to refer mothers to appropriate low/no cost health clinics for treatment of high blood pressure or diabetes (Essential Service 7). Faculty team members recruited health science students from their own didactic courses or clinical rotations to assist in the health assessments and this provided students with a unique opportunity to work side by side with faculty and develop clinical and social skills to assure competent future health care workforces (Essential Service 8). During the pre/post assessments, faculty team members were able to learn more about accessibility and quality of personal health services and the barriers single mothers with financial stress often encounter (Essential Service 9). The uniqueness of this project will provide new insights into the health effects of financial stress, as well as potentially serve as an innovative model for addressing health issues of single-mother families (Essential Service 10).

DISCUSSION

While many other financial education programs exist, the FSP is unique and highly sought after due to its three core components: an outstanding trainer, financial coaching, and an easy to use money management system. Unlike other financial education programs, where the primary focus is home ownership or small business start-ups, single mothers under financial stress need a plan to help them change their financial behaviors. The FSP focuses on the financial challenges unique to single mothers under financial stress. An outstanding trainer is essential. The trainer for the FSP has significant life experiences, including being a single mother, that complements her skills as a facilitator and allows her to talk about common financial problems faced in this population without evoking a feeling of judgment in the women enrolled.

The second core component of the FSP is the financial coaching. The FSP directors carefully distinguish the word "coach" from "mentor" for this position which ultimately directs the relationship that exists between the coaches and the single-mother participants. The coaches are to work WITH the women in the program to bring about a change in their financial behavior rather than give advice or use confrontation as a financial expert or "mentor." This technique is one example of how motivational interviewing is used by the coaches to elicit financial behavior change (20). Many of the coaches are single-mothers themselves. This attribute allows them to display greater empathy toward the women in the program and support their self-efficacy in making a positive change. Empathy and promotion of self-efficacy are two other key components to motivational interviewing and successful behavior change (20). In addition to motivational interviewing, coaches use various methods of communication to reach the FSP participants. Meetings can occur face to face, over the telephone, through email and via social media. This varied approach ensures that women are being contacted in a way that is convenient and most helpful to them.

The third and final core component of the FSP is an easy to use money management system. Program participants are given an Excel spreadsheet on a jump drive so they can input their expenses. The participants review their expense logs with their financial coaches to identify patterns or areas for improvement. By seeing where their money is being spent, the women realize they have more choices. For many women, it is the first time they feel they have some control in one aspect of their lives. This leads to the realization they also have control in other areas of their lives, including their health and wellness. A sense of internal control (as opposed to being controlled by others or circumstances beyond personal control) has been associated with a perception of being able to impact one's personal health in positive ways (21, 22). Moreover, perception of personal, internal control over stressful events can promote a mindset of less stress and a physiological diminished cortisol response to stressors (23).

For many of the women starting the FSP, being financially stressed takes precedence in their lives which limits their ability to pay attention to information or behaviors related to exercise and nutrition. Making better financial decisions gives women the ability and confidence to focus on issues other than money and empowers them to address the health and wellness of themselves and their family.

CONCLUSION

Financial stress is a non-traditional risk factor for heart disease and may be a novel target for public health interventions to improve cardiovascular risk and overall well-being. Single-mother families have higher reported rates of poverty than two parent families and endure significantly higher financial strain. The FSP is an innovative program focused on decreasing financial stress and improving money-management skills in low-income single-mother families. The program is also being evaluated for its effect on health and well-being. To date, this is the only published study assessing the impact of a financial education intervention on health. The program and study highlight a unique interprofessional partnership that bridges social sciences (business administration) with health care disciplines (pharmacy, occupational therapy, physical therapy and nursing). The collaboration allows for expert attention to both personal finances and personal health with broad public health implications. Further research will determine whether the program makes a significant impact on the health and wellbeing of the single mother families that participate.

REFERENCES

[1] DeGoma EM, Knowles JW, Angeli F, Budoff MJ, Rader DJ. The evolution and refinement of traditional risk factors for cardiovascular disease. Cardiol Rev 2012; 20(3): 118-29.
[2] Eaker ED, Pinsky J, Castelli WP. Myocardial infarction and coronary death among women: psychosocial predictors from a 20-year follow-up of women in eth Framingham Study. Am J Epidemiol 1992; 135: 854-64.
[3] Rosengren A, Hawken S, Ounpuu S, et al. Association of psychosocial risk factors with risk of acute myocardial infarction in 11,119 cases and 13,648 controls from 52 countries (the INTERHEART study): case-control study. Lancet 2004; 364: 953-62.
[4] Kunz-Ebrecht SR, Kirschbaum C, Steptoe A. Work stress, socioeconomic status and neuroendocrine activation over the working day. Soc Sci Med 2004; 58: 1523-30.
[5] Dettenborn L, Tietze A, Bruckner F, Lirschbaum C. Higher cortisol content in hair among long-term unemployed individuals compared to controls. Psychoneuroendocrinology 2010; 35(9): 1404-9.
[6] Steptoe A, Phil D, Brydon L, Kunz-Ebrecht S. Changes in financial strain over three years, ambulatory blood pressure, and cortisol response to awakening. Psychosomatic Med 2005; 67: 281-7.
[7] Gundersen C, Mahatmya D, Garasky S, Lohman B. Linking psychosocial stressors and childhood obesity. Obser Rev 2011; 12(5): e54-63.
[8] Chichlowska KL, Rose KM, Diez-Roux AV, et al. Life course socioeconomic conditions and metabolic syndrome in adults: the Atherosclerosis Risk in Communities (ARIC) Study. Ann Epidemiol 2009; 19: 875-83.
[9] Lidfeldt J, Li TY, Hu FB, Manson JE, Kawachi I. A prospective study of childhood and adult socioeconomic status and incidence of type 2 diabetes in women. Am J Epidemiol 2007; 165: 882-9.
[10] Galobardes B, Smith GD, Lynch JW. Systematic review of the influence of childhood socioeconomic circumstances on risk for cardiovascular disease in adulthood. Ann Epidemiol 2006; 16: 91-104.
[11] Careerbuilder.com. Percentage of U.S. workers living paycheck to paycheck reaches recession era low, finds careerbuilder survey[internet]. Careerbuilder.com; 2012 [cited 2013 Jul 1]. Available from: http://www.careerbuilder.com/share/aboutus/pressreleasesdetail.aspx?sd=8%2F15%2F2012&id=pr711&ed=12%2F31%2F2012.
[12] Casey T, Maldonado H. Worst off -- single-parent families in the United States: a cross-national comparison of single parenthood in the U.S. and sixteen other high-income countries [Internet]. New York; Legal Momentum; 2012 [cited 2013 Aug 26]. Available from: http://www.legalmomentum.org/sites/default/files /reports/worst-off-single-parent.pdf.

[13] Nebraska Department of Health and Human Services. Smoking among Nebraska adults, 2009. Nebraska Behavioral Risk Factor Surveillance System [internet]. 2010 Jun [cited 2013 Jul 1]; Volume 1, Issue 5. Available from: http://dhhs.ne.gov/publichealth/Documents/Vol1-Issue5.pdf.

[14] Nebraska Department of Health and Human Services Data. Overweight and obesity among Nebraska adults, 2010. Nebraska Behavioral Risk Surveillance System [internet]. 2011 May [cited 2013 Jul 1]; Volume 2, Issue 1. Available from: http://dhhs.ne.gov/publichealth/Documents/vol2-iss1-Overweight-obesity.pdf.

[15] Nebraska Department of Health and Human Services Data. Physical activity among Nebraska adults, 2009. Nebraska Behavioral Risk Surveillance System [internet]. 2010 May (cited 2013 Jul 1]; Volume 1; Issue 2. Available from: http://dhhs.ne.gov/publichealth/Documents/Vol1-Issue2.pdf.

[16] Nebraska Department of Health and Human Services Data. Behavioral Risk Factor Web Query System, 2010. Nebraska Behavioral Risk Surveillance System [internet]. 2010 [cited 2013 Jul 1]. Available from: http://public-dhhs.ne.gov/Brfss/.

[17] Nebraska Department of Health and Human Services Data. Behavioral Risk Factor Web Query System, 2009. Nebraska Risk Surveillance System [internet]. 2009 [cited 2013 Jul 1]. Available from: http://public-dhhs.ne.gov/Brfss/QueryResults.aspx.

[18] HealthyPeople.gov [Internet]. Washington: U.S. Department of Health and Human Services [updated 2013 Aug 28; cited 2013 Aug 30]. Heart Disease and Stroke. Available from: http://www.healthypeople.gov/2020/topicsobjectives2020/objectiveslist.aspx?topicId=21.

[19] Health Functions Steering Committee. 10 essential services of public health. Public Health Functions Steering Committee, 1994.

[20] Miller WR, Rollnick S. Motivational Interviewing: Preparing People for Change 2002. Guilford Press, New York.

[21] Martins RG, Carvalho IP. Breaking bad news: Patients' preferences and health locus of control. Patient Education and Counseling 2013; 92: 67-73.

[22] Sundin O, Lisspers, J, Homan-Bang C, Nygren A, Ryden L, Ohman A. Comparing multifactorial lifestyle interventions and stress management in coronary risk reduction. Int Journal of Behavioral Medicine 2003; 10(3):191-204.

[23] Bollini AM, Walker EF, Hamann S, Kestler L. The influence of perceived control and locus of control on the cortisol and subjective responses to stress. Biological Psychology 2004; 67: 245-260.

[24] Child and Adolescent Health Measurement Initiative. National survey of children's health, 2007 Data Resource Center [internet]. 2007 [cited 2013 Jul 1]. Available from: http://www.childhealthdata.org/docs /nsch-docs/nebraska-pdf.pdf.

Chapter 6

UTILIZATION OF PEER TEEN ADVOCATES TO INCREASE AWARENESS OF HUMAN PAPILLOMAVIRUS AND VACCINATION AMONG URBAN YOUTH

Denise Uyar[1,*], MD, Staci Young[2], PhD, Sarah Tyree-Francis[3] CFLE, and Mary Ann Kiepczynski[4], RN

[1] Medical College of Wisconsin, Department of Obstetrics and Gynecology, Division of Gynecology Oncology, Wisconsin, United States of America
[2] Medical College of Wisconsin, Department of Family and Community Medicine, Wisconsin, United States of America
[3] Program Manager, Adolescent Holistic Health Initiatives, Boys and Girls Clubs of Greater Milwaukee, Wisconsin, United States of America
[4] City of Milwaukee Health Department, Disease Control and Environmental Health, Public Health Nurse Immunization Program Coordinator, Milwaukee, Wisconsin, United States of America

The city of Milwaukee, Wisconsin ranks among the highest urban areas for sexually transmitted disease in the United States with human papillomavirus being one of the most common sexually transmitted infections. In 2006, the Advisory Committee on Immunization Practices recommended routine vaccination of adolescent girls at ages 11 or 12 years with 3 doses of the Food and Drug Administration approved HPV vaccination. Despite the availability, safety and demonstrated efficacy of these vaccines, only 33% of adolescent girls in the United States have received all three doses of the series. In Milwaukee, less than 30% of adolescents have received the vaccination series. Several studies have evaluated the barriers for HPV vaccination. Consistently, deficits in knowledge and education for both parents and adolescents regarding HPV and the vaccination are cited as reasons why youth did not get the vaccine. This study was created to determine if today's urban youth could successfully be engaged in a program of positive health messaging surrounding HPV and the HPV vaccination using peer educators and social media.

---

[*] Corresponding author: Denise Uyar, MD Medical College of Wisconsin, Associate Professor Department of Obstetrics and Gynecology, Division of Gynecology Oncology 9200 West Wisconsin Avenue, Milwaukee, WI 53226, United States. E-mail: duyar@mcw.edu.

Keywords: human papillomavirus, adolescents, peer teen educators

INTRODUCTION

Human papillomavirus (HPV) infection is the most common sexually transmitted infection in the United States (1). Approximately 79 million persons in the United States are currently infected with HPV and approximately 14 million will become infected each year (2). HPV is not a reported infection, but its rates are believed to mirror that of other reportable infections, such as chlamydia and gonorrhea. Prevalence rates have been documented based on seroprevalence (3-5). Human papillomaviruses (HPVs) are typically acquired within the first months of sexual initiation. The peak incidence occurs among men and women ages 15-24 years (4). Persistent HPV infection is associated with a spectrum of health concerns from condyloma and anogenital pre-cancers to cervical, vulvar, vaginal, anal, penile and some oropharyngeal malignancies (6). Cervical cancer has been entirely attributed to persistent HPV infection with high risk viral types (HPV 16 and HPV 18) (7). In the United States, approximately 11,000 cases of cervical cancer are diagnosed each year with 4,000 women dying of the disease annually despite effective screening for cervical cancer (8). The direct cost of treatment of HPV-related diseases is approximately $4 billion per year in the United States. The vaccination is not intended to replace cervical cancer screening, but combined with increased compliance with screening measures it represents a potential cost-effective dual strategy ultimately resulting in decreased HPV morbidity and mortality (9, 10). HPV infections and their associated morbidity have been found to disproportionately affect racial and ethnic minority populations in the United States (11, 12). Thus, specific subgroups of youth are at particularly high risk. Nearly one quarter of 14-19 year olds are infected with HPV but the greatest prevalence is noted among low-income minorities (13). Lack of uptake of the HPV vaccination of this subgroup has raised concerns that the current disparity seen in HPV infection morbidity and mortality will grow ever wider in the future (14). HPV infection, therefore, represents a significant health concern for all, but especially for vulnerable minority youths where rates of sexually transmitted diseases are known to be highest (15). Two prophylactic HPV vaccines are available and have been approved by the Food and Drug Administration (FDA). The Advisory Committee on Immunization Practices (ACIP) recommends vaccination for both males and females for ages 11-12 years with catch up vaccination from age 13 until age 26 years. Both the quadrivalent and bivalent vaccines protect against infection with high risk HPV 16 and HPV 18 which cause 70% of cervical cancers and the majority of other HPV-associated cancers. The quadrivalent vaccination also protects against low risk HPV 6 and HPV 11 which cause 90% of genital warts (16, 17). The efficacy and safety of the vaccination has been established with long term evaluation (16, 18, 19). Clinical trials have established 90-100% efficacy for the prevention of precancerous cervical lesions for these vaccines when given prior to initiation of sexual activity (18, 20). The potential public health impact of these vaccinations has not been realized as it depends largely on vaccination acceptability and uptake among the target youth population and especially among groups disproportionately affected by HPV within the population.

In the United States, the 2007-2012 National Immunization Survey-Teen (NIS-Teen) reported that only 54% of girls have received one or more doses of the HPV series and only

33% have received all 3 doses to complete the HPV series (2). HPV vaccination rates have unfortunately stalled in the United States with no observed increase in vaccination rates from 2011 to 2012 (2). The barriers to HPV vaccination acceptance and uptake are multifactorial and include factors such as parental acceptability of HPV vaccination, adolescent acceptability of the HPV vaccination, physician acceptability of vaccination and endorsement, and vaccine access (21, 22). Frequently, lack of knowledge, on the part of parents, adolescents and physicians, is a central theme surrounding lack of vaccination (23). Several studies have pointed out the need for more tailored approaches to increasing vaccination acceptability (14, 24).

Although there has been almost universal agreement that HPV infection is an increasing health burden, particularly affecting minority youth and that a new strategy for increasing vaccination rates is needed, there seemed to be very few strategies proposed to start addressing the current deficits. This project proposes a tailored approach to specifically address deficits in HPV and HPV vaccination knowledge among urban minority youth in Milwaukee, Wisconsin. The HPV vaccination rate in Milwaukee is less than 30% (personal communication city of Milwaukee Health Department), far below the national average and the established targets for Healthy People 2020 (25), demonstrating a large need for increased HPV knowledge and awareness in our community. A partnership led by the Medical College of Wisconsin (MCW), the Boys & Girls Clubs of Greater Milwaukee (BGCGM) and the City of Milwaukee Health Department (MHD) utilized peer teen educators and social media to achieve project objectives. Partners received funding from MCW's Healthier Wisconsin Partnership Program.

Post and Retrospective Pretest Measures

DATE: ________ **GENDER (Circle one):** Female Male Transgender **AGE:** ________

RACE/ETHNICITY (Circle one): Black/African American White/Caucasian Latino/Hispanic Native American Asian American Other: ________ **ZIP CODE:** ________

Instructions: Look at learning areas #1-8. Tell us what you knew *before* you started this program AND what you know *after* participating in this program.

BEFORE participating in this program... **AFTER participating in this program...**

Was Poor	Was Fair	Was Good	Was Excellent	Learning Areas	Is Poor	Is Fair	Is Good	Is Excellent
				1.My awareness of HPV.				
				2.My knowledge of HPV.				
				3.My understanding of the risk factors for contracting HPV.				
				4.My knowledge of the health risks associated with HPV.				
				5.My knowledge of how to protect myself against HPV.				
				6.My awareness of the need for the HPV vaccine for females.				
				7.My awareness of the need for HPV vaccine for males.				
				8. My understanding of where to get the HPV vaccine for free.				

Figure 1. Pre- and post-training survey.

METHODS

The MCW Institutional Review Board (IRB) approval was obtained prior to recruiting or consenting participants.

Recruitment and training. Youth were eligible to participate in the program if they were between 13-19 years of age. Participants were recruited from the BGCGM, a national non-profit organization that provides after school services to urban youth; Milwaukee has program sites throughout the city. BGCGM is the oldest and largest youth serving agency in the city with 43 locations. Six youth age 15 and over were recruited as team leaders for this study. Leaders participated in an age appropriate HPV informational session created by MCW and MHD about the HPV virus, sexually transmitted disease and protection from infection which included discussions about vaccination, condom use and abstinence. These team leaders then recruited up to six additional team members from BGCGM or associated programs for their group. A total of 29 team members were consented and enrolled in this study. Study participants were both male and female. Team leaders were responsible for organizing their group meetings and ensuring their group members attended the HPV training. Participants completed pre- and post-training surveys to assess their HPV knowledge following each training session (see Figure 1). All participants received stipends for their participation at specified levels of the project to increase participants desire to complete the program. Team leaders received $10 for each team member recruited and $25 for completing the extra 60-90 minute training session. Participants that completed the pre and post-tests received $25. Each participant received $25 for completion of the storyboard or preliminary design of the project. Each team member received $100 for completion of the project in its entirety. Attendance at the 2nd Annual PSA Premiere held in downtown Milwaukee was awarded $25. The winning team members of the individual campaigns in each category (PSA, billboard or brochure) were awarded $50.

Educational intervention. After the training sessions, youth participants discussed and decided their choice of media for presentation: public service announcements (PSA), brochures or city billboards. Brainstorming sessions were also performed concurrently among team members and study coordinators to discuss a "brand" for the HPV project including a logo design and website domain name. Participants completed a survey to identify their preferred social media platforms; Twitter and Facebook were the most preferred methods of communication. Participants received education on responsible social media use and signed a contract to ensure that they utilized it responsibly. Teams used Twitter, Instagram, and Facebook to coordinate their meetings and to inform their peers about the program.

Groups were assigned to one of their first two choices of media for presentation and paired with a volunteer community mentor with media expertise. Two groups created individual finished products in each category; at the completion of the program there were two PSA videos, two billboards campaigns and two brochures. Groups met at least bi-weekly for four months with mentors to create and formalize their ideas in their respective categories. Partners purchased the domain name *itsjust3hpv.org* and developed an interactive website including the logo created by the youth, rendered by a local artist (Figure 2.). Website functionality enabled our study team to track votes the first two weeks and visits on a monthly basis. All of the completed products displayed the website and logo for heightened community awareness and project visibility.

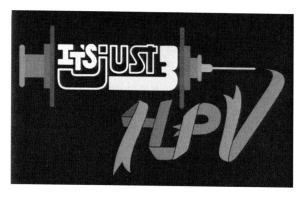

Figure 2. HPV project logo created by project participants.

RESULTS

A total of 24 of 29 youths (82%) completed this project; 19 of 24 participants (79%) were female and 5 of 24 participants (20%) were male. Ages of participants ranged from 14-18 and they all resided in the city of Milwaukee. Participants identified themselves as African American, Latino or Native American, with only one identified as "other, not otherwise specified" and one who did not designate ethnicity.

The survey results indicated that 83% of participants completed the pre- and post-training surveys (see Figure 1). The pre-training surveys indicated primarily "poor, fair or good" responses to HPV knowledge questions with only six respondents indicating "excellent" to two or more survey questions. In contrast, on the post-survey questionnaire respondents indicated universally "good to excellent" responses to the HPV knowledge questions with only two surveys with one answer in the "poor" category.

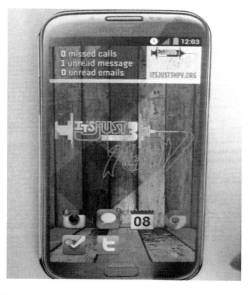

Figure 3. Winner of the HPV brochure campaign.

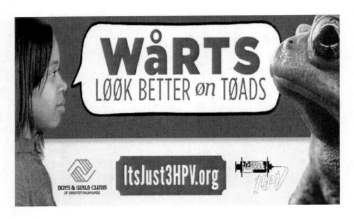

Figure 4. Winner of HPV billboard campaign.

Votes for the best project in PSAs, billboards and brochures were tracked online for a two week period and additionally with live texting at the 2nd Annual PSA Premiere, a citywide event in Milwaukee with approximately 250 youth in attendance. 557 votes were counted to determine winners in each category and the winning projects were announced and posted on the *itsjust3hpv.org* website. The unique brochure created was a tri-fold with the appearance of a cell phone which was particularly well received. The billboard exemplified the youths appeal for short messages with a striking visual. The brochure and billboard winners are shown in Figures 3 and 4. The PSA video winner is not visible in this article; videos are posted on the website and on YouTube, and have over 600 views.

The website includes information about HPV and HPV vaccinations, links or visual images of all completed projects, and the teams of youth involved and their community mentors. Between the April 2013 launch of the website and December of 2013 there have been over 4500 visits and the website metrics reveal that it is viewed on average 35 times per day. In January 2015 the average views on the website totaled 69 times per day, showing the need for on-line presence continuing well beyond the duration of the program.

The winning brochure was featured on the website with an added option for professionals to order 50 free copies for their sites needs beginning in September of 2013. Partners track brochure distribution by the recipients' postal address and a questionnaire that recipients complete that includes their organization description. To date, approximately 28 individuals representing various programs have requested brochures to distribute at their respective agency. The majority of requests are from the greater Milwaukee area but, due to the dissemination of the work at local and regional conferences, requests have come from; rural Wisconsin, Minneapolis, MN, Louisville, KY, New York, NY, New Haven, CT, Frankfort, KY, and Memphis, TN. The majority of recipients identify themselves as non-for profit organizations (27%), schools (27%), community organizations (21%), or hospital/clinics (24%). The audience for their distribution is indicated as urban (75%), youths ages 13-20, males and females and of black, white, Latino/Hispanic or multiracial ethnicities. Over half of the recipients (66%) indicate knowledge of the project from the website, social media or a colleague, while several respondents (18%) indicated a peer educator as their source for locating the project.

DISCUSSION

The concept of this study arose from the partnership's shared goal of improved reproductive health, specifically the great need to address the low HPV vaccination rate in a city where the rates of sexually transmitted diseases are among the highest in the nation. The urban community we serve is comprised predominantly of ethnic and racial minorities as evidenced by the demographics of the youth participating in this project. The literature to date reveals many barriers to HPV vaccination but few recommendations on how to approach these issues. Fernandez et al. organized potential HPV interventions into three categories: community education, provider education and improving vaccine access (24). Our study sought to address one component of this triad: community education; specifically in adolescents, utilizing peer teen educators. Fernandez et al. noted that personal perceptions of HPV risk, personal perceptions of HPV severity, perceptions of one's peers and social norms are significant factors influencing willingness to have oneself vaccinated (24). Peer perceptions have significant influence.

Several studies have demonstrated that peer education can make a significant difference among youths. Peer educators are motivated young individuals that have undergone informal education with their peers with the intent of augmenting their own knowledge and skills to enable them to make better health decisions and hopefully assist their peers in doing the same. Youth led education models have been associated with increased knowledge and self-efficacy as well as decreased levels of stigma and sexual risk taking behaviors (26-28). Cai et al. (26) even demonstrated a long-term benefit for a peer led education model after one year. Youth educators have also been associated with greater efficacy than adult educators in some settings. For these reasons, peer educators were chosen in our study as an important way to convey sensitive health messages to this targeted population.

Targeting the youth population eligible for the HPV vaccine is particularly challenging. This age group is beyond most mandatory vaccination programs and they are typically outside of the age for regular physician well examinations. Despite not fitting into these conventional groups, they are almost universal users of the internet, and as a result may obtain much of their health information from this source. A Pew Research study (May 2013) on teenage social media use revealed that 95% of those ages 12-17 years use the internet. Eight in ten online teens use some kind of social media; 77% of online teens use Facebook and about one in four online teens use Twitter. Adolescents and teens are consistently accessing information online which provides an opportunity and a venue to create positive health messages in a format that appeals to them and communicate important health information. Our group of peer educators gained the desired knowledge as indicated by their survey responses and created such messages for their cohorts. They introduced messages that appealed to their interests in the form of the videos, brochures and billboards and utilized the internet, Twitter and Facebook to promote interest. During the course of the project, their participation was Tweeted, posted on Facebook and communicated to their peers, broadening the exposure of HPV and HPV vaccination into their everyday conversation.

The youth-focused creations from this project seem to resonate well with their peers as evidenced by the visits that we continually track from the website, the viewings on YouTube and by the requests from organizations for brochures for distribution to similar populations. Tailoring the message to improve education surrounding this issue is a first step. Continued efforts to maintain the website presence and the media visibility of this project are ongoing. The long term effects of this project remain to be seen. Our goal was to ultimately increase HPV vaccination uptake in our community. Increasing the HPV vaccination rates in Milwaukee, much like many other urban areas, requires continued efforts in community education, provider education and vaccine access. We need to keep tailoring our messaging by including our target population in the creation of health marketing materials in order to make health education appealing to those we are trying to reach, if we are going to see real improvement.

REFERENCES

[1] Koutsky L. Epidemiology of genital human papillomavirus infection. Am J Med 1997;102:3-8.
[2] Centers for Disease Control and Prevention. Human papillomavirus vaccination coverage among adolescent girls, 2007-2012, and postlicensure vaccine safety monitoring, 2006-2013 - United States. MMWR 2013; 62: 591-5.
[3] Dunne EF, Sternberg M, Markowitz LE, McQuillan G, Swan D, Patel S, Unger ER. Human papillomavirus (HPV) 6, 11, 16, and 18 prevalence among females in the United States--National Health And Nutrition Examination Survey, 2003-2006: opportunity to measure HPV vaccine impact? J Infect Dis 2011; 204: 562-5. doi: 10.1093/infdis/jir342.
[4] Dunne EF, Unger ER, Sternberg M, McQuillan G, Swan DC, Patel SS, Markowitz LE. Prevalence of HPV infection among females in the United States. JAMA 2007; 297: 813-9. doi: 10.1001/jama.297.8.813.
[5] Markowitz LE, Sternberg M, Dunne EF, McQuillan G, Unger ER. Seroprevalence of human papillomavirus types 6, 11, 16, and 18 in the United States: National Health and Nutrition Examination Survey 2003-2004. J Infect Dis 2009; 200: 1059-67. doi: 10.1086/604729.
[6] Forman D, de Martel C, Lacey CJ, Soerjomataram I, Lortet-Tieulent J, Bruni L, Vignat J, Ferlay J, Bray F, Plummer M, Franceschi S. Global burden of human papillomavirus and related diseases. Vaccine 2012; 30(Suppl 5): F12-23. doi: 10.1016 /j.vaccine.2012.07.055.
[7] Bosch FX, de Sanjose S. Chapter 1: Human papillomavirus and cervical cancer--burden and assessment of causality. J Natl Cancer Inst Monogr 2003;3-13.
[8] Centers for Disease Control and Prevention. Adult vaccination coverage--United States, 2010. MMWR 2012; 61: 66-72.
[9] Taira AV, Neukermans CP, Sanders GD. Evaluating human papillomavirus vaccination programs. Emerg Infect Dis 2004; 10: 1915-23. doi: 10.3201/eid1011.040222.
[10] Coupe VM, Berkhof J, Bulkmans NW, Snijders PJ, Meijer CJ. Age-dependent prevalence of 14 high-risk HPV types in the Netherlands: implications for prophylactic vaccination and screening. Br J Cancer 2008; 98: 646-51. doi: 10.1038/sj.bjc.6604162.
[11] Freeman HP, Wingrove BK, Center to Reduce Cancer Health Disparities (U.S.) Excess cervical cancer mortality: a marker for low access to health care in poor communities: an analysis. Rockville, MD: National Cancer Institute, Center to Reduce Cancer Health Disparities, 2005.
[12] Kahn JA, Lan D, Kahn RS (2007) Sociodemographic factors associated with high-risk human papillomavirus infection. Obstet Gynecol 2007; 110:87-95. doi: 10.1097/01.AOG.0000266984. 23445.9c.
[13] Perkins RB, Brogly SB, Adams WG, Freund KM. Correlates of human papillomavirus vaccination rates in low-income, minority adolescents: a multicenter study. J Womens Health (Larchmt) 2012; 21: 813-20. doi: 10.1089/jwh.2011.3364.
[14] Downs LS, Smith JS, Scarinci I, Flowers L, Parham G. The disparity of cervical cancer in diverse populations. Gynecol Oncol 2008; 109: S22-30. doi: 10.1016 /j.ygyno.2008.01.003.

[15] Satterwhite CL, Torrone E, Meites E, Dunne EF, Mahajan R, Ocfemia MC, Su J, Xu F, Weinstock H. Sexually transmitted infections among US women and men: prevalence and incidence estimates, 2008. Sex Transm Dis 2013; 40: 187-93. doi: 10.1097/OLQ.0b013e318286bb53.

[16] Garland SM, Hernandez-Avila M, Wheeler CM, Perez G, Harper DM, Leodolter S, Tang GW, Ferris DG, Steben M, Bryan J, Taddeo FJ, Railkar R, Esser MT, Sings HL, Nelson M, Boslego J, Sattler C, Barr E, Koutsky LA. Quadrivalent vaccine against human papillomavirus to prevent anogenital diseases. N Engl J Med 2007; 356: 1928-43. doi: 10.1056/NEJMoa061760.

[17] Garland SM, Steben M, Sings HL, James M, Lu S, Railkar R, Barr E, Haupt RM, Joura EA. Natural history of genital warts: analysis of the placebo arm of 2 randomized phase III trials of a quadrivalent human papillomavirus (types 6, 11, 16, and 18) vaccine. J Infect Dis 2009; 199: 805-14. doi: 10.1086/597071.

[18] Future II Study Group. Prophylactic efficacy of a quadrivalent human papillomavirus (HPV) vaccine in women with virological evidence of HPV infection. J Infect Dis 2007; 196:1438-46. doi: 10.1085/522864.

[19] Hariri S, Markowitz LE, Dunne EF, Unger ER. Population Impact of HPV Vaccines: Summary of Early Evidence. J Adolesc Health 2013; 53: 679-82. doi: 10.1016/j.jadohealth.2013.09.018.

[20] Future II Study Group. Quadrivalent vaccine against human papillomavirus to prevent high-grade cervical lesions. N Engl J Med 2007; 356: 1915-27. doi: 10.1056/NEJMoa061741.

[21] Allen JD, Othus MK, Shelton RC, Li Y, Norman N, Tom L, del Carmen MG. Parental decision making about the HPV vaccine. Cancer Epidemiol Biomarkers Prev 2010; 19: 2187-98. doi: 10.1158/1055-9965.EPI-10-0217.

[22] Conroy K, Rosenthal SL, Zimet GD, Jin Y, Bernstein DI, Glynn S, Kahn JA. Human papillomavirus vaccine uptake, predictors of vaccination, and self-reported barriers to vaccination. J Womens Health (Larchmt) 2009; 18: 1679-86. doi: 10.1089/jwh.2008.1329.

[23] Gowda C, Schaffer SE, Dombkowski KJ, Dempsey AF. Understanding attitudes toward adolescent vaccination and the decision-making dynamic among adolescents, parents and providers. BMC Public Health 2012; 12: 509. doi: 10.1186/1471-2458-12-509.

[24] Fernandez ME, Allen JD, Mistry R, Kahn JA. Integrating clinical, community, and policy perspectives on human papillomavirus vaccination. Annu Rev Public Health 2010; 31:235-52. doi: 10.1146/annurev.publhealth.012809.103609.

[25] Centers for Disease Control and Prevention. Adult vaccination coverage--United States, 2010. MMWR 2012; 61: 66-72.

[26] Cai Y, Hong H, Shi R, Ye X, Xu G, Li S, Shen L. Long-term follow-up study on peer-led school-based HIV/AIDS prevention among youths in Shanghai. Int J STD AIDS 2008; 19:848-50. doi: 10.1258/ijsa.2008.008129.

[27] Denison JA, Tsui S, Bratt J, Torpey K, Weaver MA, Kabaso M. Do peer educators make a difference? An evaluation of a youth-led HIV prevention model in Zambian Schools. Health Educ Res 2012; 27: 237-47. doi: 10.1093/her/cyr093.

[28] Ibrahim N, Rampal L, Jamil Z, Zain AM. Effectiveness of peer-led education on knowledge, attitude and risk behavior practices related to HIV among students at a Malaysian public university--a randomized controlled trial. Prev Med 2012; 55: 505-10. doi: 10.1016/j.ypmed.2012.09.003.

In: Public Health Yearbook 2015
Editor: Joav Merrick
ISBN: 978-1-63484-514-4
© 2016 Nova Science Publishers, Inc.

Chapter 7

INNOVATIONS IN CONTINUING PROFESSIONAL EDUCATION: A MODEL TO IMPACT INTERPROFESSIONAL COLLABORATION

Linda J Mast[1,], PhD, Ateequr Rahman[2], PhD, Bard I Schatzman[1], PhD, Diane Bridges[1], MSN, RN, CCM, and Neil Horsley[3], DPM*

[1]College of Health Professions, Rosalind Franklin University of Medicine and Science, North Chicago, Illinois, United States of America
[2]College of Pharmacy, Rosalind Franklin University of Medicine and Science, North Chicago, Illinois, United States of America
[3]Scholl College of Podiatric Medicine, Rosalind Franklin University of Medicine and Science, North Chicago, Illinois, United States of America

This study addresses the critical need for innovation in public health workforce training and continuing education to foster effective interprofessional collaboration. The focus of this study was to assess the impact of interprofessional collaboration on practitioners who were charged with creating an interprofessional (IP) care model emphasizing primary and secondary prevention services specific for seniors with diabetes. The impact of interprofessional collaboration as an intervention for practitioners was assessed using a half day problem-based learning workshop and facilitated group sessions over a six month time period. Practitioner subjects representing disciplines of physician's assistant, physical therapy, pharmacy, nursing, registered dietician, and podiatry all participated in the intervention. Using an authentic task-based curriculum and guidelines for required care protocols, these practitioner subjects completed a specific workshop about IP care collaboration and four facilitated work sessions. The impact of participating in an IP team was measured using pre-test and post-test instruments including the Interprofessional Education Perception Scale (IEPS) to assess attitudes and the Concerns Based Adoption Model (C-BAM) to assess actual behaviors related to interprofessional collaboration. Results of this research provided a workforce training and facilitated team building model

---

[*] Corresponding author: Linda J. Mast, PhD, Rosalind Franklin University of Medicine and Science, 3333 Green Bay Road, North Chicago, IL 60064, United States. E-mail: linda.mast@rosalindfranklin.edu.

that can be used to enhance interprofessional collaboration. The study demonstrates a process for implementing a continuing education program that engages an interprofessional healthcare team in the creation of an effective preventive care model. This preventive care model responds to the need to develop new methods for ongoing training of the public health workforce in an interprofessional collaborative process. Initial findings are promising in that this innovative approach to continuing education resulted in both increased interprofessional collaboration behaviors and more favorable attitudes about working in interprofessional teams.

Keywords: interprofessional, collaboration, problem-based learning, continuing professional education, public health, workforce training

INTRODUCTION

Challenges exist for public health workforce development in both developing countries and wealthier countries alike. Beaglehole and Dal Poz (1) relate this challenge to the traditional emphasis on formal academic and didactic training with very limited attention being paid to training methods that are field-based continuing education where the workforce can participate in work group training that addresses the diversity and complexity of the healthcare team from a wide range of occupational backgrounds (1). Patients today have complex medical issues requiring more than one healthcare professional which calls for interprofessional collaboration (2). In 2001, acknowledging the medically challenging needs of patients, the Institute of Medicine (IOM) Committee on Quality of Health Care in America recommended that healthcare professionals be able to work in interprofessional (IP) teams (3). The research of Schofield et al. demonstrated that, especially for complex, chronic conditions, a multidisciplinary, or IP, team offers many advantages for patients and their families (4). Bringing an interprofessional focus to the development of innovative care delivery models requires collaboration among the health professions to increase learning about, from and with each other, as well as incorporation of a patient centered perspective (5). A growing consensus exists that interprofessional (IP) team-based care offers the potential to improve quality of care and lower costs (6). However, Varda et al. emphasize that even though there is growing interest in collaborative practice in public health, there is still little empirical evidence within the public health literature to support and inform this practice (7). According to Gebbie and Turnock, public health is especially challenged due to the multidisciplinary nature of services provided (8), and there is often very limited opportunities for workforce training and continuing education interventions that address the need for interprofessional collaboration. In November 2012 the Global Health Forum on Innovation in Health Professional Education convened in Washington, D.C. One of the obstacles identified for implementing IP education was "knowing how to weave IP content into meaningful clinical and community experiences" (9). Such obstacles, while challenging for students, become even more daunting when the learners are practicing clinicians where continuing education programs need to be relevant to current practice needs, and delivered in ways that encourage professional development. This study provides a model for continuing education that addresses the need to engage learners in ways that use authentic tasks to develop interprofessional collaboration.

Collaborative partnerships in practice

Bringing an interprofessional focus to the development of innovative care delivery models requires collaboration among the health professions to increase learning about, from and with each other (10), as well as incorporation of a patient centered perspective. Continuing professional education research emphasizes that educating working professionals must use authentic projects that have relevance in practice. To date, there is very limited research addressing knowledge translation or continuing professional education within the interprofessional context (11). Further, the World Health Organization (WHO) supports the development of evidence to inform best approaches to public health workforce development (1).

Interprofessional teams develop through interprofessional collaboration. Interprofessional collaboration is a "partnership between a team of health providers and a client in a participatory collaborative and coordinated approach to shared decision making around health and social issues" (12). These collaborations "create an interprofessional practice team where healthcare providers from different professional backgrounds work together with patients, families, and communities to deliver the best quality of care." (13).

Interprofessional collaborative practice encompasses the synergistic input of each individual team member's skill and knowledge through a process of effective communication and decision making (14). Blending of professional cultures, shared skills, respect, accountability, coordination, cooperation, mutual trust and autonomy are components of an interprofessional collaborative practice (13-15). According to Bromage (16), this approach to team working, known as interprofessionalism, emphasizes highly collaborative problem-solving. This interprofessional team approach allows sharing of professional expertise with the ultimate goal of improving patient outcomes while sharing resources. (2, 5). The intent of interprofessional teams is to collaborate and communicate closely with other healthcare professionals to achieve this common goal (17). However, U.S. public health workforce enumeration data suggests only 20% of the workforce had the education and training needed to work most effectively, and, therefore, a continuing education model that supports close integration of all health personnel is needed (18).

Continuing professional education (CPE) for interprofessional collaboration

The field of interprofessional education has been growing, and in May of 2011, an interprofessional panel representing the professions of allopathic medicine (AAMC), pharmacy (AACP), nursing (AANA), osteopathic medicine (AACOM), and dentistry (ADEA) established four domains for interprofessional competencies designed to guide the educational process for healthcare professionals: 1) Values/Ethics; 2) Roles/Responsibilities; 3) Interprofessional Communication; 4) Teams/teamwork (19). Although strides have been made to advance interprofessional care across the professions, there are still significant gaps between current needs for enhanced interprofessional collaboration and what is in practice in primary and preventive services (20).

Challenges exist for new graduates entering into professional practice where strong territorial cultures and barriers to interprofessional collaboration (i.e., silos) persist (19). This means that recent graduates may be prepared to engage in IP collaboration, but then find themselves immersed in healthcare delivery cultures that have not kept pace with advances in IP models of care.

There are powerful influences of professional enculturation and limited understanding of continuing professional education (CPE) and actual change in practice (21). IP collaboration must include interprofessional education, interprofessional practice and interprofessional interventions (22). Continuing education that includes interprofessional education is critical in order to prepare practicing professionals to effectively collaborate. The Institute of Medicine (IOM) Committee on Planning a Continuing Health Care Professional Education Institute completed an in depth study of continuing education for the health professions that concluded team-based health care delivery is necessary, and that effective continuing education for healthcare professionals will be grounded in ways to engage practitioners in authentic work that has patient care and population health as its focus (9).

Consequently, for this study, the Problem-based learning (PBL) model was selected for a half-day workshop because it was determined that PBL would be an ideal approach to use as a way to assess impact on interprofessional collaboration attitudes and behaviors within the context of an authentic problem and work setting.

Problem-based learning model for CPE

Problem-based learning (PBL) originated as a teaching strategy at McMaster University in the 1960s and has since been adopted throughout North America and worldwide (23). Barrows (24) developed a taxonomy of PBL types to better define the key elements of this educational format. It is generally characterized as an instructional method where small groups of learners address a specific patient problem. The PBL approach was selected as the instructional method (the intervention) for the CPE workshop because it engages participants in a small group environment and is grounded in authentic problem solving tasks.

This is supported by the theoretical foundation that adult learners prefer the use of authentic practice settings that include a problem to be solved. (25–26). PBL has been used in prior interprofessional continuing education programs where participants learned about the roles and contributions of other health professions within the context of an authentic task (26).

Continuing professional education (CPE) instructional design

This study used a PBL half day workshop and facilitated follow up group meetings led by a professional group facilitator to encourage interprofessional collaboration within the context of developing a preventive care model for older adults with Type 2 diabetes. The workshop included an authentic case study to engage the participants in an interprofessional discussion to model the expectations of PBL work. This was followed by introduction of the assigned task to develop a care model to provide primary and secondary preventive services to seniors with diabetes. Details of the instructional design for the program are provided in Table 1.

Table 1. Workshop Instructional Design

Workshop Curriculum				
Introductions and Welcome	Research Team and Participant Introductions	Welcome greetings from a recognized leader in Interprofessional education	Overview of workshop materials (includes strategically selected journal articles on IP collaboration and diabetes that were pre-selected by the researchers to give participants some foundational research sources)	Pretest surveys completed
Group Activity to Introduce the Problem Based Learning Process	Initial group work (non-directed) to engage participants in working together	Tour of facilities where care will be provided (ambulatory care clinic and a mobile care unit)	Time for relationship building among practitioner subjects	Discovery and discussion based on workshop materials and journal articles
Experiential Case relevant to benefits of IP collaboration (Specific to Diabetes and Community Needs)	Authentic case presented on a senior with diabetes	Participant subjects discuss what they identify as top priorities	Discussion on how top priorities may vary based on practitioner discipline.	Discovery and discussion on value of IP collaboration.
Authentic Task Introduction and Assignment	IP participants introduced to the authentic task to develop an IP care model for seniors with diabetes based on primary and secondary prevention	Timeline for completion and parameters of the objective are discussed	IP participants are asked to identify and appoint a group leader for their PBL team and team process	Care model is implemented at clinical location sites
Follow up collaborative sessions with guided reflection worksheets and facilitator	Participant group leader (PBL team leader) continues collaborative meetings with participants to begin developing the care model.	Professional Group facilitator coordinates follow up meetings with PBL team leader for month 3 and 6 of the six month process	Debriefing session with participant PBL team, professional group facilitator and research team.	Post-test surveys completed

The advantage of using the PBL curriculum design is that it focuses on team building and inquiry in the PBL context. This continuing education model can be customized to meet the needs of any specific community's health priorities, whether rural or urban, by selecting a focused and relevant case study that allows participants to work toward desired outcomes related to improved patient care.

METHODS

The population for potential subjects was limited to clinical practitioners working in one healthcare organization. Written informed consent was obtained from each practitioner subject following Protocol IPHS #001 as approved by the authors' Institutional Review Board. A purposive sample was obtained to represent registered nurses, physical therapists, physicians, physician assistants, registered dieticians, pharmacists, and podiatrists (the physician did not complete the study due to geographic relocation). Practitioner subjects participated in a half day PBL based workshop followed by monthly facilitated discussions with the task of developing an IP care model for seniors with diabetes.

Intervention

The half-day workshop was designed to immerse participants in experiential learning about interprofessional concepts centered on the core interprofessional competencies (19). Application of these concepts used patient simulations, debriefing discussions and team based activities using a social learning framework that have been demonstrated to be effective for team building within a professional context (28-29). The content for the workshop was developed by faculty experts in group dynamics, leading changes, and delivery of CPE programs for health care professionals. The program was delivered in an interactive conference style setting, and the assigned task for the participants in the workshop was based on community needs assessment data from the local public health department. At the workshop, the practitioner subjects were assigned the task of creating a comprehensive, patient–centered care model for delivering prevention services for seniors with diabetes.

Participation in the process of creating the interprofessional care (IP) model served as the experiential lab for the study of the participants' IP collaboration experience. The follow up facilitated group meetings were based on interprofessional protocols established by Belanger and Rodriguez (30), including significant investment in time and training, clear role development, communication strategies, trust and respect, and systems to guide cooperative practice. Participants in the study were made aware that their newly created interprofessional care model for preventive services would be implemented and used over a six month time interval to evaluate patient outcomes and to measure any changes in interprofessional collaboration perspectives among clinician participants. The intervention process was sequenced as follows for practitioner participants:

1. Pre-implementation: Collection of pre-test Concerns-Based Adoption Model (CBAM) Levels of Use (LoU) and Interprofessional Education Perception Scale (IEPS) data.
2. Half day workshop: Program introduced foundation information about the target patient population, the mobile care unit facility and interprofessional collaboration. The workshop was designed as an integrated process; the teams were supported by interprofessional faculty and by specialists in interprofessional education.
3. An overview of expectations of the project was provided. Content included experiential activities and the focus will be on team building and the four established competencies of interprofessional collaboration.
4. IP Care Model development: The practitioner subjects completed four self-directed PBL sessions of 1-2 hours to develop the interprofessional care model to be implemented for older adult patients with Type 2 diabetes. The CPE workshop content included specific guidelines for the care protocol process and established designation of assigned professionals to work with patients. Each member of the interprofessional team focused on the various aspects of the project as clinician, providing clinical care for patients as educator, and as innovator, contributing to the ongoing refinement and evaluation of the interprofessional practice model. Informal discussion and email exchanges among the team in smaller groups occurred routinely throughout the process. Goldman's work with IP group facilitation informed the design of four sessions as follows: a. Review objectives, examine clinical evidence with focus on primary and secondary prevention, explore barriers and enablers to change, needs assessment for assigned patient population; b. Review needs assessment using mind mapping to finalize an ideal delivery pathway and present to IP peers. Use evidence and literature support to support selected pathway; c. Draft interprofessional model care protocols; d. Refine protocol and organize materials to implement the IP care model (22).
5. Debriefings: Six monthly interprofessional debriefings were completed. Four were conducted by the group leader chosen by the participant subjects and two, one at mid-point and at the end, were conducted by an expert group facilitator for thirty minutes to one hour to discuss the interprofessional care model delivery as it progresses. At the end, the team came together for a final debriefing and discussion. During this time, review and assessment was done, which included a list of the issues identified and addressed as well as any outstanding concerns and a proposed management plan for these concerns.
6. Post-test data collection: Posttest CBAM-LoU and IEPS data were collected at the end of the six month IP care model intervention.

Research questions

This research project addressed the following research questions pertaining to clinical practitioner subjects:

1. Are there differences among clinical professionals' behaviors related to inter-professional collaboration?
2. Are there differences among clinical professionals' perceptions of inter-professional collaboration?
3. Does participation in an interprofessional care team impact clinical professionals' perceptions and behaviors with regard to interprofessional collaboration?

Dependent variables

Two instruments were used to collect pretest and post test data. These were the Interprofessional Education Perception Scale (IEPS), and the Concerns-Based Adoption Model-Level of Use (CBAM-LoU).
Dependent variable measures:

1. Total IEPS Scores
2. IEPS sub scores
3. CBAM-LoU scores
4. CBAM-LoU sub scores over 8 dimensions

Independent variable (practitioner):

1. Clinical profession

Measures

Data collection
The IEPS and CBAM-LoU instruments were used to collect pre- and post-test data related to attitudes about IP collaboration (IEPS) and behaviors related to IP collaboration. Pre-test data was collected at the workshop and facilitated meeting sites. Post-test data was collected at the end of the six month implementation of the IP care model.

The Interdisciplinary Education Perception Scale (IEPS)
The Interdisciplinary Education Perception Scale (IEPS) was developed by Luecht et al. (31) and has been widely used to assess attitudes about interprofessional education among graduate and undergraduate students. In this study, however, the instrument was used to assess the attitudes of professionals in practice. More recently, an alternative, remodeled twelve item instrument has been developed consolidating the four original subscales into three. The revised instrument (IEPS Model 7) with three subscales of Competency and Autonomy, Perceived Need for Cooperation, and Perception of Actual Cooperation was used for this study. Construct validity of the IEPS was confirmed in using expert feedback from interdisciplinary health care professionals for each survey item (32). The remodeled IEPS instrument is considered a stable and reliable instrument with good internal consistency of the total scale with Chronbach's alpha of 0.86 (32).

The Concerns-Based Adoption Model - Levels of Use (CBAM-LoU v1.1)

The Concerns-Based Adoption Model - Levels of Use (CBAM-LoU v1.1) is a focused interview process that has been used to describe behaviors of those engaged in an innovation or change as they progress through levels of use. It does not focus on attitudinal, motivational, or other affective aspects of the user. The CBAM LoU interview process has been widely used in studies related to change and innovation. It is based on the eight levels of use defined as: (0) Non-Use, (I) Orientation, (II) Preparation, (III) Mechanical Use, (IVA) Routine, (IVB) Refinement, (V) Integration, and (VI) Renewal. It is an ideal instrument to measure changes over time along a continuum (34). Test-retest reliability and alpha of 0.84 – 0.87 has been demonstrated (33). It has been used in many published empirical studies over the past thirty years (35). Although it has been most frequently used in education, more recently it has been adapted for research in the department of defense and health care. A limitation of the CBAM-LoU is the potential for variability in scoring among reviewers and the need for strict adherence to the focused interview protocols. In depth training for researchers conducting and scoring the focused interview ensures that scoring results are based on the prescribed process following decision points from the subject's responses.

RESULTS

Participant subjects included one registered nurse, one physician assistant, one psychiatrist (who did not complete participation due to relocation to another state), one pharmacist, one podiatrist, and one physical therapist.

Scoring

IEPS

The IEPS is a twelve item self-report survey instrument. Each of the seven practitioner subjects were asked to indicate their level of agreement with each statement using a six point Likert type scale (6 = Strongly Agree; 5 = Agree; 4= Somewhat Agree; 2 = Disagree; 1 = Strongly Disagree). The IEPS was completed prior to the half day workshop as a pre-test, and again as a post-test at the completion of the six months of facilitated group meetings that followed the workshop.

For each sub-scale (SS1, SS2, SS3) items are grouped based on a specific construct related to interprofessional team work. Highest possible scores are shown in Table 2.

Table 2. IEPS Highest Possible Scores (Total and Sub-scales)

Scale Section	Highest Possible Score
Total score	72
SS1	30
SS2	12
SS3	30

CBAM-LoU

The CBAM-LoU is an interview based assessment that assesses actual behaviors related to an innovation. For this study IP collaboration was the innovation introduced to the subjects during the pre-test and post-test private interviews. Pre-test interview results indicated that most subjects had limited or mechanical use of IP collaboration. Post-test interviews at the end of the six months of the study revealed positive trends with IP collaboration behaviors for all subjects. Some subjects behaviors related to IP collaboration advanced to refinement and integration in to their practice. Table 3 highlights results of the pre-test and post-test CBAM-LoU interviews.

Results of private interviews with a member of the research team who was trained in the CBAM-LoU interview protocol were rated by four members of the research team to ensure consistent results with ratings for levels of use. The interview process is based on a very structured and truncated interview style designed to provide consistent results as illustrated in figure 1.

Table 3. Subject Ratings of Levels of Use (of Interprofessional Collaboration)

Subject#	Pretest	Posttest
1	II	IVa
2	III	IV a
3	I	III
4	II	VI
5	IVa	V
6	III	IVa

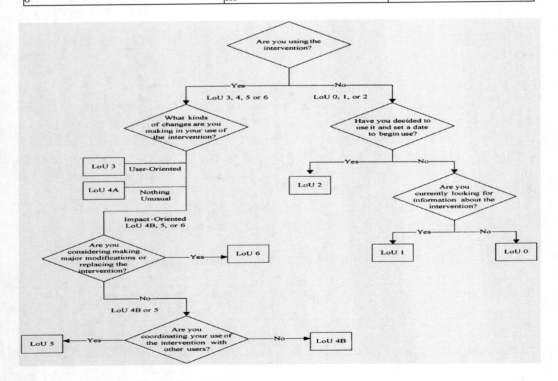

Figure 1. CBAM-LoU Branching Chart (36).

Levels of use are a behavioral phenomenon that does not address attitudes or feelings. It only addresses what subjects actually do. For this reason, it was an ideal companion to the IEPS survey that measures only attitudes in order to get a broader understanding of both attitudes and behaviors regarding IP collaboration. Levels of use include eight levels that range from nonuse to renewal as outlined in Table 4.

Analysis

IEPS

The IEPS survey instrument assesses self-reported attitudes regarding IP collaboration. Using the remodeled instrument (39), total IEPS scores and the three sub-scores were compared across practitioners for differences between professions, as well as to identify changes in scores that may have occurred over time based on the six months of facilitated collaboration following the PBL workshop. Total IEPS scores and the three sub-scores were compared across professions, prior to the workshop and following the workshop and six months of facilitated collaboration. See Table 5 for descriptive statistics.

Table 4. Levels of Use of the Innovation (36)

0	*Nonuse:* State in which user has little or no knowledge of the innovation.
I	*Orientation:* State in which the user has acquired or is acquiring information about the innovation, and is exploring its value.
II	*Preparation:* State in which the user is preparing for first use of the innovation.
III	*Mechanical Use:* State in which the user focuses most effort on the short-term day to day use of the innovation with little time for reflection.
IVA	*Routine:* Use of the innovation is stabilized. Few if any changes are being made in the ongoing use. Little preparation or thought is being given to improving the innovation.
IVB	*Refinement:* State in which the user varies the use of the innovation to increase the impact on clients within immediate sphere of influence.
V	*Integration:* State in which the user is combining own efforts to use the innovation with the related activities of colleagues to achieve a collective effect on clients within their common sphere of influence.
VI	*Renewal:* State in which the user reevaluates the quality of the use of the innovation, seeks major modifications or alternatives to the present innovation to achieve increased impact on clients.

Table 5. IEPS Descriptive Statistics

Practitioner Subject	Total Score	SS1	SS2	SS3	Total Score (Pre-test)	SS1	SS2	SS3 (Post-test)
1	58	24	11	23	57	24	10	23
2	66	27	11	28	66	27	10	29
3	58	24	10	24	65	28	12	25
4	22	7	3	12	64	26	11	27
5	61	26	9	26	66	28	12	26
6	50	22	11	17	63	26	11	26
7	Did not complete the study				Did not complete the study			
MEAN SCORES	52.5	21.7	9.2	21.7	63.5	26.5	11	26

n = 6.

Table 6. Comparison of Mean Pre-test & Post-test Scores

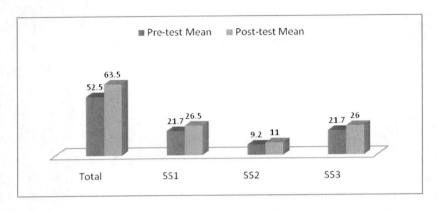

n = 6.

Total scores ranged from 22 to 66 with a mean score of 52.5. Notably the lowest score came from a subject with no prior knowledge or experience with IP collaboration. Other participants all had prior knowledge and experience with IP. Based on pre-test and post-test scores, consistent positive trends in both total scores and all sub scores were observed. See Table 6.

Comparison of pre-test and post test scores for each individual participant also resulted in positive trend with increased total scores and increases for all sub scores. Notably, the subject with no prior knowledge or experience had post test scores in similar ranges with other subjects who came to the study with prior IP knowledge and experience. See tables 7- 10.

CBAM-LoU

The pre-test results of the CBAM-LoU interviews indicated most subjects were at the Orientation or Preparation level of use. One individual was at Mechanical Use and one was at Routine level.

Table 7. Total Scores by Subject (Practitioners)

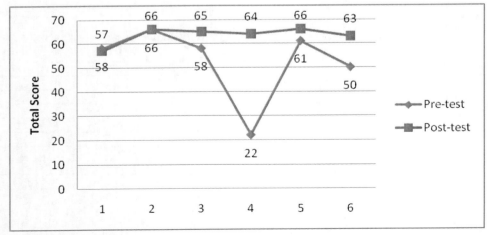

n = 6.

Table 8. Comparison of Mean Pre-test & Post-test SS1 Scores

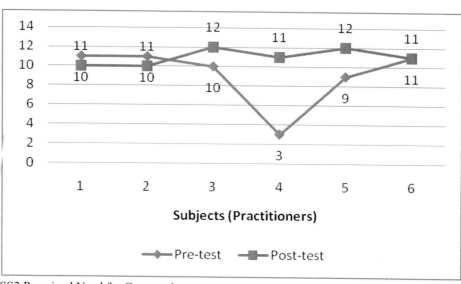

n=6. SS1; Competency and Autonomy.

Table 9. Comparison of Mean Pre-test & Post-test SS2 Scores

n = 6; SS2 Perceived Need for Cooperation.

The subject who was at Orientation level was the subject with no prior interprofessional experience and the subject at Routine level had the most prior experience and had worked previously at an organization that promoted interprofessional collaboration. Post-test results indicated positive trends with increased interprofessional collaboration behaviors. The subject with no prior experience increased from Orientation to Mechanical Use, and all other subjects were at either Routine levels of use or Integration.

Table 10. Comparison of Mean Pre-test 7 Post-test SS3 Scores

Subject	Pre-test	Post-test
1	23	23
2	28	29
3	24	25
4	12	27
5	26	26
6	17	26

n = 6; SS3 Perception of Actual Cooperation.

DISCUSSION

Recognizing the limitations of sample size, the results of the study indicate positive changes in attitude about IP collaboration, as well as moderate enhancements in behaviors regarding IP collaboration. This suggests there are potential benefits of using a defined continuing professional education process, such as PBL, to create an environment that fosters the interprofessional collaboration that will improve patient outcomes.

Evidence shows that there are powerful influences of professional enculturation and limited understanding of the relationship between continuing professional education (CPE) and actual change in practice. Team-based health care delivery is necessary and effective continuing education for healthcare professionals needs to be grounded in ways to engage practitioners in authentic work that has patient care and population health as its focus. The PBL model for the continuing professional education intervention used in this study can provide guidance for workforce training in interprofessional (IP) collaboration to develop IP care models that may improve clinical outcomes and care delivery efficiencies.

This study addresses the critical need for innovation in workforce training and professional development through continuing education. It demonstrates a process for implementing a PBL continuing education process that is grounded in adult learning theory and authentic task content. The results of this study give direction for future research with expanded populations of practitioners in public health settings.

Limitations for practitioner subject analysis are as follows: Due to the nature of the practitioner environment, totally randomized subjects will not be feasible. In addition, the research will not be able to control for dispositional factors of individual practitioners, and the relatively small sample size of practitioner subjects. Further, the one group pre-test, post-test design provides a measure of change but does not provide conclusive results about its cause.

Findings of this study may serve as a model for future research opportunities to implement this PBL based continuing educational model across larger groups of public health provider communities.

ACKNOWLEDGMENTS

This study was financially supported by the Office of Sponsored Research at Rosalind Franklin University of Medicine and Science. The contributions of Kevin Morris and Rafeda Khan, who are both students in the Doctor of Pharmacy program in the College of Pharmacy at Rosalind Franklin University of Medicine and Science, were instrumental in the implementation of the CPE workshop. The researchers would also like to express appreciation to Gene Hall, PhD, Professor of Educational Leadership at the University of Nevada in Las Vegas for his guidance on use of the CBAM-Lou and to Richard Luecht, PhD, University of North Carolina at Greensboro. Professor and Chair of the Department of Educational Research Methodology and Director of the Center for Educational Research and Evaluation (CERE), for his generous permission to use the IEPS instrument.

REFERENCES

[1] Beaglehole R, Dal Poz MR. Public Health workforce: Challenges and policy issues Hum Resour Health 2003; 1(1): 4.
[2] Lumague M, Morgan A, Mak D, Hanna M, Kwong J, Cameron C, Zener D, Sinclair L. Interprofessional education: The student perspective. J Interprof Care 2008; 20(3): 246-53.
[3] Institute of Medicine. Redesigning continuing education in the health professions. Washington, DC: National Academy Press, 2009.
[4] Schofield D, Fuller J, Wagner S, Friis L, Tyrell B. Multidisciplinary management of complex care. Aust J Rural Health 2009; 17(1): 45-48.
[5] Barker, K, & Oandasan I. Interprofessional care review with medical residents: Lessons learned, tensions aired-A pilot study. J Interprof Care 2005; 19(3): 207-14.
[6] Fisher E, Bynum J, Skinner J. The policy implications of variations in Medicare spending growth. 2009. Accessed 2012 Dec 2. URL: http://www.dartmouth atlas.org/downloads/reports/Policy_ Implications_Brief_022709.pdf.
[7] Varda D, Shoup J, Miller SA. Systematic review of collaboration and network research in the public affairs literature: Implications for public health practice and research. Amer J Public Health 2012; 102(3): 564-71.
[8] Gebbie KM, Turnock BJ. The public health workforce, 2006: New challenges. Health Aff 2006; 25(4): 923-33.
[9] IOM (Institute of Medicine). Interprofessional education for collaboration: Learning how to improve health from interprofessional models across the continuum of education to practice: Workshop summary. Washington, DC: The National Academies Press. 2013.
[10] Centre for the Advancement of Interprofessional Education (CAIPE). Accessed June 12, 2013. URL: http://caipe.org.uk/about-us/defining-ipe/
[11] Zwarenstein M, Reeves S. Knowledge translation and interprofessional collaboration: Where the rubber of evidence-based care hits the road of teamwork. J Contin Educ Health Prof 2006; 26(1): 46-54.

[12] Canadian Interprofessional Health Collaborative. A national interprofessional competency framework; February 2010. Accessed June 12, 2013. URL: http://www.cihc.ca/files/CIHC_IPCompetencies_Feb1210.pdf.
[13] Freeth D, Hammick M, Reeves S, Koppel I, Barr H. Effective interprofessional education: Development, delivery and evaluation. Oxford: Blackwell, 2005.
[14] Kasperski M. Implementation strategies: Collaboration in primary care family doctors and nurse practitioners delivering shared care. Toronto, ON: Ontario College of Family Physicians, 2000. Accessed June 12, 2013. URL: http://www.cfpc.ca/English/CFPC/CLFM/bibnursing/default.asp?s_1.
[15] Morrison S. Working together: Why bother with collaboration? Work Based Learning in Primary Care 2007; 5: 65-70.
[16] Bromage A. Interprofessional education. higher education.
[17] resources 2009. Accessed: September 15, 2011. URL: http://highereducationresources.atspace.com/interprofessional.htm.
[18] Barr H, Koppel I, Reeves S, Hammick M, Freeth, D. Effective interprofessional education: Development, delivery and evaluation. Oxford: Blackwell, 2005.
[19] USA public health workforce enumeration. Accessed December 12, 2013. URL: http://bhpr.hrsa.gov/healthworkforce/reports/publichealthstudy2005.pdf.
[20] Schmitt M et al. Core competencies for interp rofessional collaborative practice.The Interprofessional Education Collaborative (IPEC). Accessed December 12, 2013. URL: http://www.asph.org/userfiles/collaborativepractice.pdf.
[21] Young L, Baker P, Waller S, Hodgson L, Moor M. Knowing your allies: Medical education and interprofessional exposure. J Interprof Care 2007; 21(2): 155-63.
[22] 21 Umble KE, Cervero RM, Langone CA. Negotiating about power frames, and continuing education: A case study in public health. Adult Educ Q 2001; 51(2): 128.
[23] Goldman J, Zwarenstein M, Bhattacharyya O, Reeves, S. Improving the clarity of the interprofessional field: implications for research and continuing interprofessional education. J Contin Educ Health Prof 2009; 29(3): 151-6.
[24] Albanese M, Mitchell S. Problem-based learning: A review of literature on its outcomes and implementation issues. Acad Med 1993; 68(1): 52-81.
[25] Barrows H. A taxonomy of problem-based learning methods. Med Educ 1986; 20: 481-86.
[26] Cervero RM, Wilson AL, Associates. Power in practice: Adult education and the struggle for knowledge and power in society. San Francisco: Jossey-Bass, 2001.
[27] Moore DE, Pennington FC. Practice-based learning and improvement. J Educ Health Prof 2003; 23 (Spring Suppl- 1): S73-80.
[28] Mann K, Viscount P, Cogdon A, Davidson K, Langille D, MacCara M. Multidisciplinary learning in continuing professional education: The heart health Nova Scotia experience. J Contin Educ Health Prof 1996; 1 6(1):135-41.
[29] Vygotsky LS. Mind in society: Development of higher psychological processes. (Cole M, John-Steiner V, Scribner S, Souberman E, eds.). Cambridge, MA: Harvard University Press, 1978.
[30] Bandura A. Self-efficacy: The exercise of control. New York: WH Freeman, 1997.
[31] Belanger E, Rodriguez C. More than the sum of its parts? A qualitative research synthesis on multi-disciplinary primary care teams. J Interprof Care 2008; 22(6): 587-97.

In: Public Health Yearbook 2015
Editor: Joav Merrick
ISBN: 978-1-63484-514-4
© 2016 Nova Science Publishers, Inc.

Chapter 8

COMMUNITY WISE: A FORMATIVE EVALUATION OF A COMMUNITY-BASED HEALTH INTERVENTION

Liliane Cambraia Windsor[1,*]*, PhD, MSW, Lauren Jessell*[3]*, LMSW, Teri Lassiter*[2]*, PhD, and Ellen Benoit*[3]*, PhD*

[1]School of Social Work, Rutgers The State University of New Jersey, Newark, New Jersey, United States of America
[2]School of Public Health, Rutgers The State University of New Jersey, Newark, New Jersey, United States of America
[3]National Development and Research Institutes, New York, United States of America

Individuals with histories of incarceration and substance abuse residing in distressed communities often receive suboptimal services partly due to a lack of empirically supported substance abuse treatments targeting this population. Grounded in community based participatory research, we developed *Community Wise*, a manualized, 12-week, group behavioral intervention. The intervention aims to reduce substance use frequency, HIV/HCV risk behaviors, and reoffending among individuals with histories of substance abuse and incarceration. Thirty six individuals were recruited to participate in a formative evaluation of Community Wise processes and outcomes. Analysis showed significantly lower post-intervention number of cigarettes smoked per day, days using an illicit drug, money spent on illegal drugs, and rearrests. Based on the evaluation, the research team made the following changes: 1) added a session on sexuality; 2) increased the number of sessions from 12 to 15; and 3) modified strategies to help participants develop and implement capacity building projects.

Keywords: substance abuse treatment, community based participatory research, critical consciousness theory, HIV/HCV prevention, reoffending

---

[*] Corresponding author: Liliane Cambraia Windsor, PhD, MSW, 360 Martin Luther King Jr. Blvd, Hill Hall, Room 401, Newark, NJ 07102, United States. E-mail: lwindsor@ssw.rutgers.edu.

INTRODUCTION

Health disparities in the United States are well documented and result in a significant financial burden to the nation. For example, the per capita rate of new AIDS cases is 8 times higher for Blacks than it is for Whites (1). These differences, as identified by the National Healthcare Disparities Report, mandated by Congress, impose great financial and human costs. According to the Joint Center for Political and Economic Studies, health disparities cost the United States $1.24 trillion between 2003 and 2006 and this burden has only continued to grow (2). Disparities related to race and income are exacerbated in low-income African-American communities, where substance abuse and incarceration rates are high. Health indicators show that African-Americans suffer significantly harsher consequences of substance use than their White counterparts (e.g., higher rates of HIV/HCV infection), and yet, have less access to HIV and substance abuse interventions that could mitigate this disparity (3, 4).

For low-income African-Americans involved in the criminal justice system, incarceration has a significant impact on health and substance use, especially upon release. Few individuals receive substance abuse treatment and HIV/HCV prevention services while in prison and they often return to the same distressed communities in which they obtained and used drugs, engaged in related risk behaviors, and became exposed to the criminal justice system (5). Research has identified these issues as major obstacles in maintaining recovery (6, 7).

Despite increased efforts to reduce health disparities in distressed African American communities, few evidence-based interventions have been successfully adopted by these communities (8). Often substance abuse and community reentry programs focus solely on individual treatment even though community-based models have been shown to enhance effectiveness by addressing the environmental context in which problems occur (9).

This paper reports results of the formative evaluation of *Community Wise,* a community-based, manualized, multilevel health intervention designed to reduce substance use frequency, HIV/HCV risk behaviors, and reoffending among individuals with histories of substance abuse and incarceration residing in distressed communities in Newark, New Jersey. The long term goal of *Community Wise* is to reduce health disparities. Distressed communities are defined as geographic areas where rates of poverty, drug use and traffic, violence, and disease are higher than in neighboring areas (10).

Developing "*Community Wise*"

Community based participatory research (CBPR) principles were used to develop and pilot-test *Community Wise*. CBPR requires that researchers and community members work together to identify community problems and solutions through the combination of scientific and experiential knowledge. The key purpose of CBPR is to help create knowledge that can be immediately used to help the community involved in the research (11, 12).

Community Wise was developed by a team of community members, consumers (individuals with histories of incarceration and substance abuse and their families and friends), service providers, researchers, and government officials who compose the Newark Community Collaborative Board (NCCB). The NCCB has been working together using a

CBPR framework since September 2010 to develop *Community Wise*. During phase 1 of the formative evaluation, the NCCB was formed; trained; and engaged in CBPR to conduct a needs assessment as well as an ethnographic study that informed the development of *Community Wise*. The NCCB also developed the first edition of the *Community Wise* manual (13–15). During phase 2 of the formative evaluation, *Community Wise* was implemented for the first time in the Spring of 2012 with 26 individuals at a community based agency to test the feasibility of the manual and develop the first evaluation procedures (16). The current paper reports findings from phase 3 of the formative evaluation, where the NCCB implemented the revised version of *Community Wise*'s manual with 36 individuals at a community-based agency in Newark, NJ. Phase 3 aimed to examine the feasibility of the revised manual and maximize its potential efficacy. This paper discusses, in detail, the process implemented by the NCCB to evaluate the intervention's feasibility and the lessons learned in this process.

Table 1. Intervention sessions and respective goals

Session # and Theme	Overall Goals
Session 1: Icebreaker and Welcome	*To introduce participants and facilitators to one another,* *To present an overview of Community Wise* *To establish ground rules.*
Session 2: Critical Thinking	*To explore critical thinking literature and evaluate one's own thinking patterns*
Session 3: Solar System	*To use the solar system image as a metaphor to help participants explore power dynamics and the role of community building and civic engagement as empowerment tools*
Session 4: Empowerment	*To help participants development personal goals and a capacity building project as empowerment strategies*
Session 5: Funhouse Mirrors	*To use the funhouse mirrors image metaphor to help participants explore the impact of internalized and structural oppression on their communities, thinking patterns, and risk behaviors*
Session 6: Empowerment	*To help participant develop personal goals and a capacity building project as empowerment strategies*
Session 7: Walls	*To use the metaphor of confining walls image to help participants identify structural oppressive systems and appropriate strategies for overcoming them*
Session 8: Empowerment	*To provide support to participants as they attempt to implement their personal goals and capacity building project*
Session 9: Historical Trauma	*To use the historical trauma image to examine the impact of historical trauma on participants' present behaviors*
Session 10: Empowerment	*To support participants in evaluating progress and addressing challenges in their personal goals and capacity building projects.*
Session11: Family structure and dynamics	*To use the family image to explore how different family structures and dynamics may influence both positively and negatively the perpetuation of structural and internalized oppressions*

Table 1. (Continued)

Session # and Theme	Overall Goals
Session 12: Termination and Personal Evaluation	*To help participants work through feelings that arise from ending group work and to articulate orally new skills and ways of thinking acquired through their participation in Community Wise. Participants are encouraged to share how new skills and ways of thinking may help them accomplish longer term plans*
Graduation	*Participants celebrate their work, and engage with community members to raise awareness about substance abuse, HIV/HCV risk behaviors, and reoffending.*

Theoretical framework

Community Wise was informed by Paulo Freire's critical consciousness theory (17). Freire defined critical consciousness as the ability to "perceive social, political, and economic contradictions, and to take action against the oppressive elements of reality" (p. 19). Based on this theory, vulnerable populations should be encouraged to engage in critical dialogue about the oppressive elements in their lives and communities. Critical consciousness can empower these individuals to engage in social action (e.g., engage in their communities' political process) to combat the oppression they experience (e.g., lack of access to affordable and healthy food, meaningful employment, and quality health care). Oppression can be internalized, contributing to criminal activity, substance use and other risk behaviors. Using critical consciousness theory, *Community Wise* seeks to redirect the effects of oppression away from destructive, health-risk behavior into outward, positive action such as planting a community garden and/or advocating for community resources. In order to achieve this goal, the 12 group sessions that make up *Community Wise* encourage participants to think critically and engage in dialogue about the oppression they experience. At the same time, participants are encouraged to combat oppression by working with one another to create a community capacity building project and develop the skills they need (e.g., leadership) to bring about change in their community (e.g., increasing access to quality foods) (18). Table 1 displays a summary of the intervention's sessions with respective goals.

METHODS

A mixed-methods research design informed by CBPR was implemented to test *Community Wise's* feasibility. Quantitative methods consisted of process measures and a pre-posttest design to gage changes in substance use frequency, HIV/HCV risk behaviors, and reoffending before and after the intervention. Qualitative methods consisted of analyzing four focus groups with *Community Wise* participants to explore participants' feedback about the intervention and qualitative analysis of session video digital recordings to explore the development of critical consciousness and the application of *Community Wise's* key ingredients. The findings were then combined to inform revisions made to the manual and the research protocol. The current paper will focus on the qualitative component of the evaluation.

Staff and NCCB training and monitoring

The current evaluation was conducted after obtaining approval from the Institutional Review Board (IRB) at two partner universities and at the community based organization where groups were held. Social workers and research support staff were directly supervised by the Principal Investigator (PI). The staff received training on study measures, data collection, and the *Community Wise* manual. Members of the NCCB received training on CBPR principles and philosophy, ethical treatment of research participants, and research methods and procedures. NCCB members met monthly to review and approve research procedures, resolve any challenges, and make decisions about potential changes to the manual and the research protocol.

Sample recruitment

Participants were recruited by the NCCB using purposive sampling. Specifically, recruitment flyers were distributed to service providers and potential study participants who contacted the study's phone number so that people could help spread the information to friends, family members, and acquaintances.

To be eligible, participants had to have been incarcerated within the past four years, have a history of substance abuse within the past year, be 18 years of age or older, reside in Essex County, NJ, speak English and provide informed consent. Participants were screened by a masters-level social worker using standardized measures (19–22).

Participants were deemed ineligible if they were found to have a high level of suicidality, an unstabilized psychotic disorder, gross cognitive impairment or did not have a moderate to high level of drug and/or alcohol use in the past year.

Participants received $15 for completing a clinical screening. Individuals who met eligibility criteria were invited to participate in *Community Wise* and distributed into four intervention groups based on gender and availability. Study staff reviewed a written consent form, outlining the risks and benefits of participating and the certificate of confidentiality obtained from the federal government to prohibit court-ordered violations of participants' confidentiality.

In signing the consent form, participants agreed to have all *Community Wise* sessions video-taped and to use code names during the group sessions to protect their confidentiality. Seventy-nine participants completed a phone screening followed by a clinical screening to assess eligibility. Forty individuals were assigned to *Community Wise* and 36 completed the 12-week data collection follow-up.

Procedures

The qualitative evaluation included four focus groups (one focus group for each *Community Wise* group) which occurred after the *Community Wise* sessions were completed.

The purpose of the focus groups was to obtain feedback from participants. An NCCB member and a research assistant hired specifically to fulfill this role conducted the focus groups. All 40 participants who attended at least one *Community Wise* session were invited to participate. Those who participated received $20 (N = 36).

Group facilitators attended weekly clinical supervision with the project PI. Clinical supervision enhanced treatment fidelity and provided facilitators with feedback.

During supervision, the group discussed challenges, ensured that the manual was being implemented accurately, and discussed non-responsive clients. The PI watched all session videos and completed a checklist to provide feedback to facilitators.

Data analysis

Data from qualitative analyses included a random sample of 23 out of 48 digital videos of group sessions and verbatim transcriptions of focus groups. The focus group transcripts were coded and analyzed manually by one of the authors and a thematic analysis was conducted (23). This process involves reading the data several times, coding and recoding through a process of constant comparison until themes and categories become clear. The focus group data complemented quantitative measures of participant feedback. Such triangulation helps ensure completeness of data and can reveal convergence or dissonance in key themes developed in our analyses (24).

Video data was open coded by two research assistants using N-vivo qualitative data analysis software. Inter-rater reliability was calculated reaching over 90% agreement on all codes. The codes were then analyzed for common themes by the PI and two NCCB members. The research questions included: 1) What were the main *Community Wise* ingredients impacting critical consciousness, drug use frequency, HIV/HCV risk behaviors, and reoffending?; and 2) Were these ingredients successfully implemented and if not, how should they be modified?

RESULTS

A total of 36 individuals participated in this study. Ninety-four percent were African-American; most were heterosexual, single, unemployed and reported a mean household yearly income of less than $10,000. Most were not currently supervised by the criminal justice system. The charge associated with participant's last incarceration varied; the most common charges were drug possession, property and technical violations, and violent crimes. On average, participants had been released from their last incarceration 13 months prior to the intervention. All participants were either using an illicit drug or alcohol at the time of baseline or reported use within the past year. Most were smoking an average of ten cigarettes per day at the time of baseline. Ten percent reported being HIV positive and 11% reported being HCV positive. Table 2 displays participants' demographics.

Table 2. Participants' characteristics at baseline (N = 36)

Characteristic	N (%) or Mean (±SD)
Male	18 (49)
Heterosexual	32 (89)
Age	44.65 (±8.4)
Race	
Black/African American	34 (94)
White	2 (06)
Ethnicity	
Hispanic	3 (07)
Not Hispanic	33 (93)
Household yearly income	7,340.73 (±9,805.5)
Religion	
Christian	24 (67)
Muslim/Islam	8 (22)
None	4 (11)
Marital Status	
Single/never married	18 (57)
Unemployed	33 (91)
Criminal Justice System Status	
Parole	4 (10)
Probation	5 (13)
No supervision	27 (77)
Number of months since release from incarceration	13 (±13.8)
Criminal Charge at Last Incarceration	
Violent crime (assault, homicide, carjacking, robbery)	4 (12)
Property crime (burglary, fraud, shoplifting)	13 (36)
Drug Possession	13 (36)
Drug dealing	1 (02)
Sex Work	1 (02)
Warrants/technical violations	4 (12)
Reporting committing any crime(s) above since last incarceration	8 (22)
Substance Use	% (n) or mean (±SD)
Reported alcohol use in the past 90 days	21 (58)
Number of days in which alcohol was used in the past 90 days	28 (±36)
Number of heavy drinking days (past 90-days)	13 (±28.2)
Average Drinks per drinking day (past 90-days)	4.93 (±14.3)
Number of Current Smokers	31 (86)
Number of Cigarettes per day	9.2 (±8.7)
Reported illicit drug use past 90 days (cocaine/opiates/marijuana)	28 (78)
Number of days any illicit drug use past 90 days (cocaine/opiates/marijuana) Money spent on illicit drug per using day	40.52 (±34.7) 29.5 (±37.5)
HIV/HCV Status and HIV/HCV Risk/Protective Factors	
HIV +	4 (11)
HCV+	5 (14)

Table 2. (Continued)

Characteristic	N (%) or Mean (±SD)
Average number of times tested for HIV	7.5 (±9.9)
Average number of times tested for HCV	5.0 (±8.7)
Number of times engaging in risky drug use in past 30 days	0.9 (±5.1)*
Frequency of engagement in risky sexual behaviors	0.5 (±0.3)*
Psychological Distress**	
PTSD*** (responding yes to having had a near death experience)	20 (56)
PTSQ (PTSD Symptom Severity)	1.1 (±0.3)
BSI 18 Total Score	0.7 (±0.2)
Attitudes Toward Research	
Average # agreeing that research is important	31 (86)
Average # agreeing that research procedures were easy to understand	21 (58)
Average # agreeing that researchers do not always inform participants about the risks involved in health research	13 (36)

* Indicates that in average participants reported either never engaging or only engaging a few times in risky sex and/or drug use behaviors.
**Ranges from 0 to 4 (higher scores mean higher psychological distress).
***Ranges from 0 to 3 (higher scores mean higher PTSD symptom severity).

Intervention retention

Participants completed an average of 7 (± 3.85) out of 12 sessions. Participants were defined as having successfully completed the intervention if they attended six or more group sessions and showed clinical improvement.

Clinical improvement was established in clinical supervision and measured by specific progress that each participant made on personal goals, participation in capacity building projects, and improvement on distal outcomes. Seventy percent successfully completed the intervention. Completion was defined based on previous work examining other behavioral interventions in the literature (25, 26).

Specifically, successful completion included those who attended at least 7 sessions, demonstrated clinical improvement (e.g., reduced drug use, improved mental health symptoms), and engaged in capacity building projects.

Findings from focus groups

A total of 25 out of 36 participants attended the focus groups. Analysis revealed two overall themes: 1) Participant satisfaction with the intervention, and 2) Areas of strengths and areas that need to be improved. Overall, focus group participants reported that the intervention was useful, with many expressing a desire to maintain contact with the program post-graduation as a means of continuing their personal growth and development. Participants identified group facilitators and the participant's manual as key factors in their satisfaction with *Community Wise*. According to participants, the facilitators were viewed as a source of knowledge and information, as well as providing a support mechanism for some of the participants. For instance, a male participant noted that his facilitator took time from his schedule to check on him when he had no one else to turn to, which in turn provided the motivation he needed to continue the program. Participants reported the manual was useful in helping them think about the group work outside of group and it was a way to share what they were learning with others.

Participants had a few suggestions to improve the intervention. A female participant believed it is unrealistic to complete a capacity building project in twelve weeks. One of the male participants agreed and in order to address this issue in his group, they decided to meet outside of the scheduled sessions, at a participant's home, to "carry on our part of our project that we still feel we want to see through to the end." Finally, participants felt that *Community Wise* should provide them with concrete job leads and references to increase their chances of gainful employment; according to them, this should be the first priority of the intervention.

Findings from session videos

Analysis revealed Community Wise's mechanisms of change which included two overall domains: 1) Operational ingredients; and 2) active ingredients. Figure 1 displays the mechanisms of change.

Operational ingredients are intended to create a safe environment where the intervention can thrive. These included group introductions, a description of *Community Wise*'s background, and the mutual development of group guidelines. Combined, these activities served as a way for the facilitator to establish confidence, trust and commitment among the group members. For instance, in establishing group norms and expectations, the facilitators explained *Community Wise's* background to the participants, how the intervention was developed, and their personal commitment to it. Group norms and expectations were established by the participants themselves, who were encouraged during the beginning few sessions to come up with their own group guidelines. The guidelines were revisited throughout the intervention, as expectations changed and commitment to the group grew.

The active ingredients of Community Wise comprised activities that seemed to impact the development of critical consciousness and distal outcomes. These activities included 1) critical thinking; 2) identifying and discussing the link between oppression and harmful behavior; 3) taking action; 4) voicing & validating each other's feelings and experiences; and 5) sharing knowledge, experiences, and resources. Figure 1 displays *Community Wise's* mechanisms of change.

Critical thinking involved the group participants questioning information and examining the quality of their own thinking process, often as a result of the homework assignments (e.g., reading an article about Crack Baby syndrome or researching and questioning HIV conspiracy theories) and the group dialogue. In thinking critically, participants linked structural oppression to their behavior and means of coping. For example, in the women's group, participants discussed the article about crack baby syndrome and whether or not it is a real problem. Before reading the article, the group shared their experiential knowledge about this topic, with many women describing the sick babies they met in their lives. Then, they read the article and posed critical questions (e.g.,: How do you know what you know is true? What information is more reliable: Scientific? Experiential? Coming from authorities?). The discussion finally culminated with the question: What are the consequences if I believe that the crack baby syndrome is true? And what are the consequences if I believe it is not true? The group engaged in a deep discussion about the role of racism, stigma, and classism in the production of knowledge and how these macro level issues impact their individual beliefs and behaviors.

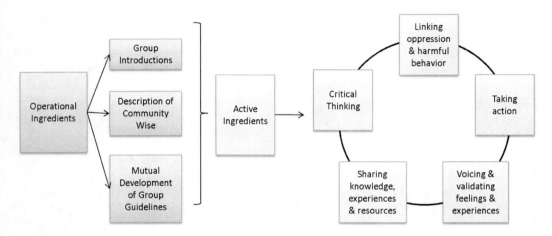

Figure 1. Community Wise's Mechanisms of Change.

Understanding and identifying the role of oppression was stressed by the group facilitators throughout the sessions. The homework, exercises and prompts from the facilitators and one another encouraged participants to connect the role of oppression to the choices that they make in relation to substance use, HIV/HCV risk behavior, and reoffending. For example, in reacting to an illustration of a person of color engaging in harmful behaviors, one participant described how the negative image he has of himself in society makes him want to drink. He explained,

"…to keep certain images out of my mind and by the time they added all up you know, they may not be all of them mirrors but there's a couple of them mirrors, not really proud of it, and in my mind it's like well don't think about that and my weakness was just, well you won't really have to think about it if you just have a few more drinks, you know?"

Taking action is another active ingredient that seemed to impact critical consciousness and distal outcomes among participants. Throughout the group sessions, participants were encouraged to respond to their experiences of structural oppression by taking action against it. They were encouraged to do this by setting and talking about personal goals and by organizing a capacity building project amongst themselves. For example, one of the participants described how no matter how hard he tries he can't find employment: "I filled out 1,000 applications, no exaggeration…" The participants in this group eventually agreed to create a community garden where they would grow vegetables and sell them in a farmers market. In taking action, this participant started to respond to the oppression in his life by supporting his community. Rather than harming himself, he was encouraged to work with other participants to react in a more positive and action-oriented way, creating his own employment opportunity.

Voicing and validating each other's experiences and anger related to structural oppression was another active ingredient of *Community Wise*. It allowed participants to give and receive support and to articulate experiences related to oppression that are not always acknowledged. Participants described the frustration they faced trying to achieve financial stability and shelter while having a criminal history. One participant talked about his steps to join a protest group in Newark, NJ representing the unemployed and another discussed getting denied low-income housing because they don't accept ex-offenders:

> "I'm just like yesterday and today I just been like real frustrated you know because like I'm trying to do what I can to you know better myself and it's like I keep hitting brick walls…"

This participant then went on to say that he can't allow himself to act on his frustration by returning to illegal activities because that will just lead him back to "prisons, institutions and death." Issues related to structural oppression were also discussed from the homework assignments and activities and again, participants received validation and the freedom to express their anger in a supportive environment. In providing one another with a means to express their anger and hardships, they were able to engage in critical dialogue to develop community engaged ways to combat the oppression they were facing.

Sharing knowledge, experiences and resources served as an additional way of responding to oppression, this time by empowering one another and exchanging information. Perhaps as a result of talking about the oppression in their lives and supporting each other throughout the group sessions, participants began working together to share resources and knowledge they had about jobs, social service benefits, housing options and other useful resources with one another. They also began using one another as resources, supporting each other through the challenges they went through during the week. As the weeks went on, participants worked together as a team, not just on the capacity building projects but also to support one another individually to make better choices related to their health and behavior. For example, participants encouraged each other to avoid substance use and other harmful behavior, asking that they call other group members before engaging in risky behavior, rather than after. One participant in the women's group talked about how she has been thinking about calling the co-facilitator who attends 12-step meetings and that she was contemplating going back to meetings and "getting clean" again:

> "I know meetings work for me, they kept me clean for multiple years, over a decade. So I know that but I dunno, I just know I've got new hope with going back to work and getting a pay check like I used to get before I got fired I got a pay check so I've got a little renewed hope."

In getting her basic needs met (e.g., obtaining a job), this participant expressed being more motivated to stop using substances. The group encouraged this participant to reach out to them and to use resources in the community, such as a detox center and 12-step meetings.

While the ingredients appeared to work and affect change in two of the groups, they did not work as well in the third. This may have been due to the facilitator's failure to establish a belief in the group's ability, such as their capacity to create and follow group guidelines.

Also, critical thinking was not explained well by this facilitator as a means to recognize oppression and the link between oppression and harmful behavior was not well established. These issues may have had a negative impact on the ingredients' ability to affect change among the participants in this group.

DISCUSSION

Findings from this process evaluation showed that *Community Wise* was acceptable to individuals with a history of substance abuse and incarceration residing in a distressed community. Participants found the intervention useful and process measures revealed strong alliance and a high retention rate in the intervention, considering this is such a hard to reach and hard to engage population (18, 27). Overall, the results suggest that participants were able to engage in treatment and viewed the intervention as beneficial, despite the multiple challenges they face (e.g., homelessness, unemployment, poverty).

Analysis of process measures indicated a high level of satisfaction with *Community Wise* through high scores in working alliance and group climate. Participants reported finding the intervention useful and reporting intent to use the skills they learned in the *Community Wise* groups (18). *Community Wise* retention rates were higher than retention rates reported in the literature from evidence-based substance abuse treatment evaluations with substance abusing individuals. Specifically, 70% of *Community Wise's* participants successfully completed treatment. Literature reporting findings from cognitive behavioral therapy evaluations with this population reveal an average of only 58% completion rates (28, 29).

The mechanisms of change identified in the qualitative analysis indicated key operational and active ingredients that, when implemented by the facilitator according to the *Community Wise* manual, seemed to affect change among the participants. Some of these activities, however, were not implemented as well as they could have been. For example, the facilitator in the third group did not implement the group introductions, critical thinking or group guidelines activities as indicated in the manual. Other problems with activities consisted of issues with the intervention itself. The NCCB worked together to modify *Community Wise* in order to resolve these issues.

For example, the "taking action" mechanism of change activity of engaging in capacity building projects still needed further development. Participants encountered challenges when developing and implementing the capacity building projects, likely causing frustration, and it was difficult to measure the impact of these projects on the community. Initially, the capacity building projects were designed to be individual projects. Approximately 3 weeks into the intervention, we realized that these should be group projects for several reasons: First, critical consciousness is developed through dialogue and group work. The focus must be on process and on the skills that are learned and developed collectively by the groups. Thus, we changed the rules midway and allowed the groups to develop group projects. The next challenge happened when participants started to develop very large ideas and struggled to break them down into small, accomplishable steps. By the time the groups were finally able to agree on a small and feasible project, the groups were ending. The capacity building projects are supposed to help participants learn group working skills, connect with others in their communities, and feel proud of the community work they accomplish. In this formative evaluation however, only one group was able to develop and implement a capacity building project.

In addition to problems with the capacity building projects, qualitative analysis of video sessions indicated a lack of content specific to sexuality issues and challenges with the design of capacity building projects. It is likely that these weaknesses in the manual are at least partially responsible for the lack of significant changes in HIV/HCV risk behavior (see the Lessons Learned/Manual Changes section below). Due to methodological limitations (e.g.,: lack of a control group), it is not possible to conclude that the intervention caused the changes in outcomes. However, pre- to post-intervention changes in outcome measures seem to indicate that *Community Wise* has the potential to be helpful as indicated by many favorable outcome changes in the expected direction. Small to large positive effect sizes were found for the overall sample in all of the outcomes. Findings were especially promising for substance abuse and reoffending outcomes as many of these variables reached statistical significance despite the small sample. However, no statistically significant changes were found in HIV/HCV risk behaviors. These findings replicate results from *Community Wise's* cohort 1(16).

Lessons learned/manual changes

Once the process evaluation data analysis was completed, findings were presented to the NCCB and discussed to determine implications and future steps. The NCCB agreed to meet for a retreat in which changes to the manual, guided by the research findings and by NCCB's experiential knowledge, would be discussed and implemented. The NCCB agreed to increase the number of sessions from 12 to 15, with two of the additional sessions dedicated to discussions about the capacity building projects and one session focused on sexuality. The goal of the sexuality session will be to explore homophobia and sexism as forms of oppression and to understand the impact of this oppression on behavioral health and HIV/HCV risk behaviors.

The NCCB also spent a great deal of time discussing the capacity building projects. Members agreed that capacity building projects must focus on process, rather than project outcomes, with step by step guidelines on how to best research and implement goals. The projects must be feasible and accomplishable in a short period of time. We are currently developing the model that participants will follow as they engage in their capacity building projects.

CONCLUSION

While data provides evidence indicating that *Community Wise* is a promising intervention, formative evaluation indicates that future development and research is needed to test the mechanisms of change and the real effect of *Community Wise* on distal and proximal outcomes. Funding is currently being sought to conduct a randomized clinical trial to test the efficacy of the revised manual of *Community Wise*.

ACKNOWLEDGMENTS

The project described was supported by the Center for Behavioral Health Services and Criminal Justice Research (CBHSR), which is funded by National Institute of Mental Health, award number P30MH079920 and by the HIV Intervention Science Training Program for Promising New Investigators from Underrepresented Groups (HISTP), funded by the National Institutes of Health (NIH), award number R25MH080665. The content is solely the responsibility of the authors and does not necessarily represent the official views of the National Institute of Mental Health, the National Institutes of Health, CBHS, Rutgers University, HISTP, or Columbia University. We would like to acknowledge the contributions made by all members of the Newark Community Collaborative Board, our statistical consultant Don Hoover, and *Community Wise* participants in the development of this work.

REFERENCES

[1] Centers for Disease Control. HIV among African Americans. Atlanta, GA: CDC, 2014.
[2] LaVeist TA, Gaskin DJ. The economic burden of health inequalities in the United States. Washington, DC: Joint Center for Political and Economic Studies, 2009.
[3] Warnecke RB, Oh A, Breen N, Gehlert S, Paskett E, Tucker KL, et al. Approaching health disparities from a population perspective: The National Institutes of Health Centers for Population Health and Health Disparities. Am J. Public Health 2008;98(9):1608–15.
[4] Allen K. Barriers to treatment for addicted african-american women. J Natl Med Assoc 1995;87(10):751–6.
[5] Weinbaum CM. Sabin KM, Santibanez SS. Hepatitis B, Hepatitis C, and HIV in correctional populations: A review of epidemiology and prevention. AIDS 2005;19(Suppl 3):S41–6.
[6] Shorkey C, Windsor L, Spence R. Assessing and developing cultural competence relevance in chemical dependence treatment organizations that serve mexican american clients and their families. J Behav Health Serv Res 2009;36(1):61–74.
[7] Windsor L, Dunlap E. What is substance use all about? Assumptions in New York's drug policies and the perceptions of drug using low-income african-americans. J Ethn Subst Abuse 2010;9(1):67–87.
[8] Schmidt L, Greenfield T, Mulia N. Unequal treatment: Racial and ethnic disparities in alcoholism treatment services. Alcohol Res Heal 2006;29(1):49–54.
[9] Trickett EJ. Multilevel community-based culturally situated interventions and community impact: an ecological perpective. Am J Commun Psychol 2009;43:257–66.
[10] Dunlap E, Golub A, Johnson BD. The severely-distressed african american family in the crack era: empowerment is not enough. J Sociol Soc Welfare 2006; 33(1):115–139.
[11] Israel B, Schultz A, Parker E, Becker A, Allen A, Guzman R. Critical issues in developing and following community based participatory research principles. In: Minkler M, Wallerstein N, Hall B, eds. Community-based participatory research for Health. San Francisco, CA: Jossey-Bass, 2008.
[12] Pinto RM, Spector AY, Valera PA. Exploring group dynamics for integrating scientific and experiential knowledge in Community Advisory Boards for HIV research. AIDS Care 2011;23(8):1006–13.
[13] Windsor L. Using concept mapping for community-based participatory research: Paving the way for community-based health interventions for oppressed populations. J Mix Methods Res 2013;7(3):274–93.
[14] Windsor L, Murugan V. From the individual to the community: Perspectives about substance abuse services. Soc Work Pract Addict 2012;12(4):412–33.
[15] Ivanova T. Due process: Breaking the cycle, 2012. Accessed 2013 Jun 05. URL: http://www.youtube.com/watch?v=0udmYxCyjw4.

[16] Windsor L, Jemal A., Benoit, E. Community wise: Paving the way for empowerment in community reentry. Int J Law Psychiatry, 2014; 37(5): 501-511.
[17] Freire P. Pedagogy of the oppressed. New York: Continuum, 1976.
[18] Windsor L, Pinto RM, Benoit E, Jessell L, Jemal A. Community wise: The development of an anti-oppression model to promote individual and community health. J Soc Work Prac Addictions, 2014; 14 (4): 402-420.
[19] Folstein MF, Folstein SE, McHugh P,R Fanjiang G. Mini-Mental State Examination user's guide. Odessa, FL: Psychological Assessment Resources, 2001.
[20] Sheehan DV, Lecrubier Y, Harnett-Sheehan K, Amorim P, Janavs J, Weiller E, et al. The M.I.N.I. International Neuropsychiatric Interview (M.I.N.I.): The development and validation of a structured diagnostic psychiatric interview for DSM-IV and ICD-10J Clin Psychiatry 1998;59:22–33.
[21] Blanchard KA, Morgenstern J, Morgan TJ, Labouvie EW, Bux DA. Assessing consequences of substance use: Psychometric properties of the Inventory of Drug Use Consequences. Psychol Addict Behav 2003;17(4):328–31.
[22] Sobell LC, Sobell MB. Timeline followback: A technique for assessing self-reported alcohol consumption. In: Litten RZ, Allen J, eds. Measuring alcohol consumption. New Jersey: Humana Press, 1992:41–72.
[23] Braun V, Clarke V. Using thematic analysis in psychology. Qual Res Psychol 2006;3(2):77–101.
[24] Farmer T, Robinson K, Elliott SJ, Eyles J. Developing and implementing a triangulation protocol for qualitative health research. Qual Health Res 2006;16(3):377–94.
[25] Pinto RM, Campbell ANC, Hien DA, Yu G, Gorroochurn P. Retention in the National Institute on Drug Abuse Clinical Trials Network Women and Trauma Study: Implications for posttrial implementation. Am J Orthopsychiatry 2011;81(2):211–7.
[26] Windsor L, Jemal A, Alessi E. Cognitive behavioral therapy: A meta-analysis of race and substance use outcomes. Cultural Diversity Ethnic Minor Psychology 2014, DOI: 10.1037/a0037929.
[27] Lewis C, Johnson BD, Golub A, Dunlap E. Studying crack abusers: Strategies for recruiting the right tail of an ill-defined population. J Psychoactive Drugs 1992;24(4):323–36.
[28] Carroll KM, Nich C, Lapaglia DM, Peters EN, Easton CJ, Petry NM. Combining cognitive behavioral therapy and contingency management to enhance their effects in treating cannabis dependence: less can be more, more or less. Addiction 2012;107(9):1650–9.
[29] Epstein DH, Hawkins WE, Covi L, Umbricht A, Preston KL. Cognitive-behavioral therapy plus contingency management for cocaine use: findings during treatment and across 12-month follow-up. Psychol Addict Behav 2003;17(1):73–82.

In: Public Health Yearbook 2015
Editor: Joav Merrick

ISBN: 978-1-63484-514-4
© 2016 Nova Science Publishers, Inc.

Chapter 9

THE PROMISING POTENTIAL ROLE OF SUSTAINABLE DEVELOPMENT AND CONSERVATION RELATED BRIDGING ORGANIZATIONS IN PROMOTING HEALTH

Paivi Abernethy[*], MSc, MRes, PhD, ABD
Department of Environment and Resource Studies,
University of Waterloo, Waterloo, Canada

Promoting health has remained strongly in the domain of the health sector, despite the ambitious rhetoric of international agreements. Complex environmental health issues, for instance, are not solvable without active collaboration of the public, private, not-for-profit, and academic sectors together with the communities in which they function. This paper explored the United Nations Educational, Scientific and Cultural Organization (UNESCO) mandated biosphere reserves as bridging organizations outside of the health sector that have begun to bring together diverse stakeholders to address public health and environmental issues as an integrated part of sustainability. A qualitative study of Canadian and British biosphere reserves revealed cross-sectoral health promoting projects ranging from individual health behavior change to those embracing wider social determinants of health. Drivers for and barriers to the integration work were analyzed. Results indicate that organizations with primary focus other than health have a potential to play a meaningful role in providing a neutral, apolitical, platform that helps bringing diverse community stakeholders to the table to promote health.

Keywords: bridging organizations, cross-sectoral collaboration, health promotion, sustainable development, biosphere reserves

---

[*] Corresponding author: Paivi Abernethy, PhD Candidate, MSc, MRes, Environment and Resources Studies, University of Waterloo, 200 University Avenue West, Waterloo, ON N2L 3G1, Canada. E-mail: pkaberne@uwaterloo.ca.

INTRODUCTION

Promoting health has remained strongly in the domain of the health sector, despite the ambitious rhetoric of international agreements such as 'Bangkok Charter for Health Promotion' (1) and 'Health in All Policies' (2) that declared health as a responsibility of all sectors. Environmental health is an area where health outcomes cannot be the sole responsibility of the health sector. Complex environmental issues are not solvable without active collaboration of the public, private, not-for-profit, and academic sectors together with the communities in which they function. Furthermore, environmental pollution and other social determinants of health, such as food security and sustainable livelihoods, are interests shared by diverse health and environmental stakeholders, as well as communities in general.

In current compartmentalized societies, however, someone needs to take the initiative to cross the disciplinary or interest-specific boundaries. Often neither health professionals nor environmental authorities see themselves as having the mandate or capacity to take the lead in addressing environmental health issues. Non-governmental organizations, however, have a greater flexibility in directing their activities. Social movements and organizations addressing specific social determinants of health are known to facilitate cross-sectoral collaborations, such as the 'Vibrant Communities' initiatives focusing on poverty reduction (3). A Dutch study (4), explored health brokers as specific agents facilitating cross-sectoral health promotion. There has been little study of organizations whose cross-sectoral mandates are only implicitly health-related, yet sufficient as a basis for bringing together diverse stakeholders to promote health. This paper explores the potential of UNESCO mandated biosphere reserves (BRs) as bridging organizations bringing together communities for health and sustainable development.

A BR is a specific region, recognized by UNESCO, guided by an organization of the same name that attempts to help people find ways to build sustainable livelihoods while maintaining the health of the ecosystem that supports their existence within the area (5). Currently, there are 621 BRs in 117 countries (6). The structure, organization and governance of BRs have been adapted to meet the local conditions and needs and therefore vary significantly from one another (7). Because of their mandate, BRs are often viewed as 'learning laboratories' for sustainable development (8-9). The purpose of BRs is to demonstrate the integration of conservation and sustainable development.

In this study, BRs were analyzed as examples of organizations outside of the health sector that have begun to bring together diverse stakeholders to address public health and environmental issues as an integrated part of sustainability. Because of the local adaptations of the mandate, only some BRs have included health promotion explicitly in their operations. This study explored how and why some BRs have explicitly integrated health into their activities, whilst others have not. Furthermore, it investigated the types of health related programming as well as drivers for and barriers to implementing health focus.

'Bridging organizations' is a new concept to health promotion and public health but is used in, for example, international development (10) and environmental governance (11-13) literatures. The term refers to local groups or associations that facilitate horizontal linkages between sectors as well as foster vertical connections across administrative layers, which allow local influence on higher level decision-making and policy development (10). The Millennium Ecosystem Assessment (14) defined their purpose as to facilitate collaboration among actors by providing "arenas for multisector and/or multilevel collaboration for conceiving visions, trust-building, collaboration, learning, value formation, conflict resolution, and other institutional innovations." Bridging organizations are often seen critical for community capacity-building (14) and for adaptive co-management of natural resources (15), because they provide both services and facilitate collaboration between non-governmental organizations, government agencies, research organizations, and other stakeholders.

The Millennium Ecosystem Assessment as well as adaptive environmental governance literature, in general, have identified BRs as bridging organizations (11-12, 14). The role of BRs as bridging organizations is to create a safe meeting forum to facilitate cross-sectoral collaboration (13, 17-18). Many BRs appear also to be functioning as bridging organizations in practice. Forty-six of 146 surveyed BR managers said their organizations were "effectively achieving developmental goals" by engaging local stakeholders, academics, politicians and government administrators in sustainable development and conservation promotion (18). This study by Schultz et al. emphasized the great potential role of BRs as bridging organization in linking ecosystem services and human well-being, which is a complex, long-term, experiment requiring continuous innovation and learning.

The factors influencing health and well-being extend from biophysical to socioeconomic elements, thus finding meaningful, sustainable solutions to the complex public health challenges requires complex solutions. Already in 1973, Rittel and Webber (19) labeled these complicated, messy challenges as 'wicked problems' and the discussion has been on-going. By their nature, environmental health issues fall under this category (20-22). They involve a great range of stakeholders, who perceive the problem and its solutions in various ways. Wicked problems can be managed, if not solved (21), but that requires natural scientific as well as social scientific understanding and solution alternatives. Because wicked problems often are created by pigeonholed problem solving attempts, tackling them demands opening up for new ways of thinking (22). This paper explores one unconventional, alternative approach to facilitating cross-sectoral collaboration to promote public health that addresses limitations of the current system.

METHODS

The research project focused on cross-sectoral bridging of health and sustainable development. This particular component of the study centered on asking: How can non-governmental organizations function as bridging agents facilitating cross-sectoral collaboration between the health and environmental sectors? The data were collected by document analyses, semi-structured interviews and, overt participant observation. The analysis was made by analytic induction (23), using sensitizing concepts based on health promotion theories to frame the investigation with the desired focus (see Table 1) (23). The research aimed to find answers to the following four questions: 1) What type of health promotion related activities and programs take place in the BRs? 2) To what extent have the BRs been able to function as bridging agents facilitating cross-sectoral collaboration between health and sustainability sectors? 3) What type of barriers to and drivers for integrating health into their programming can be identified?

Table 1. Examples of how *health* and *well-being* were addressed in Madrid Action Plan (24)

The potential role of BRs in addressing emerging challenges caused by climate change, biodiversity loss, and rapid urbanization (p.4):
• "From these challenges, several opportunities for change arise, through increased awareness at all levels of the need to maintain and secure access to ecosystem services for human **well-being**, including **health**, security and justice/equity." • "Develop mechanisms to encourage the sustainable development of BRs carried out in partnership with all sectors of society (i.e., public and private institutions, [non-governmental organizations], stakeholder communities, decision- makers, scientists, local and indigenous communities, land owners and users of natural resources, research and education centres, media) to ensure the **well-being** of people and their environment;..." [emphasis added]
The Madrid Action Plan's overall goals are to (p.5):
• "anchor the research, training, capacity building and demonstration agendas of [Man and the Biosphere-project] at the interface between the interlinked issues of conservation and sustainable use of biodiversity, mitigation and adaptation to climate change, and socio-economic and cultural **well-being** of human communities" • "enable the active use of places included in the [World Network of Biosphere Reserves] as learning sites for sustainable development, i.e., demonstrating approaches to enhance co-operation amongst epistemic (academic), political, practitioner and stakeholder communities to address and solve context specific problems to improve environmental, economic and social conditions for human and ecosystem **well-being**" [emphasis added]

This research followed the normal procedures for health research concerning human participants with full ethics clearance by the Office of Research Ethics at the University of Waterloo (ORE #18477).

Explicitly health-related projects were investigated in all Canadian (n=16) and British (n=3) BRs that follow the guidelines specified by the Madrid Action Plan (24). The Canadian analysis was based on a project database created by Helene Godmaire of the Canadian BR Association (CBRA), semi-structured interviews, and participant observation at two Annual General Meetings of CBRA, in 2011 and 2012, respectively. The British analysis was based on document analysis, semi-structured interviews, and one week of participant observation in the two established BRs.

North Devon, Dyfi, Frontenac Arch, and Georgian Bay BRs were selected for detailed case studies to identify all activities that can be considered health promotion, and to understand the collaborative relationships, drivers for, and barriers to the integration of health into programming. The selection was based on three criteria: two case studies per country; two organizations that had programming with an explicit health focus and two that did not focus on health; and comparability of their geographic profiles.

Semi-structured interviews (n = 29) were conducted at all four locations between November 2012 and May 2013. The interviewees were all experts in the field, staff, partners or Board members of the BRs, and therefore the qualitative in-depth interviews followed an inter-active style (23). The interview guide covered four specific areas: health-related projects, barriers to and drivers for health integration, available local knowledge, and cross-sectoral bridging capacity. The order and format of the questions varied depending on the flow of the discussion and the professional role of the interviewee. Interviews were conducted until saturation was observed and the same topics kept reappearing in responses.

Data analysis

All the interviews were recorded and transcribed by the author. The coding was created based on sensitizing concepts and additional codes were created when unanticipated health promotion related topics appeared. Participants were provided with a summary of all findings and specifics related to their own interviews for review and validation. Triangulation of the results was further strengthened by engaging other health promotion professionals to assess the analysis and appropriateness of coding. Because of the rural and small community context, all the results have been pooled to one single general story of BRs as bridging organizations for health and sustainable development to protect the confidentiality and relative anonymity of the participants.

RESULTS

The results come successively from the pilot project and the case studies. The pilot component of the project explored the status of health in the universal UNESCO mandate and in the activities of BRs. Attitudes towards health-related activities among BR practitioners were also explored. The pilot results provided justification to the four in-depth case studies.

Document analysis and participant observation assessing health focus in the UNESCO mandate, in general, and in Canadian and British BRs in particular.

The 3rd World Congress of BRs, held in February 2008, produced the 'Madrid Action Plan' for the BRs. It can be considered as the overall strategic mandate for BRs for 2008-2013. Building on the Seville Strategy of 1995 that shifted the focus from conservation to sustainable development, the Madrid Action Plan aimed "to raise BRs to be the principal internationally-designated areas dedicated to sustainable development in the 21st century."(24). In the document, the words health and well-being show up once and ten times, respectively (see Table 1).

Well-being is also included in both vision and mission statements for the 'World Network of BRs,' which aim:

- To foster "harmonious integration of people and nature for sustainable development through participatory dialogue, knowledge sharing, poverty reduction and human well-being improvements, respect for cultural values and society's ability to cope with change, thus contributing to the [Millennium Development Goals]"; and
- "To ensure environmental, economic, social (including cultural and spiritual) sustainability through: development and coordination of a worldwide network of places acting as demonstration areas and learning sites with the aim of maintaining and developing ecological and cultural diversity, and securing ecosystem services for human well-being."

Many BRs mention health on their website, promoting healthy economy, healthy environment, healthy society, and healthy culture (e.g., Bras d'Or Lake BR and Georgian Bay BR). However, only two out of the sixteen BRs in Canada and one out of the original two (now three) in the UK explicitly addressed human health in their activities, when the research project was embarked in 2011. When asked about their interest in integrating health in biosphere activities, organisations that did not explicitly focus on health expressed a unanimous desire to learn more about the opportunities to collaborate with the public health sector.

Only one of the studied BRs, Clayoquot Sound BR, has adopted healthy communities as one of its three core priorities and also extensively focuses on health in its activities. The BR is located on Nuu-chah-nulths First Nations' traditional lands, who represent fifty per cent of the current all-year population in the area. Originally the Western term sustainable development was replaced by healthy communities, but nowadays the terms appear interchangeably in the Clayoquot public documents.

Clayoquot Sound BR is also the only one of all the Canadian and British BRs studied that explicitly defines health on its website:

> "Health encompasses everything from walking trails and clean water to access to recreational opportunities, adequate housing and stable employment. The [Clayoquot Biosphere Trust] is committed to supporting projects that support health, in its broadest sense." (clayoquotbiosphere.org; emphasis added)

These findings were deemed sufficient to advance to the four case studies, which is the main focus of this paper.

Further document analysis, semi-structured interviews, and participant observation, focusing on the four cases studies

Almost all activities in the Canadian and British BRs depend on project specific grants from private foundations or governments. Moreover, most of the activities rely on community volunteers and are supported by in kind contributions from partnering organizations. The actual operational funding of the BRs is relatively small and reflected in the number of paid staff, which ranges from two part-time individuals to five full-time employees in the BRs in question. Only one of the four organizations has a full-time paid manager. One BR has two paid part-time managers sharing the duty, and two BRs have volunteer-based management. The staffing and funding structures vary from region to region. In 2012, federal government prematurely terminated five-year operational funding support for the Canadian BRs, as part of the broader financial cuts to the environmental sector. One of the three BRs in the UK operates autonomously under the Regional Council; the other two are essentially grassroots organizations, despite their UNESCO status. All four case study organizations perceive themselves as partnerships or networks and see the role of their staff to function as networking facilitators, who bring together partners to work on shared issues.

The following table (see Table 2) provides an overview of the types of health promotion related activities that have taken place within the four BRs, since adaptation to the Seville Strategy. Mapping all the projects and involved partners of the BRs was beyond the scope of this project, but Table 2 helps illustrate the range of identified health-related activities as well as the scope of bridging potential that this type of organizations may hold.

The sensitizing concepts were based on generally accepted health promotion categories and concepts (25-26). They acknowledge health promotion efforts needed at multiple levels of the society, from facilitating the individual behavior change to systems-wide policy change, as well as the impact of social determinants of health. Some examples could fit under multiple categories but they are included only once to illustrate the diversity. BRs aim to remain politically neutral and therefore the organizations do not engage in advocacy and direct policy development activities.

To assess the future potential of the BRs as bridging organizations bringing together health and sustainability the key drivers for and barriers to such integration processes were explored.

Table 2. Health promotion projects in BRs since the adaptation to the Seville Strategy

Health promotion category	Examples of projects related to public health	Types of partners engaged
PROMOTING HEALTHY BEHAVIOUR CHANGE		
A) Focus on individual behaviour change		
Physical activity	"Walking for Health": local walking groups that provide walks specifically tailored to support good health through exercise and social interaction; e.g., tinyurl.com/WalkingGroups [accessed 2014 Jan 15]	Public health (NHS*), local governments, ENGOs*, other NGOs*, community volunteers
Nutrition (physical activity)	"Local Flavours": a program promoting local food production and healthy, nutritious eating, combined with local art, and connecting food and nutrition with physical activity; includes over 100 local food producers, retailers, and food services; e.g., tinyurl.com/LocalFlavours & tinyurl.com/ActiveBody [accessed 2014 Jan 15]	Public health unit (nutritionist), local governments, private the private sector, ENGOs*, community volunteers
Nutrition	Free, food-related, community workshops in collaboration with local volunteers: growing own fresh food, identifying edible wild plants, raising chicken & keeping bees; e.g., tinyurl.com/BR-ActionGroup & tinyurl.com/GrowOwnFood [accessed 2014 Jan 15]	Public health unit (community health promoter); HNGO* (intellectual disabilities); other NGOs*, community volunteers
Environmental health	"Life on the Bay": guidance for healthy & sustainable septic tank management, handling of domestic toxic chemicals, drinking water & waste treatment, etc., e.g., tinyurl.com/EnvGuide [accessed 2014 Jan 15]	Federal & provincial governments (Parks Canada, Environment Canada, Ontario MNR*), the private sector, and ENGOs*
Mental health (physical activity)	"Tirwedd Dyfi": promoting well-being gained by understanding the linkages between the sense of place, language, culture, landscape and being outdoors; focus on lifestyles; "trying to get people to appreciate the importance of the outdoors in Welsh language culture, in other words tempt them to go out and to see the outside and landscape as being part of their innate culture..." (interview participant); e.g., tinyurl.com/HealthyCulture & tinyurl.com/CulturePaths [accessed 2014 Jan 15]	National & regional governments (National Park Authority & CCW*), schools, ENGOs* & other NGOs*, community volunteers

Table 2. (Continued)

Health promotion category	Examples of projects related to public health	Types of partners engaged
B) Focus on community level behaviour change		
Food security	Cookbook supporting local foods: emphasizing what people eat and how its produced leaves lasting traces in the local landscape and culture, connecting food with the living and working countryside; e.g., tinyurl.com/CookLocal [accessed 2014 Jan 15]	University of the Third Age, NGOs*, the private sector
Food security	Interactive collaborative school program to promote local food, engaging children to analyse the local food system and engage the community in their research; e.g., tinyurl.com/Food-Kids [accessed 2014 Jan 15]	Schools, university, government, ENGOs*, other NGOs*, local food producers & the private sector
Active transportation (nutrition/food security)	Interactive trails maps with health messaging & sustainable development focus; e.g., bringing together over 30 regional trail organizations; e.g., tinyurl.com/TrailNetwork & tinyurl.com/ActiveWithNature [accessed 2014 Jan 15]	Public health, federal & provincial governments (Parks Canada; Ontario Parks, MTCS*, MOE*, & MNR*), municipal governments, ENGOs*, other NGOs*, the private sector, community volunteers
Active transportation	Easy access trail mapping project to promote active transportation and outdoors experiences to mobility challenged individuals; e.g., tinyurl.com/EasyTrails [accessed 2014 Jan 15]	ENGOs*, HNGO* (physical disabilities), local governments, community volunteers
Environmental Health	"Catchment Sensitive Farming": a partnership to reduce diffuse pollution from agriculture & grant management; e.g., tinyurl.com/HealthyFarming & tinyurl.com/FarmingGrants [accessed 2014 Jan 15]	ENGOs*, national government (Environment Agency), local farmers
PROMOTING SYSTEMS LEVEL CHANGE		
Food security (poverty reduction)	Collaborating to expand the existing community gardens, providing workshops (see above example A3), arranging "Food Festivals" and a "Food Forum" to create awareness and to develop a sustainable food system as part of poverty reduction efforts & sustainable community development [in rural communities efforts are often intertwined]; e.g., tinyurl.com/LocalFood Map & tinyurl.com/LocalFoodsystem & tinyurl.com/HealthyUrbanForest [accessed 2014 Jan 15]	Public health (community health promoter), local hospital, HNGO* (intellectual disabilities); other NGOs*, municipal government, community volunteers
Healthy & sustainable community development	Initiating and organizing a "Regional Sustainability Initiative," a "Community Survey" and "Integrated Community Sustainability Plans," inviting a broad range of community stakeholders to the table; e.g., tinyurl.com/AskingCommunity & tinyurl.com/BRdrivenICSP & tinyurl.com/CrossSectoralCollaboration [accessed 2014 Jan 15]	Public health (MOH*), health professionals (family physicians), local municipalities, public library, ENGOs*, HNGO* (developmental disabilities), other NGOs*, school boards, the private sector

Health promotion category	Examples of projects related to public health	Types of partners engaged
Environmental health (Poverty reduction)	"Sustainable Energy Action Plan and Sustainable Energy Partnership": including public, private and voluntary sector interests and education/training providers; coordinating strategic planning and action towards zero carbon energy use goal (includes tackling fuel poverty); e.g., tinyurl.com/SustEnergyPlan & tinyurl.com/CommPartnerships [accessed 2014 Jan 15]	A broad range of the public & private sector stakeholders, NGOs, *schools, public housing, etc.
Environmental health	"State of the Bay": ecosystem health report card; presents information about key ecosystem health indicators along the Bay. Key indicators were selected in the areas of water quality, wetlands, fisheries, and landscape; summarizes existing scientific reports from the local perspective; e.g., preview.tinyurl.com/EnvAssessment [accessed 2014 Jan 15]	5 other local ENGOs*; federal & provincial governments (funding)

[*NGO: Non-Governmental Organization; ENGO: Environmental NGO; HNGO; Health-related NGO; MOH: Medical Officer of Health; CCW: Countryside Council for Wales, currently known as Natural Resources Wales; NHS: UK National Health Services; MNR: Ontario Ministry of Natural Resources; MOE: Ontario Ministry of Environment; MTCS: Ontario Ministry of Tourism, Culture and Sports].

Some of the main topics identified can be found in Table 3 with examples of the responses categorized under respective themes.

Table 3. Participant comments on barriers to and drivers for integrating health and sustainable development

Drivers for & barriers to integrating health	Identified themes and examples of verbatim quotes from interview responses
Health being explicit vs. implicit in mandate/ activities	• Not explicit: "It's may be in the BR's vision statement (…) – but it's not explicit in the strategic level of what the BR is doing, that it should be promoting health. I think there is a natural kind of overlap, but the priorities that have been set don't spell it out…" • Disadvantage of health not being explicit: "If we're not being pulled in a health direction, it might not be spelled out as that, it might not be identified as that, or it might not happen." • Value of making health explicit: "If you think that public health is part of sustainability, these are some of the areas that would be particularly relevant and these could maybe some of the techniques that could be used." • Supportive vs. active role: "happy to encourage [health promotion]. (…) But I don't see my role, at the moment, to initiate that sort of project."
Knowledge & awareness	• Unawareness within the health sector: "Going to health meetings where there is absolutely no interest at all – they talk about healthy foods and healthy eating – but there is no interest at all to what food is produced [here] – or no knowledge. There is no attempt at choosing local produce." • Unawareness within the BR: "It's the individuals who sort of shape the organization. Take a look at our Board, it's the same thing. If [the health researcher interviewing] were to join our Board then you would introduce new ideas and new concepts and help us explore new ideas. If it isn't there, it is not part of the organisation background – in terms of the people that are involved."

Table 3. (Continued)

Drivers for & barriers to integrating health	Identified themes and examples of verbatim quotes from interview responses
	• Understanding within the BR: "From the data point of view, if you look at the statistics of the BR, you can see that there is a lot of deprivation and disease. That data has been collected nationally, so we can compare ourselves as a region with the rest of the county or country. We can even interpolate between these data points, since it's all based on national health statistics and census data. So we can see that in the BR region there are some real critical health and economy issues for a lot of people. Superimposing another data set that explored the sense of pride people in their area, their likely health status according the stats, their income, all these three things overlap geographically and correlate really well. In other words a person will no interest in their area, is likely to be have low income, and highly likely to suffer an illness."
Perception	• Health as a driver for sustainability: "If we look at human wellbeing as the driver of sustainable development and the driver of individual's position within sustainable development, then you could say that their own personal health and economic and social wellbeing is a key factor in how a community wellbeing is built up. (…) Theoretically and strategically it's all there, but operationally it gets a bit challenging" • Lack of general awareness: "I think [the interconnectedness between health and sustainable development] is explicit but getting the awareness – how would it come?" • Polarized perspectives: "You get two camps – this is mostly the scientific measurable stuff and we do all that, and then we have a group of people who are all about process and the emotional wellbeing (…), the personal health. Obviously health is both."
Community champions and networking	• Among the professionals/practitioners: "[The Medical Officer of Health] down here has really kind of knitted together a health unit enterprise and brought diverse groups into large and more cohesive units. And her focus is to work with the community." • In the community: "People in this area don't like to push themselves. They're naturally shy and whenever you have a public meeting, you always find that the hall will fill up from the back to the front. Nobody wants to sit in the front row and this is something we have to recognise (…) You have to identify those individuals in the community who are naturally more assertive to speak up on their behalf." • Cross-sectoral bridging: "Then again [the public health staff] will decide 'what resources do we have in our area, if they can help us [reach our operational goals]. 'Oh the BR s here – what can we do to encourage people to use their trails?' (…) we can do [health promotion] together. (…) So that's how it would happen from our end. Then from their end, they might say 'we're really interested in this' and then [the 'champion' from the BR] would speak to me and I would say 'sounds like a fit with
	what we're doing. I'll give you [Z]'s name' – and he knows [Z] cause she's one of the public health nurses – 'why don't the two of you talk together if we can actually make that happen.' So it would happen both ways."
Funding/time	• Operational funding challenge: "I can go to a [granting body] and (…) probably get somebody to do healthy communities. Say if you have a contingency of three or four staff and you want to keep them going. As a manager, you are managing those folks but you are also trying to ensure that there is continuity – so that grant follows grant follows grant, so you can keep them on-board. (…) Capacity issue is a pretty significant issue. Because you're still also trying to do all that outreach. We should be able to take the organisation to another level to be able to take on-board a healthy communities coordinator. [That requires] adding some management time, but where does that money come from."

DISCUSSION

The in-depth interviews, analysis of public documents, and participant observations, summarized above, indicate that, albeit not explicit, the universal UNESCO mandate appears to support efforts promoting health and well-being. Moreover, a great range of projects undertaken by BR organizations fall under the umbrella of health promotion (see Table 2). The projects have involved both health-related activities that focus more narrowly on individual health behavior change, such as physical activity, and those that address key social determinants of health, including poverty and food security.

All the participants in the case studies saw health and sustainable development as inherently interlinked topics, although most of the interviewees felt that the connection was intuitive rather than explainable. Individual interpretations of this interwovenness were strongly influenced by professional backgrounds, but the ubiquitous perception of interconnectedness creates a promising platform potential for increased practical integration of health and sustainability.

Three out of the four case organizations have bridged health and sustainable development by engaging health stakeholders. The fourth BR has indirect engagement through its core partner organizations, which have active collaboration with the health sector. The greatest range of health promotional activities could be identified when the BR had direct collaboration with the administrative top-level of health organizations. Although it was not always explicitly expressed, all case-study BRs have health promotion programs related to both individual health behavior change and systems change addressing wider social determinants of health (see Table 2).

All participating organizations noted that the interest of local individuals is the main determining factor for addressing health-related issues. Despite the differences in organizational structures (three organizations being strictly non-governmental and one functioning as an autonomous entity within the regional council), all four biospheres have interpreted their responsibility under the UNESCO mandate as building, in an inclusive manner from bottom-up, on local assets and needs. This deliberative approach, which is supported in much of the community-based health promotion literature (27-28), fosters the local issue ownership vital for sustainable social and behavioral change. In the current resource-scarce reality of BRs, however, the approach that requires community initiation for projects also limits most activities to the topics of community partner interests.

The perceived mandates of both stakeholders and the bridging organizations appear to influence cross-sectoral collaboration in a much more complex manner than anticipated. The BR organizations that did not explicitly integrate health into their activities did not see health as part of their mandate, whereas those focusing on health did interpret the same UNESCO mandate as inherently including health. Evidently some ambiguity surrounds the term 'well-being' and whether it is about health or sustainable development. While health stakeholders see health and well-being as synonymous, other influential voices, for instance the Government of Wales, treat well-being as identical to sustainable development. This vagueness of terms can facilitate cross-sectoral collaboration, but it also may cause unnecessary variation in interpretation of the mandates.

Similarly, interpretations of the institutional mandates were important factors determining the ability of local health professionals to engage actively in BR activities. Responses indicated that frontline health practitioners often feel strictly limited by their narrow mandates, despite the personal perceptions of the relevance of cross-sectoral integrated approach to health promotion. Particularly, environmental health practitioners are often excluded from professional collaborations, because their heavy workload is strictly guided by government directives. This is precisely the problem that Rittel and Webber identified in 1973 (19), when they developed the concept of "wicked problems."

The perceptions of upper management within healthcare organizations also strongly influence how government dictated mandates are understood and to which extent innovative cross-sectoral collaboration is encouraged in practice. For instance, in Ontario, some health units are engaged with their local BRs, whereas others remain unresponsive to invitations. Moreover, some participants expressed a desire to engage primary health care providers, e.g., to issue Green Gym prescriptions (promoting outdoors activities instead of prescription drugs or inside gyms) or to discuss the potential role of nature in mental health therapy. These findings suggest that the health sector might benefit from a more open approach to stakeholder engagement. Indeed, broad cross-sectoral engagement of unconventional partners is encouraged particularly by the settings-based health promotion perspective (29).

All participants throughout the study recognized that they had limited knowledge and understanding of one another's mandates. This was evident whether or not any active cross-sectoral collaboration with the health stakeholders was taking place. The admitted ignorance illustrates how personal perceptions, interpersonal interaction, and sense of mutual trust appears to play a much greater role in the initiation of collaborative activities than actual shared knowledge. Trust has been identified as a key factor in cross-sectoral collaboration (30), but it would be interesting to explore the impact of better mutual understanding of the mandates of respective partners on potential partnership development. The lack of knowledge about others' mandates does not necessarily prevent cooperation, as long as an overall understanding of shared issues is present. It, however, appeared to cause some form of a barrier to people's ability to identify potential unconventional collaborators.

An explicit, open, cross-sectoral dialogue might enhance the integration of health and sustainable development. The potential for more extensive bridging activities was exemplified by one environmental stakeholder, who stated that: "To be totally honest, until quite recently, I haven't given the relationship with human health a great deal of thought. But when I think about it, it is actually extremely relevant, even though the management is focused on the ecosystem and habitat and species. It is actually extremely important for human health as well, because of things like water storage, carbon storage, and the other ecosystem services that the site provides." Similarly, the public health management attendance at a meeting on integrated community sustainability plans, organized by the local BR, resulted the following statement: "It was an exciting meeting and really helped me see how our work in public health fits within the sustainable community's movement."

A number of participating non-health stakeholders pointed out that many current limitations to health-related activities reflect limited understanding of possible public health matters. In general, biosphere participants recognized that the focus of activities within their respective organizations is usually directly dependent on the engaged individuals and their expertise or interests. Only where health professionals are actively participating does health promotion become an explicit component of the bridging efforts. As noted above, open cross-sectoral discussions contain the potential to stimulate action. For example, one Canadian BR was recently inspired to partner with the local health unit to arrange walking groups and invited the engaged Public Health Nurse to join their Board.

While BRs are effective bridging organizations bringing diverse stakeholders together (see Table 2), interviewees reported that it was a challenge finding the right language to attract the health sector to join meetings. Forty years after the globally recognized Lalonde Report (31) declared environment as a determinant of health, the health sector evidently remains slow to engage with environmental stakeholders. The interview results reveal that integrating health in projects outside the health sector still depends directly on individuals who take it upon themselves to bring people together. Although each BR organization clearly is driven by a group of passionate people, the current success of health stakeholder integration seems to depend on a few visionary individuals, who are good at connecting people. Some of these community champions work within the health sector and others are networkers within BR organizations who see health as an integral component of sustainable communities. Studies on effectiveness of community-based health promotion support the value of community champions in driving change (32).

Despite the barriers, BRs have had some success in developing cross-sectoral activities that promote health-related changes both at the individual behavior and the systems level (see Table 2). Not all interviewees saw the necessity of having an explicit focus on health in BRs' program development. As one participant pointed out: "I think [health] is implicit in what we're doing already." To justify the shift to explicit health focus would require, for instance, availability of some health funding consistent with the criteria set for BR activities. That said, making the implicit explicit would probably also help health practitioners justify their participation in cross-sectoral collaboration with BRs.

This study indicates that organizations with primary focus other than health have a potential to play a meaningful role in providing a neutral, apolitical, platform that helps bringing diverse community stakeholders to the table to promote health. In the case of BRs, this potential could be significantly increased by making health an explicit part of the BR mandate and exploring the mandates of potential health-related partners in greater detail. The health sector within BR regions, in turn, has an innovative opportunity not only to promote health but also to facilitate application of 'Health in All Policies' approach. In addition to ideological goals, such collaboration could strengthen the local health promotion capacity in resource-strapped rural communities. This would, however, require more proactive strategies among the health professionals. In general, BRs have a great potential role as bridging organizations that help integrate health and sustainable development in practice. The in-depth qualitative analysis reported here indicates that this type of bridging organization represents a promising new venue for meaningful solutions to wicked public health problems at the community-level.

ACKNOWLEDGMENTS

This research was partially funded by the Canadian Social Sciences and Humanities Research Council (SSHRC).

REFERENCES

[1] World Health Organization (WHO) Bangkok Charter for Health Promotion. URL: http://www.who.int/healthpromotion/conferences/6gchp/bangkok_charter/en.
[2] WHO, Government of South Australia. The Adelaide Statement on Health in All Policies: moving towards a shared governance for health and well-being. Health Promot Int 2010; 25: 258-60.
[3] Born P. Creating vibrant communities: How individuals and organizations from diverse sectors of society are coming together to reduce poverty in Canada. Toronto: BPS Books, 2010.
[4] Harting J, Kunst AE, Kwan A, Stronks K. A 'health broker' role as a catalyst of change to promote health: An experiment in deprived Dutch neighbourhoods. Health Promot Int 2011; 26(1): 65-81.
[5] UNESCO [homepage on the Internet]. What is a biosphere reserve? Paris: UNESCO Headquarters, 2014. URL: www.unesco.org/mab/doc/faq/brs.pdf.
[6] UNESCO [homepage on the Internet]. Biosphere Reserves – Learning Sites for Sustainable Development. Paris: UNESCO Headquarters, 2014. URL: http://www.unesco.org/
[7] Francis G. Biosphere reserves in Canada: Ideals and some experience. Environ 2004; 32(3): 3-26.
[8] Nguyen NC, Bosch OJ, Maani KE. Creating 'learning laboratories' for sustainable development in biospheres: A systems thinking approach. Syst Res Behav Sci 2011; 28(1): 51-62.
[9] Matysek KA, Stratford E, Kriwoken LK. The UNESCO biosphere reserve program in Australia: Constraints and opportunities for localized sustainable development. Can Geogr 2006; 50(1): 85-100.
[10] Brown LD. Bridging organizations and sustainable development. Hum Relat 1991; 44(8): 807-31.
[11] Schultz L. Nurturing resilience in social-ecological systems: Lessons learned from bridging organizations. Dissertation. Stockholm: Stockholm University, 2009.
[12] Biggs R, Westley FR, Carpenter SR. Navigating the back loop: Fostering social innovation and transformation in ecosystem management. Ecol Soc 2010; 15(2): 28.
[13] Crona BI, Parker JN. Learning in support of governance: Theories, methods, and a framework to assess how bridging organizations contribute to adaptive resource governance. Ecol Soc 2012; 17(1): 32.
[14] Malayang BSI, Hahn T, Kumar P. Responses to ecosystem change and to their impacts on human well-being. Millennium ecosystem assessment, ecosystems and human well-being: Multiscale assessments: Findings of the sub-global assessments working group. Washington, DC: Island Press, 2007: 203-28.
[15] Berkes F. Devolution of environment and resources governance: Trends and future. Environ Conserv 2010; 37(4): 489-500.
[16] Hahn T, Olsson P, Folke C, Johansson K. Trust-building, knowledge generation and organizational innovations: The role of a bridging organization for adaptive comanagement of a wetland landscape around Kristianstad, Sweden. Hum Ecol 2006; 34: 573-92.
[17] Berkes F. Evolution of co-management: Role of knowledge generation, bridging organizations and social learning. J Environ Manage 2009; 90(5): 1692-1702.
[18] Schultz L, Duit A, Folke C. Participation, adaptive co-management, and management performance in the world network of biosphere reserves. World Dev 2011; 39(4): 662-71.
[19] Rittel HWJ, Webber MM. Dilemmas in a general theory of planning. Policy Sci 1973; 4(2): 155-69.
[20] Kreuter MW, De Rosa C, Howze EH, Baldwin GT. Understanding wicked problems: A key to advancing environmental health promotion. Health Educ Behav 2004; 31(4): 441-54.
[21] Caron RM, Serrell N. Community ecology and capacity: Keys to progressing the environmental communication of wicked problems. Appl Environ Educ Commun 2009; 8(3-4): 195-203.
[22] Brown V, Harris J, Russell J. Tackling wicked problems through the transdisciplinary imagination. London: Earthscan, 2010.
[23] Patton MQ. Qualitative research and evaluation methods. Thousand Oaks, CA: Sage, 2002.
[24] UNESCO [homepage on the internet]. Madrid Action Plan. Paris: UNESCO Headquarters, 2014. URL: http://www.unesco.org/
[25] Nutbeam D, Harris E. Theory in a nutshell: a practical guide to health promotion theories. Sydney: McGraw-Hill Australia, 2004.

[26] Bartholomew LK, Parcel GS, Kok G, Gottlieb NH editors. Planning health promotion programs: an intervention mapping approach. San Francisco, CA: Jossey-Bass, 2006.
[27] Minkler M editor. Community organizing and community building for health. New Brunswick, NJ: Rutgers University Press, 1997.
[28] Kretzmann JP, McKnight J. Building communities from the inside out: a path toward finding and mobilizing a community's assets. Evanston, IL: Asset-Based Community Development Institute, Institute Policy Research, Northwestern University, 1993.
[29] Poland BD, Green L, Rootman I. Settings for health promotion: Linking theory and practice. London: Sage, 2000:1–43.
[30] Wakefield SEL, Poland BD. Family, friend or foe? Critical reflections on the relevance and role of social capital in health promotion and community development. Soc Sci Med 2005; 60(12): 2819-32.
[31] Health Canada. Lalonde Report: A new perspective on the health of Canadians: a working document. Ottawa, ON: Health Canada, 1974.
[32] Popay J, Attree P, Hornby D, Milton B, Whitehead M, French B, et al. Community engagement in initiatives addressing the wider social determinants of health: A rapid review of evidence on impact, experience and process. Soc Determinants Effectiveness Rev 2007:1-226. URL: www.nice.org.uk/nicemedia/live/11929/44494/44494.pdf.

In: Public Health Yearbook 2015
Editor: Joav Merrick

ISBN: 978-1-63484-514-4
© 2016 Nova Science Publishers, Inc.

Chapter 10

THE LUTIISI ACADEMY PRIMARY SCHOOL: USING COMMUNITY-CENTERED DESIGN AS A CATALYST FOR CHANGE

Peter J Ellery[1],, Jane Ellery[1], John Motloch[2] and Martha Hunt[2]*

[1]Fisher Institute for Wellness and Gerontology, Ball State University, Muncie, Indiana, United States of America
[2]Department of Landscape Architecture, Ball State University, Muncie, Indiana, United States of America

Universal Primary Education (UPE) in Uganda has resulted in a significant increase in student enrollment and the need for more teaching resources and infrastructure, especially in rural areas of the country. While more classrooms and schools are being built to address these needs, little attention has been directed toward the value of the landscape that surrounds school buildings. The purpose of this project was to use a community-centered, collaborative design approach to explore the potential of the landscape surrounding a school. Site concept plans and images were developed in collaboration with school participant groups consisting of students, teachers, the School Management Committee, and local community members for the Building Tomorrow (BT) Lutiisi Academy primary school in Wakiso, Uganda. These plans and images highlighted potential health and educational opportunities that exist within the landscape surrounding this school and allowed school participant groups to envision the school as being more than just a building or classrooms. The plans and images were further explored, discussed, and revised by the school participant groups. These combined efforts resulted in the community committing the financial and human resources needed for the construction of new teacher housing on the site.

Keywords: Uganda, design, landscape, sustainability, community centered, rural schools, education

---

* Corresponding author: Peter J. Ellery, BEd, MA, MLA, PhD, Fisher Institute for Wellness and Gerontology, Health and Physical Activity Building – HP 302/Room 305, Ball State University, Muncie, IN 47306, United States. E-mail: pellery@bsu.edu.

INTRODUCTION

One of the primary focal points in the United Nations Millennium Development Goals (UNMDG) is the reduction in the number of children in Africa who are uneducated by the year 2015 (1, 2). In support of this goal, the Ugandan Government introduced legislation in 1997 that mandated Universal Primary Education (UPE) (1, 3). This legislation ensures the right of every child in Uganda to a free Primary School level education and is based on the premise that education provides the nation with the literacy skills, income, health, political participation, liberty, and general welfare attributes essential to the political, social, and economic growth of Uganda as a nation (4).

In the year following the implementation of UPE, enrollment in government-owned primary schools increased by 58%. Enrollment figures at the primary school level have now stabilized and average? 86% of all children who are eligible to attend primary school (5). This rapid increase in government primary school enrollment, however, has created a significant strain on existing schools, teachers, teaching resources, drinking water, and hygienic latrine facilities. These resources are essential if children are to successfully complete their primary education and a significant concern for schools in rural areas of the country where funding for new construction or school improvements is less prevalent. More schools and schooling infrastructure are needed if the health and educational issues now being faced by the nation's primary school system are to be resolved (3, 6).

In response to these concerns, externally funded organizations and foundations, like Building Tomorrow (BT) in the United States, have begun supporting the development and construction of more school buildings and infrastructure in rural areas of Uganda. Since its inception in 2006, BT has successfully built and opened 15 new primary schools, with a further five primary schools either in the site planning or construction phases of development. Each of these schools provides teaching and learning space for 325 primary school aged students, and BT has made a public commitment to the construction of 60 more primary schools by 2016. Key to the success of BT is the development of these primary schools in partnership with the community in which the school will be located. While BT is responsible for raising the money that will pay for the construction of the school, the community is responsible for the provision of the land, the construction of the school itself, and the maintenance and continued upkeep of the school once it has been completed. As BT notes, when a community partnership approach is used, "each school serves as a source of pride and a catalyst for change within the community. We have seen roads built, gardens harvested, scholarships funded, teachers organized, and housing constructed as a direct result of communities being empowered to help themselves (7)."

While organizations like BT are working effectively to build more school facilities and buildings in rural areas of Uganda, few have utilized the potential educational, health, and social opportunities the landscape surrounding the school can provide. This consideration of the landscape is perhaps even more important as many of the educational goals sought in the Ugandan primary school curriculum are ideally suited to a practical, outdoor learning environment (8–10). Further, research has shown that education in outdoor and natural settings can have a number of benefits including increased environmental knowledge, increased environmentally appropriate behavior, improved academic performance, and gains in physical health (11–15).

From a design thinking perspective, the landscape can be used to resolve health and educational issues that currently exist, while adding elements that support and supplement the school's mission and purpose (16, 17). The additional land at a school, if designed effectively, could be used to harvest water, grow food, keep animals, house teachers, collect energy, and provide recreational space for both the children attending the school and the community surrounding it. The landscape could also promote learning opportunities through the creation of outdoor learning environments (18), and improve the appeal of the school for students, community members, and teachers through the addition of play and recreational facilities. With a significant portion of the primary school curriculum now focused on education in agriculture, community service, and health and physical education (10), the design of the school's landscape should be as important as the design and construction of the school building itself. In response to these issues, this study explored the potential of the school landscape to determine if it could be designed to better serve the needs of the students, teachers, and community members in that area.

METHODS

The site chosen for this project was the Lutiisi Academy primary school in Wakiso, Uganda. The school is located approximately 25 miles, or 40 kilometres, northwest of Kampala along the Kampala-Hoima road. The Lutiisi Academy was the first school to be built by BT. It was selected for this project because it could be accessed from Kampala on a daily basis, it was approximately 6.5 acres in size, and it had been completed and in operation since 2006. This last factor was particularly important because it meant the school had students, teachers, and a well-established, community-based School Management Committee that could also take part in this design initiative.

The study utilized a participatory approach (19) that was designed to engage the BT staff, and school participant groups like students, teachers, the Lutiisi Academy School Management Committee, and local community members in discussions about the school's landscape (20, 21). Information collected through personal discussions with the BT staff indicated they focused on school building construction and had yet to consider the role the land around the school. As such, they had no specific goals or issues that needed to be addressed but were interested to see what options might be available to them in the design and construction of future schools. Interviews were conducted with the principal and individual teachers at the school, and a focus group discussion was conducted with the School Management Committee and local community members. Notes and comments from teachers during the interview process were recorded directly as all of the teachers were able to communicate very well in English. Notes and comments from the School Management Committee and community member focus group discussion were recorded with the assistance of a translator. A translator was needed as the community members in attendance primarily spoke the local tribal language of the district, and not English. Data gathered from interviews and the group discussion were then analyzed to determine themes that could be addressed through design.

Students used an art-based activity to provide information regarding their play and recreational preferences for the school (22). This activity started with students from the school's year five (i.e., P5) class viewing images depicting a wide variety of play and recreational settings. They were then given the opportunity to discuss and draw what they would like to see as play and recreational areas at their school. Upon completion of their artwork, the students were videoed holding their pictures and describing in English what they had drawn. The student narratives were transcribed, and a word analysis showcased which terms were used most often to describe their play settings (23). The most commonly occurring terms were also identified as themes to be addressed in the design process.

The themes obtained from the teacher interviews and the School Management Committee and community member focus group discussion were combined with those from the children's art activity to develop a design program containing prioritized goals and objectives for the design process. A series of design iterations were developed to examine design opportunities for the school site. From these iterations, a concept site plan for the school was developed. This initial plan was shared with students, teachers, the School Management Committee, and community members from the school. These participants were encouraged to see the site concept plan as a starting point for discussion and revision of the design elements being suggested and to consider the feasibility of these elements actually being developed and implemented at the Lutiisi Academy primary school.

Data collection and analysis

Teachers at the Lutiisi Academy Primary School were interviewed to determine their perspectives on how the school and school landscape could be improved. The teacher interview guide consisted of 25 open-ended questions. These questions covered topics like: (1) the role of education in preparation of children for life in Uganda; (2) the school as a work environment; (3) the school teaching day as it is experienced by teachers; (4) the physical working conditions at the school; (5) the problems teachers encounter in the school; (6) those aspects of the school they felt needed improvement; (7) what they would like to see added to the school; and (8) whether they would use the school facilities if there were adult educational or in-service programs made available to them through the school.

Information was obtained from four teachers through personal interviews during lunch and non-instructional times of the day. Examples of teacher comments included:

> "We don't have a lot of equipment or play things like swings or climbing apparatus. The children do have some sporting equipment to play formal games and they play these games in the small, grassed areas alongside the school. When they play sports formally, they have to go to another place that has a full size soccer field or sport space."
>
> "Everything from basic planting of plants, watering, making a garden, compost, mulching, herbicides and spraying for disease, etc. fertilizer are taught at the school. We don't have any livestock education involving animals like goats, pigs, or chickens, because you would need someone to watch for them during the holidays or at times when school is not in session."
>
> "We collect rainwater in a tank for drinking and compost vegetation and scraps for recycling and use on crops. We treat our water by boiling it on sheets of shiny corrugated iron for 12 hours in plastic bottles. This is needed because the water tank (2000 L) tank can only provide water for a week or two before being empty. When the water tank is dry, the water we drink comes from a well. It is not a deep well and the water is not very tasty or clean. It undergoes the same process of boiling to make it fit to drink."

"The latrines are 'dry' latrines (i.e., holes in the ground that will require the moving of the latrine in time). We are lucky though in that holidays and times when the children are not at school, the waste recedes extending the life of the latrine location. We would like to have a septic tank system as there is a government service that will come and empty it. We would also like a larger set of restrooms for both boys and girls and for them to be separate rather than joined by a common wall."

An analysis of the responses taken from the teachers who were interviewed produced the following themes:

1. The children need playgrounds, sporting fields and equipment.
2. Teachers need to be housed on school grounds.
3. Barriers are needed to keep neighboring livestock off school property.
4. Agricultural experiences involving animals, the environment, and energy issues need to be developed.
5. More water collection, storage and cleaning features are needed to increase water availability during dry periods.
6. Pit latrines need to be replaced with a septic tank toilet system, with separate facilities for teachers, male, and female students.
7. Power to the school is needed for lighting and the use of educational technologies.

Focus group discussion with the school management committee and community area parents

The School Management Committee along with interested community members were invited to be part of a focus group discussion to determine issues and concerns they would like to see addressed at the school. The discussion guide for the school management committee and community members consisted of 11 open ended questions. The topics addressed in this group discussion included: (1) the role of the school within the community; (2) a description of a regular day for the children attending the school; (3) a description of the educational areas being taught to their children; (4) their overall opinion of the school's instruction, the teachers and the school as it relates to their children's education; (5) the kinds of things they would like to see added or changed at the school; and, (6) whether they would use the school facilities if adult educational or recreational programs were available to them at the school.

Information was obtained from 15 participants, some of whom had walked three miles to attend the meeting. Responses were translated into English by local BT staff and examples of the comments made by participants during the meeting included:

"We want our children to pass these basic educational skills so that they can have a skill for the future like being a teacher, or a radio presenter, etc."

"If I die and left my child 10 acres of land, and they could not farm it, then they would just sell it and take the money. This money would just last a short time. But, if they had farming knowledge, they could then farm the land and grow things. The land now has personal as well as family value to the new family owner and now has on-going value and worth to them."

"I would like my children to learn about the agriculture of their community and the heritage-based, traditional methods that the community uses" (i.e., agricultural strategies that include permaculture techniques, mulching and composting, crop rotation, and other sustainable land management practices.)

"We would like to see the school have spaces for sports like Netball, Soccer, Track and Field Athletics, Boxing, Volleyball, Basketball, and Swimming," and "more playgrounds and play equipment like swings, climbing apparatus, and slides for the children."

An analysis of the School Management Committee and Community Member responses from the participants who took part in the focus group discussion produced the following themes:

1. The school curriculum needs to be extended to include livestock, issues related to permaculture, and sustainable farming practices.
2. More water collection is needed for drinking, sanitation, and instruction in health-related behaviors and practices.
3. Playgrounds are needed for child development, and sporting fields are needed for classes like physical education and school sporting teams.
4. More plants need to be grown for food and aesthetic appeal.
5. Teachers should be housed on the school grounds, and the school should be painted school colors.
6. The school needs electricity or a power source for lighting or teaching equipment.
7. The community should be able to use the school facilities.

Student artwork and video narration activity

Students from the Lutiisi Academy's P5 classes (i.e, students approximately 10 and 11 years of age) drew pictures of the play spaces they wanted at their school. Each then described their picture while being recorded on video. Each child's video narration was then transcribed. A word count and Wordle graphic were used to identify commonly occurring terms and themes expressed by the students (see Figure 1). Examples of student artwork descriptions include:

"I have drawn a flower, I like to teaching poetry, and to playing netball, swimming pool, and swing." The student is asked, "What is the animal the children are sitting on in the picture?" The student responds, "a crocodile."

"I have drawn the shed, I have drawn the swing, I have drawn (the word cannot be understood from the recording but the child is pointing to the climbing wall)." The student is asked, "Why do you want a shelter?" The student responds, "eating porridge."

"I have drawn pictures of playing football, I have drawn a swings, I have drawn a people who are here (the student gestures to the children walking on a log)."

"I draw a swing, a flower, and a shed for drinking porridge to have for lunch."

"I have drawn a swing and fruit, a girl playing and a Uganda flag."

"The picture is of playing football. This is the goal keeper, this is the swing, this is the flag. The swing as at the top and at the bottom is a bulb – electricity, it is a light bulb."

"My name is Musisi and I want flowers for our compound. I want to see them. I want the flowers to be a border for the compound."

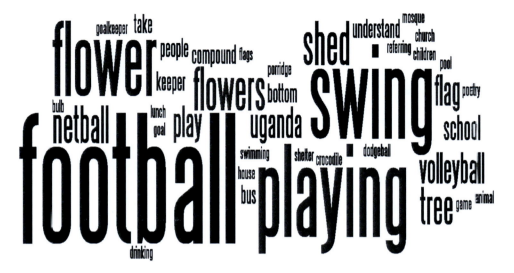

Figure 1. "Wordle," or graphical depiction of the 30 most used words used in the narratives given by students when describing their drawings (*Note: The more a word is repeated in the transcript, the larger it appears in the Wordle.

Analysis of the pictures, Wordle, and responses obtained from all of the children resulted in a number of playground elements being identified as needed for the school. These included:

1. The provision of a sporting field for games, physical education and sports like soccer, netball, volleyball.
2. The creation of play spaces with recreation equipment that includes swings, slides and climbing apparatus.
3. The addition of trees and flowers so the school is more aesthetically pleasing.
4. The addition of a shelter for shade and protection from the rain with seating and tables for lunch and getting together to talk as a group.

Physical site analysis of the Lutiisi Academy property

The school property site was evaluated for physical terrain, vegetation, water runoff patterns, transportation routes, current use, and topography. This analysis included an evaluation of current and potential issues with the site's current configuration and the identification of potential spaces that would be well suited to the suggestions made by students, teachers, and community members. The property was also evaluated at a regional and national level for soil type and quality, climate, and population. These evaluations indicated that the school was located on primarily Ferralitic and acidic (i.e., low Ph value) soil. This type of soil is dense making drainage, surface runoff, and topsoil erosion a problem in clear cut areas on slopes, but it is excellent for agriculture and for the production of food crops like plantains, coffee, tea, citrus fruit, cocoa and rubber.

Table 1. Design program for the Lutiisi Academy Primary School

Goal 1:
• Provide recreational spaces and amenities around the school that serve students, teachers and community member needs.
Design Objectives:
• Develop a sporting field area approximately 300 feet by 170 feet as a multisport playing field in close proximity to the school.
• Identify and develop play areas for children of different age groups.
• Provide a covered space that can be used for recreational and lunch purposes.
• Provide new toilets and change rooms to support the recreational areas.
• Provide additional flowerbeds, trees and vegetation to improve the aesthetic around the play areas.
Goal 2:
• Increase the collection and amount of water available to the school.
Design Objectives:
• Include water tanks and roof rainwater collection with every building on the site.
• Increase the number of water tanks used at the school to ensure the school is independent of well water needs.
• Include a solar hot water treatment process for water that is used for drinking and cooking purposes.
• Include a solar powered pump system for the solar hot water system.
Goal 3:
• Add trees and vegetation to slow water runoff from the site and increase aquifer recharge.
Design Objectives:
• Utilize permaculture and farming techniques that detain and hold water to slow runoff from the site.
• Utilize hedged shrubs for living borders and fencing
• Include an orchard and more fruit bearing trees in the landscape to increase food production on the school site as well as re-vegetate the site.
Goal 4:
• Provide an appropriate septic human waste disposal system for teachers and students at the school.
Design Objectives:
• Design and locate toilets that are located near key teacher, student, and community use areas, and that can meet the needs of community, teachers and students.
• Design and locate a septic well system for the toilets that can be easily accessed and emptied by government sanitation trucks if necessary.
Goal 5:
• Expand and develop the agricultural potential of the landscape.
Design Objectives:
• Provide design options that address concerns related to soil erosion and flooding around the school building itself.
• Provide livestock options for both instruction and food production services.
• Provide on-site teacher housing that allows for teachers to be present and monitor the animals and crops during times when school is not in session.
• Define on-site teacher crop spaces for teacher gardens and livestock accommodation.
Goal 6:
• Provide a renewable energy source and energy storage system for the school.
Design Objectives:
• Provide enough roofing Solar Panels to the school roof and surrounding buildings to create electrical energy for:
• for the lighting of a single classroom; and,
• the power needs of 10 computer systems for approximately 4 hours.
• Ensure solar panels are included as part of all new buildings (i.e., latrines, kitchen, etc.) for lighting, pumping water, etc.

Uganda lies on the equator making the climate ideal for agriculture. The average daylight time is just over 12 hours per day, varying only 15 to 30 minutes over the year, and the region experiences an average of 6 hours of direct sunlight each day making it ideal for solar energy initiatives. In contrast, however, the climate found in Wakiso includes a bimodal rain season that increases the potential for drought if rainfall is below average and an increased likelihood of crop failure.

Uganda's population distribution is most dense around major cities and along transportation corridors. While the population density in the city of Kampala is greater than 500 people per square mile, the population density in the rural central plain area is only around 50 to 75 people per square mile. The Lutiisi Academy lies on the edge of the plain area where the population is low and spread over a wide area. It should be noted that some students live two to three miles away from the Lutiisi Academy, and it is not uncommon for children living in rural areas of Uganda to spend up to 90 minutes walking to and from school each day as there is little funding or support for school student transportation.

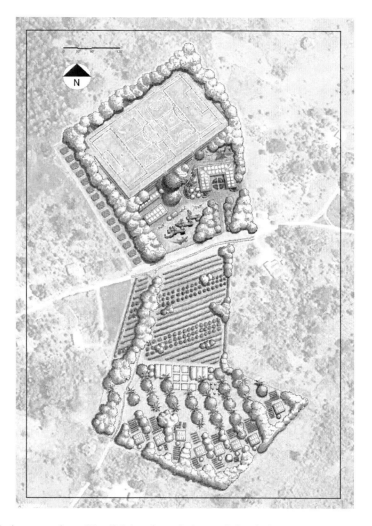

Figure 2. Aerial photo overlay of Lutiisi Academy Primary School site concept plan.

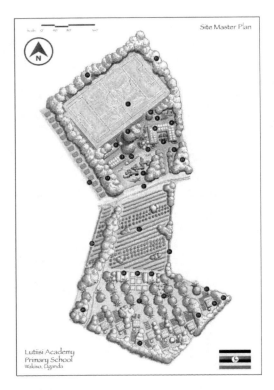

Figure 3. Lutiisi Academy Primary School site concept plan with key design elements identified.

RESULTS

The themes established from the data analysis were used to develop a design program (i.e., a list of goals and objectives that are met through the design process) (see Table 1). A series of conceptual design iterations were generated to study options that could address these goals and objectives through effective landscape design. These iterations were evaluated and consolidated into a final site concept plan for the school (see Figure 2 and 3). Those design elements that address themes and concerns identified by the students, teachers, and community members are also identified on the site concept plan and explained in the feature descriptions (see Figure 4). A series of site sections and perspective renderings were also developed to accompany the site concept plan to show how these proposed changes to the landscape might appear when completed.

A series of 24 inch by 36 inch posters were created displaying the children's artwork, site analysis, results of the data collection process, site concept plan, and associated site sections and perspectives. These posters were taken to the Lutiisi Academy primary school by the BT Foundation staff and shown to the students, teachers, School Management Committee, and community members who had participated in the site concept plan development. These participants reviewed the posters, discussed changes and revisions they thought important, and considered the feasibility of implementing these design ideas at the Lutiisi Academy primary school.

The Lutiisi Academy Primary School: Using community-centered design ... 131

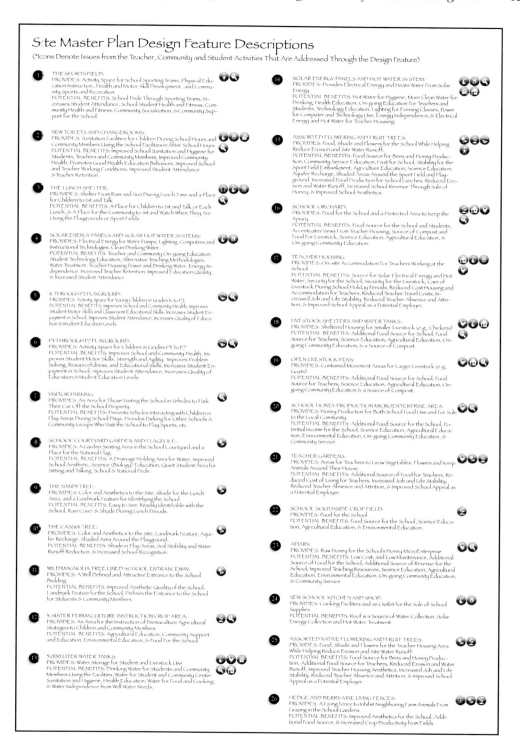

Figure 4. Lutiisi Academy Primary School site concept plan feature descriptions.

DISCUSSION

An initial site concept plan, along with images depicting what that plan might look like, was developed based on the information, activities, and conversations with the school students, teachers, School Management Committee, and community members. These plans were presented back to the participant groups so that they could envision the Lutiisi Academy primary school as more than just a building with classrooms. While some of the elements in the site concept plan, like the sporting fields, require significant capital outlay and engineering of the site, other elements like the creation of the school food gardens and orchard, would be relatively easy to create. These elements would only need the seeds or cuttings, and some human effort, to become a reality. Indeed, site concept plan elements like the school gardens could even be created by the students at the school, and infused into a science or community service lesson by their teacher. Overall, it was envisioned that these images would act as a catalyst for discussion and provide students, teachers, the School Management Committee, and community members with some potential areas in which they could initiate change.

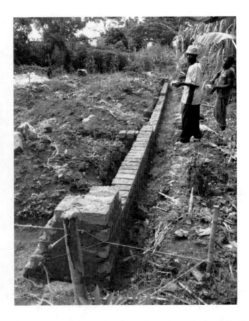

Figure 5. Lutiisi Academy Primary School teacher housing foundations being built.

The community-centered design process accomplished these goals. The initial conversations and resulting plans stimulated further discussion and ideas regarding the school's landscape. This allowed the group to explore other options in addition to those offered in the site concept plan. For example, the provision of teacher housing at the southern end of the site was of particular interest to the teachers, School Management Committee, and community members. Each of these participant groups had indicated that teacher housing should be located at the school. The inclusion of teacher housing would help address issues like teacher absenteeism and turnover rates in rural areas (24–26), and may even act as an employment incentive for good teachers to come and work at the Lutiisi Academy primary school. However, these participant groups did not think the provision of separate housing units, as displayed in the site concept plan, were necessary or feasible. While the location of the teacher housing was thought to be appropriate, the teachers, School Management Committee, and community members concluded that townhouse style accommodation (i.e., a series of apartment style homes in one large building with common dividing walls separating each home) would be more appropriate and feasible to develop financially.

Construction has now begun on the townhouse style teacher housing at the Lutiisi Academy primary school in the area proposed on the site concept plan. Further, this teacher housing construction is being completed by the Lutiisi Academy primary school community members themselves, without support or help from BT or other outside organizations (see Figure 5). At the heart of this process is the concept that design can act as a catalyst for change and that this change is most likely when community members actively participate in the process and are empowered as decision makers. As Schuman (2006) notes, neighborhood participation in the design and planning process reflects:

> "a growing recognition that neighborhood involvement produces better plans. In engenders local "ownership" of the plan that can foster long-term stewardship of public spaces. And, it values local residents as assets for their skills and knowledge. As a practical matter, community endorsement means a smoother road to implementation (27)."

ACKNOWLEDGMENTS

Our thanks to Dr Najma Dahrani at the Kenyatta University School of Environmental Studies for her assistance in the identification of native vegetation, farming, and permaculture practices in East Central Africa. Additional thanks must go to Mr. George Srour, Mr. Joseph Kaliisa, Mr. William Kajubi, and the staff of Building Tomorrow in both the United States and Uganda. This project would not have been possible without the logistical support of this organization and the on-going assistance of these individuals. Finally, I would like to express my appreciation and thanks to the principal, teachers, students, School Management Committee, and community members of the Lutiisi Academy Primary School in Wakiso, Uganda. Their thoughts, voices, and actions are the essence of this study and I wish them success as they continue to create opportunities that improve their lives, and the lives of their children at the school.

REFERENCES

[1] Grogan L. Universal primary education and school entry in Uganda. J Afr Econ 2009;18(2):183–211.
[2] United Nations General Assembly UN. Millenium Report of the Secretary-General of the United Nations [Internet]. Assembly UNG, ed. United Nations Website; 2000. URL: http://www.un.org/millennium/sg/report/index.html.
[3] Juuko FW, Kabonesa C. Universal primary education (UPE) in contemporary Uganda: right or priveledge? HURIPEC Working Paper 2007;8:55. URL; www. huripec.mak.ac.ug/working_ paper_ 8.pdf.

[4]   Nakabugo MG, Byamugisha A, Bithaghalire J. Future schooling in Uganda. J Int Coop Educ 2008; 11(1): 55–69.
[5]   Ministry for Education and Sports (MoES). A comprehensive analysis of basic education in Uganda. Ministry for Education and Sports (MoES), ed. Kampala, Uganda: Ministry Education Sports, 2005.
[6]   Chabbott C. UNICEFs child friendly schools: Case study Uganda. Child Friendly Schools. UNICEF, 2010.
[7]   Srour G. Building tomorrow, 2014. URL: www.buildingtomorrow.org.
[8]   The Republic of Uganda Ministry of Education and Sports. Primary Seven Curriculum. Sports R of UM of E, ed. Kampala, Uganda: National Curriculum Development Center, 2012.
[9]   Mucunguzi P. Environmental education in the formal sector of education in Uganda. Environ Educ Res 1995;1(2):233.
[10]   Muyanda-Mutebi P. An analysis of the primary education curriculum in Uganda including a framework for a primary education curriculum renewal. Nairobi, Kenya: ASESP, 1996: 47.
[11]   Blair D. The child in the garden: An evaluative review of the benefits of school gardening. J Environ Educ 2009; 40(2): 15–38.
[12]   Thompson CW, Aspinall P, Montarizino A. The childhood factor: Adult visits to green places and the significance of childhood experience. Environ Behav 2008; 40(1): 111–43.
[13]   Moore RC, Cooper Marcus C. The importance of designing spaces that support children's contact with nature. In: Keller S, Heerwagen J, Mador M, eds. Biohpic design: Theory, science and practice. Hoboken, NJ: John Wiley, 2008.
[14]   Wells NM, Lekies K. Nature and the life course: Pathways from childhood nature experiences to adult environmentalism. Child Youth Environ 2006;16(1):1–24.
[15]   Trudeau F, Shephard RJ. Physical education, school physical activity, school sports and academic performance. Int J Behav Nutr Phys Act 2008;5:10.
[16]   Rowe PG. Design thinking. Boston, MA: MIT Press, 1987.
[17]   Motloch J. Introduction to landscape design, 2nd ed. New York: John Wiley, 2001.
[18]   Dillon J, Rickinson M, Teamey K, Morris M, Choi MY, Sanders D, et al. The value of outdoor learning: Evidence from research in the UK and elsewhere. Sch Sci Rev 2006;87:107–11.
[19]   Minkler M, Wallerstein N. Community based participatory research for health; From process to outcome. San Fransisco, CA: Jossey-Bass, 2008.
[20]   Woolner P, Clark J, Hall E, Tiplady L, Thomas U, Wall K. Pictures are necessary but not sufficient: Using a range of visual methods to engage users about school design. Learn Environ Res 2010;13(1):1–22.
[21]   Woolner P, Hall E, Wall K, Dennison D. Getting together to improve the school environment: User consultation, participatory design and student voice. Improv Sch 2007; 10(3): 233–48.
[22]   Carlson M. Kids know their school best. Educ Facil Plan 2010;44(4):13–6.
[23]   McNaught C, Lam P. Using wordle as a supplementary research tool. Qual Rep 2010; 15(3): 630–43.
[24]   Shiotani A, Barber M, Vermeersch C. Teacher absenteeism and teacher accountability. USAID Educ Startegy Dev 2009; 2(6410): 1–10.
[25]   Chaudhury N, Hammer J, Kremer M, Muralidharan K, Rogers FH. Missing in action. Teacher Health 2006; 20(1): 91–116.
[26]   Ariba C. Uganda: Teacher absenteeism in Teso stands at 50 percent. New Vision 2013 May 01. URL: http://allafrica.com/stories/201305010681.html.
[27]   Schuman AW. The Pedogogy of Engagement. In: Hardin MC, Eribes R, Poster C, eds. From the studio to the streets. Sterling, VA: Stylus, 2006.

In: Public Health Yearbook 2015
Editor: Joav Merrick

ISBN: 978-1-63484-514-4
© 2016 Nova Science Publishers, Inc.

Chapter 11

USING CONCEPT MAPPING TO MOBILIZE A BLACK FAITH COMMUNITY TO ADDRESS HIV

Magdalena Szaflarski[1,2,], PhD, Lisa M Vaughn[3], PhD, Daniel McLinden[4], PhD, Yolanda Wess[5], RN, BSN, ACRN, and Andrew Ruffner[6], MA, LSW*

[1]Department of Sociology and Center for AIDS Research (CFAR),
University of Alabama at Birmingham, Birmingham, Alabama, United States of America
[2]Department of Environmental Health,
University of Cincinnati College of Medicine, Cincinnati, Ohio, United States of America
[3]Department of Pediatrics, University of Cincinnati and Division of Emergency Medicine, Cincinnati Children's Hospital Medical Center, Cincinnati, Ohio, United States of America
[4]Division of General and Community Pediatrics, Cincinnati Children's Hospital Medical Center, Cincinnati, Ohio, United States of America
[5]Department of Internal Medicine, Division of Infectious Diseases, University of Cincinnati, Cincinnati, Ohio, United States of America
[6]Department of Emergency Medicine, University of Cincinnati, Cincinnati, Ohio, United States of America

Research that partners with community stakeholders increases contextual relevance and community buy-in and maximizes the chance for intervention success. Within a framework of an academic-community partnership, this project assessed a Black faith-community's needs and opportunities to address HIV. We used concept mapping to identify/prioritize specific HIV-related strategies that would be acceptable to congregations. Ninety stakeholders brainstormed strategies to address HIV; 21 sorted strategies into groups and rated their importance and feasibility. Multidimensional scaling and cluster analysis were applied to the sorting to produce maps that illustrated the stakeholders' conceptual thinking about HIV interventions. Of 278 responses, 93 were

---

[*] Corresponding author: Magdalena Szaflarski, PhD, Department of Sociology, University of Alabama at Birmingham, HHB 460Q, 1720 2nd Ave S, Birmingham, AL 35294-1152, USA, Email: szaflam@uab.edu.

used in the sorting task. The visual maps represented eight clusters: church acceptance of people living with HIV; education (most feasible); mobilization and communication; church/leaders' empowerment; church involvement/collaboration; safety/HIV prevention; media outreach; and, stigma (most important). Concept mapping clarified multifaceted issues of HIV in the Black faith community. The results will guide HIV programming in congregations.

Keywords: HIV, human immunodeficiency virus, AIDS, acquired immunodeficiency syndrome, Black faith community, concept mapping, HIV intervention strategies

INTRODUCTION

Faith communities, especially African American churches, have been suggested as a key partner to address HIV (1-3). HIV, or human immunodeficiency virus, can lead to a terminal condition known as AIDS (acquired immunodeficiency syndrome). African Americans are disproportionately affected by HIV (4). The Black church (evangelical congregations predominantly made up of African American members) has been a powerful voice in communities of color, but its role in shaping HIV-risk behaviors and HIV prevention/care has been mixed (1). A national study estimated that 5.6% of U.S. congregations provide programs or activities to people living with HIV (PLWH), which were facilitated by presence of PLWH in the congregation, formal community needs assessment activities, religious tradition (Black Protestantism), and openness to gays/lesbians (5). Another study has shown that only a third of Black Protestant congregations offer HIV prevention/counseling programs (2). The literature has identified stigma linked with religious doctrines and moral positions as a key barrier to effective HIV prevention/care (6). Even churches willing to address HIV in their communities defer from discussing specific HIV-risk behaviors (7). How to tackle doctrinal stances on HIV remains unclear, but mobilization and input directly from faith leaders and faith communities in specific local contexts are emerging as useful approaches (8).

Involving community members in the process is considered as crucial to improving the success of health interventions (9). Research that partners with community stakeholders increases contextual relevance and community buy-in and therefore maximizes the chance for intervention success. As one strategy to HIV prevention, federal agencies have been funding Black churches as partners in HIV prevention (10). Most of this work has been capacity-building and HIV-related training. The development of community-based coalitions and partnerships is another effective strategy (11). Such connections have been seen as major opportunities for faith leaders to gain support and garner resources for faith communities' HIV involvement. Some faith institutions have been implementing HIV programs and services that they find acceptable within the context of their religious doctrine (12). Researchers have also begun engaging directly with faith leaders to learn about factors that facilitate or inhibit effective HIV prevention/care in at-risk communities (8).

Unfortunately, data from such studies sometimes lack rigor because traditional research and evaluation methods are difficult to implement on a large scale and in "fluid" community settings. There are also several potential barriers to implementing health programs and in particular those addressing HIV within religious settings. These include the presence of mistrust and a reciprocal lack of understanding of the values, norms, and customs between religious organizations and their partners in science, public health, or academia (13). Therefore, innovative methodologies rooted in social sciences, not widely used within public health, are urgently needed. Furthermore, demonstrations and exploratory studies need to be repeated in a broad range of environments and might even be uniquely important in areas outside of epicenters in which relatively more motivations/resources are available. Finally, community mobilization with a focus on HIV can be effective, but such interventions are most effective when they occur spontaneously and emerge directly from communities (rather than being "implemented" by an outside agent) (14). There are few studies describing programs that emerge in such "organic" fashion.

The purpose of the current study was to generate and then prioritize specific strategies to address HIV in a Black faith community. The intent was to inform the design of HIV intervention strategies based on the lived experience of the broader community of stakeholders -- providers, faith-community stakeholders (faith leaders, health ministers, and congregants), community advocates, and health researchers. Necessary here was a method that included the voice of the many and diverse perspectives of the total community and provided a process for meaning to emerge. Notably, this is the first study to examine a faith-community driven approach to HIV in the southern Midwest.

METHODS

This study was conducted in Cincinnati/Hamilton County, Ohio. Hamilton County is considered a low-to-moderate HIV prevalence area with an estimated 274 per 100,000 residents living with a HIV diagnosis (15). Most (57%) of these cases are among non-Hispanic black/African Americans, and two of three Blacks with HIV in Ohio reside in Hamilton County.

A previous study has identified about 450 religious congregations in the Greater Cincinnati area, with over 100 located in the City of Cincinnati (2). About a third of Black Protestant congregations in Greater Cincinnati have offered HIV prevention/counseling programs, compared to 3-4% of other types of congregations. However, the differences in the provision of HIV programs by theology-polity have been linked to urban location, organizational resources, and broader community service (2).

The current study was conducted in the context of an academic-community partnership and a community project that involved a selected group of Black churches serving high HIV-risk neighborhoods. The program aimed to educate faith leaders about HIV and assist churches with the development of suitable, faith-based HIV stigma reduction and prevention programs. Participants in the current study were recruited from members of the faith and other community members who attended a town hall meeting organized by the academic-community partners. The target audience was faith and community leaders, health professionals, and HIV-infected or at-risk individuals. The study was approved by the University of Cincinnati Institutional Review Board.

Study design

We used *concept mapping* to generate and then prioritize specific strategies to address HIV in a Black faith community. *Concept mapping* is a mixed-method, participatory research methodology. Through brainstorming and sorting steps followed by multidimensional scaling and hierarchical cluster analysis, concept mapping results in a structured, data-driven visual representation of thoughts or ideas of a group (16). Concept mapping is an ideal participatory framework for the study of community health issues, and an extensive methodological work has demonstrated both its validity and utility. Concept mapping has been used to address substantive issues in culturally competent intervention services and health disparities (17, 18). The aim of the current study was to apply concept mapping to identify contextually relevant HIV interventions in the Black faith community and expand on prior research by involving community members in the process.

Procedure

Step 1: Brainstorming

As part of an evaluation at a community town hall meeting about HIV sponsored by our partnering community organization, attendees were asked to generate items that completed a partial statement (*focus prompt*) relevant to HIV in their community—*"To address HIV/AIDS in the Black faith community, I believe we need to...."* In concept mapping methodology, the intent of the focus prompt is to focus respondents on a specific issue, addressing HIV within the Black faith community in this case, and then ask them to provide brief responses that complete the prompt. The focus prompt was administered as part of the town hall meeting evaluation, and as such was included on a questionnaire given out at the beginning of the meeting. Attendees responded anonymously in writing with 3-5 brief responses that completed the focus prompt.

Step 2: Statement editing

Items generated in Step 1 were edited by the research team in order to reduce the number of items to a manageable set of less than 100 responses (18). The research team eliminated items not consistent with the focus prompt or items expressing similar ideas. Further editing was done for grammar and clarity of expression without altering the original meaning of the responses. The outcome of the editing process was a manageable number of items for the sorting task in Step 3.

Step 3: Sorting and rating

A smaller number of stakeholders from the same broad categories of attendees (i.e., professionals, community/church, and those personally affected by HIV) sorted the items into groups of similar ideas (19, 20). Sorters were asked to identify their involvement within the HIV community (e.g., clinicians, researchers, service providers, community members, community agency, a person with HIV, and/or family member of a person with HIV. Sorters could identify with more than one category. The sorters received a deck of cards and were directed to complete the sorting task. Each card contained one item generated in response to the focus prompt along with an identification number. The sorters were asked to individually sort cards into groups based on their perception of similar ideas. Next, the sorters were directed to place each group of cards into separate envelopes. On the front of the envelope, the sorters were asked to provide a label/name for each group of cards and to rate each group of cards in terms of importance and feasibility on a 5-point Likert scale.

Data analysis

Sorting data from each individual resulted in a symmetric matrix with a column and row for each of the responses. Cells in the matrix represented the intersection of each item with every other item and contained a 1 if the intersecting items were placed in the same group by the respondent or a zero if not placed in the same group. A dataset of all of the respondents' matrices was analyzed using multidimensional scaling (21) to create x, y coordinates and position the ideas as points in a two-dimensional map. Items that were often sorted together by different respondents shared a conceptual similarity in the minds of the sorters and, as a result, these items had x, y coordinates close to each other. Cluster analysis was applied to the x, y coordinates of the points to determine where boundaries could be drawn around groups of items (22). A judgment had to be made about the appropriate number of clusters because cluster analysis results in as many clusters as there are sorted responses. The goal in this interpretive process was to describe the issue in the map with as few clusters as possible but express sufficient detail. In this case, the academic-community partnership team reviewed multiple cluster solutions and determined the appropriate number of clusters. A final step was to create a label for each cluster that succinctly expressed the theme for a cluster while remaining grounded in the meaning provided by respondents. As such, the academic-community partnership team reviewed the labels used by respondents as a guide for creating final names for the clusters.

Concept maps illustrate what a group thinks about a particular issue. While the group involved in concept mapping is composed of individuals with an informed perspective, members of the group often represent multiple and diverse perspectives on the issue under consideration.

An additional step that can be applied to the concept maps is to elicit the value system of the various stakeholder groups to determine the extent to which groups are in agreement. This step is accomplished by comparing value ratings provided by different stakeholder groups and then displaying and comparing the pattern of value among different groups. Termed "pattern matching" (16), the intent is to focus on the differences and similarities in the patterns of value across all of the concepts/clusters. The value that a sorter gave each group of items was assigned to all items in that grouping. The mean value for each item was then calculated across all raters, and the average value of all items in a cluster was calculated from the item means. The pattern of results was examined across all participants and within three stakeholder groups by rank-ordering the final clusters on a vertical number line for importance and feasibility. The three stakeholder groups were categorized as: 1) professionals (e.g., clinicians, researchers, service providers, etc.); 2) community (e.g., members, churches, agencies); and/or, 3) individuals personally affected by HIV (e.g., self/HIV-infected or at-risk, family members).

RESULTS

A total of 90 attendees to a community town hall meeting identified themselves via self-report (attendees could select more than one option) as church members/leaders associated with the project (42%), community members and members of agencies interested in addressing HIV/AIDS (45%), PLWH (8%), family member of PLWH (11%), clinician/researcher working with PLWH (20%), and other (students, visitors from another city, etc., 13%). As part of the town hall meeting, the participants completed an evaluation that included a question about strategies to address HIV/AIDS in the Black faith community. A smaller group of stakeholders from the same broad categories (n = 21) worked individually to complete an unstructured sorting of these strategies into groups of similar ideas.

Brainstormed items

Stakeholders brainstormed a diverse set of 278 items from multiple perspectives that were relevant to addressing HIV in the Black faith community. After editing to eliminate redundant ideas and deleting items that did not respond to the focus prompt, 93 items were used in the sorting task.

Concept maps

The multidimensional scaling results (Figure 1) show how the 93 items are arranged in relation to each other; points close together represent items that the sorters considered as similar. The results also show how the 93 items coalesce into groups in the cluster analysis.

Ignoring for the moment the boundaries drawn around groups of points and the labels for those boundaries, the points alone illustrate the most detailed perspective. Based on the x,y coordinates produced by multidimensional scaling, the locations of items and the distance between items can be explored because distance between points has meaning. For example, two statements located in the lower right portion, cluster 6, are item 69, *"practice safe sex,"* which is close to item 15, *"have condoms more available,"* but neither of these items are close to item 47, *"give people with HIV/AIDS love - God loves them - we should too"* located on the opposite left hand top corner of the map. The location of these points indicates that the sorters more often sorted items 69 and 15 into the same group which signifies that they thought the ideas expressed in these two items were conceptually similar. The sorters never sorted items 69 and 15 together with item 47 because the sorters saw these items as conceptually dissimilar. The multidimensional scaling routine takes the multiple data from multiple sorters and finds a single solution with best location for all points in a two-dimensional arrangement by placing the conceptually similar items closer together and the dissimilar items further apart. Because the sorting process was done individually, the sorters varied in how they organized items. For instance, items 69 and 15 may have been sorted into the same group by different sorters, but each sorter may have had different other items in the group in which 69 and 15 were placed, so these other points are nearby and still conceptually related. However, there is not complete agreement on all responses from all sorters. This illustrates a methodological nuance that is important in concept mapping -- it is not necessary to facilitate consensus in the group and thereby eliminate individual differences. Individual sorters provided their individual perspective, and the process enabled a single picture to emerge that shows where consensus exists (e.g., items 69 and 15) and where slight differences emerge (e.g., items near 69 and 15 in nearby clusters).

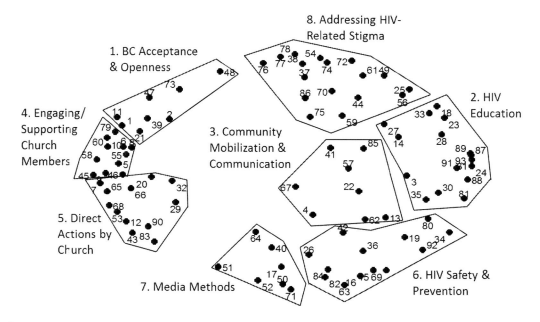

[a] Clusters:
Black churches' acceptance of and openness to PLWHs.
Education about HIV among Black youth, families, and communities.
Black community mobilization and honest communication about HIV.
Engaging and supporting church members and leaders in talking about HIV.
Direct actions churches can take in addressing HIV.
Suggested strategies for HIV safety and prevention.
Media methods to increase awareness about HIV.
Addressing sexual and other stigmas about HIV.

Figure 1. Point and cluster map -- strategies to address HIV in a Black faith community[a] (BC = Black church).

While understanding the nuance of point location is useful, it is also useful to see the bigger picture -- that is, applying cluster analysis to determine how multiple individual ideas represented by points coalesce into a smaller number of key concepts (*clusters*) in a map. The academic-community partnership team agreed that an eight-cluster map illustrated the key issues. Each cluster was named through a consensus process; for example, Cluster 1 was given the title, "*Black Churches' Acceptance and Openness to PLWHs*" which consisted of related responses about the church accepting PLWH (e.g., "*allow faith to evolve and progress in order to become more accepting of different lifestyles*"; Table 1).

Table 1. Example responses in each cluster

Cluster 1: Black churches' acceptance of and openness to people living with HIV (PLWH) *Help the churches become more accepting of men that have sex with men*
2. *Allow faith to evolve and progress in order to become more accepting of different lifestyles*
21. *Address the issue in church - we know abstinence is not the message, so let's get real*
Cluster 2: Education about HIV among Black youth, families, and communities
30. *Educate the public on the risks involved with unprotected sex*
89. *Get young people talking about HIV/AIDS and educate them*
14. *Acknowledge that this epidemic is impacting our community*
Cluster 3: Black community mobilization and honest communication about HIV
13. *Mobilize community to talk about the issue (prevention, social and population behaviors)*
57. *Encourage HIV/AIDS at home conversations with families or at family reunions*
85. *Discuss contextual factors that affect African American women and female adolescents such as SES, negotiation skills, etc.*
Cluster 4: Engaging and supporting church members and leaders in talking about HIV
8. *For the church leadership to proclaim their support of HIV/AIDS prevention and pass this on to their congregations*
46. *Listen to members of the church and how they deal with HIV/AIDS*
79. *Address it openly and lovingly in church - no shame! Within the church (pastor and family included)*

Pattern matching

The importance and feasibility of the eight strategies were compared for each of the three stakeholder groups (i.e., professionals, community/church, and those personally affected by HIV). Keeping in mind that all items and clusters are important and to some extent feasible, pattern analysis visually orients stakeholders' priorities and beliefs about importance and feasibility. For example, across all the sorters, Cluster 8, *Addressing HIV-Related Stigma*, was rated as most important while Cluster 4, *Engaging /Supporting Church Members*, was rated as least important (Figure 2). Cluster 2, *HIV Education*, was rated as most feasible, and Cluster 1, *Black Church Acceptance and Openness*, as least feasible (Figure 2).

Pattern analysis was also used to explore the beliefs about importance and feasibility within stakeholder groups. For example, the professionals rated Cluster 8, *Addressing HIV-Related Stigma*, as most important and Cluster 5, *Direct Actions by Church*, as least important (Figure 3). They rated Cluster 6, *HIV Safety & Prevention*, as the most feasible and Cluster 1, *Black Church Acceptance and Openness*, as the least feasible strategy. The community group rated Cluster 3, *Community Mobilization & Communication*, as most important and Cluster 5, *Direct Actions by Church*, as least important (Figure 4). The community group rated Cluster 2, *HIV Education*, as most feasible and Cluster 1, *Black Church Acceptance and Openness*, as least feasible. Finally, the group personally affected by HIV rated Cluster 6, *HIV Safety & Prevention*, as most important while Cluster 4, *Engaging/Supporting Church Members*, was rated as least important (Figure 5). For those personally affected by HIV, Cluster 8, *Addressing HIV-Related Stigma*, was rated as most feasible, and Cluster 1, *Black Church Acceptance and Openness*, was rated as least feasible.

DISCUSSION

There is increasing interest and research activity on African American faith community's involvement in HIV prevention. Concept mapping was used in the current study to identify and prioritize contextually relevant HIV-related strategies within a local Black faith community. Community-based approaches are recognized for their utility in disparities reduction efforts, due to their emphasis on inclusion of those communities most directly affected by the disparity to identify problems and potential solutions. Without these perspectives, professionals in public health, HIV treatment, and research fields may not identify the complexity of issues that could have an impact on outcomes. To develop the concept maps, we sought to obtain diverse perspectives on faith-based HIV prevention by including church members and leaders who were currently involved in an HIV prevention project, PLWH and their family members, HIV clinicians/researchers, and other community members who had expressed interest through their attendance at a community town hall meeting on HIV in the African American faith community. In doing so, we were able to represent views from both inside and outside of the social systems that might be involved in a community response to HIV. By maximizing the diversity of the respondents, the resulting concept maps can be placed in the context of stakeholders' collective experience and values.

Like any methodology, concept mapping has limitations including nonrandom sampling, small sample size, and the time and labor-intensive process required to involve multiple stakeholders. However, concept mapping provides researchers and practitioners with a unique, participatory data collection and intervention design process that allows for individual-level responses (brainstorming) and group-level wisdom (sorting and data analysis). In addition, this study was specific to one geographic location and a selected group of individuals within a specific faith community and that group's particular concerns; thus, the content of the results may not be applicable to other contexts.

These limitations notwithstanding, this study offers useful insights into the faith community's perspective on how faith leaders and congregations can engage in public health efforts to address HIV among African Americans. One key finding in our study was the high importance of addressing HIV-related stigma in faith settings and some problems with (lower feasibility of) this strategy. Previous research has shown that faith communities have frequently shunned persons at risk of HIV, such as men who have sex with men and drug users, because of strict doctrinal interpretations of religious texts and a culture of silence, stigma, and homophobia (1). Indeed, representatives of various groups, including faith leaders, HIV activists, and researchers, have claimed for over a decade that homophobia is the key factor blocking the Black church's response to HIV (23, 24). These attitudes hinder effective HIV prevention and care in at-risk communities (10). Many studies have identified stigma as a specific barrier to congregational involvement in HIV prevention (25).

The fact that the faith community in our study considered addressing stigma as less feasible than some other strategies suggests that the Black church is not as well equipped to tackle HIV stigma versus delivering HIV education or mobilizing. However, although HIV stigma is typically an issue within conservative churches, some denominations and churches have been able to address stigma despite conservative theologies (25). For example, congregations can donate resources to support HIV-related programs, such as condom distribution and clean needle exchanges, as part of their service mission, without engaging in such activities directly (26). Other congregations simply follow their ideology of welcoming *all* people, regardless of their lifestyles (e.g., homo-/bi-sexuality) or disease (e.g., HIV) states or risks (27). Research shows that presence of PLWH in the congregation and openness to gays/lesbians, among other factors, helps to enhance congregational HIV programming (5).

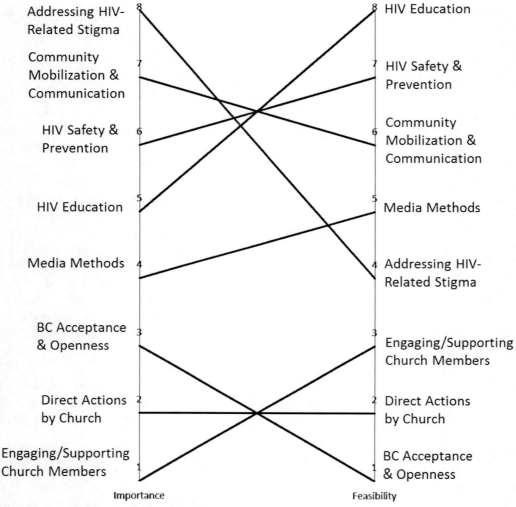

[a] Higher values indicate greater importance and greater feasibility.
[b] Professionals, community, and individuals personally affected by HIV (i.e., HIV-infected and at-risk individuals; family/friends of people living with HIV [PLWH]).

Figure 2. Pattern matching of rank-ordered clusters by importance and feasibility[a]: all sorters[b] (BC = Black church).

Using concept mapping to mobilize a black faith community to address HIV 145

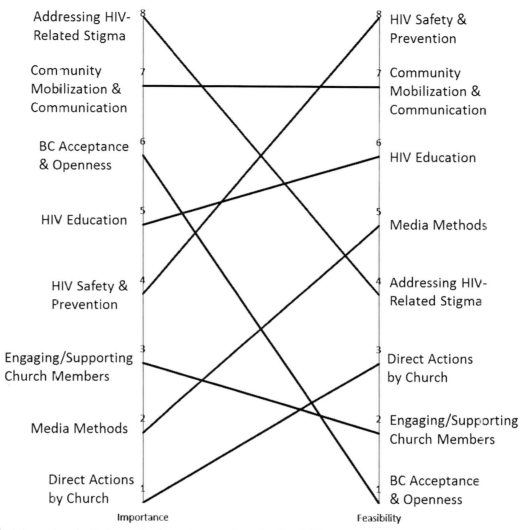

[a] Higher values indicate greater importance and greater feasibility.

Figure 3. Pattern matching of rank-ordered clusters by importance and feasibility[a]: professionals (BC = Black church).

In our study, addressing stigma and community mobilization were identified as distinct strategies (i.e., different clusters). However, the literature suggests that they are more intertwined. For example, Tyrell and colleagues (28) propose that the faith community history of shaming and blaming deters HIV prevention efforts, and the way to address this is by engaging faith leaders who are historically the community mobilizers in the Black community. The impact of stigma on behaviors and self-perceptions of PLWH is important because those who are stigmatized are less likely to display health-seeking behavior. Stigma can make people less likely to seek an HIV test, less likely to disclose HIV status if they are positive, and more likely to engage in high-risk sexual activities (28), further emphasizing the importance of our study in aiding the Black church in choosing interventions that can lessen HIV-related stigma.

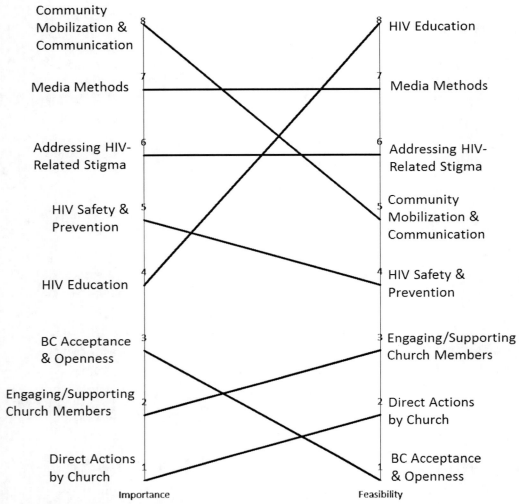

[a] Higher values indicate greater importance and greater feasibility.

Figure 4. Pattern matching of rank-ordered clusters by importance and feasibility[a]: community (BC = Black church).

Interestingly, people affected by HIV rated tackling stigma lower in importance than the other groups in our study while they rated this strategy as the most feasible. One potential explanation for such views is the perception that attitude change does not require resources. Another explanation could be that people affected by HIV often participate in settings that welcome them, and stigma appears not to be a significant problem in those settings. Further research will need to clarify the perspectives of people affected by HIV on the stigma problem within faith communities.

Another cluster of strategies proposed by the faith community in our study focused on the need for community outreach. Previous research has shown that faith leaders and congregations are often unaware of the extent of the HIV epidemic in their surrounding communities and thus feel no sense of need or urgency (25). If an intervention can rectify this issue, churches may be willing to engage in HIV-related activities. For example, in one project, data were presented to churches on various health problems, including HIV, in the geographic communities surrounding the churches, and the congregations chose themselves to target HIV and youth sexual risk behaviors in their health programming (29). Research at the national level shows that formal community HIV-related needs assessments facilitate the provision of HIV programming (5). Raising awareness through dissemination of data about the local epidemic is also one strategy to change attitudes about and increase compassion for persons with or at high risk of HIV in the faith communities (30).

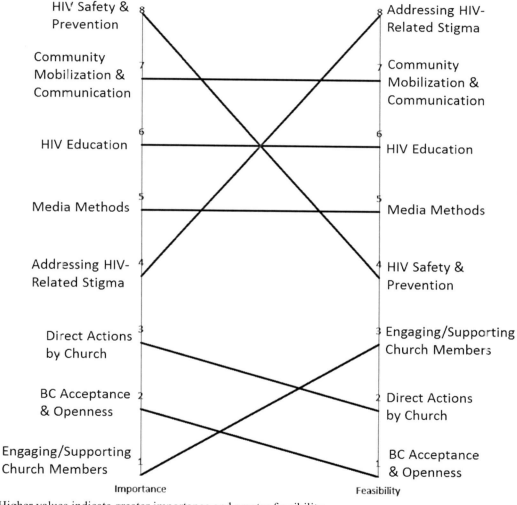

[a] Higher values indicate greater importance and greater feasibility.

Figure 5. Pattern matching of rank-ordered clusters by importance and feasibility[a]: individuals personally affected by HIV (BC = Black church).

Our data suggest that faith-community mobilization is a key component of HIV-related community outreach and that supporting the Black faith community mobilization efforts is highly feasible as well as highly important. Many Black churches around the country have taken a stance on homophobia and have led efforts locally and nationally to address HIV stigma, for example, the Trinity United Church of Christ, a Black-mega church; the Balm in Gilead, an organization based in New York City that has championed HIV awareness and intervention for three decades; the Regional AIDS Interfaith Network in North Carolina; and, Unity Fellowship Churches based in several large metropolitan areas (24, 31). Partnerships between faith-based, public health, and academic institutions have emerged all across the country. Some of these coalitions engage large numbers of churches; for example, a Michigan program engaged more than 40 congregations (32). The evidence suggests that with resources and multiple stakeholders at the table, faith-based community outreach is highly feasible. Although sustainability of programs remains limited, community-driven interventions have unique potential vis-à-vis other types of interventions because they capitalize on strengths of communities and attain community trust needed to address HIV (32).

The findings from our study also indicate the high importance and feasibility of faith-based educational and media campaigns. The use of faith communities as both agents and target audiences in the dissemination of HIV-related information and messages is innovative and can supplement traditional educational and media approaches. The need for HIV safety and prevention knowledge dissemination in this faith community was rated among the top three items in importance and feasibility. However, the literature suggests that only certain messages tend to be acceptable in faith-based settings. For example, one study showed that faith leaders have a strong preference for abstinence-based sex education, and they are not willing to discuss specific behaviors associated with HIV transmission (7). Furthermore, engaging and supporting church members in discussing HIV at the congregational forum were rated low in importance and feasibility among our community stakeholders. These findings indicate limited readiness of this community to address the faith/doctrinal aspects related to HIV. The community partners in our project repeatedly stressed the importance of "meeting the churches where they are" -- that is, offering congregations options for HIV involvement that would not compromise or negate their religious doctrine.

In our sample, respondents were able to identify and had fair levels of agreement about specific strategies to address HIV within the Black church, as evidenced by content areas involved in the clusters. Next steps include forming action groups at the participating churches composed of church members who are interested in developing specific interventions to address HIV based on the identified clusters. The eight-cluster concept maps will be used to guide the process and ensure that all viewpoints are considered, rather than the individual church or one group of stakeholders having a dominant voice. Specific brainstormed responses underlying the clusters can be consulted alongside existing models and research about how to best address HIV within this Black faith community. The concept maps can also facilitate considerations of various levels which need to be addressed (e.g., church, broader community, society) within the design of an HIV-related intervention or program.

The eight clusters identified in this study can serve as a roadmap for an improved understanding of the types of HIV approaches that are most promising and those that are less likely to be acceptable to this Black faith community for implementation. Without input from and inclusion of all relevant stakeholders, interventions may be void of the lived experience and daily lives of those affected. Efforts to eliminate or reduce HIV-related disparities must involve local communities and consider their views, thereby increasing individual and community ability to address the existing concerns in the community.

ACKNOWLEDGMENTS

The project described was supported by the National Center for Research Resources and the National Center for Advancing Translational Sciences, National Institutes of Health, through Grant 8 UL1 TR000077-05. Preliminary work for this project was supported by the *Eunice Kennedy Shriver* National Institute of Child Health and Human Development, through Grant 5R21HD050137-02. The content is solely the responsibility of the authors and does not necessarily represent the official views of the National Institutes of Health. Specifically, the project was funded through a Community Health Grant from the University of Cincinnati Center for Clinical and Translational Science and Training (CCTST). The grantee was *IV-CHARIS*, a faith-based non-profit HIV service agency in Cincinnati, Ohio. Dr. Szaflarski and Dr. Vaughn were the academic co-principal investigators on the project. This research was presented at the University of Alabama at Birmingham 8th Annual Health Disparities Research Symposium, where it received the Charles Barkley Health Disparities Investigator 1st Place (Oral Presentation) Award from the Minority Health Disparities Research Center.

We thank the following collaborators for their contributions: Ms. Mamie Harris, CDCA, and Camisha Chambers, BA of *IV-CHARIS*, Cincinnati, Ohio, for leading the community mobilization and program implementation effort and assistance with data collection; Nancy Peter, BA of the University of Cincinnati Local Performance Site, Pennsylvania/ MidAtlantic AIDS Education and Training Center (PAMAAETC), for her assistance with educational programming and partnership-building activities; Chandra Smith, MSW, LISW and the Cincinnati Queen Chapter of Delta Sigma Theta Sorority, Inc. for their community mobilization efforts and in-kind support; and, LaSharon Mosley, PhD for assistance with data design and collection. Also, special thanks to the CCTST leaders: Joel Tsevat, MD, MPH, for senior advice and research ethics support, and Monica Mitchell, PhD, for linking us with the CCTST Community Engagement Core and its resources. We also thank P. Neal Ritchey, PhD for guidance on coalition-building and program evaluation; Ruchi Bawa, MPH for research assistance at the onset of the project; Cathy Siemer (PAMAAETC) for administrative support; and, Teresa Smith, BA (CCTST) for grant-related assistance.

Last, but not least, we would like to acknowledge and commend the following congregations and faith leaders for their participation in the project and in-kind support (e.g., meeting space): Zion Global Ministries – Pastor Freddie T. Piphus; Gaines United Methodist Church – Pastor Curnell Graham; St. Mark Missionary Baptist Church – Pastor Dr. Cecil Ferrell; Corinthian Baptist Church – Pastor KZ Smith; New Prospect Baptist Church – Pastor Damon Lynch III; Lincoln Heights Missionary Baptist Church – Pastor Dr. Elliott Cuff; Turning Point Church of Zion – Pastor James Bready; Light of the World Ministries – Pastor Mike Scruggs; St. Mark A.M.E. Zion - Pastor Jermaine Armor; Bethel Baptist Church - Pastor Wayne Davis; Tryed Stone New Beginnings - Pastor Jerry Culbreth; Inspirational Baptist Church - Pastor Victor Couzens; World Outreach Christian Center - Pastor Gregory Chandler; and, Second Trinity Church - Pastor Kenneth Bibb.

REFERENCES

[1] Sutton MY, Parks CP. HIV/AIDS prevention, faith, and spirituality among Black/African American and Latino communities in the United States: strengthening scientific faith-based efforts to shift the course of the epidemic and reduce HIV-related health disparities. J Relig Health 2013; 52(2): 514-30.

[2] Szaflarski M, Ritchey PN, Jacobson CJ, Williams RH, Baumann Grau A, Meganathan K, et al. Faith-based HIV prevention and counseling programs: findings from the Cincinnati Census of Religious Congregations. AIDS Behav 2013; 17: 1839-54.

[3] Szaflarski, M. Spirituality and religion among HIV-infected individuals. Curr HIV/AIDS Rep 2013; 10(4): 324-32.

[4] Centers for Disease Control and Prevention. HIV among African Americans. 2013. URL: http://www.cdc.gov/hiv/pdf/risk_HIV_AfricanAmericans.pdf.

[5] Frenk SM, Trinitapoli J. U.S. congregations' provision of programs or activities for people living with HIV/AIDS. AIDS Behav 2013; 17(5): 1829-38.

[6] Williams JK, Wyatt GE, Wingood G. The four Cs of HIV prevention with African Americans: crisis, condoms, culture, and community. Curr HIV/AIDS Rep 2010; 7(4): 185-93.

[7] Francis SA, Lam WK, Cance JD, Hogan VK. What's the 411? Assessing the feasibility of providing African American adolescents with HIV/AIDS prevention education in a faith-based setting. J Relig Health 2009; 48(2): 164-77.

[8] Nunn A, Cornwall A, Chute N, Sanders J, Thomas G, James G, et al. Keeping the faith: African American faith leaders' perspectives and recommendations for reducing racial disparities in HIV/AIDS infection. PloS One 2012; 7(5): e36172.

[9] Minkler M, Wallerstein N. Community-based participatory research for health: from process to outcomes, 2nd ed. San Francisco, CA: Jossey-Bass, 2008.

[10] Eke AN, Wilkes AL, Gaiter J. Organized religion and the fight against HIV/AIDS in the black community: the role of the Black Church. In: McCree DH, ed. African Americans and HIV/AIDS: understanding and addressing the epidemic. New York: Springer, 2010: 53-68.

[11] Centers for Disease Control and Prevention. CDC executive summary: CDC consultation on faith and HIV prevention. 2006. URL: http://www.cdc.gov/hiv//resources/other/PDF/faith.pdf

[12] Derose KP, Mendel PJ, Palar K, Kanouse DE, Bluthenthal RN, Castaneda LW, et al. Religious congregations' involvement in HIV: a case study approach. AIDS Behav 2011; 15(6): 1220-32.

[13] Campbell MK, Hudson MA, Resnicow K, Blakeney N, Paxton A, Baskin M. Church-based health promotion interventions: evidence and lessons learned. Ann Rev Public Health 2007; 28: 213-34.

[14] Blankenship KM, Friedman SR, Dworkin S, Mantell JE. Structural interventions: concepts, challenges and opportunities for research. J Urban Health 2006; 83(1): 59-72.

[15] Ohio Department of Health. HIV/AIDS integrated epidemiological profile for Ohio: 2011 edition. Columbus, OH: Ohio Department of Health, 2012.

[16] Trochim WMK, Kane M. Concept mapping: an introduction to structured conceptualization in health care. Int J Qual Health Care 2005; 17(3): 187-91.

[17] Jackson KM, Trochim WMK. Concept mapping as an alternative approach for the analysis of open-ended survey responses. Organ Res Meth 2002; 5(4): 307-36.

[18] Vaughn LM, Jacquez, F, McLinden, D. The use of concept mapping to identify community-driven intervention strategies for physical and mental health. Health Promot Pract 2013: 14(5): 675-85.

[19] Rosenberg S, Moonja Park K. The method of sorting as a data gathering procedure in multivariate research. Multivar Behav Res 1975; 10(4): 489-502.

[20] Weller SC, Romney AK. Systematic data collection. Newbury Park, CA: Sage, 1988.

[21] de Leeuw J, Mair P. Multidimensional scaling using majorization: SMACOF in R. J Stat Softw 2009; 31(3): 1-30.

[22] Kane M, Trochim WMK. Concept mapping for planning and evaluation. Thousand Oaks: Sage, 2007.

[23] Fullilove MT, Fullilove RE. Stigma as an obstacle to AIDS action: the case of the African American community. Am Behav Sci 1999; 42(7): 1117-29.

[24] Ward EG. Homophobia, hypermasculinity and the US black church. Cult Health Sex 2005; 7(5): 493-504.

[25] Williams MV, Palar K, Derose KP. Congregation-based programs to address HIV/AIDS: elements of successful implementation. J Urban Health 2011; 88(3): 517-32.
[26] Koch JR, Beckley RE. Under the radar: AIDS ministry in the bible belt. Rev Relig Res 2006; 47(4): 393-408.
[27] Leong P. Religion, flesh, and blood: re-creating religious culture in the context of HIV/AIDS. Sociol Relig 2006; 67(3): 295-311.
[28] Tyrell CO, Klein SJ, Gieryic SM, Devore BS, Cooper JG, Tesoriero JM. Early results of a statewide initiative to involve faith communities in HIV prevention. J Public Health Manag Pract 2008; 14(5): 429-36.
[29] Kruger DJ, Lewis Y, Schlemmer E. Mapping a message for faith leaders: encouraging community health promotion with local health data. Health Promot Pract 2010; 11(6): 837-44.
[30] Bluthenthal RN, Palar K, Mendel P, Kanouse DE, Corbin DE, Derose KP. Attitudes and beliefs related to HIV/AIDS in urban religious congregations: barriers and opportunities for HIV-related interventions. Soc Sci Med 2012; 74(10): 1520-7.
[31] Cohen C. The boundaries of Blackness: AIDS and the breakdown of Black politics. Chicago: University of Chicago Press, 1999.
[32] Griffith DM, Pichon LC, Campbell B, Allen JO. YOUR Blessed Health: a faith-based CBPR approach to addressing HIV/AIDS among African Americans. AIDS Educ Prev 2010; 22(3): 203-17.

Chapter 12

BUILDING INTERPROFESSIONAL CULTURAL COMPETENCE: REFLECTIONS OF FACULTY ENGAGED IN TRAINING STUDENTS TO CARE FOR THE VULNERABLE

Joy Doll[*], Ann Ryan Haddad, Ann Laughlin, Martha Todd, Katie Packard, Jennifer Yee, Barbara Harris and Kimberly Begley

Department of Occupational Therapy, Department of Pharmacy Practice, College of Nursing, Department of Exercise Science, Department of Social Work, Creighton University, Omaha, Nebraska, United States of America

Interprofessional education (IPE) necessitates that both educators and students need to engage in a process that requires learning and reflecting upon professional identity, both their own and those of the other professionals on the healthcare team. Despite thinking team skills are inherent, it has become apparent that health professions students need to be taught the skills of how to communicate and negotiate as part of a team to provide collaborative care. These skills demand that health care providers need to not only learn discipline-specific clinical reasoning but team-based clinical reasoning as well. The Interprofessional Education Collaborative Expert Panel has clearly identified team-based skills as a core skill to health care practice. Teamwork and team-based skills become even more critical in health care delivery for vulnerable patients and populations. Vulnerable patients present with complex health issues that benefit from a team-based approach to care. This manuscript will describe the development and implementation of a pilot IPE course preparing students for health care with vulnerable patients. The authors discuss the importance of developing interprofessional cultural competence for the faculty team of educators in order to execute such complex IPE. Reflections on the challenges to developing and implementing such an innovative IPE experience will be discussed.

---

[*] Corresponding author: Joy Doll, OTD, OTR/L, Vice Chair, Director of Post Professional OTD Program, Associate Professor, Department of Occupational Therapy, School of Pharmacy and Health Professions, Creighton University, 2500 California Plaza, Omaha, Nebraska, United States. E-mail: joydoll@creighton.edu.

Keywords: interprofessional education, interprofessional collaboration, vulnerable population

INTRODUCTION

Scholars, educators and health care organizations all agree: interprofessional education (IPE) and collaborative health care practice are essential to provide quality, holistic care for patients across health care settings (1). Health care providers today are faced with challenges including complex diagnoses and limited resources along with providing care in a diverse team environment to maximize care. The importance of team care becomes more evident when working with patients who are vulnerable. Collaborative care and team-based practice are now being recognized as skills that need to be taught and enhanced (1). Health care team interactions that are negative or ineffective can profoundly impact patient outcomes and the overall success of a health care organization (2). Team development, both for the individual health care practitioner and the health care team, is also critical to the success of collaborative care (2). Interprofessional education (IPE) has emerged as a pedagogical approach to train health care students to be prepared for health care practice. Within the context of IPE, a variety of pedagogies have been shown to teach collaborative, team skills. The overall intent of IPE is to move students beyond thinking within one's own health care discipline and to expand clinical reasoning to a team-based approach (3).

Accreditation bodies have now included interprofessional practice as a core skill for many health care professions (4, 5). Students from across the health sciences will now be learning skills including collaborative ethical decision making, how to engage in successful team interactions, appropriate team communication and team problem solving (1). Pecukonis, Doyle, and Bliss (6) propose that the best way to prepare students to build the skills necessary for collaborative care in practice is to develop interprofessional cultural competence. Despite an effort in IPE to build team-based care skills, health care education is largely "profession-centric" which leads to the development of ethnocentrism held by professionals creating barriers to collaborative health care practice (6).

According to Pecukonis et al. (6), even the social construction of the term "professionalism" does not promote collaboration but instead leads to competition among health care providers. Due to the social construct of being part of a profession, collaborative care faces challenges and requires health professions educators to alter their thinking to develop and implement appropriate IPE. In order to break down existing social constructs to promote increased collaborative care, Pecukonis et al. proposed that educators follow the concept of IDEA: Interaction, Data, Expertise and Attention (6). The authors of this manuscript will use the mnemonic of IDEA to describe the development of an IPE course focused on preparing students, both as individuals and as part of a team, to provide care to vulnerable populations and/or individuals. The premise of IDEA provides a foundation for building interprofessional cultural competence not just among students but professionals and educators as well. Experts in interprofessional education have long argued the importance of faculty development for successful IPE (7).

Table 1. IDEA constructs for interprofessional cultural competence

Construct	Description
Interaction	**Educators will:** Expose to students and professionals from different health professions to develop knowledge about professional practices across professions • Have students learning in collaboration with other professions forcing students to challenge professional beliefs and move towards interprofessional cultural competence
Data	**Educators will:** Facilitate students to ask and seek information about other health care professions to understand their profession's role in accordance with the roles of other professions on the health care team • Help students explore stereotypes and biases they hold about professions' roles including their own • Provide activities that allow students to develop relationships with students from other professions to see them not just as professionals, but a person
Expertise	**Educators will:** • Encourage the development of skills in collaborative communication and reflective practices in order to develop an increased awareness of others in order to promote collaborative care
Attention	**Educators will:** • Provide opportunities for students to reflect both personally and as a team on their own beliefs about professions' roles and team-based care

Any team of educators implementing IPE need to develop their own interprofessional cultural competence in order to be effective in designing and implementing successful IPE for students. This manuscript will describe the journey of a team of educators in developing interprofessional cultural competence while facing the challenges of developing an IPE course focused on vulnerable populations.

INTERSECTING INTERPROFESSIONAL EDUCATION AND VULNERABILITY

Simulation centers, service-learning, case analysis, and patient safety have all been exemplars in teaching health professions students the skills necessary to engage in collaborative health care practice (3, 4, 10). However, as identified by Dow et al. (9), one area of interprofessional education still in need of development is the preparation of the interprofessional team for working with vulnerable and/or underserved populations. According to Dow et al. (9) "a student planning to practice in a resource-poor, primary care setting needs specific skills in teamwork, leadership, and followership that bolster collaboration by allowing all health care professionals to practice at the top of their licensed abilities" (9).

In fact, these leaders in IPE identify the skills for working as part of an interprofessional team with a vulnerable population as one of the existing challenges facing current interprofessional education (9). But a question remains: how do we prepare health professions students to graduate prepared with the skills to collaborate in a team specifically focused on the needs of a vulnerable and/or underserved population? Dow, et al., suggest that educational institutions need to partner with health care organizations where both entities work together "to devise curriculum and measure outcomes" (9). Based on this identified gap in IPE, educators are called to develop educational opportunities to prepare students to practice in underserved areas.

Vulnerability can be described in a multitude of ways and is confounded in health care by factors such as chronic disease, poverty, low health literacy rates, uninsured and underinsured health care insurance coverage, and health disparities. These issues are further exacerbated by limited English proficiency, cultural beliefs and underrepresentation of minorities in health care provision (10, 11). Multiple factors related to vulnerability can result in increasing the complexity of health care decision making for the individual health professional and the health care team. Eamon (12) defined a vulnerable population as "a group possessing a disproportionate amount of societal resources and influence." Vulnerable populations are "at risk of discrimination, oppression, possessing few social and economic resources and exclusion from decision-making processes" (12). Across the literature, there are examples of IPE experiences have taken place with ethnic minorities and rural populations where community leaders and educators have felt that interprofessional practice is necessary to address the needs of vulnerable populations. These experiences often focus on identified "underserved populations," who experience vulnerability due to health disparities and geographic isolation (13).

Student-run clinics in underserved communities have been one avenue for exposing students to IPE with vulnerable populations (14). Students report enjoying these experiences as a way to collaborate and meet community needs (15). Educational experiences with underserved populations also allow students the opportunity to learn the importance of overlapping roles and how to collaborate with limited resources to meet patient needs (16). However, to develop and sustain these interprofessional experiences for students, academicians have to be committed to collaborative work, crossing professional boundaries and possess a willingness to grow as a team (17). It bears stating that any team of educators implementing IPE need to experience team development and effective collaboration in order to effectively educate teams of health professions students (18). In other words the team of faculty developing and implementing IPE needs to develop interprofessional cultural competence among its member and the team as a whole. To achieve IPE, each faculty member must confront and identify how to distribute "power within the work environment, how training should proceed within the clinical setting, the level, and nature of inter-profession communication, resolution of conflicts and management of relationships between team members and constituents" (6).

When developing a team, educators and students alike are called to explore their own vulnerabilities in order to identify and develop interprofessional cultural competence. Although this vulnerability is different than the vulnerabilities of the underserved, the exposure to these feelings can be a catalyst to the openness needed by both the educators and the students to effectively work as a team with vulnerable patients. Furthermore, the members of a health care team should experience their own vulnerability in order to reflect and grow into a strong collaborative team. All of these elements are critical in order for an individual and a team to develop interprofessional cultural competence (18).

Interaction: Formulating the course design

According to Pecukonis et al. interaction "is the process during which the student has the opportunity to work and learn directly with individuals from other health disciplines" (6). The same principle is as true for health sciences educators, as it is for students. The educators involved in developing the interprofessional course exemplar discussed here had a longstanding relationship with one another. Prior to the course development and implementation, these educators had collaborated on the execution of an interprofessional clinic for the underserved in a low socioeconomic area lacking in health care services. The clinic resulted from a group of passionate and committed faculty who were compelled to interact to make the clinic a successful reality. Through these interactions surrounding the clinic, faculty engaged in collaborative communication, role negotiation, knowledgeable transition about professions on the team, and developed a sense of advocacy for all the various professions involved. These activities are critical in the process of developing interprofessional cultural competence (6).

To maintain the demands of the clinic, faculty and student volunteers took responsibility for the day-to-day management of the clinic. From the faculty experience with the students, the educators identified a need to formalize the education occurring at the community partner site to structure learning experiences and prepare students for the realities of the needs and desires of vulnerable clients. Faculty observations and conversations revealed a significant lack of knowledge demonstrated by students regarding how to address the needs of the vulnerable population being served at the clinic. Furthermore, the students were observed to have a lack of clear awareness of how to act and interact as part of a health care team. From these observations and discussions, the idea of an interprofessional course focused on developing the skills necessary to provide collaborative care for vulnerable populations emerged. It is significant to point out that the interprofessional team of faculty had to collaborate and engage in open dialogue in order to clearly identify the educational needs of the students. The interactions from the clinic established clear team interactions and allowed the team to identify the need to grow interprofessional education experiences for the students.

Data: Course design and implementation

In the IDEA mnemonic, Data focuses on "obtaining accurate information from health professions" (6). In order to cultivate the IPE course, the faculty began to meet and collaborate on the course design which included the development of the course syllabus and exploration into the administrative infrastructure for the approval of such a course. The course was designed by the team of faculty involved in the clinic from the professions of exercise science, occupational therapy, nursing, pharmacy and social work. Each faculty member then recruited students from these professions to engage in the course. As part of the process, faculty developed a strong understanding of the roles of other team members to formulate how the course would be presented. To role model collaborative care to students, the educators, themselves, had to learn about one another and negotiate their own collaborative process.

The team of faculty was also required to navigate the institutional infrastructure required to implement an IPE course which necessitated the team members to acquire new knowledge.

For the course to be approved and categorized as IPE, a copy of the syllabus had to be reviewed and accepted by the curriculum committees of each profession involved at the institution. The team of faculty designing the course was responsible for contacting the appropriate representatives and garnering support to receive approval from all the curriculum committees. In one discipline, the curriculum committee did not approve the course so students from this discipline had to be excluded from the enrollment. Furthermore, IPE courses are a workload add-on at the institution and not currently recognized in a faculty's current teaching duties. This situation forced the team members to negotiate with administrators and those on the team to identify a time to hold the course sessions that worked for all involved, both students and instructors. Due to workload issues, the team decided to limit the enrollment of students to 8 health professions students in order to pilot the course and ensure its successful implementation. Team members also took responsibility for teaching certain modules in an effort to manage faculty workload. In overcoming logistical challenges, the team members had to understand all team members' roles advocating for one another to ensure the course could take place. Understanding the roles of each member on the team was critical to ensure successful collaboration and a positive course experience for all involved.

Another component of data is "developing both insight and understanding about the person one is working with" (6). The successful design and implementation of this course was generated out of the passion of a group of faculty who care for one another and those who are vulnerable, not only as professionals and patients, but as people. These underpinnings of teamwork can be misconstrued as too qualitative and are often undervalued (19). However, the authors of this manuscript feel that the elements of compassion and empathy are sorely underscored in many IPE endeavors (20). This compassion among team members led to the consideration of many small, yet important, elements in the course design like the need to implement the course off campus. The rationale for holding the course in the community was to ensure the students gained a "real world" experience outside the sheltered context of the university.

Upon designing the course, faculty had to obtain administrative approval from the university to offer a full course off campus and also coordinate with the community site to choose a time that worked for the partner, the students' and the educators' schedules. In order to allow collaboration and address schedule conflicts, the course was designed as a hybrid learning experience requiring some learning in the community and some in an online environment. The instructors found both interactions to be rich in nature demonstrating the importance of care for team members in all contexts. Although often undervalued, caring for one another allowed the team, both of faculty and students, to interact effectively and maintain momentum despite some arduous barriers. This led to Expertise, the next component in cultivating interprofessional cultural competence.

Expertise and attention: Build competence to implement successful IPE

Expertise entails "the ability to communicate clearly, and effectively with other disciplines concerning the values and processes of patient care" (6). In order to develop and implement the course, the educators had to be efficient collaborators which included communicating with team members and beyond. In addition to Expertise, the team had to engage in extensive critical reflection, both individually and as a team, which addresses the aspect of Attention of the IDEA mnemonic. Attention "involves the in-depth exploration of one's personal, professional and cultural background" along with recognizing and trying to understand the biases and assumptions carried by others on the team (6).

Negotiating workload concerns was an issue that required significant communication among the faculty team members in planning the course. Discussing team members' perceptions and assumptions was an important part of the process to help the team collaborate. These negotiations required the team to engage in both Expertise and Attention to develop team competence. During the class sessions, all the instructors involved in the course made a concerted effort to be on site to role model interprofessionalism to the student interprofessional teams. Once students were given their case and charged with meeting in their teams to develop care plans, the instructors were available for both discipline-specific and interprofessional interactions as consultants. This infrastructure was necessary in order to role model and help the students build skills in communication for the progress of their own interprofessional cultural competence.

It is important to note that ventures, such as the design and implementation of an IPE course of this nature, require significant faculty time commitment and passion. Furthermore, the development and maintenance of the team aligns with the concept of Expertise which "requires compromise, embracing the others perspectives" (6). To design the course framework, the team of faculty met many times to discuss the course lessons. There were zealous discussions about course content and how it should be delivered. Critical to the success of this collaborative design was the prior establishment of a strong team of interprofessional faculty where members felt free to voice their thoughts and opinions. The process of dialogue and compromise led to the development of a course that met the requirements of multiple health professions and the passions of the team of faculty involved in the course. The ultimate goal of implementing IPE to train future health professions for intervening with vulnerable populations was realized due to the faculty team's concerted effort to foster and build interprofessional cultural competence.

IDEA: Student formation of interprofessional cultural competence

Eight students were selected to be enrolled in the pilot IPE course focused on vulnerable populations. Upon completion, the course was entitled "Developing Care for a Vulnerable Population: An Interprofessional Collaborative Approach for Health Promotion." Health professions students from the disciplines of nursing (n = 2), occupational therapy (n = 2), pharmacy (n = 2), social work (n = 1) and exercise science (n = 1) were recruited by faculty investigators in the semester prior to starting the course. In some professions, there was a large interest in the course and the faculty had to gather to choose the students for the course. When this was the case, the instructors selected students whom they felt would be committed to the course and held a strong desire to serve with vulnerable populations as part of their future professional practice.

The course met for eight weeks focused on acclimating students to their discipline. The students were divided into two 4-member teams mixing up the disciplines. Prior to collaborating with clients, students also engaged in course activities learning about the role of their discipline with a vulnerable population, the role of the other disciplines on the team, exploring the context of vulnerability, evaluating case scenarios, and promoting interprofessional dialogue and interactions between both students and faculty. The students engaged in learning activities, discussed team skills, and developed a collaborative agreement for how the team would interact to serve the vulnerable client.

In partnership with the community, two community members who had been reoccurring users of the clinic and currently experiencing complex health issues were invited to participate as the clients for the course. The community members were each invited to a live classroom session at the community partner site to share their experience with the health care system and their health concerns with both teams. The teams were then each assigned one of the community members who were considered part of their team. Students, with faculty supervision, conducted further assessment of the community member with their consent and developed a collaborative care plan for the client. Students were encouraged to reflect both individually and as a team. In group reflection discussions, students reported surprise at the complexities of the issues, both health and social, experienced by the community members who volunteered to work with the students.

In order to gauge the impact of the course and focus on the growth in interprofessional cultural competence, the faculty spent time reflecting on this pilot both during and after the course, which led to course modification and the formation of this manuscript. Quantitative data was also collected from the student participants to assess the impact of the course on their learning. This data was important to evaluate the effect on the learning of the group of interprofessional health professions students enrolled in the course. It was hypothesized that after completing the course, student perceptions about working as part of a team would improve. The study was reviewed and approved by the University Social/Behavioral Institutional Review Board.

At the beginning and end of the course, students completed the Team Skills Scale (21). Questions for the Team Skills Scale were drawn from the John A Hartford Foundation, Geriatric Interdisciplinary Team Training Program (GITT) kit (22). The scale measures perception of capabilities for effective team interactions and consists of 17 questions at 5 points each, for a maximum score of 85 points. The scale was originally designed to measure three key areas: interpersonal skills, profession-specific skills, and geriatric care skills. Questions are answered on a Likert scale measuring 1 = poor, 2 = fair, 3 = good, 4 = very good, and 5 = excellent.

Data from the pre- and post- student surveys were analyzed using Microsoft Excel using paired student's t tests. A p-value less than .05 was considered statistically significant. There was a non-significant increase in the mean Team Skills Scale score (70.0 ±11.1 pre versus 75.9 ±13.0 post, p = 0.09) (Table 2).

Table 2. Team Skills Scale data

	Pre-Course	Post-Course
Mean ± SD	70.0 ± 11.1	75.9 ± 13.0
P value	0.09	

Though the data show trends in perceived improvement of skills needed to work as part of an interprofessional team, statistical significance may not have been achieved due to small sample size (n = 8). Likewise, it has been shown that students new to interprofessional experiences often overestimate their baseline team skills, which may explain why several of the students showed a decrease in their overall score post intervention (23). These data show that a semester long interprofessional course in caring for vulnerable populations may improve students' perceptions of their abilities to work as part of an interprofessional team. It may begin the journey for health professions students in gaining interprofessional cultural competence. As the course is replicated in subsequent semesters, the sample size will increase to determine if this is a significant finding. Despite the lack of significance, the faculty involved in the course feel that the lessons learned about implementing such an IPE experience cannot be undervalued. The authors feel that the journey to interprofessional cultural competence is a story worth telling to demonstrate the complexities and intricacies of IPE for vulnerable populations.

DISCUSSION

In this pilot experience of developing and executing an IPE course focused on preparing students for team-based practice with vulnerable individuals, faculty educators set out focusing on the students and student learning outcomes. However, as the team of faculty reflected back on the experience in preparation for future offerings with a larger class size, it became apparent that the structure of the faculty team is a critical component to the success of such IPE ventures.

As the authors engaged in reflection considering lessons learned, the need to develop and maintain interprofessional cultural competence was discussed and identified as a foundation for success (6). The process of engaging and developing interprofessional cultural competence seems especially true when many professional and institutional barriers exist and collaboration is not a norm. As presented here, there exists an opportunity for interprofessional teams of educators to foster and maintain interprofessional cultural competence. When this process is successful, educators can design significant IPE learning experiences for students. The faculty team can also role model to students the interprofessional cultural competence needed for collaborative care as identified in the mnemonic IDEA.

Furthermore, there remains a significant need for health professions students to gain proficiency in both team skills and preparation for vulnerable patients and populations (9). Integrating team skills with knowledge of how to effectively serve the underserved can prepare a health professional with the aptitude to practice in many health care arenas and address complex issues seen in patient care. Further exploration into the impact of IPE with vulnerable populations is needed. This article also highlights the importance of the passion and compassion of interprofessional faculty to cultivate and devise such complex IPE experiences and the growth needed for such a team when engaging in this type of innovative pedagogy. It further demonstrates that even when facing significant professional and institutional barriers, a passion for social justice and helping those who are vulnerable will prevail. IPE experiences with vulnerable populations will require strong faculty development and institutional support to be successful. But it also cannot be ignored that human nature and care for others remains a critical piece to developing interprofessional cultural competence among faculty which can, in turn, be passed onto students.

REFERENCES

[1] Interprofessional Education Collaborative. Core competencies for interprofessional collaborative practice: Report of an expert panel. Washington, DC: Interprofessional Education Collaborative, 2011.

[2] Sargeant J, Loney E, Murphy G. Effective interprofessional teams: "contact is not enough" to build a team. J Contin Educ Health Prof 2008; 28(4): 228-34.

[3] Reeves, S, Zwarenstein, M, Goldman, J, Barr, H, Freeth, D, Koppell, I, et al. The effectiveness of interprofessional education: Key findings from a new systematic review. J Interprof Care 2010; 24: 230-41.

[4] Hammick, M. Interprofessional education: evidence from the past to guide the future. Med Teacher 2000; 22: 461-7.

[5] Zorek, J, Raehl C. Interprofessional education accreditation standards in the USA: A comparative analysis. J Interprof Care 2013; 27: 123-30.

[6] Pecukonis E, Doyle O, Bliss DL. Reducing barriers to interprofessional training: Promoting interprofessional cultural competence. J Interprof Care. 2008; 22(4): 417-28.

[7] Steinert, Y. Learning together to teach together: interprofessional education and faculty development. J Interprof Care 2005; 19: 60-75.

[8] Oandasan, I, Reeves, S. Key elements for interprofessional education. Part 1: The learner, the educator and the learning context. J Interprof Care 2005; 19: 21-38.

[9] Dow A, Blue A, Konrad SC, Earnest M, Reeves S. The moving target: outcomes of interprofessional education. J Interprof Care 2013; 27(5): 353-5.

[10] Brach, C, Fraserirector, I. Can cultural competency reduce racial and ethnic health disparities? A review and conceptual model. Med Care Res Rev 2000; 57: 181-217.

[11] Andrulis, DP, Brach, C. Integrating literacy, culture, and language to improve health care quality for diverse populations. Am J Health Behav 2007; 31: S122-33.

[12] Eamon, MK. Empowering Vulnerable Populations. Chicago, Illinois: Lyceum Books, 2008.

[13] Royeen CB, Jensen GM, Harvan RA. Leadership in interprofessional health education and practice. Boston, MA: Jones Bartlett, 2011.

[14] Moskowitz D, Glasco J, Johnson B, Wang G. Students in the community: an interprofessional student-run free clinic. J Interprof Care 2006; 20(3): 254-9.

[15] Bridges DR, Davidson RA, Odegard PS, Maki IV, Tomkowiak J. Interprofessional collaboration: three best practice models of interprofessional education. Med Educ Online 2011; 16. doi:10.3402/meo.v16i0.6035.

[16] Toner JA, Ferguson KD, Sokal RD. Continuing interprofessional education in geriatrics and gerontology in medically underserved areas. J Contin Educ Health Prof 2009; 29(3): 157-60.

[17] Hall, P. Interprofessional teamwork: Professional cultures as barriers. J Interprof Care 2005; 19: 188-96.

[18] Gilbert, JH. Interprofessional learning and higher education structural barriers. J Interprof Care 2005; 19: 87-106.

[19] Xyrichis, A, Lowton, K. What fosters or prevents interprofessional teamworking in primary and community care? A literature review. Int J Nurs Stud 2008; 45: 140-53.

[20] Lindqvist, SM, Reeves, S. Facilitators' perceptions of delivering interprofessional education: a qualitative study. Med Teacher 2007; 29: 403-5.

[21] Grymonpre, R, van Ineveld, C, Nelson, M, Jensen, F, De Jaeger, A, Sullivan, T, et al. See it – Do it – Learn it: Learning interprofessional collaboration in the clinical context. J Res Interprof Pract Educ 2008; 1(2): 127-144.

[22] Miller, BK, Ishler, JK The rural elderly assessment project: A model for interdisciplinary team training. Occupat Ther Healthcare 2001; 15: 13-34.

[23] Coster, S, Norman, I, Murrells, T, Kitchen, S, Meerabeau, E., Sooboodoo, E et al. Interprofessional attitudes amongst undergraduate students in the health professions: A longitudinal questionnaire survey. Int J Nurs Stud 2008; 45: 1667-81.

In: Public Health Yearbook 2015
Editor: Joav Merrick

ISBN: 978-1-63484-514-4
© 2016 Nova Science Publishers, Inc.

Chapter 13

BUILDING A CO-CREATED CITIZEN SCIENCE PROGRAM WITH GARDENERS NEIGHBORING A SUPERFUND SITE: THE GARDENROOTS CASE STUDY

Monica D Ramirez-Andreotta[1,], PhD, Mark L Brusseau[1,2], PhD, Janick Artiola[1], PhD, Raina M Maier[1], PhD, and A Jay Gandolfi[3], PhD*

[1]Department of Soil, Water and Environmental Science,
The University of Arizona, Tucson, Arizona, United States of America
[2]Department of Hydrology and Water Resources Department,
The University of Arizona, Tucson, Arizona, United States of America
[3]Department of Pharmacology and Toxicology,
The University of Arizona, Tucson, Arizona, United States of America

A research project that is only expert-driven may ignore the role of local knowledge in research, often gives low priority to the development of a comprehensive communication strategy to engage the community, and may not deliver the results of the study to the community in an effective way. Objective: To demonstrate how a research program can respond to a community research need, establish a community-academic partnership, and build a co-created citizen science program. Methods: A place-based, community-driven project was designed where academics and community members maintained a reciprocal dialogue, and together, we: 1) defined the question for study, 2) gathered information, 3) developed hypotheses, 3) designed data collection methodologies, 4) collected environmental samples (soil, irrigation water, and vegetables), 5) interpreted data, 6) disseminated results and translated results into action, and 7) discussed results and asked new questions. Results: The co-created environmental research project produced new data and addressed an additional exposure route (consumption of vegetables grown in soils with elevated arsenic levels). Public participation in scientific research improved environmental health assessment, information transfer, and risk communication efforts. Furthermore, incorporating the community in the scientific process produced both

---

[*] Corresponding author: Assistant Professor Monica D Ramirez-Andreotta, MPA, PhD, Department of Soil, Water and Environmental Science University of Arizona, 1177 E Fourth Street, Rm. 429, Tucson, AZ 8572, United States. E-mail: mdramire@email.arizona.edu.

individual learning outcomes and community-level outcomes. Conclusions: This approach illustrates the benefits of a community-academic co-created citizen-science program in addressing the complex problems that arise in communities neighboring a contaminated site. Such a project can increase the community's involvement in risk communication and decision-making, which ultimately has the potential to help mitigate exposure and thereby reduce associated risk.

Keywords: arsenic, capacity building, citizen science, community-academic partnership, contaminated sites, gardening, public participation in scientific research, risk communication, environmental exposure assessment

INTRODUCTION

Typically community members living in contaminated communities are the ones who initially identify adverse ecological and health outcomes associated with toxic exposures (1), although a state agency, regional US Environmental Protection Agency (USEPA) office, or the responsible party may make this discovery. The USEPA may add the site to the Comprehensive Environmental Response, Compensation, and Liability Information System, which can lead to a cascade of regulatory and/or remedy events. Typically at National Priorities List (NPL) sites with groundwater contamination, the time from discovery to remedy implementation can go beyond 20 years, and long-term management (i.e., decades to centuries) is needed at many sites (2). As time passes, site managers are responsible for monitoring the progress of remediation and engaging the community to inform them of the cleanup progress and describe potential risks associated with the site.

Traditionally, site managers engage the community in a one-way communication model that solely aims to inform, change behavior, and assure populations that the determined risk is acceptable and that cleanup is underway (3, 4). This communication strategy has a low rate of success, primarily because it excludes those most affected (3) and fundamentally does not aim to increase environmental education or involve the community in the decisions about their risk. Historically, because communities were not involved in the decision-making process, mistrust often eroded the relationships between scientists, regulatory officials, and the affected communities (5, 6).

The lack of public participation at contaminated sites is a great loss, as community members have been contributing to science since the 17th century (7, 8) and in general, volunteerism is considered critical to civic life in the United States (9, 10). Volunteers have monitored watershed health in more than 700 programs in the US, involving over 400,000 local stakeholders (11) and most ecological research once fostered public participation in most or all of the steps in the scientific process (8). However, due to the professionalization of science, the role of the amateur scientist has diminished (8). The value of public participation in addressing environmental and health issues has received renewed attention in the past couple of decades through efforts such as public participation in scientific research (PPSR)/ citizen science (12), community based participatory research (CBPR) (13), popular epidemiology (14), and street science (15).

Public participation in scientific research, often termed citizen science, is a form of informal science education, and is broadly defined as a partnership between scientists and non-scientists in which authentic data are collected, shared, and analyzed (12, 16, 17). Citizen science projects are meant to increase a participant's scientific literacy (12), to collect field data to monitor a variety of environmental conditions (7), and as a framework to support and enhance decision-making in modern society (17, 18). Previous research in science education and sociology has demonstrated the need to engage communities in scientific research and that this level of engagement can be successfully facilitated via community-academic partnerships. Members of a community neighboring a contaminated site are typically intrinsically motivated to learn more about the issues regarding the contaminated site in their community and in most cases, have already begun to gather additional scientific data hypothesize other potential routes of exposure and areas that need additional monitoring. Research related to inquiry-based education has elucidated how people have a greater motivation to engage and learn when the subject matter is directly related to their lives and if the learning process is interactive (19). Popular epidemiology, a community-driven practice, was proposed after observing the activities of communities experiencing contamination and entails community initiation of investigations, gathering of scientific knowledge, and, if necessary, recruiting of scientific professionals (14). "Street Science" is an approach for environmental health justice that joins local knowledge with professional techniques, re-values forms of knowledge that professional science has traditionally excluded (15).

To date, only a limited number of co-created PPSR projects, which are jointly developed by members of the public and scientists and designed to actively involve community members in most or all steps of the scientific process, have been initiated at contaminated sites and none in conjunction with risk communication as described herein. This paper will outline the methods and activities employed to build a community-academic partnership that resulted in the co-created citizen science project entitled *Gardenroots: The Dewey-Humboldt, Arizona Garden Project* (hereafter, *Gardenroots*). In order to foster PPSR, it is essential to establish a community–academic partnership via a CBPR approach to research, which shares power with community partners in all aspects of the research process and benefits communities via interventions and policy change (13).

The enhanced CBPR approach presented herein is based upon the belief that PPSR in conjunction with CBPR can improve site assessment and risk communication efforts. Public participation can be a vehicle to address concerns regarding environmental contaminants and exposure routes that might not be addressed in a typical expert-only-led site and risk assessment. Lastly, PPSR provides a unique opportunity for informal science education and for the community to learn more about environmental science, human health research, and risk assessment.

METHODS

The Gardenroots approach followed recommended CBPR practices (13). The co-created citizen science project will be described in terms of PPSR (see Table 1), demonstrating community involvement in most phases of the research (12). The traditional CBPR/PPSR steps have been enhanced and the methods described herein also include: building a transdisciplinary team, bidirectional communication with government agencies, an informal science education learning continuum, and a substantial risk communication component. Lastly, this project received Institutional Review Board approval.

Background

Gardening and consuming edible plants grown in contaminated soils presents a health hazard that may affect home gardeners neighboring contaminated environments. The town of Dewey-Humboldt is in an arsenic endemic region of Arizona and is adjacent to the Iron King Mine and Humboldt Smelter Superfund site (Iron King). The site serves as a persistent source of pollution, introducing a host of potential human-health risks and concomitant risk communication challenges. Such contamination (natural or human-made) can affect humans directly via the inadvertent consumption of soils, through the consumption of crops grown under contaminated conditions, and/or the consumption of contaminated water.

How a research program can respond to a community research need

Beginning in 2007, the University of Arizona (UA) Superfund Research Program Research Translation Coordinator (UASRP-RTC) and the USEPA Region 9 Superfund and Technology Liaison began executing a two-pronged communication mechanism consisting of a webinar hosted by National Institute of Environmental Sciences (NIEHS) and USEPA and a "Live at R9" in-person seminar to foster regional partnerships (20). During a "Live at R9" visit in June of 2007, an USEPA project manager mentioned that an abandoned mining site located in rural Arizona would be added to the NPL and that UA and EPA might be able to assist in some capacity at the site. The USEPA kept the UASRP-RTC up-to-date on the status of the site and on August 3, 2008 the Iron King Mine Superfund site was listed on the NPL. On August 20, 2008, the USEPA organized their first community "Kick-Off Meeting" after the official listing to discuss the Superfund process and that they were initiating the field investigation portion of the Remedial Investigation and Feasibility Study. Forty-six community members, two members of UASRP-RTC, the USEPA Project Manager and Community Involvement Coordinator, a member of the Arizona Department of Environmental Quality, and the Dewey-Humboldt mayor attended the meeting.

During the meeting, several community members asked whether the site has impacted their soil and if they may continue to grow vegetables. At the end of the meeting, members of the Dewey-Humboldt, community specifically asked the UASRP-RTC "Is it safe to garden and consume vegetables from my home garden? And if so, how much can I eat from my garden?" Without any specific data to conclusively answer the question, a representative of the UASRP-RTC, stated that she was interested in this research question as well, and whether they (the people who expressed concern) were interested in participating in a research project. Residents agreed and in less than two years an academic-community partnership came into fruition that took the form of a co-created citizen science project, *Gardenroots*. The goals of *Gardenroots* were to bring scientists from various disciplines together within the UA and to work in collaboration with the affected community to: (1) determine the uptake of arsenic in garden vegetables grown by the Dewey-Humboldt, AZ community, and (2) conduct an exposure assessment and characterize the potential risk posed by gardening and consuming vegetables from residential home gardens.

Establishing a community academic partnership

The community members who originally posed the research question and the lead UA investigator became the point of contact and "champions" (21) for the research project within their affiliations. They were persistent, promoted the project, and networked to obtain the involvement of a broader representation of residents in the area. In addition, the UA Investigator made a point to maintain a consistent presence in the community by attending town council, USEPA meetings and community events and was in the area at a minimum frequency of once every two months throughout the duration of *Gardenroots*. It was this type of promotion and dedication that truly fused and generated the community-academic partnership. In addition to promotion, continuity is crucial. To date, the RTC continues to maintain bidirectional communication between the community, EPA, Arizona Department of Environmental Quality (ADEQ), Arizona Department of Health Services, and Agency for Toxic Substances and Disease Registry, via teleconferences and meetings to ensure transparency and unified messaging to the community.

Building a research team

A transdisciplinary team was created involving the Dewey-Humboldt community and the UA including researchers in the disciplines of environmental chemistry and microbiology, soils, hydrology, public health, and visual communications. The UA Cooperative Extension Director of Yavapai County was recruited as part of the team to provide home gardening expertise. Interactions with USEPA Region 9 representatives were ongoing to ensure that this research question was aligned with their current research challenges at the Iron King site.

Building a co-created citizen science research program: public participation in environmental research

As stated above, the UA Investigator maintained a consistent presence in the community by attending town council, USEPA and community meetings and events and was frequently in the Dewey–Humboldt area. Through the continuity of community engagement, the UA investigator built trust and learned a great deal about the nuances and idiosyncrasies of the area. This knowledge facilitated implementation of a place-based communication strategy (22) to recruit other community members into *Gardenroots*. The recruitment and design of recruitment and educational materials was informed by the social context and community ecology of Dewey-Humboldt, Arizona. The majority of the recruitment for *Gardenroots* was done via personal interaction at local community events through the following activities:

- Handing out informational bookmarks (Figure 1) at community festivals, EPA community meetings, and Town Council meetings.
- Follow-up mailings, telephone calls and emails to community members
- A County Cooperative Extension Press Release
- An announcement in the Dewey-Humboldt town newsletter
- A website

Greenhouse study

Collecting soils from a residential area in Dewey-Humboldt, AZ was fundamental to conducting the controlled greenhouse study. Since the USEPA had already begun the site investigation, members of the community had been given their residential soil results. Based on their results, a community member offered their soils for the greenhouse study and assisted in identifying the appropriate locations to collect soils in their yard based upon the USEPA data and their understanding of the neighboring watershed. In addition, this community member provided detailed historical information regarding their property and the Superfund site areas of interest.

Field study

After all recruitment activities discussed above were completed, those who signed up for *Gardenroots* were asked to attend a 1.5-hour training session wherein they were provided information on how to properly collect soil, water, and vegetables samples from their home garden for laboratory analysis. Two trainings were formally offered and community members that participated in the training took home an instructional manual (Figure 2A) and a tool kit with all supplies required for sample collection from their home garden. Several community members were unable to attend a scheduled training. An additional less formal training was offered and in some instances, kits were personally delivered to community member's homes at their request.

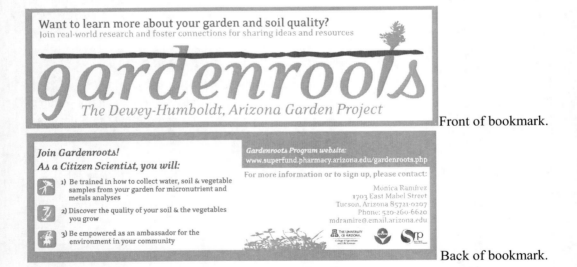

Figure 1. Front and back of promotional bookmark distributed at community events to recruit gardeners.

Table 1. The components of Gardenroots: The Dewey-Humboldt, Arizona Garden Project

Steps in Scientific Research	Participant Participation	Community Roles and Benefits	Challenges Associated with Step
Choose or define question(s) for study	√	• Community members posed research question at the EPA Superfund Site Kick Off Meeting in August 2008	• It took a year to secure funding for the project
Gather information and resources	√	• Community member provided soils for greenhouse study • Yavapai and Pima County Master Gardeners in the area assisted with what to grown in the greenhouse. • Participants were asked to describe how he or she amends their soils.	• Reaching all community members in the area interested in vegetable gardening
Develop explanations (hypotheses)	√	• At trainings, community members developed hypotheses regarding what they expected to observe in their household results and for the entire study. For example, several participants hypothesized that the closer to the tailings a home was, the higher the arsenic concentration would be in the soils.	• Setting and maintaining expectations. It was important to restate goals and what type of data could truly be expected from *Gardenroots*. • Explaining that the number of samples was not sufficient to truly characterize the spatial distribution of arsenic as well as the complexity and uncertainty related to the atmospheric distribution of arsenic. • For example, wind direction in the area changes seasonally, the area has naturally occurring arsenic and has been affected by both smelting and mine tailings, which produce different sized particles that can experience different levels of transport by wind.
Design data collection methodologies	√	• Participants decided where to collect soils from their residential property (garden and yard) and what vegetables they wanted analyzed	• Since there was not one predetermined vegetable grown in every garden, it was challenging to compare across households. Regardless, it was important to have participants grow what they wanted to make sure the study was relevant and applicable to everyone. • Explaining that the one area they sampled might not be representative of their entire yard and that arsenic soil concentrations may vary in a relatively small spatial area.
Collect samples and/or record data	√	• Participants collected their soil, vegetable and irrigation samples	• No major challenges to report.

Table 1. (Continued)

Steps in Scientific Research	Participant Participation	Community Roles and Benefits	Challenges Associated with Step
		• Participants labeled all samples	
Analyze samples	x	• Community did not participate in this step, although at community gatherings, analytical methodology was described in great detail	• Due to the nature of the sample analyses and formal laboratory procedures, the participants did not get to prepare their samples via acid digestion or analyze samples via inductively coupled plasma mass spectrometry.
Analyze data	x	• Community did not participate in this step, UA investigator analyzed all the data. • At the "Results for Lunch" and other community gatherings, the methods and mathematical equations used to interpret the data was described in great detail and participants were given the opportunity to recalculate their potential exposure and risk and change the variables to suit their behavior.	• No challenges to report.
Interpret data and draw conclusions	√	• Participants were given the results from their individual soil, water, and vegetable samples, exposure assessment and risk characterization results. • At community gatherings and meetings, the aggregated results were presented	• Determining whether their soil and water arsenic concentrations may be due to naturally occurring and/or from anthropogenic sources like the mine and smelter.
Disseminate conclusions/translate results into action	√	• Participants shared data with others outside of the *Gardenroots* project • Using their data, participants have translated the results into personal action and have modified their gardening practices.	• Even though *Gardenroots* informed and invited USEPA and ADEQ to all report-back and community events, it was challenging to maintain bidirectional communication between the project and all government agencies working at the site.
Discuss results and ask new questions	√	• At the "Results for Lunch" and other community gatherings, results were discussed in detail, participants compared their results to their neighbors and friends and new questions were posed.	• Since *Gardenroots* was an environmental monitoring project, inquiries regarding potential health outcomes were outside the feasibility of *Gardenroots*. In these cases, the expectations and goals of *Gardenroots* were restated and the inquiries were forwarded to health scientists at the UA.

During the five-month period from when participants received their kit and during the Spring/Summer growing season, participants were asked to deliver their samples to the local Cooperative Extension office. The in-person training, designing a user-friendly manual, and collaborating with the local extension office assured sample quality. In the end, participants actively contributed to the field study portion of *Gardenroots*. Table 1 outlines the steps in scientific research, level of public participation, the community's role and benefits, and challenges associated with each step.

Capacity building and continuity

In order to properly and effectively manage community expectation and involvement throughout the entire *Gardenroots* project (from the posing of the research question to the final community report-back events), ongoing communication was maintained via phone, email and mail correspondence, and informal science educational experiences were offered. Based upon what the community wanted to learn, and in efforts to further understand their concerns regarding the Iron King site, the *Gardenroots* Learning Continuum was designed to provide participants with responsive, unique, and informal learning opportunities (Figure 2) throughout the course of the *Gardenroots* project. *Gardenroots* culminated in a large report-back gathering "Results for Lunch: Your Soil, Water and Vegetable Outcomes" (Results for Lunch). After the Results for Lunch gathering (Figure 2B), participants requested an overall summary of results and presentations that would be open to the broader community. In response, three additional presentations were given and a "Summary of Results" booklet was generated and distributed to participants and other community members in the Dewey-Humboldt, Arizona area.. In addition to the *Gardenroots* Learning Continuum, and as stated in the Field Study section above, participants were actively involved in most steps of the scientific process (Table 1) and this high level of participation was instrumental in building capacity and maintaining continuity.

Risk communication

Once all community samples had been analyzed, results were reported back to the participants to answer questions such as: Can I consume vegetables from my garden? If so, how much is safe? To do this, participants were invited to the Results for Lunch gathering, where they were given an informal presentation on the: 1) methodologies used to prepare and analyze their household samples, 2) exposure assessment and risk characterization calculations used to interpret their data, and 3) an introduction to the format in which their results would be presented. Next, they were given tailored personalized booklets (Figure 2B) that contained the "raw" confidential data (i.e., milligrams of arsenic per kilogram of vegetable) as well as a table that outlined the quantity of vegetables they could consume at various target risk levels compared to the US Department of Agriculture recommended amounts (Supplemental Fig. 1). It is important to emphasize that intake rates based on the site-specific characteristics of their individual garden were calculated for each participant to consider. Additionally, the concentrations observed in the vegetables were compared to the concentrations of arsenic reported in the U.S. Food and Drug Administration Total Diet Study Statistics on Element Results based on the 2006–2008 Market Basket Study.

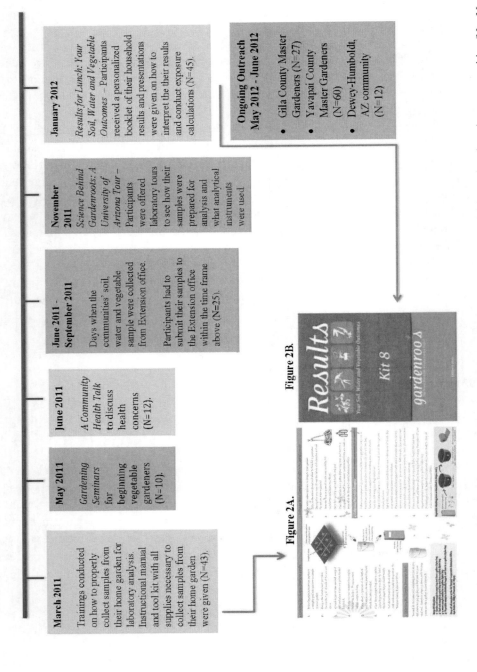

Figure 2. *Gardenroots* Learning Continuum and collection times. The time line demonstrates the activities and co-learning opportunities (N = Number of participants at each event) provided throughout the program.

The Market Baskets Study involved purchasing samples of food throughout the U.S., preparing the food as it would be consumed, and analyzing the foods to measure the concentrations of selected elements and compounds. This provided a valuable frame of reference and is considered an acceptable risk comparison (5). This reporting method was designed to give participants all the information they requested and allow them to decide for themselves the target risk they wanted to achieve (Table 2).

Table 2. Comparing report-back efforts and what information *Gardenroots* participants were provided throughout the project

Typical participant questions about personal exposure results, Brody et al., 2007	Information provided to *Gardenroots* participants
Description	
What did you find?[1] What did you look for?	Concentration of arsenic (contaminant of concern) and 19 other elements of potential interest
How much?[1]	Concentrations for all 20 elements were presented in a chart for all their vegetables, soil and water samples analyzed.
Analysis/Comparison	
Is that high?[1]	Arsenic concentrations observed in vegetables from the USDFA Market Basket Study were used for comparison. Regional soil screening levels and the maximum contaminant levels in water was provided.
Is that safe?[1]	Chart exhibiting how much of the vegetable can be consumed from their garden at various excess target risks
What should I focus on?	Participants were able to compare the risk posed from each exposure route (water, soil, vegetable) and the arsenic concentration in each vegetable to then decide where to focus mitigation efforts
Where did the chemical come from?	Participants identified their gardens as potential sources of arsenic and initially asked the research question
Recommendation	
What can/should I do?[1]	Exposure reduction/precautionary strategies were provided such as: recommended gardening practices handouts were generated to guide gardeners, "Arizona Know Your Water" and "Arizona Know Your Well Water" guides*

[1] These question were also posed by the Dewey-Humboldt, AZ community in the initial stages and of the study. All report back materials were designed to provide answers to participant's specific questions and coincide with those observed by Brody et al., 2007.

* All handouts and guides were distributed at community gatherings and are available at: http://www.superfund.pharmacy.arizona.edu/projects/community-engaged-research/gardenroots/home.

The risk associated with consumption of garden vegetables was also compared to risks associated with other potential exposure routes, such as ingestion of potable water and incidental soil. It was strongly recommended that home gardeners: sample their private wells regularly, test their soils prior to gardening, and modify their gardening behavior to reduce incidental soil ingestion (23). Based upon these findings, three waterproof handouts were developed to disseminate the recommended behavioral modifications necessary to reduce arsenic exposure from incidental soil ingestion and vegetable consumption (Supplemental Figure 4, available at http://superfund.pharmacy.arizona.edu/projects/community-engaged-research/gardenroots/home).

RESULTS

Forty-three individuals attended the training and received a *Gardenroots* toolkit and instructional manual, 58% or 25 participants actually completed the *Gardenroots* project, and of the participants, 18 completed the survey. Eighty-four percent of the population has some type of education beyond high school, 44% had been living in the area for 8 or more years, and 94% of the participants were Caucasian (Supplemental Table 1). Based on the most recent US Census Bureau, the demographics are reflective of the area, except 28% of the *Gardenroots* participants had a bachelor's degree or higher compared to 13.5% for the general population.

Outcomes

It has been suggested that citizen science learning outcomes can best be evaluated by observing three levels: individual learning, programmatic, and community-level outcomes (24). This is very similar to the evaluation strategies used to report CBPR program successes in the Northern California Household Exposure Study (25) and in 54 National Institute of Environmental Health Sciences funded environmental justice projects (26). Below, we apply this new framework and describe the results and outcomes of the *Gardenroots* project.

Individual learning outcomes – what community members learned and new research questions posed

The results of *Gardenroots* indicated that for the Dewey-Humboldt community mitigating arsenic exposure from potable water and incidental soil ingestion (not even considering vegetable consumption) would significantly reduce daily arsenic intake. The challenge in communicating these results was the fear that the participants, realizing that their water and soil arsenic levels were high, would no longer want to garden or consume vegetables from their garden, regardless of the comparatively low arsenic exposure from their raw vegetables. Fortunately, the majority of the participants stated that they would continue to eat home-garden vegetables, but would modify their gardening practices. This demonstrates that the scientific findings were understood and that the community could put into action behavioral changes necessary to reduce their arsenic exposure from water and soil. This capacity demonstrated by participants is similar to what has been previously reported, where community members demonstrated a capacity to understand and contend with the complexity and uncertainty associated with the results (27).

Analysis of individual learning also showed that *Gardenroots* prompted curiosity and an increased understanding of soil contamination, food quality, and the scientific process. Several participants asked to have their chicken eggs sampled to determine the concentrations of arsenic and heavy metals. They hypothesized that the deaths of some of their chickens were due to the arsenic and heavy metal concentrations observed in their potable water, soil, and vegetables Further, they wanted to determine if there was a correlation between the exposure pathways and the concentrations found in the eggs. Another participant inquired whether cinder blocks in a raised garden bed contributed arsenic to their soil, and if samples from the local river or the soil from a local farm had been tested. Participants' questions were answered and the chicken eggs were analyzed. Results were reported back to the participants, who then shared the results with others. These inquiries signify the increase in capacity within the community and could also constitute a community-level outcome.

When comparing report-back methodologies by Brody et al. (2007) and those used for *Gardenroots*, one can observe many similarities in what participants want to know and how to make the information meaningful for action (see Table 2). In summary, the UA scientists learned the importance of reporting individual results with an understanding of what people want and need to know to guide action, as witnessed in other studies (29). Additionally, it is important to present specific steps that the community can take to assert some level of control in their lives and methods in which they can implement to reduce their exposure to potential environmental hazards (5).

Programmatic outcomes

The *Gardenroots* project has contributed to the fields of environmental science, environmental health, and research translation. Currently, there is limited information regarding combined arsenic exposure from water, soil, and homegrown vegetables neighboring hazardous waste sites. This PPSR project has improved understanding of: 1) the uptake of arsenic in common homegrown vegetables grown in soils near a mining site (28); and 2) the amount of arsenic introduced to an individual via the ingestion of homegrown vegetables, soils (incidental), and water, and potential risks posed by those exposure routes (23). This data has been published and demonstrates that community members can successfully participate in environmental science investigations. Lastly, *Gardenroots* participants reviewed this manuscript to ensure the integrity of the project and representation of the partnership.

Community-level outcomes – redefining the question and policy implications

Gardenroots increased social capital and community capacity by serving as a platform for participants to learn more about environmental contamination in general and the Iron King site. It was a catalyst to generate environmental communication efforts amongst the participants and the rest of the community. As a result, participants increased their community networking in resource-related issues and participated in other resource-related projects. Based on conversations with participants, there was interest in leveraging the results to pressure government officials to take action and be more stringent in their cleanup efforts. This is similar to other work in contaminated areas (27).

For example, the *Gardenroots* project revealed that the local public water system was serving water that exceeded the arsenic drinking water standard (0.010 mg/L). *Gardenroots* participants worked together to identify and notify additional households that were connected to the public water supply. They also reported their test results to USEPA and ADEQ, advocating that this issue needed to be addressed (*Gardenroots* also notified and sent the results to the USEPA). As a result, the municipal water suppler was issued seven Notices of Violation by the ADEQ, one for exceeding the arsenic drinking water standard. In the words of a *Gardenroots* participant: "The people in Humboldt served by Humboldt Water System are deeply indebted to Mrs. Ramirez-Andreotta's study which served to reveal a serious problem with the municipal water." Additionally, arsenic concentrations in water exceeded the drinking water standard for several participants who rely solely on their private wells for potable water. UA personnel worked closely with those households to provide information regarding water treatment technologies that could be implemented to reduce their arsenic concentrations. Now, the community is reporting that they are regularly testing their private wells, and are pressuring ADEQ to ensure that water entering their home is at or below the arsenic drinking water standard.

Furthermore, *Gardenroots* built trust between the UA scientists and the Dewey-Humboldt, Arizona community. This trust has set the groundwork for a long-term community-academic partnership. Due to the efforts discussed above, three additional research projects have been initiated to address pressing remediation and characterization challenges posed by the Iron King site. For example, the Metals Exposure Study in Homes was designed to determine the levels of metal exposure in children ages 1-11 years. Two former Gardenroots participants have been hired as UA employees to be part of the local field team. This is evidence that the Gardenroots community-academic partnership has enhanced social capital and community capacity and has even had a small economic impact in the community. Lastly, the Metals Exposure Study in Homes established a community advisory board to guide the research endeavor, maintaining the community-academic partnership.

DISCUSSION

Several limitations were observed throughout the project and these are also presented in table 1. First, setting and maintaining the expectations was a challenging. For example, *Gardenroots* could provide environmental monitoring and potential soil, water and vegetable exposure data, but could not provide specific data related to health outcomes. It was important to restate the goals and what type of data could truly be expected from the project. Second, due to the nature of the sample analyses and formal laboratory procedures, the participants did not get to prepare and analyze their own samples. In response, participants were invited to a laboratory tour called "The Science Behind *Gardenroots*" at the UA to learn the methodologies. Unfortunately, the attendance was low, and this was most likely due to the travel distance (~200 miles) and large time commitment. Lastly, even though *Gardenroots* informed the USEPA and ADEQ on all activities, it was challenging to maintain bidirectional communication between the *Gardenroots* project leader and all government agencies working at the site. At one point, EPA did not agree with the communication methodology, was uncomfortable with a few community member's responses and activism (Ramirez-Andreotta et al., forthcoming).

Reflecting on the process

Gardenroots satisfied the concepts of a co-created citizen (co-created PPSR) project based upon the level of participation throughout the scientific research process (Table 1), as compared to a contributory project (where participants solely collect samples) or a collaborative project (were participants may be involved in five or more additional steps) (12). In addition, *Gardenroots* was a CBPR project that, as originally outline by Israel et al., 1998, recognized the community as an unit of identity, facilitated collaborative, equitable involvement of all partners in most phases of the research, integrated knowledge and intervention for mutual benefit of all partners, promoted a co-learning and empowering process, and disseminated findings and knowledge gained to all partners. There are more components involved in CBPR, but not all projects require or are functionally set up to involve each and every component. It is important to be flexible and adapt to what is actually feasible, while successfully meeting and maintaining the expectations of the community-academic partnership.

In addition to describing risk, practitioners must also put the risk into perspective and in terms of consumption behavior. Converting the raw risk data into a personalized, more relatable format, specifically the quantity of vegetables they could consume at various target risks, and comparing this exposure route to water and soil ingestion was instrumental in translating the *Gardenroots* results. It is recommended that participants be given all of their personal data to review so that they can then decide for themselves which risk level is comfortable for them. This act can also facilitate inquiry and knowledge synthesis where participants compare and combine the results with their existing knowledge, furthering their inquiry-based learning.

Location	Target Risk 1/1,000,000	Target Risk 1/100,000	Target Risk 1/10,000	USDA Recommended Amount (cups/week)
Onion				
Your Garden	3/4	7	70	4 cups/week total of "Other Vegetables"
Lettuce				
Your Garden	1/2	5	50	3 cups/week total of "Raw Leafy Dark Green Vegetables"
Tomato				
Your Garden	1-1/2	15	150	5 cups/week of red and orange vegetables

This is just an example; no actual community member results are shown.

Supplemental Figure 1. Amount you can eat from your garden based on a varying cancer target risk. An example of the risk communication and graphical layout selected to inform and properly answer the research question posed by the community: "How much can I eat from my garden?"

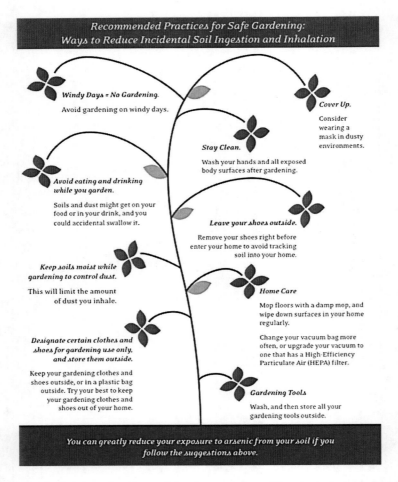

Supplemental Figure 2. An example of one of the three waterproof handouts that were made to disseminate the recommended behavioral modifications necessary to reduce arsenic exposure.

Public participation methods have been used for a few exposure assessment and health studies, but not in conjunction with risk communication at a Superfund site. This case study demonstrates that risk communication efforts can be effective when the affected community is involved in the research project and in determining the content of the risk analysis. In addition, evaluating program outcomes at the individual, programmatic, and community levels is a useful and creative way to capture the successes of citizen science and community-academic partnerships. In summary, the project design clearly justifies public participation in scientific research projects, may influence national policy regarding environmental science education practices for the general public, and definitely redefines who may generate environmental monitoring data in site assessments.

Acknowledgments

The authors would like to give a special thanks to all the Gardenroots participants for their participation and assistance in the project and for reviewing this manuscript. Additionally, the authors would like to thank the town of Dewey-Humboldt, Arizona, Dewey-Humboldt Town Librarian, Jeff Schalau, UA Yavapai Cooperative Extension Director, Mike Kopplin (UA Superfund Research Program's Hazard Identification Core) and Dr. Atasi Ray-Maitra (UA Water Quality Laboratory). Lastly, thank you to Phil Brown for his comments on this manuscript.

This research was funded by the US EPA Office of Research and Development and NIEHS' Superfund Research Program (Grant P42 ES04940). The first author gratefully acknowledges financial support by the NASA Space Grant Program, UA TRIF Water Sustainability Program, and the Alfred P. Sloan Foundation that funds the National Action Council for Minorities in Engineering Scholarship program.

LIST OF ACRONYMS

US Environmental Protection Agency	USEPA
National Priorities List	NPL
Community based participatory research	CBPR
Public participation in scientific research	PPSR
University of Arizona Superfund Research Program Research Translation Coordinator	UASRP-RTC
National Institute of Environmental Sciences	NIEHS
The Universality of Arizona	UA
Arizona Department of Environmental Quality	ADEQ
Iron King Mine and Humboldt Smelter Superfund Site	Iron King

REFERENCES

[1] Brown P, Mikkelsen EJ. No safe place. Toxic waste, leukemia, and community action. Berkeley, CA: University California Press, 1990.

[2] National Research Council. Alternatives for managing the nation's complex contaminated groundwater sites. Washington, DC: National Academy Press, 2012.

[3] Chess C, Purchell K. Public participation and the environment. Do we know what works? Environ Sci Technol 1999; 30(16): 2685-92.

[4] Cox R. Environmental communication and the public sphere. Thosand Oaks, CA: Sage, 2013.

[5] Galvez MP, Peters R, Graber N, Forman J. Effective risk communication in children's environmental health. Lessons learned from 9/11. Pediatr Clin North Am 2007; 54: 33-46.

[6] Senier L, Hudson B, Fort S, Hoover E, Tillson R, Brown P. The Brown Superfund Research Program. A multistakeholder partnership addresses real-world problems in contaminated communities. Environ Sci Technol 2008; 42(13): 4655-62.

[7] Silbertown J. A new dawn for citizen science. Trends Ecol Evol 2009; 24(9): 467-71.

[8] Miller-Rushing A, Primack R, Bonney R. The history of public participation in ecological research. Front Ecol Environ 2012; 10(6)285-90.

[9] Thoits PA, Hewitt LN. Volunteer work and well-being. J Health Soc Behav 2001; 42: 115–31.

[10] Wilson J, Musick M. The effects of volunteering on the volunteer. Law Contemp Probl 1999; 62(4): 141–68.

[11] Flemming W. Volunteer watershed health monitoring by local stakeholders. New MexicoWatershed Watch. J Environ Educ 2003; 35(1): 27–32.

[12] Bonney R, Ballard H, Jordan R, McCallie E, Phillips T, Shirk J, Wilderman CC. Public Participation in Scientific Research: Defining the Field and Assessing Its Potential for Informal Science Education. Washington, DC: Center Advancement Informal Science Education (CAISE), 2009.
[13] Israel BA, Schulz AJ, Parker EA, Becker AB. Review of community-based research. Assessing partnership approaches to improve public health. Annu Rev Public Health 1998; 19: 173–202.
[14] Brown P. Popular epidemiology and toxic waste contamination. Lay and professional ways of knowing. J Health Soc Behav 1992; 33(3): 267-81.
[15] Corburn J. Street science. Community knowledge and environmental health justice. CAmbridge, MA: MIT Press, 2005.
[16] Brossard D, Lewenstein B, Bonney R. Scientific knowledge and attitude change. The impact of a citizen science project. Int J Sci Educ 2005; 27(9): 1099–121.
[17] Evans C, Abrams E, Reitsma R, Roux K, Salmonsen L, Marra PP. The Neighborhood Nestwatch Program. Participant outcomes of a citizen science ecological research project. Conservation Biol 2005; 19(3): 589-94.
[18] Trumbull DJ, Bonney R, Bascom D, Cabral A. Thinking scientifically during participation in a citizen-science project. Sci Educ 2000; 84: 265–75.
[19] Falk JH, Storksdieck M, Dierking LD. Investigating public science interest and understanding. Evidence for the importance of free-choice learning. Public Underst Sci 2007; 16: 455-69.
[20] Ramirez-Andreotta MD, Brusseau ML, Artiola JF, Maier RM, Gandolfi AJ. Environmental research translation. Enhancing interactions with communities at contaminated sites, forthcoming.
[21] Gallagher DR. Advocates for environmental justice. The role of the champion in public participation. Local Environ 2009; 14(10): 905-16.
[22] Green L, Fullilove M, Evans D, Shepard P. "Hey, Mom, thanks!" Use of focus groups in the development of place-specific materials for a community environmental action campaign. Environ Health Perspect 2002; 110(2): 265–9.
[23] Ramirez-Andreotta MD, Brusseau ML, Beamer P, Maier RM. Home gardening near a mining site in an arsenic-endemic region of Arizona. Assessing arsenic exposure and risk via ingestion of home garden vegetables, soils and potable water. Sci Total Environ 2013; 454-455: 373–82.
[24] Jordan RC, Ballard HL, Phillips TB. Key issues and new approaches for evaluating citizen-science learning outcomes. Front Ecol Environ 2012; 10(6): 307-9.
[25] Brown P, Brody JG, Morello-Forsch R, Tovar J, Zota AR, Rudel RA. Measuring the success of community science. The Northern California Household Exposure Study. Environ Health Perspect 2012; 120(3): 326-31.
[26] Baron S, Sinclair R, Payne-Sturges D, Phelps J, Zenick H, Collman GW, et al. Partnerships for environmental and occupational justice. Contributions to research, capacity and public health. Am J Public Health 2009; 99(Suppl 3): S517–25.
[27] Adams C, Brown P, Morello-Frosch R, Brody JG, Rudel R, Zota A, et al. Disentangling the exposure experience. The roles of community context and report-back of environmental exposure data. J Health Soc Behav 2011; 52(2): 180–96.
[28] Ramirez-Andreotta MD, Brusseau ML, Artiola JF, Maier RM. A greenhouse and field-based study to determine the accumulation of arsenic in common homegrown vegetables. Sci Total Environ 2013; 433: 299-306.
[29] Brody JG, Morello-Frosch R, Brown P, Rudel RA, Altman RG, Frye M, et al. Improving disclosure and consent: "is it safe?": new ethics for reporting personal exposures to environmental chemicals. Am J Public Health 2007; 97(9): 1547-54.

In: Public Health Yearbook 2015
Editor: Joav Merrick

ISBN: 978-1-63484-514-4
© 2016 Nova Science Publishers, Inc.

Chapter 14

COMMUNITY-ENGAGED RESEARCH AND HOMELESS ADOLESCENTS: CAPTURING PERCEPTIONS OF HEALTH CARE AND BUILDING LASTING RELATIONSHIPS WITH THE COMMUNITY

Ricky T Munoz[1],, JD, MSW, Jeremy S Aragon[2], MSW, and Mark D Fox[1], MD, PhD, MPH*

[1]Center for Health Outcomes and Improvement Research, University of Oklahoma, School of Community Medicine, Section of Medicine/Pediatrics, Department of Pediatrics, Oklahoma, United States of America

[2]Anne and Henry Zarrow School of Social Work, University of Oklahoma, Tulsa, Oklahoma, United States of America

Research has demonstrated that homeless adolescents have poorer health than their housed counterparts. We theorize that poor health outcomes are partially related to the perceptions homeless adolescents have of receiving care and the adverse effects of those perceptions on health seeking behaviors. Objective: To report on homeless adolescents perceptions regarding obtaining health care and to use the data to expand care for the homeless adolescent community whom we sampled. Participants: English-speaking adolescents aged 16-24 years who were receiving services from a homeless adolescent outreach agency located in the south central United States. Methods: Community-engaged qualitative research consisting of semi-structured interviews and focus groups. The narrative data from our focus groups and individual interviews were analyzed for content that was grouped into themes. Results: 30 adolescents participated, with 21 electing focus groups and 9 electing individual interviews. Themes include 1) homeless adolescents report feeling dehumanized when receiving health care; 2) the dehumanizing effect is related to the profit driven structure of the US Health Care System; 3) homeless adolescents react to dehumanizing care by avoiding care or turning to informal care networks; and 4) active efforts are needed by health care providers to gain the trust of homeless adolescents. Conclusion: The perception among homeless adolescents that

---

* Corresponding author: Ricky T Munoz, JD, MSW, University of Oklahoma – Tulsa, 4502 East 41st Street, Tulsa, Oklahoma 74135, United States. E-mail: rmunoz@ou.edu.

receiving health care is dehumanizing may be a contributing factor to poorer health outcomes for this population. We conclude with a discussion of how we translated results into practice with our community of interest consistent with the principals of community engaged research.

Keywords: homeless adolescents, community-engaged research, health care delivery

INTRODUCTION

According to the most recent US federal data, nearly 1.7 million adolescents annually experience a "runaway/thrown away" episode, resulting in homelessness or placing them "at risk" for homelessness (1). It is well established that homelessness is associated with poorer health, with homeless adolescents exhibiting disproportionately higher rates of illegal substance abuse, sexually transmitted infections, unwanted pregnancies, mental illness, and insufficient access to health care than housed adolescents (2-6).

Many of such poor health outcomes are a logical consequence of the conditions of homelessness, such as poor nutrition and hygiene, crowding, violence, and the need for survival sex (3, 5).

The social and environmental determinants of poor health for homeless adolescents are complex, with comprehensive solutions being a matter of public policy beyond what can be affected solely in clinical settings. Nevertheless, despite the seemingly intransigent barriers to good health for homeless adolescents, we believe there is room for health care providers to mediate the impact of these barriers by creating better models of health care delivery. Our goal with our current effort was to use community engaged research to develop a testable theory on the relationship between the perceptions of homeless adolescents of health care delivery and the impact of those perceptions on homeless adolescents' health seeking behavior. Our goal was to create transferable principals that can be used by other practitioners in the development improved models of health care delivery uniquely suited for homeless adolescents.

METHODS

We employed a community-engaged research model to engage homeless adolescents in contributing to the development of a new program for health care delivery to meet their unique needs. Community-engaged research has been championed as a method to further reduce health inequalities, (7) through emphasizing the development of lasting relationships between researchers and the community of interest (8, 9). To that end, we spent time throughout the research process cultivating a lasting relationship with the staff and clients of a street outreach program of a local social services agency. Our goal from our community engaged approach was not simply to collect data; while data collection was important, we also wanted to simultaneously demonstrate our commitment to addressing health issues of the local homeless adolescent population through the development of programs that arose directly from our research. Thus, our data were intended to serve not only academic purposes, but to provide an immediate benefit to the homeless adolescents we sampled.

Sampling

Study participants included clients (ages 16-24 years) receiving services from the homeless adolescent program of a social services agency in medium-sized city in the south-central United States. All participants were identified by the partnering agency as either homeless or "at risk" for homelessness. Potential participants were informed of the nature of the study and invited to participate in either focus groups or individual interviews based on individual preference. Participants were provided a consent information sheet that explained the the purpose of the study was to gauge the perceptions of homeless adolescents regarding health care for their community. Participants were offered a $10 gift card for their time and modest refreshments. Consent was expressed through their participation in either a focus group that lasted 60-90 minutes or an individual interview that ranged from 30-60 minutes. The study protocol was approved by the Institutional Review Board of the University of Oklahoma Health Sciences Center.

Focus groups and individual interviews were semi-structured to promote conversational, two-way communication (10). Researchers followed question guidelines based on community- and health-related themes, but were free to follow conversation trajectories based on topics that participating adolescents deemed significant. As part of our philosophy of community engagement, the question guides were reviewed by agency staff prior to implementation and agency staff participated in focus groups and interviews when they desired. All focus groups and interviews were conducted in English.

Thirty adolescents, 19 males and 11 females, met our sampling criteria and completed the study. Of those 30, 21 elected to participate in focus groups and 9 choose individual interviews. The mean age of participants was 20.3 years of age the gender make-up consisting of 65% male and 35% female. Race distribution was 50% White, 28% African American, 11% Multi-racial, 5% American Indian /Alaskan Native, 3% Hispanic, and 3% other.

Analysis

All focus groups and individual interviews were audio-recorded, transcribed, and supplemented by notes taken by the research team. Once transcription was completed, NVIVO software was used to perform a content analysis to group the narrative data into themes. The final decision regarding the total number of interviews was made according to the principal of saturation, with sampling discontinued once we made the judgment that no new themes were emerging (11). Results were then used to develop a testable theoretical model for future research (11).

RESULTS

A major theme was homeless adolescents' perceive a lack of respect from health care providers that comes from being poor and homeless. For instance, when asked about how well health care providers understood the unique health care needs and challenges for homeless patients, one focus group collectively burst into laughter, with a female participant capturing the group sentiment:

> It doesn't seem like they want to (laughter subsiding) … I mean they don't care . . . most of the time because we go to the ER, they just want us in and out. They don't care to find out about the situation.

The following quote also indicates a perception that receiving health care is dehumanizing:

> I would rather see a doctor that cares more than go to the ER and be treated like you're the stupidest person on the planet, or a fungus,…treated like you have no intelligence at all…I'm better than you because I went to medical school.

Consistently, participants indicated that health care providers devalue their health care needs because they are homeless and poor.

Dehumanization is a systematic: "It's all about the money"

Participants were relatively aware of the structural challenges within the health care system associated with financing. A second major theme was profit-driven models of care leave no room for the needs of homeless adolescents. The following excerpts are exemplary of homeless adolescents who felt health care is "all about money":

> I was sitting there arguing with him over that it's not a sprain, it's broke and it's swelled up over twice its normal size…And because I didn't have insurance he was just telling me it was just sprained. He's going to wrap it with an ace wrap.
> They're gonna get the ones that's got insurance first and then you know they'll worry about the ones that don't, and I don't think it's right…
> I've actually had an ER doctor tell me 'You need this test but since you don't have insurance, we can do without it'…Their decisions are all based on money.

One participant was even aware of the concept of "single payer" model, and suggested a health care financing model like the one in "France" is needed to help reduce health disparities.

The impact of perceptions on health seeing behavior: "Toughing it out"

The perceptions that health care providers in the US dehumanize homeless adolescent because of the financial drivers of health delivery appears to influence homeless adolescent's health seeking behaviors. The following themes capture what homeless adolescent describe as their strategies for dealing with the perceived barriers to receiving good care noted above.

First, the desire to avoid unpleasant interactions with health care providers contributes to homeless adolescents' reluctance to seek care, which one described as the "toughing it out" approach to better health. A female homeless adolescent's comment epitomizes this view:

> If we can't pay, we can't afford it, so we don't go unless it's a major emergency. Unless there is really something wrong … If you're puking up blood then yeah, you need to go to the hospital. I've got bad ankles… If those are hurting, oh well, they've been

hurting for two weeks. If I can't stand them anymore then I need to go to the hospital. So it's deal with it until you have no other choice.

Further, to reduce the need to seek care from an insensitive, formal health care delivery system, homeless adolescents in our sample reported turning to informal peer networks for alternative care. For example, one male participant shared:

> Well, me, I'm probably different than most people ... I can take and make splints; I know how to splint my fingers. I can splint my arm if I really had to, if it's broken. Basically I do the best I can, if somebody I know needs help, or if they've broke their leg or ankle, I help them.

Respondents who reported turning to other homeless adolescents for health care also reported a sense of community that increases their trust for those in their informal peer networks.

Solutions from a homeless adolescent perspective: "Be a little more understanding"

Although homeless adolescents exhibited distrust of health of the health care system, participants also held hope that health care delivery could be improved. For instance, one female homeless adolescent suggested more egalitarian partnerships with providers that incorporate shared decision making would help increase trust:

> Be a little more understanding...At least consider some of my ideas in the treatment plan instead of shoving me off like I don't know what I'm talking about. I don't know everything just like he don't know everything, you know, but the difference is I can admit it.

Another homeless male adolescent described a particular encounter he had with a health care provider during which the provider valued his perspective and incorporated it into the care plan:

> I went to the hospital because I couldn't deal with the pain anymore, and the first time in my entire life, I had a doctor actually look at me and go, what kind of medicine do you want?...that's the first time I ever had them ask my opinion. There's a doctor that cares...

While deliberate efforts to better engage homeless adolescent will not change the financing model of the US health care system, such practice improvements may have a degree of positive impact on homeless adolescents' perceptions and their associated health seeking behaviors.

Community-engaged research as relationship building

A key element of community engaged research is to use data collection as a means to build lasting relationship with study participants (9). In our case, data collection allowed for the strengthening of a social connection between the researchers and the homeless adolescent being studied. We found evidence of this with reports from homeless adolescents that they appreciated the opportunity to have their opinions heard, with one adolescent stating "You seem different, like you care about what we think." This response was brought on by the engagement associated with the research effort, which opened a door to us to further a clinical relationship with the homeless adolescents. The positive response to our data collection efforts suggests that homeless adolescents' negative perceptions of health care providers are not dispositional traits; rather, such perceptions are subject to interventions that build trust and encouragingly, community engaged research can be such an intervention.

DISCUSSION

Our results add to the literature by producing results similar to other research that shows that the interpersonal aspect of health care delivery is important to homeless adolescents (12-13). More specifically, our study makes generalizability claims stronger on conclusions that homeless adolescents feel dehumanized by the health care system (12-13). Our research also adds to the literature by offering a theoretical link between perceptions of dehumanizing care and health care seeking behaviors of homeless adolescents.

Theory development

While a portion of our current study reinforces earlier findings, the strength of qualitative research is that it offers the opportunity to create testable hypotheses. In our case, our data suggests a theoretical model for poorer health outcomes for homeless adolescents that traces to perceptions by homeless adolescents of health care providers. Our model begins with the perceptions of homeless adolescents that health care providers do not respect them for financial reasons. Because of this perception, the resulting behaviors of homeless adolescents include avoidance of health care and/or the utilization of informal peer networks of care. We hypothesize the end result of the relationship between these variables is poorer health as depicted in Figure 1.

Before continuing, in the United States it is important to note that Patient Protection and Affordable Care Act (PPACA) expands insurance opportunities for homeless adolescents in some states (14). In the state in which the research was conducted, that had not yet occurred at the time of writing. However, this disparity in expanded access does offer an opportunity for comparison research to determine if homeless adolescents' in states that have expanded insurance opportunities exhibit changes in perceptions of the health care system associated with the possession of health insurance. It may be that the introduction of health insurance moderates the relationship between the variables we depict in our model.

Ongoing community engagement

An additional contribution to the literature by our study is a description of how community engaged research can be used to build a lasting relationship with a community of interest. We think effective community engaged research involves approaching the research with a commitment to the principal of *reciprocity*, meaning a commitment by the researchers to return to the community a tangible benefit in exchange for their time (15). To do otherwise could be considered a form of *academic imperialism*, reminiscent of archaeologists of old that carried artifacts from exotic places back to their homelands for display without tangible return to the community from which the artifacts were obtained (15). To offer guidance on how we delivered reciprocity in our study, we elected to also report how our research effort directly contributed to ongoing relationships between the research team, the agency, and the homeless adolescents we seek to serve better.

Expansion of clinical activities

At the local level of our community of interest, the data was used to obtain grant funding to expand clinic services to the homeless adolescents population from which our sample was drawn. In this way, the data was used to further a lasting relationship with the community. Moreover, the practices outlined in the following paragraphs describe how results were used to inform our clinic's practice models for better service to the local homeless adolescent community.

As noted above, several participants reported that the act of interacting through interviews was a trust-building exercise. Carrying this model into our clinical practice, we now deliberately spend time conversing with homeless adolescents in locations they frequent, such as the homeless adolescent "drop-in" area located near our clinic. The goal is to interact with homeless adolescents in an egalitarian, non-clinical manner in comfortable social environments that promotes increased trust (16). Furthermore, the egalitarian communication style that starts outside the clinic continues once adolescents enter. We minimize the interactions that occur "across the exam table," through learning the adolescents' preferred street names and engaging in social conversations (16). Our clinic staff also dresses informally to create a relaxed, collegial environment designed to reduce the psychological barrier between provider and homeless adolescents (16).

An additional element of research team incorporated into the clinic includes the use of community health workers (CHWs) (17). CHWs are members of the clinic staff that are drawn from the homeless adolescent population. We based our CHW program on respondents' reports that they feel comfortable turning to peers for assistance. As of this writing, we have two members of the community who work with us to help homeless adolescents navigate the clinic and the health care system more broadly.

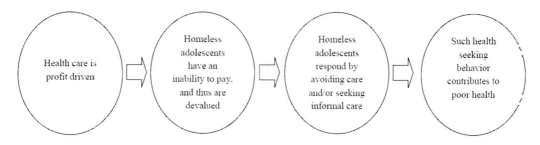

Figure 1. Proposed Relationship Model of Poorer Health Outcomes for Homeless Adolescents Based on their Perceptions of Health Care Delivery (N = 30).

Limitations and future research

The limitations of our study are those found in all qualitative research, in that our small sample does not allow for a statistical generalization of our results to the entire population of homeless adolescents. Despite that limitation, our study adds to a developing body of research on homeless adolescents' and health care by offering a testable theory of the linkage between homeless adolescents' perceptions of health care providers, health seeking behavior, and health outcomes. While it is certain that ecological variables such as a lack of adequate nutrition, housing, stress, etc. play a significant role in producing poor health care outcomes for homeless adolescents, future research should explore how much of a contribution poor perceptions of health care providers makes to health seeking behaviors for homeless adolescents and how those health seeking behaviors affect health outcomes. Our research also suggests a need for additional intervention research to test specific practice models to determine exactly which qualify as best practices for reducing distrust by homeless adolescents of the health care delivery system.

CONCLUSION

Our community engaged research approach collected qualitative data that suggests homeless adolescents' health access behaviors are driven by their negative perceptions of their treatment by health care providers and that these health seeking behaviors may be a contributor to poorer health outcomes for this population. Our approach also met the twin aims of community engaged research of not only producing data that is transferable to other health care providers, but also reciprocating to the community being studied by expanded clinical services based on the data and relationships made via the research. We are honored to have the opportunity to work with the homeless adolescent participants in our study and believe that similar research models in other communities will help realize the goals of reducing health disparities like those experienced by the homeless adolescents of our community.

ACKNOWLEDGMENTS

Our research was supported by the National Center for Research Resources and the National Institute of General Medical Sciences of the National Institutes of Health through Grant Number 8P20GM103447. The authors also would like to acknowledge Cordell Baker, BS, for his assistance with this research. All authors certify that we have no conflicts of interest in relation to this study.

REFERENCES

[1] Hammer H., Finkelhor D, Sedlak AJ. National incidence studies of missing, abducted, runaway, and thrownaway children. Runaway/thrownaway children: National estimates and characteristics.

[Internet]. Washington, DC, US: Department of Justice, Office of Justice Programs, Office of Juvenile Justice and Delinquency Prevention, 2002. URL: https://www.ncjrs.gov/pdffiles1/ojjdp/196469.pdf.

[2] Ammerman SD, Ensign J, Kirzner R, Meininger ET, Tornabene M, Warf CW, Zerger S, Post P. Homeless young adults 18-24: Examining service delivery adaptations. [Internet]. Nashville, TN, US: National Health Care for the Homeless Council, 2004. URL: http://www.nhchc.org/Publications/younghomelessadult1.pdf.

[3] Feldmann J, Middleman AB. Homeless adolescents: common clinical concerns. Semin Pediatr Infect Dis 2003; 14: 6–11.

[4] Nyamathi AM, Christian, A, Windokun F, Jones T, Strehlow A, Shoptaw S. Hepatitis C virus infection, substance use and mental illness among homeless youth: a review. AIDS 2005; 19(Suppl 3): S34–S40.

[5] Rew L, Taylor-Seehafer M, Fitzgerald ML. Sexual abuse, alcohol, and other drug use, and suicidal behaviors in homeless adolescents. Issues Compr Pediatr Nurs 2001; 24: 225–40.

[6] Roy E, Haley N, Leclerc P, et al. Mortality in a cohort of street youth in Montreal, JAMA 2004; 292: 569-74.

[7] Schmittidiel J, Grumbach K, Selby J. System based participatory research in health care: an approach for sustainable research and quality. Ann Fam Med 2010; 8(3): 256-9.

[8] Lasker RD, Weiss ES. Broadening participation in community problem solving: a multidisciplinary model to support collaborative practice and research. J Urban Health 2003; 80(1): 14-47.

[9] Mulligana M, Nadarajah, Y. Working on the sustainability of local communities with a "community-engaged" research methodology. Local Environ Int J Justice Sustain 2008; 13(2): 81-94.

[10] Lindlof, TR, Taylor, BC. Qualitative communication research methods, 2nd ed. Thousand Oaks, CA: Sage, 2002.

[11] Patton MQ. Qualitative research and evaluation methods. Thousand Oaks, CA: Sage, 2002.

[12] Ensign, J. Quality of health care: the views of homeless youth. Health Serv Res 2004; 39: 695–708.

[13] Hudson AL, Nyamathi A, Greengold B, Slagle A, Koniak-Griffin D, Khalilifard F, Getzoff D. Health-seeking challenges among homeless youth. Nurs Res 2010; 59: 212-8.

[14] Rudowitz, R. & Stephens, J. Analyzing the Impact of State Medicaid Expansion Decisions. [Internet]. Washington, DC: The Henry J. Kasier Family Foundation, 2013. URL: http://kff.org/medicaid/issue-brief/analyzing-the-impact-of-state-medicaid-expansion-decisions/.

[15] Glazer, M. The threat of the stranger: Vulnerability, reciprocity, and fieldwork. In: Sieber, J, ed. Ethics of social research: fieldwork, regulation, and publication. New York: Springer, 1982:49-70.

[16] Barry PJ, Ensign J, Lippek SH. Embracing street culture: fitting health care into the lives of street youth. J Transcult Nurs 2002; 13: 145-52.

[17] Martin M, Hernandez O, Naureckas E, Lantos J. Improving asthma research in an inner-city Latino neighborhood with community health workers. J Asthma 2005; 42(10): 891-9.

In: Public Health Yearbook 2015
Editor: Joav Merrick

ISBN: 978-1-63484-514-4
© 2016 Nova Science Publishers, Inc.

Chapter 15

BRIDGE TO CARE FOR REFUGEE HEALTH: LESSONS FROM AN INTERPROFESSIONAL COLLABORATION IN THE MIDWEST

Ruth Margalit[1,*], Laura Vinson[1], Christine Ngaruiya[2], Kara Gehring[3], Pam Franks[4], Caci Schulte[5], Andrew Lemke[5], Joshua Blood[5], Tyler Irvine[1], Chelsea Souder[1], Deeko Hassan[5], Andrea Langeveld[6], Carolyn Corn[5], Thu Hong Bui[5] and Ann Marie Kudlacz[7]

[1]Inter-Professional Service Learning Academy, College of Public Health, University of Nebraska Medical Center (UNMC), Omaha, Nebraska, United States of America US
[2]Department of Emergency Medicine, Yale New Haven Hospitals, New Haven, Connecticut, United States of America
[3]Public Health Project Coordinator, CityMatCH, Omaha, Nebraska, United States of America
[4]Embrace the Nations, Omaha, Nebraska, United States of America
[5]College of Pharmacy, UNMC, Omaha, Nebraska, United States of America
[6]College of Medicine, UNMC, Omaha, Nebraska, United States of America
[7]Southern Sudan Community Association, Omaha, Nebraska, United States of America

The United States resettles tens of thousands of refugees annually, with hundreds placed in mid-sized Midwestern cities such as Omaha, Nebraska. Prior to resettlement, refugees have limited access to health services and arrive with inadequate knowledge on basic hygiene practices, general healthcare issues, and minimal understanding of the American healthcare system. Additionally, current training for healthcare practitioners in the United States on issues related to refugee populations and their unique health needs is

---

[*] Corresponding author: Ruth Margalit MD; Associate Professor and Director, Inter-Professional Service Learning Academy, Maurer Center for Public Health, Rm 2038; College of Public Health, Health Promotion, Social and Behavioral Health, University of Nebraska Medical Center, 986075 Nebraska Medical Center, Omaha NE 68198-4375, United States. E-mail: rmargalit@unmc.edu.

insufficient. The enormous need coupled with inadequate preparation, poses great challenges for both newly resettled refugees and health professionals, and provides opportunities for improvement with creative initiatives. The Bridge to Care (BTC) project is a unique partnership between health professions students, leaders from city and state refugee service organizations, and refugee leaders. It is a student-led/community-engaged organization overseen by the Service Learning Academy (SLA) in the College of Public Health at the University of Nebraska Medical Center. The SLA facilitates campus wide interprofessional community-based experiences like Bridge to Care. Through BTC, students take the forefront in communicating directly with leaders from community organizations and engaging with refugee leaders to determine all relevant service activities. Bridge to Care provides opportunities for students to engage in experiences that are not otherwise available in their standard curriculum. While providing essential services, students are able to enhance cultural and communication skills and gain experience working with an interprofessional team, building an understanding of the vital role each profession plays within the full spectrum of care for patients and communities.

Keywords: interprofessional education, refugees, health, community engagement

INTRODUCTION

According to the United Nations High Commissioner for Refugees (UNHCR), a refugee is defined as someone who "owing to a well-founded fear of being persecuted for reasons of race, religion, nationality, membership of a particular social group or political opinion, is outside the country of his nationality, and is unable to, or owing to such fear, is unwilling to avail himself to the protection of that country" (1). "Secondary Migrants" are those refugees who have originally resettled in one part of the country and have subsequently moved to another location. There are approximately 15 million refugees around the world (1).

Refugees begin the process of seeking resettlement after fleeing their home countries to seek safety in neighboring nations. When refugees arrive at the nation providing asylum or temporary residence, they face three possible endpoints, one of which is resettlement in a third country such as the United States (1). This process often times takes more than 5 years while refugees live in harsh conditions within the refugee camps (1). The President of the United States sets the ceiling for refugee admission to the United States (U.S.) each fiscal year (2), for which the U.S. averages more than 50,000 refugee resettlements per year (1). Many of these refugees choose to resettle in mid-sized Midwestern cities given low costs of living and low rates of unemployment (2). Refugees are also placed in locations where existing family ties are already established (2).

REFUGEE RESETTLEMENT IN NEBRASKA

Currently, there are an estimated 25,000 refugees in Nebraska, with 15,000 in Omaha alone, according to Omaha resettlement agencies (personal communications) and federal resettlement reports (2, 3). In fiscal year 2013, there was a record high of 1,006 refugees resettled, and the number is expected to increase in 2014 (4). Over the years, refugees from Sudan, Somalia, Burma, Bhutan, Nepal, Iraq, Afghanistan, Ethiopia, Liberia, Congo, and

Burundi have been resettled in Nebraska. As of 2006, it is estimated that over 50% of the Sudanese population in the U.S. settled in Nebraska (5, 6). In more recent years, the majority of resettled refugees are those who have fled to camps in Thailand from nearby Burma (Myanmar) (7).

The three primary refugee resettlement agencies that provide services to these refugees in Nebraska are Lutheran Family Services (LFS), Southern Sudan Community Association (SSCA), and Catholic Charities (4). The agencies provide various services such as: English classes, cultural orientation, employment assistance, fair housing education, financial literacy and household budgeting, as well as training programs for churches and civic organizations that wish to sponsor refugees and immigration legal assistance. Agencies also help coordinate access to healthcare services while in the U.S (8).

REFUGEE HEALTH ISSUES

Prior to arrival in the U.S., the refugee receives inadequate preparation regarding health and health-related issues (3). Refugees also lack basic understanding about navigating the healthcare system, Western hygiene practices, preventive practices, and Western disease management (9). As a result of their circumstances, it is not unusual to find individuals with complicated health issues upon arrival and for years following resettlement. Past history of poor nutrition, poor sanitation, exposure to on-going violence and lack of adequate medical care also contribute to poor health (1).

One particular area of concern is the high rates of undiagnosed infectious conditions such as tuberculosis, malaria, hepatitis C, Human Immuno-deficiency Virus (HIV), as well as skin and intestinal parasites (9-11). Mental health disorders also affect a large portion of the population including a high prevalence of depression, drug and alcohol abuse (7, 11). Individuals who experienced persecution, terrorization by violent groups, imprisonment, and torture, may suffer from somatization disorders, psychosocial distress, post-traumatic stress disorder, anxiety and depression (1, 9-11). Another source of health concern is injury at the workplace (4). The majority of refugees in Omaha, Nebraska work in meat packing plants performing physically demanding jobs which puts them at high risk for injury (8).

Lastly, cultural differences distinguish America from many of the countries from which refugees originate, and these differences extend to healthcare (12). For example, in Somalia, only 2% of births take place in a health facility whereas in America, women are expected to deliver in the hospital. In addition, numerous Somali women have undergone female circumcision, which can make birthing more complicated (12).

Bridge to Care (BTC) was founded on principles of community-based participatory research (CBPR) and service learning after identifying a gap in refugee health and healthcare needs. In addition to the language barrier, numerous refugees lack the cultural constructs to understand life in this country. Timely, appropriate healthcare acculturation is frequently unmet and much needed (9, 10). Refugees receive inadequate preparation prior to resettlement regarding fundamentals such as running a 'Western home,' family roles, job distribution, the legal system, and navigating the education system (2).

The program is designed to prioritize the vast needs of the refugee populations, link refugees to existing services, and increase provider competence for refugee care. When working with refugees, BTC refers to health as "a state of complete physical, mental and social well-being and not merely the absence of disease or infirmity" (13). Few other programs have been set up to address refugee health issues through collaboration with community organizations.

The purpose of the work described in this manuscript is to illustrate the unique setup between community, interprofessional health professions students and refugee leaders to enhance refugee health in Omaha and surrounding communities. With the number of interactions through BTC currently approaching 4,000 and continuing to grow, the organizational leaders seek to share this novel initiative to impact other communities that interact with refugee populations. The Institutional Review Board of the University of Nebraska Medical Center approved parts of this project that involve research, such as implementation of surveys for the health education sessions.

METHODS

Bridge to Care (BTC) was established in April 2010 as an interprofessional organization supported by the interprofessional Service Learning Academy (SLA), College of Public Health at the University of Nebraska Medical Center (UNMC). It is a partnership involving students from the colleges of medicine, nursing, pharmacy, public health, and allied health, faculty, healthcare providers and community refugee service agencies. The goal is to facilitate positive healthcare outcomes for refugees by teaching them how to navigate the healthcare system, enhancing knowledge and cultural skills necessary for successful assimilation, and developing strong relationships with their communities.

This is achieved by: discerning group specific health needs from each refugee community; providing health education, linkage to healthcare and services; and improving cultural awareness and knowledge regarding resettled refugees among healthcare providers

BTC has three initiatives to accomplish this mission; monthly health education sessions, monthly mentoring sessions, and health fairs/linkage to care events. Each of these initiatives requires collaboration with the community. Table 1 lists the partners of this project.

Health education sessions

Health education sessions are developed with each refugee community (Sudanese, Somali, Burmese /Karen, and Bhutanese) for a period of three consecutive months. Health professions student leaders with respective refugee community leaders, work on building relationships, identifying health needs, planning the education opportunities in community settings and linking the refugee community to appropriate health services. Typically 15-40 participants attend each session.

Health education session topics have included pain management, hypertension, stroke, addiction, mental health, suicide prevention, immunizations, autism, healthy eating, using over the counter medications, and navigation of the U.S. healthcare system.

Table 1. Bridge to Care Partners

BTC Partners	Role
University of Nebraska Medical Center, College of Public Health, Service Learning Academy	Oversees the Bridge to Care program and assists in sustaining and expanding the program; Provides evidenced-based models of theory and community development, research methods for tracking and identifying evaluation process and outcomes
Southern Sudan Community Association (SSCA)	Resettlement Agency
Lutheran Family Services (LFS)	Resettlement Agency
Embrace the Nations	Faith-based organization providing cultural awareness training to Bridge to Care volunteers; Assists refugees in multiple areas of need and assists the public in better understanding and interacting with refugee populations
Omaha Public Schools, ESL Program	Partners for the mentoring program offered to refugee youth grades 5-12
Nebraska Department of Health and Human Services	Responsible for coordinating and administering the Refugee Resettlement Program on the state level
Alegent-Creighton Florence Clinic	Federally designated clinic assigned to provide initial health screenings/healthcare services to refugees; participates in annual health fair and various educational sessions, while linking refugees to long term healthcare
One World Community Health Center	Provides clinical supplies for health fairs and flu shots for multiple 'Flu Shot Clinics'
Douglas County Health Department	Providing health education resources and support
Walgreens Pharmacy	Provides clinical supplies and personnel for health fairs and flu shots for multiple 'Flu Shot Clinics'

When health needs are selected, refugee community leaders play an important role in identifying an appropriate session format (presentation by students or experts versus discussion groups), venue (faith gathering place – Church/mosque, community center, the familiar resettlement organization office), and time/day for the session, recruitment of interpreters, as well as recruitment of refugee community members to attend. The health education sessions occur once every 2-4 weeks in the community.

BTC leadership recruits health profession students to participate in the sessions.

The majority of students participating in health education sessions have no previous experience with refugees prior to their involvement with BTC. Hence, increasing the foundation of knowledge is important to foster appropriate interactions with and understanding of the populations being served. As an introduction, at every health education session prior to the arrival of the refugees, student and faculty volunteers are required to participate in cultural awareness training about refugees and their health needs. The training is designed to enhance cultural sensitivity, increase knowledge and ensure that participants are better equipped to effectively interact with the refugees. The training covers topics such as: the unique characteristics of the various refugee groups arriving in the U.S. and Omaha; the specific health needs of refugees; the importance of and tips on communicating effectively with various cultures regardless of race, ethnicity, culture or language proficiency.

Health-fairs/Linkage-to-care

In addition to health education and focused services (like flu-shot clinics for specific refugee communities), two major health fairs/linkage to care events are organized each year in response to the needs of the refugee community. These large events (up to 500 participants) offer a wide range of education opportunities, offering over 35 different resource booths in 2013, including information relating to proper hygiene, nutrition, immunizations, chronic disease management, and child health. Prescription and over the counter medication counseling is also available. Free preventative services like flu shots, screening for hypertension, diabetes, obesity, vision and dental services are also provided.

Mentoring program

In 2012, BTC expanded its engagement by adding the BTC Mentoring Program, partnering with Omaha Public School's English as a Second Language (ESL) program for refugee students. Younger, school-aged children often find it easier to acculturate into the American lifestyle and can act as a great resource for their families. Health professions students can become mentors following successful completion of a background check and training. Mentors are randomly assigned mentees and engage with them on selected Saturdays throughout the academic year, at least 12 times, covering topics concerning wellness and health. BTC has identified this venue as another way to improve communication with refugees. In Fall 2013, 352 refugee students participated with 20 health profession student mentors.

RESULTS

Since the inception of BTC (April 2010), over 700 students and over 4,000 refugees engaged together to address health needs.

Unlike other venues for volunteering, Bridge to Care is a relatively new model of healthcare outreach in the community. The track record, albeit short, has been consistent and positive. Different refugee groups throughout the city have benefitted from relevant education sessions and services. While progressing through their rigorous programs of excellence, students acquire skills and knowledge that will help them excel in their field. Such skills as compassionate care, cross cultural communication and multi-cultural care, can impact their future patients who are likely to come from various cultural backgrounds. These skills are best learned through experiential real-life learning, and the unique setting provided by BTC undoubtedly forges the place for the learning while facilitating potential better care for refugee populations in the future. Table 2 presents qualitative data illustrating community partners, refugees and students' perspectives.

In addition to asking refugees about relevant health topics and appropriate logistics to facilitate BTC programming, refugees are all asked to provide feedback through systematic evaluations through all three BTC programs; health education sessions, mentoring sessions, and health fairs/linkage to care events. For example, following each health fair, refugees are asked to complete an oral evaluation. Of the 350 refugees who attended the past Fair, 131 completed the survey of which 99% indicated that the event was 'most useful' (rated 10 on a scale of 1-10 the usefulness of the health fair - 1 being least useful and 10 being most useful), and that the information was presented in a way that they could understand. Additional responses from the refugees include the desire to have more clinical services offered and an indication of the variety of 'favorite booths' such as, basic health screenings, nutrition, over-the-counter medication, free vaccinations, dental care and vision screening with eye glasses.

Student perspectives

With each health education session, students take part in a pre/post assessment to determine knowledge, skills, comfort, and beliefs of the student's cultural competency.

Table 2. Perspectives of partners in the Bridge to Care Program

	Community partner	Refugees	Student
Positive	"Thank you for providing information to a population that may have otherwise not received anything." "Th partnership with the university helps us dream big and involve individuals that otherwise are not interested in refugees in our city." "The program provides services that we do not have resources for. At the same time students get to learn in a real-world setting. It's a win/win!" "Innovative; sustainable program!"	"My favorite part of the Fair is that my kids know more about health and healthy food." "I will tell my people to come and attend the next event." "The session helped me understand why I may need to have a flu-shot." "It's a really good experience for me to get to know more about health, improve my health." "I respect the students who care about me."	"It has really opened my eyes to refugees in Omaha to better understand the various challenges they face." "The most important part was to gain trust and build relationships with strangers: refugees and other health profession students." "I developed appreciation and awareness to the notion that nothing should be taken for granted." "I learned how important is cultural awareness and competent cultural practice."
Negative	"Shorten refugee evaluations they are hard to understand." "Make sure you use language that is simple and clear."	"They ran out of flu shots and I didn't get one!" "I want them to offer more dental care and glasses."	"I need more cultural training to be effective." "Needed interpreters, but lacked sufficient funding."

The aggregate analysis of the pre and post assessments, administered to a total of 29 students over three consecutive sessions in 2013 with the Bhutanese population concluded the following in regard to knowledge, skills and cross cultural competence: following the cultural awareness training, 80% of students reported an *increase in knowledge* of cultural challenges that face refugees in U.S. and an *increase in skills* with student's ability to communicate effectively with different cultures regardless of race, ethnicity, culture or language (increase from 2 to 4 on a Likert scale [1-least, 5-most].

Students have also consistently reflected positively on their experiences through BTC. For example, following a Somali health education session, a student stated, "It has really opened my eyes to the refugee population in Omaha and the various challenges they face." Another student reflected "....It was a rewarding experience and I felt like I was doing something that really mattered for the community. The Bridge to Care organization is a great way to interact with the diverse community that lives within Omaha. It was very beneficial to learn about a different culture as well as use skills we have learned from our time at UNMC towards those in need. I will be able to use what I learned on Sunday for the rest of my career. I would encourage anyone to help out with a Bridge to Care event[s] because not only are you helping others, you are also bettering yourself as a person as well as a professional."

DISCUSSION

The work with refugees has been often challenging, complex, and at the same time very rewarding. In various listening sessions during the past 2 years, refugees in Omaha identified the following needs: housing, health, employment, education, transportation and public safety/community awareness. Bridge to Care focused on healthcare issues, while taking into consideration the host of challenges the community face. The major lessons learned are listed below:

1. *Understanding of US healthcare system* - many members of the American society struggle to fully understand the ins and outs of the U.S. healthcare system, especially at a time of major changes in insurance coverage. Refugees have little foundational understanding of this complex system and often fall victims to misunderstandings and incur startling costs for minor services obtained outside of insurance coverage or in an inappropriate manner (for example - use of ER for simple upper respiratory infection). Refugees hold a unique understanding of health and sickness, embracing a holistic approach to treatment of diseases (American medicine is deeply embedded upon scientific data and physical exam, when other cultures look at the environment, cultural customs and traditions, and rely heavily on healers for cures). The BTC program has to be both efficient in assisting with the understanding of the healthcare system while maintaining sensitivity to the traditional approach when presenting strategies for diagnosis and management of diseases.
2. *Understanding preventive care* - Students learned firsthand how individuals from diverse populations, cultural practices and beliefs have very different perceptions and understanding regarding health. A striking example was preventive health services, discussed at an education session as an important part of maintaining good health. Yet, 'preventive care,' regarding cancer in the Bhutanese community, was found to be a new concept and a problematic one: "if you talk about or schedule screening for colon or cervical cancer you will bring it upon yourself." BTC has learned that more education and time is needed for preventive practices to be understood and embraced

by refugees. This finding was an important one shared with the practice clinical community.

3. *Refugee participation in sessions:* Almost all refugees, regardless of geographic location, tend to avoid drawing attention to themselves. Asian refugees, especially, tend to be quite reserved. This means remaining silent rather than speaking up, not asking questions, not asking for clarification and essentially agreeing with whatever is said or done. Because time is limited in the education sessions, it is difficult to check for understanding, to assess how much of the presented material is comprehended, and how useful it was for the refugees. With consistent repetition of health topics presented at health education sessions, the hope is that the information will eventually be absorbed.

4. *Sensitive topics:* Another challenge has been the discussion of more sensitive topics such as women's health, torture and abuse, mental illness and subjects related to sex (i.e., sexually transmitted diseases). Generally speaking, these topics are discussed very little in the community or in the home and special measures must be taken in order to successfully address them. Due to matters of sensitivity and confidentiality, interpreters coming from the community are especially unsuitable when discussing these personal issues. The interpreters need to correctly communicate the health needs of their respective populations, and be of an appropriate age with adequate knowledge. Medically-certified interpreters are in very high demand, and as a result, are quite expensive and often unavailable. Finding competent medical interpreters was a challenge for BTC as it was for the practice community, and many of the sensitive topics could not be addressed. New initiatives designed to address mental health and other sensitive topics in group settings are currently being developed.

5. *Logistics of the program* - The general logistics for the BTC program have been a challenge and a great lesson to all involved. Scheduling planning meetings, session dates/times, session venues, refugee recruitment and selecting appropriate food have all required on-going open communication, flexibility, leadership and good problem solving skills. Refugees often work the first (7-4) and second (1-9) shifts 6-7 days a week, have limited access to transportation, and prefer gatherings in places of worship or at the housing complexes where most of the community members live. Since weekends tend to work best for the refugees, students, community organization leaders and faculty extended their commitment to meet these needs, scheduling most activities on the weekends. Several sessions have been held following the conclusion of an existing ESL class or after faith-based activities to reach a larger number of refugees. In addition, students from the various health professions, have to coordinate between the various professional curricula to ensure student participation (avoiding dates prior to major exams etc.). In addition, for each activity, interpreters need to be recruited. They are expected to disseminate information about the activity, recruit individuals to attend, and be present at the session. As stated earlier, interpreters are in high demand and need to be contacted long in advance.

Timely communication has also been an enduring challenge; perhaps the different perception of 'time, the lack of access to electronic communication, or the difference in norms and expectations for follow-up and response. In any case, the expectation of prompt reply to phone messages and emails is unrealistic and adds another layer to coordination.

6. *Funding and sustainability* - Each of the BTC's activities, especially the bi-annual health fairs, require resources (i.e., medical supplies, transportation, food, translated materials, and many other relevant items). Funding for BTC activities has been secured through an ongoing effort by the SLA, through applications to local and national grants and for in kind contributions. Since its inception in 2010, over $20,000 cash funding were secured with over $100,000 in-kind services. Although tedious and very time consuming, through this process, BTC has formed numerous partnerships with local businesses and service providers.

New opportunities: The Refugee Health Collaborative

As a direct result of the BTC program, the Nebraska Refugee Health Collaborative (RHC) was formed, with the goal to improve health of the refugees who are a part of the fabric of the community. Twelve organizations joined together: UNMC, College of Public Health, (including the Service Learning Academy and Bridge to Care), Southern Sudan Community Association, Lutheran Family Services, Embrace the Nations, Omaha Together One Community, the Institute of Public Life, Nebraska Department of Health and Human Services (Refugee Coordinator and Refugee Health Coordinator), Douglas County Health Department, Ready in Five, Alegent-Creighton Florence Clinic, One World Community Health Centers, Omaha Public Schools, and to date, over 250 refugee leaders and key community members have participated in the monthly meetings.

Much like BTC, the larger RHC embraced the following goals: to develop mutual understanding and trust among the group, to determine major perceived barriers to service (i.e., economic, cultural, language, financial, organizational, navigation of the health system, insurance), to identify culturally appropriate methods of engagement and to determine priorities and opportunities for action.

The two sub-committees working under the RHC: The first is the Engagement Team, which looks at methods of engaging the refugee community in order to build capacity, improve existing and develop new services and empower the targeted populations to improve their own health. The second is the Data Team, which works a. to help clarify the number of refugees and their respective culture groups living in Omaha. Existing data sources were identified and will be linked to create a usable database that will support future activities including engagement and research; b. Since major funding is needed to ensure the sustainability of BTC and the RHC, the data team is working on developing scientific research grant applications. In addition, the RHC is diligently working to develop a community health worker program with the refugee communities. The RHC encourages refugee involvement at all levels including refugee leaders from all groups who are represented in the city. This is not merely a project; the RHC is committed to long-term goals and implementation. With diverse team players from academia, local refugee organizations and refugee community leaders, the potential for successful outcomes is promising.

As we identify and embrace the different refugee groups in Omaha NE, we can better understand health-related needs, develop effective interventions, enhance cultural sensitivity and track outcomes. All are bound to benefit from this endeavor.

Limitations

The limitations of this project center on the assessment of its effectiveness. Currently, due to language barriers, limited resources, slow coordination among agencies, and limited data-sharing agreements, we are unable to better track how the program is making a difference in the community.

With a $50,000 grant recently obtained for linkage of data and the development of a comprehensive data system for the city, we hope to better capture the impact on health and other related outcomes in the near future.

Conclusion

The definition of Health as referred by the World Health Organization (WHO) is especially important when considering the refugee populations (13). Started in 2010 from an initiative of a caring student (author CN) the interprofessional student-led/community-engaged Bridge to Care project expanded its activities into 2014. It created great ripples for further collaborative action and capacity building to improve the health of the refugee community. Students are rewarded with an exceptional real-life community based experience, while community needs are addressed, local capacity is built, and sustainability is built.

Acknowledgments

We are deeply grateful for the work of all of the Bridge to Care student leaders, the faculty volunteers who supervise and mentor the students, refugee community leaders; and to the refugee service organizations leaders who trust and nurture this partnership.

References

[1] UNHCR: The UN Refugee Agency. A pocket guide to refugees 2008. URL: http://www.unhcr.org/pages/49c3646c4b8.html.
[2] US Office of Refugee Resettlement. Refugee arrival data 2000-2012. URL: http://www.acf.hhs.gov/programs/orr/resource/refugee-arrival-data.
[3] US Department of State Refugee Resettlement in the United States 2013. URL: http://www.state.gov/j/prm/releases/factsheets/2013/203578.htm.
[4] Department of Health and Human Services-Nebraska, 2012-2013 Minority Health Initiative Annual Report. URL: http://dhhs.ne.gov/Pages/srd_srdindex.aspx.
[5] Lainof CA, Elsea SJ. From Sudan to Omaha: how one community is helping African refugees find a new home. Am J Nurs 2004; 104: 58-61.
[6] Tompkins M, Smith L, Jones K, Swundell S. HIV-education needs among Sudanese immigrants and refugees in the midwestern United States. AIDS Behav 2006; 10: 319-23.
[7] Benner MT, Townsend J, Kaloi W, Htwe K, Naranichakul N, Hunnangkul S, et al. Reproductive health and quality of life of young Burmese refugees in Thailand. Confl Health 2010; 4: 5.
[8] Campbell DS. Health hazards in the meatpacking industry. Occup Med 1999; 14(2): 351-72.

[9] World Health Organization. Overcoming migrants' barriers to health. URL: http://www.who.int/bulletin/volumes/86/8/08-020808/en/.
[10] Morris MD, Popper ST, Rodwell TC, Brodine SK, Brouwer KC. Healthcare barriers of refugees post-resettlement. J Commun Health 2009; 34: 529-38.
[11] Carswell K, Blackburn P, Barker C. The relationship between trauma post-migration problems and the psychological well-being of refugees and asylum seekers. Int J Soc Psychiatry 2011; 57: 107-19.
[12] Herrel N, Olevitch L, Dubois DK, Terry P, Thorp D, Kind E, el al. Somali refugee women speak out about their needs for care during pregnancy and delivery. J Midwifery Womens Health 2004; 49: 345-9.
[13] World Health Organization. Preamble to the Constitution of the World Health Organization 1946. URL: http://www.who.int/about/definition/en/print.html.
[14] Israel BA, Schulz AJ, Parker EA, Becker AB. Review of community-based research: assessing partnership approaches to improve public health. Annu Rev Public Health 1998; 19: 173-202.

Section Two - Substance abuse

In: Public Health Yearbook 2015
Editor: Joav Merrick

ISBN: 978-1-63484-514-4
© 2016 Nova Science Publishers, Inc.

Chapter 16

COMORBIDITY AND TREATMENT IN SUBSTANCE USE DISORDERS

Brieana M Rowles[*], MA, Aaron Ellington, PhD, Andrew R Tarr, BS, John L Hertzer, MD, and Robert L Findling, MD, MBA

Clinical Research Services, UPMC Cancer Center, Pittsburgh, Pennsylvania, United States of America

Substance use disorders frequently co-occur with other psychiatric disorders in adolescents and young adults. Diagnosing these comorbid conditions can be challenging in young populations. If these conditions are left untreated, the prognosis for youths with comorbid conditions may be particularly poor. This is, in part, owing to the fact that the presence of a comorbid psychiatric disorder in young patients with a substance abuse disorders increases the likelihood for problems with family and school, criminal involvement, risky behaviors, and poor treatment adherence and outcomes. Fortunately, evidence-based treatments for these co-occurring conditions have emerged from recent intervention research. This paper describes the general principles of assessment, diagnosis, and treatment for young patients with co-occurring substance use and psychiatric disorders and outlines recent treatment research for this vulnerable population.

Keywords: substance abuse, psychiatry, co-morbidity, assessment

INTRODUCTION

Substance use disorders (SUDs) are fairly common among adolescents and young adults in the United States, with prevalence rates ranging from approximately 8% (1) to approximately 35% (2). Not only are SUDs common, but they also frequently co-occur with other psychiatric disorders. The National Survey on Drug Use and Health reported that in 2010,

---

[*] Corresponding author: Brieana M Rowles, MA, Regulatory Specialist, Clinical Research Services, UPMC Cancer Center, 5150 Centre Avenue, Suite 301, Pittsburgh, PA, 15232, United States. E-mail: brieana52@gmail.com.

22.1% of adolescents aged 12 to 17 (N = 379,000) with substance dependence or abuse in the past year also had a major depressive episode during the same time period (3). Additionally, the most recent practice parameter from the American Academy of Child and Adolescent Psychiatry reported that up to 50% of adolescents with SUDs in clinical populations have a comorbid psychiatric disorder (4).

COMMON COMORBID PSYCHIATRIC CONDITIONS

Studies of community-based samples of children and adolescents generally report attention-deficit/hyperactivity disorder and disruptive behavior disorders as the most commonly occurring comorbid psychiatric conditions in SUDs, at rates just under 70% (5, 6). In addition, ADHD complicated by co-occurring oppositional defiant disorder or conduct disorder is associated with significant risk for developing SUDs (7). The next most frequently reported comorbid psychiatric conditions at approximately 20-30% are mood disorders (both depressive disorders and bipolar disorders) (5, 8). Anxiety disorders occur at a rate of approximately 20% in children and adolescents with SUDs (5).

Clinical samples

Similar to data from community samples, clinical samples of children and adolescents report rates suggesting that ADHD and disruptive behavior disorders are the most common conditions comorbid with SUDs (9-12). Approximately 40-50% of young patients diagnosed with an SUD meet diagnostic criteria for comorbid ADHD (9, 10, 12). It has been suggested that ADHD during childhood/adolescence is a significant risk factor for developing an SUD (13). Further, longitudinal assessments of the relationship of ADHD in adolescence to later SUD have found that not only are co-occurring oppositional defiant disorder or conduct disorder significant predictors of SUD (13,14), but also that comorbid conduct disorder predicts SUD in pediatric ADHD (15, 16). Conduct disorder has been reported to co-occur in approximately 50% of children and adolescents with an SUD (10-12).

Mood disorders also are commonly comorbid with juvenile SUDs in clinical settings (9, 12). Approximately 20% to more than 50% of children and adolescents with SUDs suffer from major depressive disorder (4, 11, 17, 18). Bipolar disorders (BPD) occur in 15% to 30% of juvenile SUD cases (19, 20). Further, juvenile BPD has been found to be a predictor of later SUD (21), and preliminary data suggest that co-occurring BPD and post-traumatic stress disorder increase the risk of subsequent SUD (22). Post-traumatic stress disorder and other anxiety disorders occur at rates of approximately 10% to 40% in juvenile SUD in clinical settings (4, 12, 18).

While psychotic disorders are not uncommonly comorbid with SUDs, the onset of the psychotic disorder generally occurs in late adolescence to early adulthood (23). Thus, clinical sample data are generally limited to adults. Of note, substance use and SUDs, particularly cannabis use, are associated with earlier age of onset of psychotic symptoms (24-28). Accordingly, adolescents with SUDs may be at increased risk for developing a comorbid psychotic disorder.

GENERAL PRINCIPLES OF ASSESSMENT AND DIAGNOSIS

Considering the serious risks associated with SUDs and co-occurring psychiatric conditions, and high rates of comorbid individuals, proper assessment is critical. Although validated psychometric instruments are used frequently in scientific investigations, research has shown that only a small number of treatment providers report using formal assessment measures (e.g., self-reports, structured interviews, etc.) when determining proper treatment referrals (29). Lichtenstein et al. (29), for instance, found that the standard practice in mental health settings to generate diagnostic information and determining a basic treatment plan is to conduct an informal or unstructured "clinical interview."

There also has been concern regarding the proper training of clinicians on how to properly diagnose comorbidity in youths with SUDs. Training clinicians to accurately assess comorbid individuals is critical because of the complexities in deciphering various symptoms that overlap in presentation. Clinicians are generally trained to assess and treat one segment: either SUDs or mental health disorders. Additionally, state and federal funding sources for treating comorbid individuals typically pay for one or the other disorder, but generally not both simultaneously (30). Accordingly, patients or clinicians are forced to decide what gets treated first (i.e., sequential treatment), or choose to treat both separately at the same time (i.e., parallel treatment). Research has yielded that both sequential and parallel treatment are less effective and have a higher cost than an integrative approach with properly trained staff (30-33). Jensen-Doss and Weisz (34) also found that when studying children and adolescents in an outpatient facility, in the absence of "diagnostic agreement" (i.e., the difference between the clinician-given diagnosis and a research-generated diagnosis), there were greater no-shows, cancellations, and drops-out from treatment. When SUD and depression are involved – both high risk factors for suicide in adolescents – diagnostic disagreement can have serious treatment ramifications (29).

According to *Addiction Counseling Competencies: The Knowledge, Skills, and Attitudes of Professional Practice, Technical Assistance Publication (TAP) Series 21* published by the Substance Abuse and Mental Health Services Administration (SAMHSA) (35), appropriate assessment should include a process sensitive to age, gender, racial and ethnic culture, and disabilities that includes, but is not limited to: (1) history of alcohol and drug use; (2) physical health, mental health, and addiction treatment histories; (3) family issues; (4) work history and career issues; (5) history of criminality; (6) psychological, emotional, and worldview concerns; (7) current status of physical health, mental health, and substance use; (8) spiritual concerns of the patient; (9) education and basic life skills; (10) socioeconomic characteristics, lifestyle, and current legal status; (11) use of community resources; (12) treatment readiness; and, (13) level of cognitive and behavioral functioning. These comprehensive assessment procedures combined with a comprehensive mental health assessment can aid in assessing comorbidity with appropriate precision.

GENERAL PRINCIPLES OF TREATMENT

Even when using an integrated treatment approach and a qualified treatment team, treating this population is difficult owing to the multiple issues unique to these patients. Children and adolescents with comorbid disorders are at greater risk for problems with family and school, criminal involvement, and suicidal behaviors than youths with SUDs alone (4). Also, problems related to substance use tend to persist over a longer period of time when the patient has a co-occurring mental health disorder (36). Further, comorbid patients tend to be at increased risk for non-adherence with treatment, poorer treatment outcomes, and greater use of system resources when compared to patients with just a SUD (37). As noted earlier, psychiatric comorbidity with SUDs is the rule, rather than the exception, and it seems to be essential to treat these co-occurring psychiatric conditions together (4). What follows is an overview of recent treatment research for children and adolescents with SUDs and a co-occurring psychiatric condition (see Table 1).

Attention-deficit/hyperactivity disorder (ADHD)

In general, the rates of substance use are elevated for youths with ADHD, and the presence of oppositional defiant disorder or conduct disorder has been shown to further increase the risk and frequency of illicit alcohol and/or drug use (7, 38, 39). As previously noted, ADHD is one of the most common psychiatric comorbidities in young patients with SUD (9, 10, 12). Only a few trials have studied the effectiveness of FDA-approved ADHD medications for the treatment of comorbid ADHD and SUD in children and adolescents.

Recently, atomoxetine, a selective norepinephrine reuptake inhibitor, was studied in combination with motivational interviewing (MI)/cognitive behavioral therapy (CBT) for the treatment of co-occurring ADHD and SUD in adolescents. Thurstone et al. (11) randomized 70 adolescents (aged 13-19 years) meeting diagnostic criteria for ADHD and at least one non-tobacco SUD, as well as scoring ≥22 on the DSM-IV ADHD Rating Scale (ARS-IV), to double-blind treatment with atomoxetine + MI/CBT or placebo + MI/CBT for up to 12 weeks. Participants weighing <70 kg initiated double-blind medication treatment at a dose of 0.5 mg/kg/day to 0.75 mg/kg per day. The dosage was increased 25 mg per week until the total daily dose reached 1.1-1.5 mg/kg/day. Participants weighing ≥70 kg initiated atomoxetine versus placebo at 50 mg/day.

Dosage for these patients was increased to 75 mg/day during the second week of treatment and to 100 mg/day during the third week. Adverse events were generally mild; however, participants treated with atomoxetine experienced vomiting more frequently than those treated with placebo, while treatment with placebo was associated with muscle cramps and sadness. Both treatment groups experienced significant reductions in ADHD symptoms during the 12 weeks of treatment, based upon total scores on the ARS-IV. Further, based upon clinician-administered Timeline Follow back (TLFB) procedures, there was an overall significant decrease in non-nicotine substance use from baseline to week 12 for both treatment groups. Of note, the two groups did not significantly differ from one another in reduction of ADHD symptoms ($p = 0.298$) or in decrease in substance use ($p = 0.110$). Owing to the lack of a significant between-group difference, the authors concluded that the MI/CBT may have contributed to the large treatment response in both the placebo- and atomoxetine-treated groups.

Table 1. Selected Treatment Studies of Substance Use Disorders and Comorbid Psychiatric Conditions in Children and Adolescents

Study	N	Age range	Inclusion criteria/ Psychiatric diagnosis	Design	Medication and mean dose, mg/day*	Outcome**
Attention-Deficit/Hyperactivity Disorder (ADHD)						
Thurstone et al. (11)	70	13-19	ADHD + SUD; DSM-IV ADHD checklist score ≥22	12-week DB-RPCT; ATX + MI/CBT vs. PCB + MI/CBT	PT weight <70 kg = 1.19 mg/kg/day ATX; PT weight ≥70 kg = 88.8 mg/day ATX	↓ DSM-IV ADHD Checklist scores: ATX + MI/CBT = PCB + MI/CBT; ↓ substance use: ATX + MI/CBT = PCB+MI/CBT
Riggs et al. (40)	303	13-18	ADHD + SUD	16-week DB-RPCT; OROS-MPH + CBT vs. PCB + CBT	Maximum dose: 72 mg OROS-MPH	↓ ADHD-RS scores: OROS-MPH+CBT = PCB + CBT; ↓ substance use: OROS-MPH + CBT = PCB + CBT
Depressive Disorders						
Findling et al. (42)	34	12-17	Depressive Disorder + SUD; CDRS-R score ≥ 40	8-week DB-RPCT	Maximum dose: 20 mg FLX	↓ CDRS-R scores; FLX = PCB; # of positive urine drug screens: FLX = PCB
Hides et al. (43)	60	15-25	MDD + SUD	20-week open trial, 44-week follow-up	N/A	Week 20: 82.7% full or partial remission of MDD; Week 44: 84.0% full or partial remission of MDD
Riggs et al. (44)	126	13-19	MDD + CD + SUD	12-week DB-RPCT; FLX+CBT vs. PCB+ CBT	Maximum dose: 20 mg FLX	↓ CDRS-R scores: FLX + CBT > PCB + CBT; Treatment response (CGI-I ≤ 2): FLX + CBT = PCB + CBT; ↓ substance use: FLX + CBT = PCB + CBT; ↓ CD symptoms: FLX + CBT = PCB + CBT
Cornelius et al. (45)	70	14-25	MDD + CUD	12-week DB-RPCT; FLX + CBT/MET vs. PCB + CBT/MET	Maximum dose: 20 mg FLX	↓ depressive symptoms: FLX + CBT/MET = PCB + CBT/MET; ↓ CUD DSM-IV criteria: FLX + CBT/MET = PCB + CBT/MET
Cornelius et al. (46)	50	15-20	MDD + AUD	12-week DB-RPCT; FLX + CBT/MET vs. PCB+ CBT/MET	Maximum dose: 20 mg FLX	↓ depressive symptoms: FLX + CBT/MET = PCB + CBT/MET ↓ alcohol consumption: Fl X + CRT/MFT = PCB + CBT/MET

Table 1. (Continued)

Study	N	Age range	Inclusion criteria/ Psychiatric diagnosis	Design	Medication and mean dose, mg/day*	Outcome**
Bipolar Disorder (BP)						
Geller et al. (48)	25	12-18	*DSM-III-R* BP*** + *DSM-III-R* SDD	6-week DB-RPCT; Li⁺ + IPT vs. PCB + IPT	Mean = 1769 (401) mg/day Li⁺; Target serum levels = 0.9-1.3 mEq/L	↓ *DSM-III-R* mood symptoms: Li⁺ + IPT = PCB + IPT; ↓ *DSM-III-R* SDD symptoms: Li⁺ + IPT = PCB + IPT; ↑ CGAS scores: Li⁺ + IPT > PCB + IPT
Psychotic Disorders						
Green et al. (49)	262	16-40	First-episode psychosis; Lifetime SUD: n = 97	12-week DB-RCT; OLZ vs. HPL	Mean modal dose OLZ = 10.2 mg/day; Mean modal dose HPL = 4.8 mg/day	Treatment response:**** Lifetime SUD: 27%; No SUD: 35%
Sevy et al. (51)	49	16-40	First-episode psychosis + CUD	16-week DB-RCT; OLZ vs. RIS	Mean modal dose OLZ = 15 (6) mg/day; Mean modal dose RIS = 4 (2) mg/day	Response rate: OLZ = RIS

* If applicable.
** An "=" sign in the Outcomes column indicates no significant difference between treatments.
*** *DSM-III-R* BP = bipolar I disorder, bipolar II disorder, mania, or major depressive disorder with at least one of the adolescent predictors of future BP.
**** (1) ratings ≤ 3 on the Positive and Negative Syndrome Scale (PANSS) items P1, P2, P3, P5, and P6; (2) ≥30% reduction from baseline PANSS score; and (3) a CGI-S score < 4.
↓ = decrease; ADHD = attention-deficit/hyperactivity disorder; ADHD-RS = ADHD Rating Scale; ATX = atomoxetine; BP=bipolar disorder; CBT = cognitive behavioral therapy; CD = conduct disorder; CDRS-R = Children's Depression Rating Scale-Revised; CUD = cannabis use disorder; DB = double-blind; FLX = fluoxetine; HPL = haloperidol; IPT = interpersonal therapy; Li⁺ = lithium; MDD = major depressive disorder; MET = motivation enhancement therapy; MI = motivational interviewing; OLZ = olanzapine; OROS-MPH = osmotic-release methylphenidate; PCB = placebo; PT = patient; RCT = randomized controlled trial; RPCT = randomized placebo-controlled trial; RIS = risperidone; SDD=substance dependence disorder; SUD = substance use disorder.

In a similar fashion, Riggs et al. (40) randomized 303 adolescents (aged 13-18) meeting diagnostic criteria for ADHD and at least one non-tobacco SUD to double-blind treatment with osmotic-release methylphenidate (OROS-MPH) + CBT or placebo + CBT for up to 16 weeks. Medication treatment was initiated at 18 mg/day of OROS-MPH versus placebo and increased to a maximum daily dose of 72 mg during the first two study weeks. Measures, including the ADHD Rating Scale (ADHD-RS) and the Clinical Global Impressions-Improvement (CGI-I) scale, were used to assess for improvements in ADHD symptoms. Substance outcome measures included the TLFB and urine drug screens. In both treatment groups, ADHD symptoms and substance use decreased (all p values < 0.001). However, no significant between-group differences were found. Some secondary outcomes did favor treatment with OROS-MPH, including lower parent ADHD-RS scores and more negative urine drug screens. The authors concluded that CBT for SUD may contribute to ADHD treatment response.

Warden et al. (41) explored potential associations of co-occurring MDD with baseline demographic/clinical characteristics, treatment response, and adherence/retention in a subset of the study participants with ADHD and SUD from the Riggs et al. (40) study. After comparing the 38 patients with comorbid MDD, ADHD, and SUD to the 265 patients without comorbid MDD, the authors found that the adolescents with co-occurring MDD were more likely to have more severe substance use at baseline and during study participation. As a result, the authors concluded that adolescents with ADHD, MDD, and SUD may also require interventions targeting depression.

In summary considering the large treatment responses in the groups not receiving active medication in the studies described above, it is possible that psychotherapeutic interventions for substance use that were provided concomitantly with the placebo or active medication may have contributed to the abating of ADHD symptomatology in children and adolescents with ADHD and an SUD in these clinical trials. Further exploration into the effectiveness of psychotherapy in this population appears to be warranted.

Depressive disorders

Both fluoxetine and escitalopram are FDA-approved for the treatment of MDD in young patients. However, for some time, fluoxetine was the only approved antidepressant medication for children and adolescents with MDD. Likely for this reason, fluoxetine is the most commonly studied antidepressant medication in young patients with MDD and co-occurring SUD, whether as monotherapy or in combination with psychotherapy.

Antidepressant monotherapy
Findling et al. (42) randomized 34 participants (12-17) meeting diagnostic criteria for a depressive disorder (MDD, dysthymic disorder, or depressive disorder not otherwise specified) and an SUD to double-blind treatment with either fluoxetine (n = 18) or placebo (n = 16) for up to 8 weeks. It is important to note that the study's final sample size was modest due to that fact that enrollment was terminated following a planned interim futility analysis. In this study, participants were initially given 10 mg of fluoxetine /placebo and could have their dose increased to 20 mg after four weeks, based on the discretion of the treating physician. Any participants and their families who were not currently receiving

psychotherapy were offered referrals to community-based resources for substance use disorders during study participation.

The primary efficacy measure was the Children's Depression Rating Scale-Revised (CDRS-R). Although both treatment groups had a reduction in CDRS-R scores, at the end of study participation, placebo-treated patients experienced a greater mean reduction in CDRS-R score than fluoxetine-treated patients. There were no statistically significant between-group differences in treatment-emergent adverse events; one patient in the placebo group and one patient in the fluoxetine group discontinued study participation owing to suicidal ideation. Further, there was not a significant difference in rates of positive urine drug toxicology results between treatment groups.

CBT monotherapy

Hides et al. (43) treated 60 participants (15-25 years) with MDD and co-occurring substance misuse or an SUD with individual integrated CBT treatment. Over 20 weeks, study participants received 10 CBT sessions plus case management. Measures used to assess symptoms of depression and anxiety included the Mood and Anxiety Symptom Questionnaire (MASQ), the Hamilton Depression Rating Scale (HAM-D), the Hamilton Anxiety Rating Scale (HAM-A), the Clinical Global Impression (CGI) scale, and the Social and Occupational Functioning Scale (SOFAS). Substance use measures included the TLFB, Alcohol Use Disorders Identification Test (AUDIT), Severity of Dependence Scale (SDS), Readiness to Change Questionnaire (RTCQ), Drug Use Motives Measure (DUMM), and urine drug screens. Study participants were assessed mid-trial (10 weeks), post-trial (20 weeks), and at six month follow-up (44 weeks). After 20 weeks, 82.7% of the study participants achieved partial or full remission of MDD. Overall, CBT was associated with significant improvements in depression, anxiety, and social and occupational functioning. Additionally, treatment with CBT resulted in significant reductions in the presence and number of SUDs, substance use, severity of dependence on substances, and increased days of abstinence.

Combination CBT and antidepressant therapy

Riggs et al. (44) examined the effects of fluoxetine and CBT on adolescents (13-19 years) with MDD, at least one non-tobacco SUD, and conduct disorder (CD). One hundred-twenty six participants were randomized to double-blind combination treatment with either fluoxetine (20 mg/day) or placebo and CBT for up to 16 weeks. Individual one-hour CBT sessions were administered at each study visit. For MDD, the main outcome measures were the CDRS-R and the CGI-I, while CD was assessed via self-report of number of symptoms in the past 30 days. Substance use was measured by self-report and urine drug screens. While fluoxetine combined with CBT had greater efficacy than placebo combined with CBT on change from baseline CDRS-R score, no between-group differences were noted on the CGI-I.

Further, both treatment groups reported an overall decrease of self-reported substance use and number of CD symptoms. However, the placebo-CBT group had a significantly higher proportion of substance-free weekly urine screen results than the fluoxetine-CBT group. The authors noted that adverse events in both groups were generally mild and transient. Suicidal ideation (assessed by CDRS-R item #13) decreased overall in both groups, however five study participants (fluoxetine + CBT n = 4; placebo + CBT n = 1) were evaluated or hospitalized for concerns of worsening suicidality during the study. The authors concluded that treatment with CBT, rather than with fluoxetine, may be associated with both depressive symptom improvement and decreased substance use in children and adolescents with MDD, SUD, and CD, considering the mixed efficacy findings and significant treatment response.

The 12-week efficacy of fluoxetine versus placebo in combination with CBT and motivation enhancement therapy (MET) for the treatment of depressive symptoms and cannabis use was studied by Cornelius et al. (45). Seventy adolescents and young adults (14-25 years) meeting DSM-IV criteria for a cannabis use disorder (CUD) and for MDD were randomized to double-blind treatment with either fluoxetine or placebo plus CBT/MET. To maximize participant safety and to minimize the risk of medication side effects, treatment with fluoxetine was initiated at 10 mg/day during the first two weeks of study participation and increased to 20 mg/day thereafter. Study participants received nine sessions of CBT/MET.

Both treatment groups showed significant improvements in both self-reported depressive symptoms, based upon the Beck Depression Inventory (BDI), and clinician-rated depressive symptoms, based upon the Hamilton Rating Scale for Depression (HAM-D). However, no between-group differences were found. Further, a significant decrease of approximately 40% was noted across both treatment groups in the number of DSM criteria for cannabis dependence during the study. Cornelius et al. (45) concluded that the lack of between-group differences in both depressive symptoms and cannabis-related symptoms may result from the efficacy of CBT/MET or from limited fluoxetine efficacy.

Similarly, Cornelius et al. (46) explored the acute efficacy of fluoxetine plus CBT/MET versus placebo plus CBT/MET in 50 adolescents and young adults (15-20 years) with MDD and an alcohol use disorder (AUD). Study participants were randomized in a double-blind fashion to either condition for up to 12 weeks of treatment. Treatment with fluoxetine was initiated at 10 mg/day during the first two weeks of study participation and increased to 20 mg/day thereafter. Study participants received nine sessions of psychotherapy. Analysis of the BDI and the HAM-D demonstrated significant reductions in depressive symptoms in both treatment groups. Per the Structured Clinical Interview for the DSM (SCID) and TLFB, the number of DSM-IV AUD symptoms significantly decreased, and the number of days of heavy alcohol use significantly decreased as well in both treatment groups. There were no serious adverse events, and fluoxetine was well-tolerated. Of note, the number of days of heavy alcohol use was significantly associated with the lack of remission of BDI depression scores (BDI < 8) at study week 6 and study week 12/end of study.

Similar to Cornelius et al. (45), the authors concluded that the lack of between-group differences in both depressive symptoms and drinking may result from the efficacy of CBT/MET or from limited fluoxetine efficacy. At two-year follow-up, both treatment groups demonstrated continued improvements in both depressive and alcohol-related symptoms compared to a group of adolescents with MDD and AUD that received naturalistic treatment (47). Again, no significant difference was noted between fluoxetine and placebo, thus suggesting that CBT/MET may be efficacious for the long-term treatment of MDD and AUD in adolescents and young adults.

Summary for depressive disorders

In each of the trials outlined above, both depressive symptoms and substance use decreased during study participation, regardless of treatment intervention. Considering the lack of difference between treatment with fluoxetine and placebo when combined with psychotherapy, it is possible that psychosocial treatments for substance disorders may be beneficial for young patients with MDD and an SUD. Further study of psychotherapeutic interventions in the absence of pharmacotherapy appears to be warranted in this population.

Bipolar disorder

Treatment research for children and adolescents with co-occurring bipolar disorders and an SUD is quite limited. In the only published trial we could identify, under the auspices of a randomized, double-blind, placebo-controlled study in this population, Geller et al. (48) treated 25 study participants (12-18 years) meeting diagnostic criteria for a DSM-III-R criteria for a bipolar disorder with either lithium or placebo for up to 6 weeks. Target lithium serum levels during the study were set to 0.9 to 1.3 mEq/L. Both treatment groups received weekly interpersonal therapy modified for use with families. Based upon mood and substance dependence item scores on the Schedule for Affective Disorders and Schizophrenia for School-Age Children (K-SADS), there were no significant differences between the two treatment groups with regard to symptomatic improvement.

However, Children's Global Assessment Scale (CGAS) scores were significantly higher at the end of study participation in participants randomized to lithium. Further, study participants randomized to lithium had significantly fewer positive random urine drug screens when compared to participants randomized to placebo ($p = 0.028$). Treatment with lithium was well-tolerated. Despite the administration of interpersonal therapy to all study participants, outcomes for this psychosocial treatment were not measured. Because lithium appears to be efficacious for the treatment of both bipolar disorders and SUD, longer-term and replication studies may be warranted.

Psychotic disorders

There are limited data regarding the treatment of young patients with psychotic disorders and comorbid SUDs, despite the association between substance use and early-onset psychotic symptoms (24-28). However, a few studies exploring clinical outcomes of patients with SUDs and psychotic disorders have included participants under the age of 18 years.

Green et al. (49) reported on the rates and effects of co-occurring SUDs in 262 patients (16-40 years) with first-episode psychosis (meeting DSM-IV criteria for schizophrenia, schizoaffective disorder, or schizophreniform disorder) receiving double-blind treatment with either olanzapine or haloperidol for up to 12 weeks. Of the 262 study participants, 97 (37%) had a lifetime DSM-IV SUD: 74 (28%) with a cannabis use disorder, 52 (21%) with an alcohol use disorder (AUD), 17 (6%) with a cocaine use disorder, 12 (5%) with a hallucinogen/PCP disorder, and 3 (1%) with a opioid use disorder. Treatment response was defined by: (1) ratings ≤3 on the Positive and Negative Syndrome Scale (PANSS) items P1, P2, P3, P5, and P6; (2) ≥30% reduction from baseline PANSS score; and (3) a CGI-S score < 4.

In both treatment groups, patients with a comorbid SUD were less likely than those without an SUD to meet criteria for response (27% versus 35%). In the olanzapine group, patients with an AUD were significantly less likely to respond to treatment than patients without an AUD ($p < 0.02$). Patients with an SUD and treated with haloperidol were significantly less likely to complete study participation compared to patients without an SUD and treated with haloperidol ($p < 0.04$). In the olanzapine group, SUD did not affect length of study participation, a finding in contrast to other adverse outcomes associated with the presence of SUD. Green et al. (49) concluded that first-episode psychosis patients are likely to have a co-occurring SUD, and that the presence of these disorders may negatively influence treatment response.

Secondary analysis of data from the acute treatment phase of a prospective, randomized trial of patients (16-40 years) with first-episode psychosis (meeting DSM-IV criteria for schizophrenia, schizoaffective disorder, or schizophreniform disorder) (50) compared the efficacy of olanzapine and risperidone in patients with co-occurring cannabis use disorders (CUDs) (51). Forty-nine patients with first-episode psychosis and CUD were randomized to treatment with either olanzapine (n = 28) or risperidone (n = 21) for up to 16 weeks. Sevy et al. (51) found that, in this subset of patients with CUD, neither rates of study completion nor rates of response differed between treatment groups. Additionally, there were no significant differences between treatment groups for the proportion of study participants with CUD using alcohol or cannabis during the trial.

Summary for psychotic disorders

In the absence of data, it is difficult to draw definitive conclusions specific to the treatment of young patients with psychotic disorders and comorbid SUDs. Considering a lack of difference between antipsychotic agents with regard to amelioration of psychotic symptoms and effects on substance use, other factors such as side effect profiles of individual agents may help determine antipsychotic medication selection for young patients with psychotic disorders and comorbid SUDs. However, it appears that the presence of SUDs is associated with worse outcomes, and, accordingly, specific evidence-based treatments for this population are needed.

Anxiety disorders

Despite an association between higher rates of anxiety disorders in those with substance use disorders (4, 12, 18), treatment research for children and adolescents suffering from co-occurring anxiety disorders and SUDs is lacking. However, there is evidence to suggest that children and adolescents with anxiety disorders (generalized, separation, and social anxiety disorders) who receive and respond positively to long-term treatment with CBT are less likely to engage in substance misuse in the future compared to patients who do not respond positively to CBT (52).

TREATMENT RECOMMENDATIONS AND PROGNOSIS

In both community and clinical populations of children and adolescents, SUDs are common and frequently co-occur with other psychiatric conditions. Further, children and adolescents who suffer from both SUDs and psychiatric disorders are more likely to experience negative outcomes when compared to youths with SUDs and no psychiatric comorbidities (4). Fortunately, there are emerging evidence-based treatments for these co-occurring conditions. Recent intervention research suggests that combining psychotherapeutic and pharmacotherapeutic interventions are perhaps the most effective methods of treating this patient population. However, further exploration into effective treatments is warranted, particularly with regard to treatment approaches for patients who do not initially respond to psychotherapy.

In general, prognosis for untreated comorbid patients can be poor. Nevertheless, prognosis can be improved if the following steps are adhered to during the assessment, diagnosis, treatment, and maintenance of these patients: (1) use of validated assessment tools; (2) assessment and treatment by qualified and trained clinicians; (3) making accurate diagnoses of both the SUDs and the mental health disorders; and (4) use of evidence-based and integrated treatment protocols.

ACKNOWLEDGMENTS

Dr. Findling receives or has received research support, acted as a consultant, received royalties from, and/or served on a speaker's bureau for Abbott, Addrenex, Alexza, American Psychiatric Press, AstraZeneca, Biovail, Bristol-Myers Squibb, Dainippon Sumitomo Pharma, Forest, GlaxoSmithKline, Guilford Press, Johns Hopkins University Press, Johnson & Johnson, KemPharm Lilly, Lundbeck, Merck, National Institutes of Health, Neuropharm, Novartis, Noven, Organon, Otsuka, Pfizer, Physicians' Post-Graduate Press, Rhodes Pharmaceuticals, Roche, Sage, Sanofi-Aventis, Schering-Plough, Seaside Therapeutics, Sepracore, Shionogi, Shire, Solvay, Stanley Medical Research Institute, Sunovion, Supernus Pharmaceuticals, Transcept Pharmaceuticals, Validus, WebMD and Wyeth. Drs. Ellington and Hertzer, Ms. Rowles, and Mr. Tarr have no financial ties to disclose. Ms. Rowles completed this project as part of her position as Communications and Analysis Specialist at Case Western Reserve University. This paper is a revised and adapted version of an earlier publication in the book "Substance abuse in adolescents and young adults. A manual for pediatric and primary care clinicians" edited by Donald E Greydanus, Gabriel Kaplan, Dilip R Patel and Joav Merrick with Walter de Gruyter in Berlin, 2013.

REFERENCES

[1] Kessler RC, Avenevoli S, Costello EJ, Georgiades K, Green JG, Gruger MJ, et al. Prevalence, persistence, and sociodemographic correlates of DSM-IV disorders in the National Comorbidity Survey Replication Adolescent Supplement. Arch Gen Psychiatry 2012; 69: 372-80.

[2] Copeland W, Shanahan L, Costello EJ, Angold A. Cumulative prevalence of psychiatric disorders by young adulthood: a prospective cohort analysis from the Great Smoky Mountains Study. J Am Acad Child Adolesc Psychiatry 2011; 50: 252-61.

[3] Substance Abuse and Mental Health Services Administration. *Results from the 2010 National Survey on Drug Use and Health: mental health findings*. Rockville, MD: Substance Abuse and Mental Health Services Administration, NSDUH Series H-42, HHS Publication No. (SMA) 11-4667, 2012.

[4] Bukstein OG, Work Group on Quality Issues. Practice parameter for the assessment and treatment of children and adolescents with substance use disorders. J Am Acad Child Adolesc Psychiatry 2005; 44: 609-21.

[5] Kandel DB, Johnson JG, Bird HR, Weissman MM, Goodman SH, Lahey BB, et al. Psychiatric comorbidity among adolescents with substance use disorders: findings from the MECA study. J Am Acad Child Adolesc Psychiatry 1999; 38: 693-9.

[6] Armstrong TD, Costello EJ. Community studies on adolescent substance use, abuse, or dependence and psychiatric comorbidity. J Consult Clin Psychol 2002; 70: 1224-39.

[7]   August GJ, Winters KC, Realmuto GM, Fahnhorst T, Botzet A, Lee S. Prospective study of adolescent drug use among community samples of ADHD and non-ADHD participants. J Am Acad Child Adolesc Psychiatry 2006; 45: 824-32.

[8]   Lewinsohn PM, Klein DN, Seeley JR. Bipolar disorder in a community sample of older adolescents: prevalence, phenomenology, comorbidity, and course. J Am Acad Child Adolesc Psychiatry 1995; 34: 454-63.

[9]   Latimer WW, Stone AL, Voight A, Winters KC, August GJ. Gender differences in psychiatric comorbidity among adolescents with substance use disorders. Exp Clin Psychopharmacol 2002; 10: 310-5.

[10] Dennis M, Godley SH, Diamond G, Tims FM, Babor T, Donaldson J, et al. The Cannabis Youth Treatment (CYT) study: main findings from two randomized trials. J Substance Abuse Treat 2004; 27: 197-213.

[11] Thurstone C, Riggs PD, Salomonsen-Sautel S, Mikulich-Gilbertson SK. Randomized, controlled trial of atomoxetine for ADHD in adolescents with substance use disorder. J Am Acad Child Adolesc Psychiatry 2010; 49: 573-82.

[12] Wu L, Gersing K, Burchett B, Woody GE, Blazer DG. Substance use disorders and comorbid Axis I and II psychiatric disorders among young psychiatric patients: findings from a large electronic health records database. J Psychiatr Res 2011; 45: 1453-62.

[13] Wilens TE, Martelon MK, Joshi G, Bateman C, Fried R, Petty C, et al. Does ADHD predict substance-use disorders? A 10-year follow-up study of young adults with ADHD. J Am Acad Child Adolesc Psychiatry 2011; 50: 543-53.

[14] Harty SC, Ivanov I, Newcorn JH, Halperin JM. The impact of conduct disorder and stimulant medication on later substance use in an ethnically diverse sample of individuals with attention-deficit/hyperactivity disorder. J Child Adolesc Psychopharmacol 2011; 21: 331.

[15] Gau SSF, Chong MY, Yang P, Yen CF, Liang KY, Cheng ATA. Psychiatric and psychosocial predictors of substance use among adolescents: longitudinal study. Br J Psychiatry 2007; 190: 42-8.

[16] Brook DW, Brook JS, Zhang C, Koppel J. Association between attention-deficit/hyperactivity in adolescence and substance use disorders in adulthood. Arch Pediatr Adolesc Med 2010; 164: 930-4.

[17] Birmaher B, Ryan ND, Williamson D, Brent DA, Kaufman J, Dahl RE, et al. Child and adolescent depression: a review of the past 10 years. Part I. J Am Acad Child Adolesc Psychiatry 1996; 35: 1427-39.

[18] Lubman DI, Allen NB, Rogers N, Cementon E, Bonomo Y. The impact of co-occurring mood and anxiety disorders among substance-abusing youth. J Affect Disord 2007; 103: 105-12.

[19] Wilens TE, Biederman J, Kwon A, Ditterline J, Forkner P, Moore H, et al. Risk of substance use disorders in adolescents with bipolar disorder. J Am Acad Child Adolesc Psychiatry 2004; 43: 1380-6.

[20] Goldstein BI, Strober MA, Birmaher B, Axelson DA, Esposito-Smythers C, Goldstein TR, et al. Substance use disorders among adolescents with bipolar spectrum disorders. Bipolar Disord 2008; 10: 469-78.

[21] Wilens TE, Biederman J, Adamson JJ, Henin A, Sgambati S, Gignac M, et al. Further evidence of an association between adolescent bipolar disorder with smoking and substance use disorders: a controlled study. Drug Alcohol Depend 2008; 95: 188-98.

[22] Steinbuchel PH, Wilens TE, Adamson JJ, Sgambati S. Posttraumatic stress disorder and substance use disorders in adolescent bipolar disorder. Bipolar Disord 2009; 1: 98-204.

[23] American Academy of Child and Adolescent Psychiatry. Practice parameter for the assessment and treatment of children and adolescents with schizophrenia. J Am Acad Child Adolesc Psychiatry 2001; 40: 4S-23S.

[24] Veen ND, Selten JP, van der Tweel I, Feller WG, Hoek HW, Kahn RS. Cannabis use and age at onset of schizophrenia. Am J Psychiatry 2004; 161: 501-6.

[25] Barnes TRE, Mutsatsa SH, Hutton SB, Watt HC, Joyce EM. Comorbid substance use and age at onset of schizophrenia. Br J Psychiatry 2006; 188: 237-42.

[26] Sevy S, Robinson DG, Napolitano B, Patel RC, Gunduz-Bruce H, Miller R, et al. Are cannabis use disorders associated with an earlier age of onset of psychosis? A study in first-episode schizophrenia. Schizophr Res 2010; 120: 101-7.

[27] DeHert M, Wampers M, Jendricko T, Franic T, Vidovic D, De Vriendt N, et al. Effects of cannabis use on age at onset in schizophrenia and bipolar disorder. Schizophr Res 2011; 126: 270-6.
[28] Dragt S, Nieman DH, Schultze-Lutter F, van der Meer F, Becker H, de Haan L, et al. Cannabis use and age of onset of symptoms in subjects at clinical high risk for psychosis. Acta Psychiatr Scand 2012; 125: 45-53.
[29] Lichtenstein DP, Spirito A, Zimmermann RP. Assessing and treating co-occurring disorders in adolescents: examining typical practice of community-based mental health and substance use treatment providers. Comm Ment Health J 2010; 46: 252-7.
[30] Petersen CL, Zettle RD. Treating inpatients with comorbid depression and alcohol use disorders: a comparison of acceptance and commitment therapy versus treatment as usual. Psychol Rec 2002; 59: 521-36.
[31] Drake RE, Mueser KT, Clark RE, Wallach MA. The course, treatment, and outcome of substance disorder in persons with severe mental illness. Am J Orthopsychiatry 1996; 66: 42-51.
[32] Havassy BE, Shopshire MS, Quigley LA. Effects of substance dependence on outcomes of patients in a randomized trial of two case management models. Psychiatric Serv 2000; 51: 639-44.
[33] Mueser KT, Torrey WC, Lynde D, Singer P, Drake RE. Implementing evidence-based practices for people with severe mental illness. Behavior Modification 2003; 27: 387-411.
[34] Jensen-Doss A, Weisz JR. Diagnostic agreement predicts treatment process and outcomes in youth mental health clinics. J Consult Clin Psychol 2008; 76: 711-22.
[35] Substance Abuse and Mental Health Services Administration. Report to congress on the prevention and treatment of co-occurring substance abuse disorders and mental disorders. Washington, DC: U.S. Government Printing Office, 2002.
[36] Cosci F, Fava GA. New clinical strategies of assessment of comorbidity associated with substance use disorders. Clin Psychol Rev 2011; 31: 418-27.
[37] Pray ME, Watson LM. Effectiveness of day treatment for dual diagnosis patients with severe chronic mental illness. J Addict Nurs 2008; 19: 141-9.
[38] White HR, Xie M, Thompson W, Loeber R, Stouthamer-Loeber M. Psychopathology as a predictor of adolescent drug use trajectories. Psychol Addict Behav 2001; 15: 210-8.
[39] Molina B, Pelham W. Childhood predictors of adolescent substance use in a longitudinal study of children with ADHD. J Abnorm Psychol 2003; 112: 497-507.
[40] Riggs PD, Winhusen T, Davies RD, Leimberger JD, Mikulich-Gilbertson S, Klein C, et al. Randomized controlled trial of osmotic-release methylphenidate with cognitive-behavioral therapy in adolescents with attention-deficit/hyperactivity disorder and substance use disorders. J Am Acad Child Adolesc Psychiatry 2011; 50: 903-14.
[41] Warden D, Riggs PD, Min SJ, Mikulich-Gilbertson SK, Tamm L, Trello-Rishel K, et al. Major depression and treatment response in adolescents with ADHD and substance use disorder. Drug Alcohol Depend 2012; 120: 214-9.
[42] Findling RL, Pagano ME, McNamara NK, Stansbrey RJ, Faber JE, Lingler J, et al. The short-term safety and efficacy of fluoxetine in depressed adolescents with alcohol and cannabis use disorders: a pilot randomized placebo-controlled trial. Child Adolesc Psychiatry Ment Health 2009; 3: 11.
[43] Hides L, Carroll S, Catania L, Cotton SM, Baker A, Scaffidi A, et al. Outcomes of an integrated cognitive behaviour therapy (CBT) treatment program for co-occurring depression and substance misuse. J Affect Disord 2010; 121: 169-74.
[44] Riggs PD, Mikulich-Gilbertson SK, Davies RD, Lohman M, Klein C, Stover SK. A randomized controlled trial of fluoxetine and cognitive behavioral therapy in adolescents with major depression, behavior problems, and substance use disorders. Arch Pediatr Adolesc Med 2007; 161: 1026-34.
[45] Cornelius JR, Bukstein OG, Douaihy AB, Clark DB, Chung TA, Daley DC, et al. Double-blind fluoxetine trial in comorbid MDD-CUD youth and young adults. Drug Alcohol Depend 2010; 112: 39-45.
[46] Cornelius JR, Bukstein OG, Wood S, Kirisci L, Douaihy A, Clark DB. Double-blind placebo-controlled trial of fluoxetine in adolescents with comorbid major depression and an alcohol use disorder. Addict Behav 2009; 34: 905-9.

[47] Cornelius JR, Douaihy A, Bukstein OG, Daley DC, Wood DS, Kelly TM, et al. Evaluation of cognitive behavioral therapy/motivational enhancement therapy (CBT/MET) in a treatment trial of comorbid MDD/AUD adolescents. Addict Behav 2011; 36: 843-8.

[48] Geller B, Cooper TB, Sun K, Zimerman B, Frazier J, Williams M, et al. Double-blind and placebo-controlled study of lithium for adolescent bipolar disorders with secondary substance dependency. J Am Acad Child Adolesc Psychiatry 1998; 37: 171-8.

[49] Green AI, Tohen MF, Hamer RM, Strakowski SM, Lieberman JA, HGDH Research Group, et al. First episode schizophrenia-related psychosis and substance use disorders: acute response to olanzapine and haloperidol. Schizophr Res 2004; 66: 125-35.

[50] Robinson DG, Woerner MG, Napolitano B, Patel RC, Sevy SM, Gunduz-Bruce H, et al. Randomized comparison of olanzapine versus risperidone for the treatment of first-episode schizophrenia: 4-month outcomes. Am J Psychiatry 2006; 163: 2096-102.

[51] Sevy S, Robinson DG, Sunday S, Napolitano B, Miller R, McCormack J, et al. Olanzapine vs. risperidone in patients with first-episode schizophrenia and a lifetime history of cannabis use disorders. Psychiatry Res 2011; 188: 310-4.

[52] Kendall PC, Safford S, Flannery-Schroeder E, Webb A. Child anxiety treatment: outcomes in adolescence and impact on substance use and depression at 7.4-year follow-up. J Consult Clin Psychol 2004; 72: 276-87.

In: Public Health Yearbook 2015
Editor: Joav Merrick

ISBN: 978-1-63484-514-4
© 2016 Nova Science Publishers, Inc.

Chapter 17

SUBSTANCE ABUSE AND ADOLESCENT GIRLS

Ruqiya Shama Tareen, MD*
Women's Behavioral Health, Department of Psychiatry,
Western Michigan University School of Medicine,
Kalamazoo, Michigan, United States of America

ABSTRACT

Clinicians who treat young adolescents are concerned about the rising rates of initiation of substance abuse in younger adolescents for obvious reasons. Traditionally, we have treated substance abuse as one entity without paying attention to the specific needs based on age, gender, and psychosocial makeup of the particular population. Adolescent and pre-adolescent girls in their early formative years are abusing alcohol and other substances at a much higher rate than ever before posing a unique challenge for substance abuse providers. This paper discusses some of the often over looked complications of substance abuse that are unique to the adolescent female population, including substance abuse associated sexual activity, resultant pregnancies, and associated obstetric/gynecological psychiatric complications such as perinatal mood disorder.

Keywords: substance abuse, adolescence, females, girls

INTRODUCTION

This paper considers recent trends, risk factors, and consequences for substance abuse in adolescent females. The rate of substance abuse is on the rise in US youth. According to the Substance Abuse and Mental Health Services Administration (SAMHSA), substance abuse trends are changing dramatically with initiation rates highest in young age and a dramatic shift in gender trends (1, 2). The most recent data collected in 2009 showed that 730, 228

---

* Correspondence: Ruqiya Shama Tareen MD, Associate Professor of Psychiatry, Director of Women's Behavioral Health, Department of Psychiatry, Western Michigan University School of Medicine, 1717 Shaffer Road, Kalamazoo, MI 49048, United States. E-mail: shama.tareen@med.wmich.edu.

patients twelve years and older reported using alcohol and other drugs requiring an admission to an alcohol or drug treatment program.

Alcohol remains the most commonly abused substance in adolescents with the highest use among 19 year olds; in this group about 15% reported using alcohol. The rates starts declining from there to 12.8 percent in persons aged 18 to 25 years of age (1, 2).

Out of these, about 23% were only using alcohol while 39% reported using other drugs without alcohol, and about 37% reported using both alcohol and at least one other drug at the time of admission (3). Figure 1 depicts the recent trends in choice of substances in US adolescents.

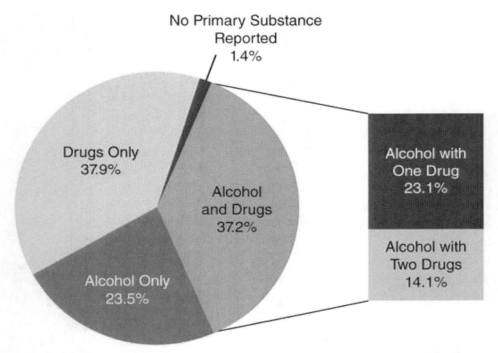

Source: Substance Abuse and Mental Health Services Administration (SAMHSA) Treatment Episode Data Set (TEDS), 2009, based on data received through November 3, 2010.
Permission. The *Data Spotlight* may be copied without permission. Citation of the source is appreciated. Find this report and those on similar topics online athttp://www.samhsa.gov/data/.

Figure 1. Substance Abuse and Mental Health Services Administration Treatment Data Set 2009.

GENDER DIFFERENCES IN SUBSTANCE ABUSE

Traditionally, substance abuse is considered to be a more common problem in male adolescents but in the last decade or so young girls slowly approached the same level. According to the SAMSHA 2000 report, when looking at the gender distribution in all age groups, males were more than twice as likely (7.7%) compared to their female counter parts (3.3%) to be abusing or being dependent on alcohol (1). While this may appear to support the general assertion that substance abuse is mainly a disease afflicting men, once one sifts through these data and breaks it out by age group, the picture changes considerably. For instance, in adolescents 12-17 years of age, the rate of alcohol abuse and dependence were very similar in both genders - 5.2% in boys versus 5.1% in girls (1).

The majority of new substance users, however, were younger and 56.2% of new initiators were female (1). Moving 5 years forward on this timeline, and in 2005, SAMSHA reported that -for the first time- adolescent girls age 12-17 years admitting to current alcohol use surpassed their male peers at the rate of 17.2% females versus 15.9% of males (2). The same pattern was seen in adolescents who started using illicit drugs other than alcohol. Over 55% were younger than age 18 when they first used, and 56.2% were female (2).

RISK FACTORS FOR SUBSTANCE ABUSE IN FEMALE ADOLESCENTS

Non-gender specific risk and protective factors have been identified that affect substance abuse predisposition in adolescents. The literature shows, in addition, that young adolescent girls have factors specific to their gender and age (see Figure 2). Early identification of these risk and protective factors is important because continuation of risks can worsen prognosis and enhancement of protective aspects can improve the course of illness. Figure 2 gives a brief overview of some of these risk factors.

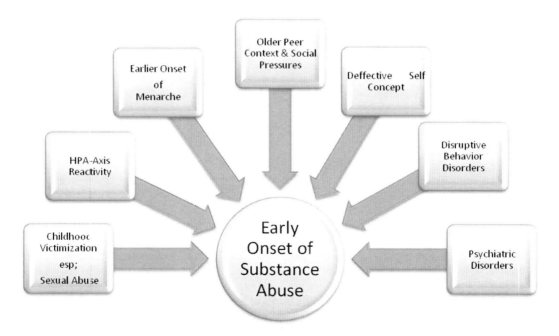

Figure 2. Risk Factors Predisposing to Early Onset of Substance Abuse in Female Adolescents.

Puberty status and timing

Attainment of puberty has been associated with a significant rise in smoking tobacco and cannabis, drinking alcohol, and abusing other substances independent of other variables such as school grade and age (4). Several researchers have suggested a role of pubertal changes and their possible link to this behavior. The age of menarche has been declining at a rate of 1–3 months per decade for more than last 175 years. For instance, in the United States in recent years, puberty has generally been occurring between the ages of 8 and 13 years of age in girls (5). It is well known that adolescents seldom start abusing substances before puberty (4). It has also been established that the earlier the onset of substance abuse, the worse the prognosis (4). The relationship between onset of puberty and initiation of substance abuse has been studied closely (5).

Puberty in this context is examined in two different developmental stages: Pubertal status and pubertal timing. Pubertal status refers to morphological changes or development of secondary sexual characteristics, defined in terms of Tanner stages of puberty (5). Puberty timing, on the other hand, is a comparison of one's pubertal standing relative to the same age and same gender peers (5). Girls who mature earlier have a higher risk of starting to abuse substances at an earlier age than their counterparts who are not as sexually matured (4, 5). Girls attaining menarche later have shown lesser risk of initiating substance abuse in early teen-age years.

There is no definite evidence of more precisely how pubertal status and timing are linked to addiction. It has been hypothesized, however, that pubertal timing affects the initiation of substance abuse. For instance, girls who attain puberty earlier than their peers are much more likely to start abusing alcohol or tobacco before age 13 years, which is itself a predictor of developing long term substance abuse and dependency (6).

Dick et al. followed five consecutive cohorts of Finnish twin girls and surveyed them at 16, 17, and 18 years of age (6). The data revealed that the twin sisters who were discordant for onset of menarche were also discordant in age of onset of substance abuse. The sisters with earlier onset of puberty were about 40% more prone to start abusing substances by age 13 when compared to their twin who achieved menarche later on (6). Attainment of puberty initiates a hormonal cascade that initiates specific changes in cognitive patterns reflective of adolescent behavior. This gives rise to ambivalence and contradictions in an adolescent who might feel out of place among age-matched peers. The initiation of substance abuse earlier in adolescents who mature earlier then age-matched peers may also be due to their identifying and associating with older persons, and their efforts to try to fit within that group by trying to engage in similar types of behavior (7).

HORMONAL CHANGES AND EMOTIONAL REACTIVITY

The hormonal cascade, which is responsible for Hypothalamic-Pituitary Axis (HPA) governs the pubertal development, can be divided into two separate processes; the early phase or adenarche and the later phase or goandarche. Adenarche can start as early as 6-9 years of age and is responsible for development of secondary sexual characteristics such as changes in skin and axillary and pubic hairs. This phase is characterized by release of dehydroepiandrosterone (DHEA) from the adrenal cortex without any changes in secretion of cortisol or adrenocorticotropic hormone (ACTH) (8).

Gonadotropin-releasing hormone (GnRH) induces release of luteinizing hormone (LH) and follicle stimulating hormone (FHS) from the pituitary gland. FSH and LH orchestrate the release of estradiol and progesterone from the gonads, which contributes to the development of secondary sexual development. Simultaneously the linear growth burst is taking place under the influence of growth hormone and insulin like growth factor-1 (IGF-1); also, cortisol is involved indirectly in this process. The challenge of physical and sexual development puts the adolescent body and mind under significant stress. Cortisol is critically important in enabling the adolescent to adapt to deal with the challenges of puberty (8).

It has been postulated that HPA-axis reactivity can be compromised in times of puberty, especially in adolescent girls. When adolescent girls during different stages of puberty were challenged with cortisol-releasing hormone (CRH), an increase in cortisol secretion was seen, suggesting a higher stress reactivity and vulnerability to stress (9). These girls not only showed increasing levels of total cortisol secretion following CRH challenge, they also had slower reactivity to cortisol, prolonged time to reach peak cortisol levels, and showed slower rate of recovery and return to base line cortisol levels (90. The baseline cortisol levels continue to increase over the course of different stages of puberty. In comparison adolescent boys actually showed a decline in baseline level of cortisol over the course of different stages of puberty (9).

This may suggest a gender specific HPA-axis dysregulation or inefficient response when girls are trying to adapt to stress of puberty (9). This HPA-axis dysregulation predisposes the adolescent females to dysphoria, irritability, and anxiety during the course of puberty (8, 9). This may also explain the significant gender divergence in incidence of psychiatric disorders such as depression and anxiety that emerges around puberty. This increased predisposition to psychiatric disorders at the time when the girls are already under pubertal stress can also predispose to substance abuse (9).

CHILDHOOD SEXUAL ABUSE

There are several different pathways that may lead to the early initiation of substance abuse in victims of sexual abuse. It has been proposed that psychological trauma suffered by these children alter the normal course of emotional, social, and cognitive development. This, in turn, creates significant hurdles in the already difficult path of mastering age appropriate normal developmental tasks. These developmental tasks include beginning to define one's own identity, constructing and consolidating self-concept, outlining normal interpersonal boundaries, and figuring out one's place in context of social context. A sexually traumatized young girl, while coping with this added burden, cannot negotiate appropriately with other normal developmental tasks at hands. It is likely that she may succumb to this overpowering psychological liability. Many children and adolescents who are sexually victimized struggle with issues of self-control, behavioral dysregulation and then engage in risky behaviors such as early substance abuse initiation (10).

Bailey et al. reported higher potential of initiation of early substance abuse in sexually abused young girls while controlling for all other confounding factors such as age, co-occurring physical abuse, childhood psychopathology (as depression and aggression), family history of alcohol and drug abuse (especially in mothers), and family dysfunction including income level, domestic violence, and parenting practices. The authors concluded that being sexually abused causes these girls to have a depressed self-concept, which leads to behavioral consequences that mediate early onset of substance abuse (10).

CONSEQUENCES OF SUBSTANCE ABUSE IN FEMALE ADOLESCENTS

Substance abuse is on rise in all adolescents but what is more worrisome is that adolescent females are smoking and using other substances much more than previously ever reported. In 2005 among all adolescents aged 12 to 17 years, the percentage of females who were currently drinking alcohol was first time higher than their male peers of same age group at 17.2% versus 15.9% (11). Onset of substance abuse in early age predisposes to lifelong emotional and physical struggles irrespective of gender; also, it poses some very unique challenges for female adolescent as depicted in Figure 3.

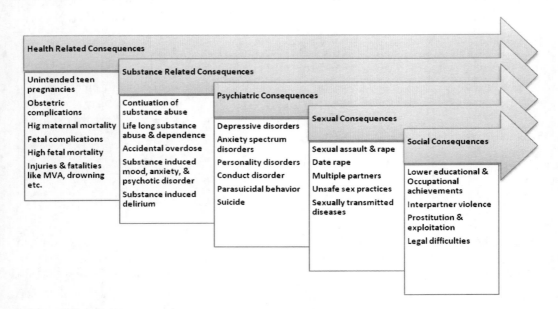

Figure 3. Consequences of Early Onset Substance Abuse in Female Adolescents.

SUBSTANCE ABUSE AND SEXUAL ACTIVITY

According to the US Centers for Disease Control and Prevention (CDC) data collected in 2009, about 9.1% adolescent female students enrolled in US high schools in 11th grade reported to be the victim of physical dating violence (PDV) and about 10.5% of adolescent girls in grades 9-12 reported being forced into a sexual encounter involving intercourse against their wishes (12). This was slightly higher from the PDV rates reported in a similar CDC survey report of 2003, at 8.8% (13). Both surveys reported higher prevalence of PDV and sexual victimization in African American and Hispanics females versus Caucasian females. From 2002 to 2004, pregnancy-related hospitalizations accounted for 49% of all hospital discharges for adolescent females. During the same period, injury related visits accounted for one third of all visits to emergency department for young girls and this rate increased by 70 percent for the groups aged 12-13 and 18-19 years of age (14).

Early initiation of substance abuse of any kind predisposes an adolescent girl to a higher risk of becoming involved in a sexual encounter and a much higher risk of becoming pregnant as a result of it. Cavazos-Rehg et al. studied the connection between the incidence of substance abuse in young high school female students (9th through 12th grades), and examined the link between initiation and intensity of substance abuse with engagement in sexual behavior resulting in teen pregnancies (15). They concluded that irrespective of the type of substance being abused (i.e., tobacco smoking, alcohol or cannabis), initiation of any type of substance abuse was associated with higher risk of sexual activity which resulted in a higher incidence of teen pregnancies. They also found a dose dependent relationship in that higher amounts of substances used posed a higher risk of getting pregnant (15). This correlation was true for even tobacco use in girls who started smoking at age 12 or younger and smoked on a daily basis (15).

Some of the risk factors are common and predisposes to both of these high-risk behaviors. In a cross sectional national survey of high school females which was conducted as part of the National Youth Surveillance System, about 10% of the 3000 participants reported having been pregnant at the time this survey was conducted. The rate was higher for Hispanic girls at 13.8% compared to White girls at 7.2% and there was a much significant difference in African American girls at 21.3% (15).

It is believed that the causes of initiating substance abuse early on and engaging in other risky behaviors such as sexual activity are due to lose of an external locus of self-control along with lack of development of an internal inhibitory control that usually is compounded by low parental monitoring and lack of positive role modeling. Also, it is not necessary for one of these behaviors to always precede the other. For instance, the initiation of substance use may be a direct cause of disinhibition resulting from substance use as well as an indirect cause of engaging in sexual behavior because of one sexual partner introducing the other one to substance abuse. Alternatively, substance use may precede sex because of an outside factor or process that includes history of childhood sexual abuse and other forms of victimizations, abnormal family dynamics, family history of substance use, and easy availability of drugs (16).

SUBSTANCE ABUSE AND UNWANTED PREGNANCY

The United States has seen a gradual decline in adolescent pregnancy rates since 1990 that more importantly includes a 34% decline in teen pregnancies in the 15–19 year age group over this period of time. However the 2007 birth rate for adolescences females increased by 4% from 2005 to 2007 or 42.5 births per 1,000 in 15–19 years. The rate was 22.2 births per 1,000 in those 15–17 years of age and 73.9 per 1,000 or 6% higher in those 18–19 year of age when compared to rates from 2005. For the 10–14 years of age group, however, the birth rates were unchanged at 0.6 per 1,000 (17).

One can extrapolate that the increasing trend of initiation of substance abuse earlier in youth may predispose young girls to other risky behaviors including sexual activity leading to an increase in birth rate and pregnancy as well as birth related health risks. In the US, adolescent girls aged 15-19 years who became pregnant reported that for 81% of them, pregnancy was unintended (18). About 40% of these pregnancies end in termination (18).

SUBSTANCE ABUSE AND PSYCHIATRIC DISORDERS

The relationship between psychiatric disorders and substance abuse is bidirectional. On the one end of this spectrum, psychiatric disorders are a risk factor for developing and continuing substance abuse; on the other hand, adolescents may present with psychiatric disorders as a short or long term sequelae of the substance abuse itself. Research has demonstrated that pubertal development may have a different impact on the psychological development of girls versus boys. The ratio between testosterone and estradiol changes during pubertal stage, and while this happens in all adolescents in same way irrespective of gender, somehow it affects the emotional tone differently according to gender. In pubertal girls the impact on emotional tone is more negative predisposing them to mood disorders while in boys it has a more protective effect (19).

Puberty is the key age where divergence in the prevalence of depressive disorders between the two genders will start and eventually reach a 2:1 ratio. This ratio remains steady throughout the rest of the female reproductive span until it declines and become equal to men around menopause. Girls score higher on a standardized depression scale between ages 12 and 16 while in pre-puberty years, the scores stayed steady from ages 8 to 11 years (20). Likelihood of co-occurrence of psychiatric and addictive disorders in adulthood increases significantly if both disorders start early on in life (20).

The prevalence of depressive disorders in adulthood increases from 10% in the general population to 30-50% in the presence of a co-occurring substance abuse disorder; also, this rate may be much higher in adolescents (21). In efforts to elucidate links between depression and addictive processes in the adolescent population, Rao et al. discussed three different ways in which both psychiatric and addictive disorders appear to have a common origin (21). Genetic studies have shown a strong predilection for both psychiatric and substance abuse disorders in probands if there is a history of either one type of disorder in the family of origin (see chapter 2). Family history of substance abuse or psychiatric disorders also predispose to an earlier onset of either depressive or addictive disorder (21). Both types of disorders also appear to have involvement of reward and motivation pathways located in the mesocorticolimbic dopamine system (MCD) of brain (see chapter 1) (21).

Depression presents as a down regulation of this pathway when a person develops anhedonia, low energy, withdrawal from activities, and amotivation. On the other hand, a drug addicted individual may desperately be trying to activate these pathways by repeatedly and increasingly using higher amounts of substances to avoid a dysphoric state (21). Many depressive symptoms are encountered in withdrawal states from many substances of abuse including but not limited to nicotine, alcohol, and other psychostimulants (see chapters 6,8, 10, and 15). The MCD system reinforces many of the euphoric or stimulating effects of drugs of abuse so that withdrawal from these substances is associated with lower levels of dopamine in this system and associated structures such as the nucleus accumbens and amygdale (21). Functional neuroimaging of brains of depressed people have shown loss of volume and decreased activity in these areas, suggesting a role of the MCD system.

There is also an increase in dopamine level in the striatum following treatment with antidepressants, indicating a role of dopamine in both types of disorders. Serotonergic deficiency, which is a major neurotransmitter in the pathophysiology of depression, is also shown to be deficient in alcohol withdrawal states whereas resuming alcohol intake is associated with increase in serotonin level (21). There are also findings that support a common role of cholinergic and GABA-ergic systems in depressive and addictive disorders (21). The fact that many co-occurring disorders respond to treatment with psychotropic medication support this common underlying origin of both disorders (21).

PERINATAL MOOD DISORDERS

In adolescent girls, substance abuse may pose unique challenges that include the added burden of unwanted pregnancy and its psychiatric sequelae. Girls who become pregnant are at a major risk to develop depressive disorders while pregnant and major psychiatric problems after delivery. They usually also have many other psychosocial risk factors which further make them more vulnerable for developing perinatal mood disorders (see Table 1 and Figure 4).

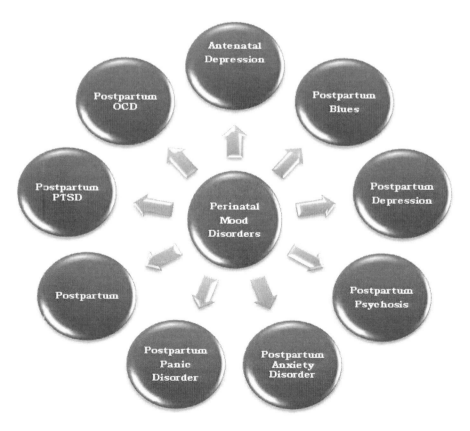

Figure 4. Spectrum of Perinatal Psychiatric Disorders.

Table 1. Common Risk Factors Predisposing to Pregnancy and Perinatal Mood Disorders

Some Common Risk Factors Predisposing to Teen Pregnancy and Perinatal Mood Disorders
Previous history of depression or anxiety spectrum disorders
Substance abuse
Family history of substance abuse
Family history of depression
Major life stressors
Childhood sexual abuse and history of other forms of trauma
Inter-partner violence
Poor social support

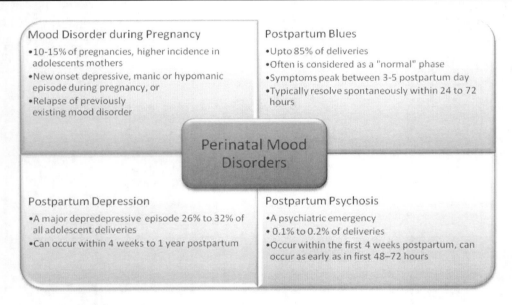

Figure 5. Types of Perinatal Mood Disorders.

Adolescent mothers are at much higher risk of becoming depressed or have a relapse of preexisting mood disorders whether unipolar or bipolar disorder. However, sometimes perinatal mood disorders in this age group may not present as a full-blown major depressive or bipolar disorder, and symptoms may be ill defined making the diagnosis difficult. Perinatal depression predisposes these adolescent to increased risk of obstetric complications including pre-eclampsia, low fetal weight gain, premature delivery, and a higher risk of cesarean section.

The perinatal period is also known as a period when adolescents with a history of other psychiatric disorders including various anxiety spectrum disorders (especially obsessive compulsive disorder [OCD] and posttraumatic stress disorder [PTSD]), may show worsening of symptoms or resurgence of a dormant problem. Perinatal depression is highly comorbid with symptoms of generalized anxiety, OCD, and panic disorder.

Adolescent mothers who were subjected to sexual abuse as children may have a sudden relapse of PTSD symptoms such as nightmares and flashbacks along with a tendency for avoidance and hyper vigilance. Adolescent mothers with history of eating disorder may have a very difficult time during pregnancy. Pregnancy related weight changes may lead to serious issues with their body image, causing them to starve, binge, purge, or restrict particular foods in order to preserve their ideal body image characteristic of eating disorders.

Depression may worsen during the third trimester, and the severity of depressive symptoms may be directly proportional to younger age as well as drug abuse (including nicotine and alcohol) along with other psychosocial stressors. Young mothers with depression are at an increased risk for giving birth prematurely, having instrument-assisted vaginal deliveries, and cesarean sections. Adolescent mothers have much lower resilience ability than older women impacting their ability to develop a positive adaption to pregnancy and to be able to cope with the responsibilities of motherhood (22). Figure 5 outlines various psychiatric disorders that may complicate the perinatal period.

SPECTRUM OF PERINATAL MOOD DISORDERS

Clinicians often consider this as a normal phase of the post-partum period. The symptoms peek between 3-5 days postpartum. The new mothers feel fatigued and complain of having no energy or appetite. They are irritable, acutely hypersensitive to any emotional stimuli, excessively worried about the baby, and easily overwhelmed. At times they feel they have no feelings for the baby. No treatment is necessary as the blues' phase is usually over within a week (23).

Postpartum psychosis

This is very rare but serious disorder complicating about only 0.1% to 0.2% of deliveries. Women with a history of bipolar disorder have a 50% chance of developing a postpartum psychotic episode. The risk is much higher in the first pregnancy but if they had a psychotic episode, this increases the risk of having another psychotic episode in subsequent pregnancies by 57% (24). The symptoms start within the first 4 weeks postpartum but may occur as early as in the first 48–72 hours (24). Most cases of postpartum psychosis are a severe manic or depressive episode of bipolar disorder with psychotic features. Symptoms can be of varied nature, including auditory and visual hallucinations, delusions of religious nature or involving an evil versus good struggle. Delusions with a focus on the infant can be quite dangerous as these mothers can harm their infants. In essence this is a true psychiatric emergency requiring immediate psychiatric admission and management (24).

Postpartum depression (PPD)

Postpartum depression (PPD) complicates about 4.8% to 15% of deliveries and this wide range depends on the different diagnostic criteria used. These adolescent mothers are at a much higher risk of developing PPD, as high as 47% of the adolescent deliveries (24). Diagnosis of PPD may not occur in a timely manner for some of them - predisposing these young mothers and their babies to various complications. Even when diagnosed, up to 15% of these women continue to have active symptoms lasting for as long as 24 weeks after the onset of the index episode (24). The Diagnostic and Statistical Manual of Psychiatric Disorders (DSM-IV-TR) defines postpartum depression as occurring within 4 weeks postpartum; however, recent research suggest that a PPD episode can occur within one year postpartum with a peak incidence at 12 weeks postpartum (25). PPD symptoms include sleep disturbances, low energy, lack of appetite, anhedonia (especially lack of interest in the baby and impaired responses to the infant's cues), persistent depressed mood with frequent crying spells, suicidal ideation, and at times infanticide ideation (24, 25).

SUBSTANCE ABUSE AND SUICIDE RISK IN YOUNG GIRLS

The link of substance abuse to suicidality is complex due to the multiple compounding psychosocial factors involved in most of these cases and also the fact that at times, it is very difficult to discern which came first. Is it the suicidality that leads to daredevil behavior including substance abuse or it is substance abuse that leads to depressive symptoms and suicidality? Behnken et al. looked at alcohol abuse as a mediator between forced sexual activity and suicidality in young girls (26). About 28% of girls reported binge drinking and this behavior was found to be highly associated with suicidal behavior in this sample. About 11% of these girls also reported being a victim of forced sexual intercourse. The study indicated a link between binge drinking to both forced sexual intercourse and suicidality (26). The association between alcohol and suicidal ideation remained strong even when one controls for sexual assault.

The pathway of mediation from forced sexual activity to suicidality was weakened when alcohol was taken out of the equation. These associations remained constant when examined across races in Caucasian, Hispanic, and African American girls. The risk of going from suicidal ideation to attempting and even completing suicide in this group of girls was much higher in the adolescent group (26). Substance abuse predisposed them to impulsivity, disinhibition, aggression, and above all poor decision making - a perfect combination for suicidal behavior. It has also been reported that when substance abuse is not involved in a sexual assault, the victim is more likely to have better coping skills and better ability to deal with stress related to trauma (26).

IMPACT OF SUBSTANCE ABUSE ON ADOLESCENT MOTHER AND OFFSPRING

Many psychoactive drugs are known to produce deleterious maternal and fetal effects in young pregnant women. The most notable one is alcohol in the well documented Fetal Alcohol Syndrome (FAS). FAS is comprised of a constellation of phenotypic features of various degrees along with developmental delays and cognitive difficulties (27). Expression of FAS occurs on a wide spectrum ranging from fetal alcohol effects, to an alcohol related neuro-developmental disorder, and to a fetal alcohol syndrome. The physical features vary significantly among affected children, ranging from mild deformities to about 8% of the infants having microcephaly; furthermore, 28% show growth retardation and 16% typical facial features (27).

The features of FAS include mid facial hypoplasia, short upturned nose, and other facial features, limb and joints anomalies, sensorineural hearing loss, and cardiovascular defects. Behavioral and cognitive effects include hyperactivity, attention problems, sensory integration difficulties, frequent temper tantrums, and fine motor difficulties. Approximately 75% of these children fall in the mild to moderate range of mental retardation (27).

Smoking tobacco increases the risk of spontaneous miscarriage in a dose dependent fashion, with risk increasing when 5 or more cigarettes a day are being smoked (28). Other maternal fetal risks observed in pregnant women smoking cigarettes are appetite suppression, low birth weight, higher plasma levels of carbon monoxide in mothers and fetus, decreased placental blood circulation, higher heart rate and decreased heart rate variability in the fetus, and much higher level of nicotine and it's byproducts in amniotic fluid. The role of hundreds of carcinogens and other toxic substances found in cigarettes is not very well defined at this time. Survey of 173,687 children with congenital malformation showed that smoking was associated with higher risks of developing cardiovascular, musculoskeletal, and gastrointestinal malformations as well as many other types of congenital malformations involving almost all systems.

Neurodevelopmental delays associated with nicotine exposures include language delays, lower global cognitive scores, and externalizing behaviors such as agitations, aggression, conduct disorder, and future risk of developing antisocial behavior (29). Temperamental difficulties and internalizing behaviors have also been documented. Increased risks of developing childhood cancer and infertility in the children exposed to smoking *in utero* as well as second hand smoke have been reported (29).

Other drug abuse has been on the rise in adolescent girls including cocaine abuse (see chapter 10). Cocaine abusing pregnant girls are at high risk for the development of spontaneous abortion, abruptio placenta, and preterm delivery. Fetal exposure to cocaine results in decreased birth weight and head circumference. Neurodevelopmental effects of cocaine are not very well understood; however, children exposed *in utero* to cocaine achieve lower scores on standardized tests (30).

SUBSTANCE ABUSE AND UNINTENTIONAL INJURIES

Alcohol is found to be responsible for about 36% of accidental deaths in adolescents from 15 to 20 years of age, while 20% of these were in children under age 15 years. Alcohol is also associated with 51% of traumatic brain injuries suffered in the adolescent age group (31). Alcohol related fatal and nonfatal injuries are a major problem in the adolescent age group. In 2005, about 13% of adolescents 12 years or older reported driving under the influence of alcohol at least once in the preceding year 2005, this corresponds to 31.7 million adolescents (31).

PREVENTION AND TREATMENT STRATEGIES SPECIFIC FOR ADOLESCENT GIRLS

The first step in devising any long-term treatment plan is to identify risk and protective factors and to devise a prevention strategy. The United States has seen a relative decline in substance abuse since the 1970s but this decline has not been seen in the female population; in fact in some age groups, it has been on rise, especially rates of earlier initiation of substance use in preteen girls (32). Studies have shown that even in age-matched controls when boys and girls are managed with the same protocols, the response rate in girls is more likely to be dependent on the risk factors predisposing them to substance abuse in first place (32).

Some of the risk factors are not gender specific such as poor psychosocial support, low socioeconomic conditions, lack of self-control, low academic achievement, and current home environment. Girls are more likely to report gender specific risk factors such as negative self-image, low self-worth, anxiety, depression, tendency to internalize stress, negative body image and dieting, and eating disorders (32). Physical and sexual abuse was also twice as commonly reported in girls than boys. These gender differences in risk factors were most prominent in the 12-13 year old age group but the difference dissipates slowly as age progresses (32).

Traditionally substance abuse programs have not focused on gender, racial, and ethnic differences in the population served. There is growing evidence that in order to be effective, existing substance abuse programs need to identify the specific risk and protective factors in the population they are serving especially in adolescent and female patients. Some of the previously used models can be modulated to address more gender-related issues such as gender specific issues in cognitive or social-ecological theory. In addition, recent gender specific theories are emerging which can be implemented to improve the outcomes and prognosis in adolescent females (32). Some of these theories are briefly described below.

Self-in-relation theory of women development

It has been proposed that good attachment is central to developing a girl's self-development in the context of the world around them. This is in contrast to the traditional model that all individuals strive for developing their own identity by separation and individuation, which was considered a critical milestone of this age group (32). Adolescent girls are more likely to become self-sufficient adults with a better worldview if they are interdependent on strong positive relationships. These strong healthy interpersonal connections give rise to greater knowledge of self and others, understanding of self-worth, confidence in self, zest, and motivation. It is important to develop programs specifically for preadolescent and adolescent girls that foster stronger, healthier connections within the family, teachers, or counselor, or through programs where such relationships can be fostered with peers and older women (32).

Social-structural model

There are several theories under this model that identify that men and women have different societal roles; also, socialization experiences are perceived and experienced vastly differently by preadolescent girls and boys (32). Any deviant social behavior such as substance abuse that is learned during this stage of development is the product of learned social behavior. In our society; peers, parents, teachers, and culture expect young girls to conform to societal gender specification. Girls are assigned this gender role very early on in life, limiting their abilities of self-actualization. They may feel suffocated in this traditional mold and this may lead to internalization behaviors including but not limiting to substance abuse.

Theory of gender and power

This theory focuses on the gender-based differential in heterosexual relationships and how they impact on the social and cultural context of women's health practices. The theory identifies three important areas of struggle for women in such dyadic relationship: division of labor, division of power, and structure of social norms as well as affective responses (32). This is a very important framework for understanding the high risk of substance abuse in adolescent girls who are physically and sexually abused and emotionally controlled.

A substance abuse program that constructs the rehabilitation and recovery framework around this model is going to help these adolescent girls to move forward from a passive to a more assertive role. When we empower young girls in this way, they learn better coping skills and will not have to rely on substance abuse to overcome such learned helplessness because of the abuse they have endured (32).

Gender informed or gender specific substance abuse treatment programs should provide treatment plans that focus on the following several important areas (32) (see Figure 6):

- *Improving self-efficacy:* This involves employing strategies to develop and enhance self-esteem as well as improve self and body image in these young girls.
- *Developing competencies:* Coach preadolescent and adolescent girls on how to change existing self-destructive behaviors and engage them in learning better coping strategies which they can use in problem solving in different areas of their lives, including interpersonal communications.
- *Promoting healthy life style:* Educating about how the risk taking behavior (such as substance abuse, unsafe sex, others.) impact the emotional and physical well-being and how to overcome this with healthy life style choices.
- *Improving family functioning:* Family therapy is part of most of traditional substance abuse programs but this needs to be more tailored towards female adolescent issues by facilitating better interpersonal communications and strengthening the family bonds by identifying power imbalances.
- *Treatment of comorbid psychiatric illness:* Given that a large number of female adolescents suffer from dual diagnosis, it is imperative to incorporate psychiatric care while they are in substance abuse rehabilitation programs to enhance compliance with the program and to improve outcomes.

- *Identifying unique challenges in treating pregnant adolescents:* This is often neglected and many programs have difficulties with providing care aiming to improve pregnancy outcomes and teaching parenting skills.

In essence, several gender-informed psychosocial models are now available and need to be incorporated in our traditional system of providing substance abuse treatment. If we choose to ignore gender differences, long term outcomes and prognosis could worsen. Gender specific programs are important to alter the course and prognosis of substance abuse disease in young women. Also, if they become pregnant while abusing substances and continue to do so during pregnancy, their children are also at high risk for negative outcomes (32).

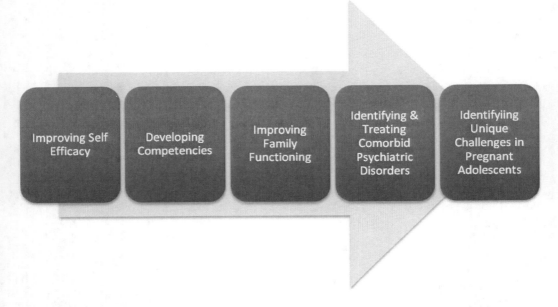

Figure 6. Substance Abuse Prevention and Treatment Strategies Specific for Adolescent Girls.

TREATMENT OF COMORBID PSYCHIATRIC ILLNESS

The bidirectional relationships of psychiatric comorbidities make it difficult to ascertain what level of treatment is necessary at a given time. It is very challenging to make a clinical distinction between primary psychiatric disorders with comorbid substance abuse and substance-induced psychiatric disorders. Taking time to obtain a careful history and to construct a chronological account of emergence of psychiatric disorders with substance abuse may help a clinician to devise an individualized plan, which may incorporate targeted treatment of both disorders.

Once it is established that a comorbid psychiatric disorder will benefit from treatment, efforts should be made to initiate it while also paying equal attention to encourage abstinence from substance abuse. The initial approach to treating most psychiatric disorders should be a psychotherapeutic approach (see chapters 4 and 5). Individual supportive therapy and cognitive behavioral therapy (CBT) have been shown to be effective in treating mild uncomplicated cases of depression as well as personality, and anxiety spectrum disorders. CBT focuses on eliciting negative schemas that patients may have developed about themselves, their relationships with family and friends, and their general worldview. CBT attempts to challenge these negative schemata and help patients change them in a positive direction. This helps these adolescents to develop a better understanding of their illness, improve compliance with their substance abuse treatment, and improve overall prognosis as well as long term abstinence.

Use of psychotropic medication will be necessary in patients with severe anxiety spectrum or depressive disorders who have failed to respond to psychotherapeutic interventions (see chapter 5). The decision to treat a comorbid psychiatric illness depends on the nature and severity of illness, and its impact on co-occurring substance abuse disorders. More likely than not, a comorbid psychiatric illness decreases compliance with the goals of substance abuse treatment programs and leads to a relapse and recovery revolving door. *Selective serotonin reuptake inhibitors* (SSRIs) are now considered the first line medications for the management of anxiety and depression in these patients. All SSRIs are considered equal in efficacy but only a few are officially approved for use in the pediatric population (32). At present fluoxetine is approved for use in children ≥8 years of age for depression and in those ≥7 years for obsessive compulsive disorder (OCD). Fluvoxamine is approved in patients ≥8 years, sertraline in patients ≥6 years, and escitalopram for adolescents ≥12 years of age for OCD (33). See chapters 5 and 13.

Once a decision is made to treat, the choice of an SSRI depends on various factors such as the specific side effect profile, whether this medication has produced good results in this patient previously or even has shown a good response in a family member, contraindications, the availability of acceptable formulations (i.e., solution or suspension), and its cost (33). Cost is an important factor as some of the newer SSRIs are not covered by major formularies or insurance plans. One should also take into account every measure possible to improve compliance with these medications. For instance, prescribing a medication with single daily dosing is usually preferable to two or three times a day dosing (33).

The United States Food and Drug Administration (FDA) has issued an advisory and black box warning about emergence of suicidal ideation during the initial phase of SSRI treatment; this development has changed the prescribing behaviors of many primary care physicians and pediatricians in recent years leading to a reluctance in some to prescribe SSRIs. It is, however, recommended that the use of SSRIs in children and adolescents be taken in consideration in situations where it is indicated and these pediatric patients should be followed closely, especially in the earlier phase of treatment, to monitor for any suicide risk (33).

TREATMENT OF SUBSTANCE ABUSE IN PREGNANT ADOLESCENTS

The cocaine epidemic of the 1980s in the United States was the first time that pregnant substance abusing women became a focus of medical attention. Most of attention, however, revolved around the obstetrical emergencies and complications in these women, and little attention was paid to the unique challenges these females posed for the existing traditional rehabilitation and recovery programs (34). Most substance abuse programs still continued to focus on traditional male-focused models when treating pregnant adolescents and failed to take in account that these young women are "not alone" in their struggle for recovery. They have to deal with the added psychological and physical burden of pregnancy while working on their recovery. While going through the rigors of abstinence, they have to take care of their children and deal with a multitude of related psychosocial stressors and often scarce resources that available to them (34).

Most researchers in the area of substance abuse management agree that screening for substance abuse should be done early on for all pregnant women irrespective of age, socioeconomic background, and their presentation (see chapter 3). Brief screenings tools such as the 4P-Plus questionnaire have been shown to be very effective and can be easily administered in a busy primary care or obstetrics practice (34). Engaging pregnant substance abusers in a substance abuse program is challenging. These young girls are usually facing many other psychosocial stressors and may lack the supportive and empathetic network needed to enhance their chances of long-term recovery.

Most young women do not divulge their substance abuse to their obstetric providers fearing the consequence of losing their children. Creating a safe and trusting environment for these women is important to build a therapeutic relationship. Developing a comprehensive program where these mothers can keep their children with them while engaging in recovery with the involvement of local child protective services has demonstrated a better retention rate (35). Pregnant women who successfully complete a comprehensive residential rehabilitation program of sufficient duration were shown to be more likely to remain abstinent, have fewer psychiatric comorbidities, be gainfully employed, and have better parenting skills and attitudes. More recently, motivational interviewing and computer-based motivational intervention have revealed good results in this high risk group (35).

Most pharmacological interventions used for substance abuse disorders are not well studied in pregnant population for obvious reasons. Two notable exceptions are the use of methadone and buprenorphine. A recently published prospective multicenter study compared 90 women taking buprenorphine versus 45 women who were managed on methadone, considered a gold standard in treating pregnant women with opioid dependence (36). The study reported no significant differences between these two strategies; both drugs showed equal efficacy and there were no differences in outcome measures such as pregnancy outcomes, birth outcomes, or severity of neonatal abstinent syndromes (36). This is of special significance in the adolescent population because opioid abuse and dependence is on the rise in this age group, mostly in form of prescription opioid abuse.

FUTURE ASPECTS

In last few years, there has been growing awareness of the lack of focus on the female population in the existing system of substance abuse management programs. SAMSHA has recognized this concept and in March of 2009, a panel started developing the competencies for substance abuse health care providers, specifically for adolescent girls and women. The task was to identify some overarching core concepts as a foundation to develop the competencies to address the specific needs of this population group (37).

Table 2. Core Competencies for Delivery of Gender Specific Substance Abuse Treatment

Competencies	Description
Gender Difference	Differences in physiology, cognition, emotions, social development, communication patterns, roles, socialization, risks, and resiliency affect the prevention, treatment, and recovery needs
Biopsychosocial & Spiritual	It is critical that staff delivering substance abuse care understand how sociocultural identities differ among women and girls and may lead to different health outcomes.
Violence and Trauma	Vulnerability to violence and trauma must be addressed in prevention efforts as well as other mental health and substance abuse services.
Physical & Medical Problems	Higher risk of physical and medical problem in women & girls and identifying the risk factors like intimate partner violence, rape/sexual abuse, and childhood abuse and neglect
Societal expectations & Sexuality	Acceptance and inclusion of women with lived experiences of mental health problems, substance abuse, and trauma in the delivery of comprehensive, gender-responsive services and recovery-oriented care.
Bounderies	Acceptance and inclusion of women in the delivery of comprehensive, gender-responsive services where staff delivers care with self-awareness and appropriate boundaries
Physiological Demands	Demands of puberty, pregnancy, perimenopause, menopause and accompanied physiological, psychological, and developmental changes, with changing risks, opportunities, and support needs.
Parenting and Family Context	Consideration of culturally sensitive, family-centered work with a woman's family is critical to her wellness and recovery, including working with children, intimate partners and other family members.
Socio-economic Considerations	Navigation, access, use, and coordination among community resources and systems may be necessary for women's success in prevention and treatment programs.
Stigma	Address the impact of stigma and stereotypes on recovery for women and girls, as well as the skills and attitudes required to address these challenges.

Adopted from Substance Abuse and Mental Health Services Administration (2011). Addressing the Needs of Women and Girls: Developing Core Competencies for Mental Health and Substance Abuse Service Professionals. HHS Pub. No. (SMA) 11-4657. Rockville, MD.

CONCLUSION

Rapidly rising rates of substance abuse in young girls pose unique challenges that are not commonly understood by health care providers. Substance abuse rehabilitation and recovery programs usually provide a male-oriented approach which fails to recognize the specific needs of the female population. There is a growing need to focus on understanding the protective and risk factors of preteen and teenage age girls early on to provide prevention, timely intervention, and abstinence efforts within a gender-specific treatment approach. Investment in developing comprehensive substance abuse and recovery programs will not only result in positive outcomes in these adolescent girls but will also decrease the likelihood of negative outcomes in their offspring.

ACKNOWLEDGMENTS

This paper is a revised and adapted version of an earlier publication in the book "Substance abuse in adolescents and young adults. A manual for pediatric and primary care clinicians" edited by Donald E Greydanus, Gabriel Kaplan, Dilip R Patel and Joav Merrick with Walter de Gruyter in Berlin, 2013.

REFERENCES

[1] SAMHSA, Office of Applied Studies, National Household Survey on Drug Abuse, 2000. Accessed 2013 Dec 02. URL: http://www.icpsr.umich.edu/icpsrweb/SAMHDA/studies/3262?q=national+house+hold+survey+2Date.

[2] Substance Abuse and Mental Health Services Administration. Results from the 2005 National Survey on Drug Use and Health: National Findings. Rockville, MD: Office of Applied Studies, NSDUH Series H-30, DHHS Publication No SMA 06-4194, 2006.

[3] Substance Abuse and Mental Health Services Administration (SAMHSA) Treatment Episode Data Set (TEDS), 2009, based on data received through Nov 3, 2010. Accessed 2013 Dec 02. URL: http://www. store.samhsa.gov/list/series?name=Treatment-Episode-Data-Set-TEDS.

[4] Patton GC, McMorris BJ, Toumbourou JW, Hemphill SA, Donath S, Catalano RF. Puberty and the onset of substance use and abuse. Pediatrics 2004;114:300-6.

[5] Ganong WF. Physiology of reproduction in women. In: DeCherney AH, Nathan L. Current diagnosis & treatment obstetrics and gynecology, 10th ed. New York: McGraw-Hill, 2007.

[6] Dick DM, Rose RJ, Viken RJ, Kaprio J. Pubertal timing and substance use: Associations between and within families across late adolescence. Dev Psychol 2000;36:180-9.

[7] Al-Sahab B, Ardem CI, Hamadeh MJ. Age at menarche and current substance use among Canadian adolescent girls: results of a cross-sectional study. BMC Public Health 2012;12:195-03.

[8] Blumenthal H. Relations among pubertal maturation, cortisol reactivity, pubertal timing, and social anxiety symptoms among female adolescents. ProQuest Dissertations and Theses, Univ of Arkansas, 2009.

[9] Stroud LR, Papandonatos GD, Williamson DE. Sex differences in cortisol response to corticotropin releasing hormone challenge over puberty: Pittsburgh Pediatric Neurobehavioral Studies. Psychoneuroendocrinol 2011;36(8):1226-38.

[10] Bailey JA. McCloskey LA. Pathways to adolescent substance use among sexually abused girls. J Abnorm Child Psychol 2005;33(1):39-53.

[11] Substance Abuse and Mental Health Services Administration. Results from the 2005 National Survey on Drug Use and Health: National Findings. Rockville, MD: Office of Applied Studies, NSDUH Series H-30, DHHS Publication No. SMA 06-4194, 2006.

[12] Shaw FE, Casey CG. Centers for Disease Control and Prevention. Surveillance Summaries. MMWR 2010;59:SS-5.

[13] Black MC, Noonan R, Legg M, Eaton D, Breiding MJ. Physical dating violence among high school students-United States. MMWR 2006;55:532-5.

[14] MacKay, Duran C, Andrea AP. Adolescent health in the United States. Hyattsville, MD: National Center Health Statistics, 2008-1034, 2008.

[15] Cavazos-Rehg PA, Bierut LJ, Cottler LB. Substance use and the risk for sexual intercourse with and without a history of teenage pregnancy among adolescent females. J Stud Alcohol Drugs. 2011;72(2):194-8.

[16] Palen LA, Smith EA, Cladwell LL, Mathews C, Vergnani T. Transitions to Substance Use and Sexual Intercourse Among South African High School Students. Subst Use Misuse 2009;44(13):1872-87.

[17] Hamilton BA, Martin JA, Ventura SJ. Births: Preliminary Data for 2007. Natl Vital Stat Rep 2009;57:12.

[18] Finer LB, Henshaw SK. Special Tabulations, commissioned by the national campaign to prevent teen and disparities in rates of unintended pregnancy in the United States, 1994 and 2001, Perspect Sex Repro H 2006;38(2):90-6.

[19] Angold A, Costello EJ, Worthman CM. Puberty and depression: the roles of age, pubertal status and pubertal timing. Psychol Med 1998;28(1):51-61.

[20] Twenge J, Nolen-Hoeksema S. Age, gender, race, socioeconomic status, and birth cohort differences on the Children's Depression Inventory: a meta-analysis. J Abnorm Psychol 2002;111(4):578-88.

[21] Rao U. Links between depression and substance abuse in adolescent's neurobiological mechanisms. Am J Prev Med 2006;31(6):S161-74.

[22] Salazar-Pousada D, Arroyo D, Hidalgo L, Pérez-López FR, Chedraui P. Depressive symptoms and resilience among pregnant adolescents: a case-control study. Obstet Gynecol Int 2010:1-7.
[23] O'Keane V, Lightman S, Patrick K, Marsh M, Papadopoulos AS, Pawlby S. Changes in the maternal hypothalamic-pituitary-adrenal axis during the early puerperium may be related to the postpartum 'blues.' J Neuroendocrinol 2011;23(11):1149-55.
[24] Doucet S, Dennis C, Letourneau N. Differentiation and clinical implications of postpartum depression and postpartum psychosis. J Obstet Gynecol Neonatal Nurs 2009;38(3):269-79.
[25] American Psychiatric Association. Diagnostic and Statistical Manual of Mental Disorders, Fourth Edition-Text Revision. Washington, DC: APA, 2000.
[26] Behnken MP, Le YCL, Temple JR. Forced sexual intercourse, suicidality, and binge drinking among adolescent girls. Addict Behav 2010;35:507–9.
[27] Jones MW, Bass WT. Fetal Alcohol Syndrome. Neonatal Netw 2003;22(3):63-70.
[28] Economides D, Braithwaite J. Smoking, pregnancy and the fetus. J R Soc Health 1994;114(4):198-201.
[29] Melo M, Bellver J, Soares SR. The impact of cigarette smoking on the health of descendants. Expert Rev Obstet Gynecol 2012;7(2):167.
[30] Loebstein R, Koren G. Pregnancy outcome and neurodevelopment of children exposed in utero to psychoactive drugs: The motherisk experience. J Psychiatry Neurosci 1997;22(3):192-6.
[31] Sleet DA, Ballesteros MF, Borse NN. A review of unintentional injuries in adolescents. Annu Rev Public Health 2010;31:195-212.
[32] Amaro H, Blake SM, Schwartz PM. Developing theory-based substance abuse prevention programs for young adolescent girls. J. Early Adolescence 2001;21(3):256-93.
[33] Kamboj MK, Tareen RS. Management of nonpsychiatric medical conditions presenting with psychiatric manifestations. Pediatr Clin North Am 2011;58:219-41.
[34] Chasnoff IJ, McGourty RF, Bailey GW. The 4P's Plus screen for substance use in pregnancy: clinical application and outcomes. J. Perinatol 2005;25(6):368-74.
[35] Lester BM, Twomey JE. Treatment of substance abuse during pregnancy. Womens Health 2008;4:67-77.
[36] Lacroix I, Alain Berrebi A, Garipuy D. Buprenorphine versus methadone in pregnant opioid-dependent women: a prospective multicenter study. Eur J Clin Pharmacol 2011;67(10):1053-9.
[37] Substance Abuse and Mental Health Services Administration. Addressing the needs of women and girls: Developing core competencies for mental health and substance abuse service professionals. Rockville, MD: Substance Abuse Mental Health Services Administration, HHS Pub No. (SMA) 11-4657, 2011.

Submitted: August 05, 2013. *Revised:* October 01, 2013. *Accepted:* October 10, 2013.

In: Public Health Yearbook 2015
Editor: Joav Merrick

ISBN: 978-1-63484-514-4
© 2016 Nova Science Publishers, Inc.

Chapter 18

COLLEGE STUDENTS, PRESCRIPTION STIMULANT, AND OTHER SUBSTANCE ABUSE

Brandon Johnson, MD, and Jeffrey H Newcorn, MD*
Mount Sinai School of Medicine, New York, United States of America

ABSTRACT

Substance abuse among college students has been the focus of considerable recent attention, given the high prevalence of use/abuse in this population, the nature of the drugs that are abused, the specific contextual issues that fuel abuse in this population, and the potentially dire outcomes of substance use in this population. It is hoped that better understanding the types of substance abuse that most often occur in the college age population, the specific contextual factors that support substance abuse in this population, and the various available methods of prevention and treatment of substance abuse that have been developed for college students will contribute to more informed approaches to managing this problem.

Keywords: substance abuse, college, students

INTRODUCTION

Substance abuse among college students requires specific attention because of the unique circumstances and characteristics of drug-taking behavior in this population. In 2011, the rate of illicit substance use among full-time college students was 22% (1). In addition to frank substance abuse, there are significantly higher rates of binge alcohol use among full-time college students as opposed to others aged 18-22 years. The risk of substance use in the college population is potentiated by decreased parental supervision, a new and complex social

---

[*] Correspondence: Jeffrey H Newcorn MD, Associate Professor of Psychiatry, Icahn School of Medicine at Mount Sinai, Department of Psychiatry, One Gustave L Levy Place Box 1230, New York, NY 10029, United States. E-mail: jeffrey.newcorn@mssm.edu.

structure that often includes communal living, and a view of substance intoxication as being relatively normative.

Consequences of substance use can have a profound impact on young adults, and are a major public health concern in the United States. Alcohol related deaths alone in college students reached 1,825 in 2005. In 2001, 10.5% of college students reported being injured because of drinking, 12% were hit or assaulted by another college student, and 2% reported sexual assault related to alcohol. Furthermore, 28.9% of college students reported driving while under the influence of alcohol, suggesting there is a significant risk of alcohol-related motor vehicle accidents (2). Another significant aspect of substance abuse in college students is its relation to comorbid mental health disorders and suicide. One study found that suicidal ideation was higher in students with nicotine dependence, alcohol related problems, and illicit drug use (3). Prevention and treatment of substance use disorders in college students may help to diminish these adverse outcomes and reduce the public health burden from this population.

Certain trends highlight the environmental influences of college life and their role in substance use. For example, college-bound 12th graders were found to have a lower than average use of all illicit substances while they were in high school compared to those who did not attend college. However, the eventual use of illicit substances by this group when they reached college was found to equal or in some cases exceed the use of their non-college peers. This "catching up" effect may in part be related to important contextual issues; the fact that college students often leave the parental home for the first time and tend to defer marriage leaves them more independent than they were in high school, but also not grounded in either their family of origin or a new family (4).

Increased academic demands and pressure to succeed may drive some college students to use substances as a coping mechanism, or even to misuse substances in an attempt to enhance academic performance. Of note, a national health survey found that college students reported the highest use in the past year of Adderall (i.e., mixed amphetamine salts, a stimulant medication prescribed for attention-deficit/hyperactivity disorder; see below) compared to several other demographic groups. This increased use among college students may be attributable to the desire to stay awake and focused during study time, as well as completion of course work (Johnston, 2011). Issues related to abuse of prescription stimulants will be covered in detail below.

The goals of this chapter are to discuss use of various licit and illicit substances of abuse by the college student population, including demographics and recent trends of use, relationship to use of other substances, co-occurrence of psychiatric disorders, consequences of using specific substances, and implications for prevention and treatment.

ALCOHOL

In addition to the types of alcohol abuse seen in other populations, binge drinking is particularly common in the college age population. Binge drinking is usually defined as having 5 or more drinks in a row on a single occasion for men, or 4 or more drinks for women (5). As this type of drinking is one of the main forms of alcohol use during the college years, it should be specifically queried in clinical assessment.

Prevalence and demographic features

Drinking increases rapidly during the young adult years and alcohol use peaks during these years (i.e., ages 18-24). The prevalence of alcohol abuse and dependence also peak during this age range. Roughly 38% of college students meet criteria for an alcohol use disorder – 31.6% meet criteria for alcohol abuse and 6.3% meet criteria for alcohol dependence (6). In one survey of college students (5), the prevalence of binge drinking in the 2 weeks prior to the survey was 50% in men and 39% in women. In the same study, more than one-fifth of college students binged 3 or more times in the two week period queried. Risk factors for higher rates of binge drinking in this population include male gender, Caucasian race, residing in a fraternity, being involved in athletics, binge drinking as a high school senior, and viewing parties as very important (5). In support of the above, results of another study indicate that high school drinkers are three times more likely to meet criteria for alcohol dependence during the first year of college than non-drinkers (7).

There is not a consensus about whether college students drink more than their non-college peers. Carter et al. found that college students drink more and with increased frequency compared to their non-college peers, however, these differences were thought to be due to factors other than college attendance itself (8). One such factor is the nature of the living situation; alcohol dependence was highest in men and women living in dormitories, while the highest levels of alcohol abuse were by men living off campus. Age was also determined to be an important factor in drinking habits. Increased frequency of drinking was found in younger college students, and tended to decrease later in college. The latter finding is in contrast to drinking patterns of non-college drinkers, whose drinking continues to increase throughout young adulthood.

Consequences

The frequent occurrence and potentially dire consequences of alcohol use disorders in college students illustrate that this problem is a major public health concern. Compiling data from multiple national public health resources, Hingson et al. reported that in 2005 college drinking accounted for 1,825 student deaths, 599,000 injuries, and 97,000 instances of sexual assault or date rape (2). Factors associated with adverse consequences from drinking include participation in athletics, living in dormitories, being a member of a fraternity/sorority, and spring break trips (9, 10).

New methods of ingestion

Alcohol is consumed and abused by college students in several non-traditional ways. One new method of consumption involves combining alcohol with energy drinks. Energy drinks are highly marketed to the young adult population, and it is estimated that 51% of college students consume them. Studies attempting to elucidate the reasons for mixing energy drinks with alcohol have concluded that college students mix the two in order to quicken the onset of intoxication, reduce fatigue after drinking, and because they don't like the taste of alcohol (11).

Dangers associated with the combination include: misjudgment of level of intoxication, the drinker's erroneous belief that he/she is able to perform tasks that require fine motor control, and increased intent of drinkers to drive home (12). Also of concern are findings that college students who consume alcohol mixed with energy drinks are significantly more likely to report marijuana, cocaine, and ecstasy use. Increased rates of high-risk sexual behaviors were also found in this population (12).

Another alarming recent development involves ingestion via the so-called "alcohol enema." This method involves placing a tube in the consumer's rectum and pouring beer through the tube, directly into the rectum. This practice is extremely dangerous as it avoids first-pass metabolism by the liver and increases the blood alcohol concentration very rapidly. A handful of cases of dangerous intoxication or death by this method have made national headlines in the U.S. No studies have yet been conducted to determine the prevalence of this method of ingestion.

Prevention and treatment

Nelson et al. examined the rate of college binge drinking and the rate of adult binge drinking by state, and found the two to be highly correlated (13). This study also showed an inverse relationship between the rates of college binge drinking and the number of laws in a state that restrict the promotion and sale of high quantities of alcohol. The rate of adult binge drinking and number of regulatory laws were determined to be independent predictors of college binge drinking. It is therefore reasonable to conclude that stricter regulation of alcohol sales may result in decreased binge drinking among college students.

Parental involvement is another important factor mediating alcohol use disorders in college. Kaynak et al. found that higher levels of parental monitoring during high school correlated with a decreased risk for alcohol dependence in the first year of college (7). Several parent-based interventions attempt to educate parents of incoming freshmen about the risks of college drinking, with the goal of increasing discussion between parents and students about alcohol use and abuse, and decreasing parental permissiveness regarding drinking. Measures of program effectiveness document a decrease in the frequency of alcohol use and the occurrence of high risk drinking in participants (7).

The specific circumstances and culture of college campuses may contribute to the high rates of alcohol use disorders in college students in important ways, and these can be targeted in prevention and treatment programs. Of note, amendments to the Higher Education Act of 1965 which specify policies to prevent the use of illicit drugs and abuse of alcohol are often not stringently enforced on college campuses. These regulations mandate that colleges share information with students and employees about the dangers of drug and alcohol consumption as well as available treatment options.

In 2012, the US Department of Education's Office of the Inspector General published a report indicating that enforcement of the substance use policies in the Higher Education Act has been almost nonexistent (14). Better enforcement of, and compliance with, these policies may help change the culture of college campuses, where many students report that drinking is an expected aspect of college life.

Treatment of alcohol use disorders in college students requires the same steps as treating alcohol use disorders in other age groups. Prochaska and DiClemente's Stages of Change (15) are especially pertinent to this population, and Motivational Interviewing (16) is accepted as the gold standard for therapeutic intervention. Particular problems in implementing these interventions in the college population include the inconsistent availability of resources, and ongoing uncertainty as to how best to deliver the treatments.

Early intervention, via brief structured interventions administered before or shortly after the onset of negative consequences of alcohol consumption, has been found to be particularly effective in reducing the frequency and consequences of alcohol use disorders. One example of such a program is the Brief Alcohol Screening Intervention for College Students (BASICS). This intervention involves two face-to-face interviews. The first encounter is a motivational interview, and the second gives personalized feedback based on student drinking behavior. Students undergoing this intervention were found to have a significant reduction in alcohol consumption as well as alcohol-related problems (17). The method of delivering alcohol education services may also influence the success of the outcome. Fachini found that face-to-face interventions, as opposed to computerized interventions, may be better received by the student and may create a stronger commitment to change (17).

NICOTINE

Despite extensive public health initiatives and costly government taxes on cigarettes, 18.1% of the U.S. population continues to smoke (18). Among college students, rates are at least as high or even higher; one recent study found that 35.3% of college students smoke cigarettes to varying degrees. Factors found to correlate with higher smoking level include having more friends that smoke, drinking, binge drinking, and more "other" tobacco use (19). Of note, many students in the latter study were non-daily smokers, who represent a growing subgroup of the smoking population. Despite the previous belief that non-daily smoking is a pathway to daily smoking, or conversely to quitting, evidence suggests that non-daily smoking behavior can be sustained for long periods of time, and poses serious health risks (20).

One important subset of non-daily smokers in college is the group of "social smokers." These individuals tend to smoke almost exclusively in the presence of peers – usually at parties, bars, or nightclubs. Schane et al. found that social smokers tend not to label themselves as smokers, do not consider themselves addicted, and often do not understand the negative consequences of their smoking (20). Consequently, this type of smoker shows little interest in quitting and believes he/she can quit at any time.

In addition to cigarettes, other means of smoking have become popular among college students – e.g., smoking tobacco through a hookah. As many as 50% of students who smoke tobacco with a hookah do not smoke cigarettes, and they tend to view hookah smoking as safer than cigarette smoking (21). However, smoking tobacco via a hookah one time delivers 20 times the number of carcinogens than one cigarette (22). Cigar use is also on the rise among college students, and there are a significant number of students who smoke cigars who do not smoke cigarettes (21). Consequently, smoking prevention efforts need to highlight the risks tobacco products other than cigarettes.

Important relationships exist between nicotine addiction and mental illness. Nearly every known psychiatric disorder has been shown to be associated with increased smoking rates, including affective disorders such as major depressive disorder and bipolar disorder, and psychotic disorders such as schizophrenia. In particular, nicotine use and depression are highly comorbid, and can each potentiate the other (23). Multiple anxiety disorders including post-traumatic stress disorder, panic disorder, generalized anxiety disorder, social anxiety disorder, and specific phobia have also been associated with increased risk of smoking (24). The link between smoking and psychiatric disorder is even clearer with regards to ADHD. A review by McClernon et al. highlighted that patients with ADHD have a higher rate of smoking, initiate smoking earlier, smoke larger quantities of cigarettes, and are less likely to quit compared to their non-ADHD counterparts (25). This strong association may be related to overlap in neurobiological and/or genetic substrates that underlie ADHD and smoking. In particular, both dopaminergic and nicotinic systems are implicated in the two disorders (25).

Treatment

Smoking cessation continues to be a major U.S. public health priority. Traditional methods of smoking cessation include the use of nicotine patches and gums, behavior modification therapies, or the combination. Pharmacologic agents influencing reward circuits in the brain, such as bupropion and varenicline, have shown efficacy in clinical trials; both of the above medications are FDA approved for smoking cessation. More recent data suggests that a combination of varenicline, bupropion, and a serotonin reuptake inhibitor may be more effective than varenicline alone in enhancing smoking cessation (26).

Due to the fact that non-daily smoking and binge drinking are highly comorbid behaviors in college students, concomitant treatment of alcohol use disorders may be an important strategy for smoking cessation in this population (27). Targeting comorbid non-substance abuse psychiatric disorders can also play an important role. As an example, a variety of psychopharmacologic therapies have been studied as possible adjunctive treatments for smoking cessation in patients with ADHD. In one study, OROS-methylphenidate (OROS MPH; a long-acting, sustained delivery form of the stimulant methylphenidate) was found to decrease ADHD symptoms, but did not impact smoking cessation (28).

However, another study (29) found that non-Caucasian patients had a statistically significant increase in smoking cessation when treated with adjunctive OROS MPH compared to Caucasian patients. Further study is necessary to better understand the apparent discrepancies across the latter two studies. Treatment of nicotine dependence can also overlap with treatment for mood and anxiety disorders. As discussed above, bupropion, a medication that can be used for smoking cessation, is also a commonly used treatment for depression and anxiety, and is also a recognized off-label treatment for ADHD.

MARIJUANA

Marijuana is second only to alcohol in frequency of use among college students. A survey of college students across the US found that 37.6% had tried marijuana at least once, and 15.9% had used in the prior month (30). Another study found that among past-year college users, 25% met DSM-IV criteria for a cannabis abuse disorder (31).

One factor which seems to influence marijuana use among college students is the perception of how much their peers use the substance. The ACHA survey cited above found that college students perceived that 81.8% of their peers had used marijuana in the last month (30). There is concern that the perception by abstainers that a vast majority of their peers are using may compromise their ability to maintain abstinence (31).

One tool for correcting misconceptions regarding peer use is the eCHECKUP TO GO (e-TOKE), a web-based marijuana intervention for college students currently abstaining from marijuana. In a pilot study using this instrument, e-TOKE was found to aid in decreasing the misperception of exaggerated use among peers. While there was no significant difference in initiation of marijuana use between the e-TOKE group and the control group, students who used this tool did report less perceived disapproval from their peers regarding their abstention (31).

Consequences

Marijuana use can be associated with a variety of adverse outcomes, both acutely and as a function of chronic use. Difficulties with psychomotor function, attention, memory, and learning have been associated with acute cannabis intoxication, and may persist after a short period of abstinence (33). In a study of at-risk marijuana users in college (≥5 times in the past year), the most common marijuana-related impairments were concentration problems, driving while high, missing class, and putting oneself at risk for physical injury (31). Many of the at-risk users in this study did not meet the criteria for a cannabis use disorder according to DSM-IV criteria. This finding underscores the importance of recognizing and targeting students for treatment even if they do not have a formal cannabis use disorder diagnosis (31).

Association with other conditions and implications for prevention and treatment

While marijuana use can have negative health consequences on its own, it is also important to consider the potential for comorbidity of marijuana, tobacco and alcohol use. Among college students who smoked marijuana in the last 30 days, 38% also smoked cigarettes, and 69% binge drank (34). Due to the high level of comorbid use of these substances, treatment and prevention measures which target multiple substance use may prove to be more effective than targeting any single drug of abuse.

In addition to established behavioral treatments for cannabis dependence (e.g., motivational enhancement, 12 step programs, CBT), there is new research on pharmacological agents that may be effective in promoting cannabis cessation (35). Gray et al. studied the over-the-counter agent N-acetylcysteine (NAC) as a possible treatment for cannabis use in adolescents between the ages of 15 and 21, based on the ability of this agent to up-regulate the cystine-glutamate exchanger in the nucleus accumbens (36). The cystine-glumate exchanger has been shown in animal models to be down-regulated during chronic administration, and administration of NAC has been shown to reduce drug-seeking behavior (37). Results of the Gray study were encouraging; there was a significant reduction in positive urine toxicology in the NAC-treated group versus the placebo group (36).

COCAINE

According to statistics collected by the Substance Abuse and Mental Health Services Administration, cocaine abuse is most prevalent among young adults in the United States and has been on the rise in recent years (38); 2.6% of college students reported last-year use in 1996 compared with 5.1% in 2007 (39). A high rate of exposure to opportunities for cocaine use has been shown to correlate with increased rate of use. Bythe end of their fourth year of college, as many as 36% of students have had the opportunity to use cocaine at least once, and 13% have used cocaine at least once. Of those students who reported having the opportunity, 37% used cocaine at some point during four years of college (40). Cocaine users are more likely to be male, Caucasian, and meet criteria for a comorbid alcohol or cannabis use disorder.

Possible gender differences should be considered; in the Kasperski study there was a non-significant trend for female college students who use cocaine to be more likely than their male peers to meet criteria for cocaine abuse (8.4% vs 5.4%) and cocaine dependence (9.3% vs 2.5%) (40). Although alcohol use and related consequences receive the most attention from college administrators, cocaine use also poses a serious health risk for college students, since cocaine use is relatively common and often concurrent with other substance use.

PRESCRIBED STIMULANTS

A growing and particularly pernicious problem in the college age population is the misuse, diversion and abuse of prescription stimulants, which are prescribed for attention-deficit hyperactivity disorder (ADHD). ADHD is a neuropsychiatric disorder that affects between 2% and 8% of the U.S. college student population (41). Stimulant medications are considered the gold standard treatment for ADHD, though a variety of non-stimulant medications and psychosocial treatment options are also available.

Recent emphasis on the frequent continuation of this disorder into adulthood has contributed to increasing use of prescription stimulant medications in the college population. However, accompanying the appropriate and justified increase in use of prescription stimulants in this population are important concerns about nonmedical use, diversion and abuse potential (42). In one study, specific risk factors for the nonmedical use of prescription stimulants among college students included being male, Caucasian, Jewish, affiliated with a fraternity or sorority, and having a lower grade-point average (42).

College students may misuse prescription stimulants to improve concentration, increase alertness and energy, as a study aid, and to attain euphoria (43). The communal nature of college living and the relatively visible nature of daily living habits in this setting likely represent additional important risk factors for diversion of stimulants in this population.

Of note, not all stimulant medications carry the same risk of misuse. College students are more likely to misuse short or intermediate acting formulations than long-acting formulations. This is particularly true for students who report using the medication to get high (43, 44). One possible reason for this difference in abuse potential is that the short acting stimulants produce a more immediate upsurge in stimulant blood level and resultant dopamine release, and thereby induce more of a euphoric effect than their longer-acting counterparts. Also of interest is the route of administration of stimulants when they are misused. One study found that nearly all misusers used an oral route of administration (95.3%), but 38.1% did report snorting the medication (44). Several studies have shown that mixed amphetamine salts (MAS; i.e., Adderall) and MAS-XR are the most commonly diverted stimulants in the college population (43, 44).

ADHD is the most frequent FDA-approved indication for stimulant medication use. The increasing number of prescriptions written, however, has led many to question the appropriateness of the ADHD diagnosis in an as yet undefined subgroup of individuals who are prescribed stimulants. Musso et al. noted that the base rate of malingering in the face of external incentives is 10.2% (45). Possible incentives for feigning ADHD and thereby receiving prescriptions for stimulant medications include the potential for improved performance, recreational use, and selling the medication illicitly. In addition, feigning a diagnosis of ADHD can result in receiving academic accommodations that may further improve performance. How to more carefully determine which students should be legitimately prescribed stimulants and academic accommodations for ADHD and weeding out those with malingering behavior remains the subject of much discussion.

Examples of misuse of prescription stimulants include using more of the drug than has been prescribed, mixing the drug with alcohol or other drugs, or using the drug to intentionally get high. In one study among college students using prescribed stimulants for ADHD, 40% reported misuse of some kind in the last year; 36% reported using too much of their stimulant, 19% reported general misuse, and 19% reported intentionally using their stimulant with other drugs (43). Another study found that 25% of college students who were prescribed stimulants for ADHD used the medication to get high (46). In the Sepulveda study, college students who initiated use of prescribed stimulants for ADHD during college were more likely to misuse their medications than those who initiated treatment at an earlier age (43).

A similar but somewhat different problem is the diversion of prescription stimulants; i.e., providing access to those who do not have a prescription. Data from one study showed that more college students report illicit use of prescription stimulants than medical use, and that the leading source of obtaining the medication was through friends or peers. In the same study, 54% of college students who were legitimately prescribed stimulants for the treatment of ADHD were approached to sell, trade, or give away their medication each year (42). Diversion of medication occurred in 36% of students who had received a prescription for stimulants. Among those who reported personal misuse of their stimulants, the rate of diversion was even higher (57%) (43). Similarly, Upadhyaya found that 29% of students prescribed stimulants reported that they had given or sold their medication to someone else at some point in time (46).

Associations/risk factors for misuse and diversion

Multiple studies have linked the misuse of prescription stimulants with increased use of other substances, including cigarette smoking, binge drinking, marijuana use, and other drug use (43, 46). Students with ADHD who had active ADHD symptoms were more likely to use tobacco or drugs other than alcohol or marijuana (46). While the relationships among ADHD symptoms, stimulant treatment and use of other substances is intriguing, it is unclear what the nature of the associations are; does misuse of ADHD medications lead to other substance abuse, or vice versa? One theory posits that nicotine use among students with active ADHD symptoms represents self-medicating, since nicotine is known to enhance dopaminergic neurotransmission and has been shown to improve attention in individuals with ADHD (47). Due to the increased level of other substance use in students who misuse prescription stimulants, one must consider these individuals to be at increased risk for the negative outcomes associated with those other substances as well.

Prevention and treatment

Prevention and treatment strategies include: 1) better control of ADHD symptoms, which will likely decrease risk for subsequent drug abuse; 2) considering the full range of therapeutic options (i.e., not just stimulant medications) for treating youth with ADHD; 3) counseling college students about the potential personal and legal risks of misuse and diversion; and 4) impressing on college students that safety of prescribed stimulants can only be assured within the designated therapeutic range and in patients who have been adequately screened for risk of adverse effects (including potentially lethal cardiovascular adverse effects). Following from the above, counseling college students should include specific discussion about the likelihood of being asked to share their prescription stimulants with friends, methods of properly storing their medication, and potential safety issues that can occur if individuals who have not been screened medically use their drugs.

Educating physicians who treat ADHD in college students is an important strategy for several reasons. As previously noted, short-acting stimulant formulations are more likely to be misused than long-acting formulations; therefore, use of long-acting stimulants as a first choice option when stimulants are prescribed is likely to decrease the amount of stimulant misuse. In addition to altering the pharmacokinetic distribution curve (i.e., generally slower onset of effect and distribution of drug over a longer period of time), some of the long-acting formulations offer additional protection in that the medication can't be crushed and delivered in an alternative form.

Another option for restricting the use of immediate release stimulants is to consider the use of approved non-stimulant medications where appropriate (i.e., atomoxetine for ADHD (FDA approved for this indication in this age group (48); bupropion for depression with ADHD symptoms (approved for depression in this age group and documented off-label efficacy in ADHD (49, 50); long-acting alpha-2 agonists (FDA approved in children under 18 years but likely useful in at least some older patients) (51). In addition, it is important to consider evidence-based psychosocial approaches, which teach and support improved organizational skills (52, 53).

As noted above, several studies have shown that mixed amphetamine salts (MAS; i.e., Adderall) and MAS-XR are the most commonly diverted stimulants in the college population (43, 44). While further study is required to determine whether this is due to higher rates of prescription and availability of these formulations, or other factors related to the formulations themselves, use of methylphenidate compounds (i.e., a different class of stimulants) preferentially might be potentially useful. When using amphetamine compounds, preferentially prescribing the long-acting amphetamine formulation lisdexamfetamine (i.e., dextro-amphetamine which is covalently bound to the naturally occurring amino acid, l-lysine, which renders it inert until metabolized gradually in the blood stream) would also seem to minimize risk of diversion. However, the above suggestions have not been formally studied and therefore cannot be recommended as evidence-based.

Finally, as it has been shown that college students can easily feign ADHD symptoms, it is important to educate physicians to use structured rating scales and validated interviews in making the diagnosis, and to consider the possibility that at least some individuals inappropriately seeking prescription stimulants know the diagnostic criteria and feign positive responses (54). Consequently, it is important to collect information regarding other contextual and developmental characteristics of the disorder, and also consider whether there is sufficient impairment to warrant treatment.

Conclusion

Substance abuse among college students has been the focus of considerable recent attention, given the high prevalence of use/abuse in this population, the nature of the drugs that are abused, the specific contextual issues that fuel abuse in this population, and the potentially dire outcomes of substance use in this population. It is hoped that better understanding the types of substance abuse that most often occur in the college age population, the specific contextual factors that support substance abuse in this population, and the various available methods of prevention and treatment of substance abuse that have been developed for college students will contribute to more informed approaches to managing this problem.

Acknowledgments

This paper is a revised and adapted version of an earlier publication in the book "Substance abuse in adolescents and young adults. A manual for pediatric and primary care clinicians" edited by Donald E Greydanus, Gabriel Kaplan, Dilip R Patel and Joav Merrick with Walter de Gruyter in Berlin, 2013.

References

[1] Substance Abuse and Mental Health Service Administration, Results from the National Survey on Drug Use and Health: Summary of national findings. Rockville, MD: Substance Abuse and Mental Health Service Administration, NSDUH Series H-44, HHS Publication No (SMA) 12-4713, 2012.

[2] Hingson RW, Zha W, Weitzman ER. Magnitude of and trends in alcohol-related mortality and morbidity among U.S. college students ages 18-24, 1998-2005. J Stud Alcohol Drugs 2009;16(Suppl):12-20.

[3] Skala K, Kapusta ND, Schlaff G, Unseld M, Erfurth A, Lesch OM, et al. Suicidal ideation and temperament: An investigation among college students. J Affect Disord 2012;141(2-3):399-405.

[4] Johnston LD, O'Malley PM, Bachman JG, Schulenberg JE. Monitoring the future national survey results on drug use, 1975–2011: Volume II, College students and adults ages 19–50 years. Ann Arbor: Institute Social Research, University Michigan, 2012.

[5] Wechsler H, Dowdall G, Davenport A, Castillo S. Correlates of college student binge drinking. Am J Public Health 1995;85:921-6.

[6] Knight JR, Wechlser H, Kuo M, Seibring M, Weitzman ER, Schuckit MA. Alcohol abuse and dependence among US college students. J Stud Alcohol 2002;63:263-70.
[7] Kaynak O, Meyers K, Caldeira KM, Vincent KB, Winters KC, Arria AM. Relationships among parental monitoring and sensation seeking on the development of substance use disorder among college students. Addict Behav 2012;38:1457–63.
[8] Carter AC, Brandon KO, Goldman MS. The college and noncollege experience: A review of the factors that influence drinking behavior in young adulthood. J Stud Alcohol Drugs 2010;71:742-50.
[9] Lee CM, Maggs JL, Rankin LA. Spring break trips as a risk factor for heavy alcohol use among first-year college students. J Stud Alcohol 2006;67:911-6.
[10] Presley CA, Meilman PW, Leichliter JS. College factors that influence drinking. J Stud Alcohol 2002;14(Suppl):82-90.
[11] Marczinski CA. Alcohol mixed with energy drinks: Consumption patterns and motivations for use in U.S. college students. Int J Environ Res Public Health 2011;8(8):3232-45.
[12] Snipes DJ, Benotsch EG. High-risk cocktails and high-risk sex: Examining the relation between alcohol mixed with energy drink consumption, sexual behavior, and drug use in college students. Addict Behav 2012;38:1418-23.
[13] Nelson TF, Naimi TS, Brewer RD, Wechsler H. The state sets the rate: The relationship among state-specific college binge drinking, state binge drinking rates, and selected state alcohol control policies. Am J Public Health 2005;3:441-6.
[14] Kelly TA, McGuinness TM. Treatment of alcohol-dependent college students. J Psychosoc Nurs Ment Health Serv 2012;50(10):15-8.
[15] Prochaska JO, DiClemente CC. Stages of change in the modification of problem behaviors. Prog Behav Modif 1992;28:183-218.
[16] Miller WR. Motivational interviewing. In: Hersen M, Rosqvist J, eds. Encyclopedia of behavior modification and cognitive behavior therapy, Vol 1. Adult clinical applications. Thousand Oaks, CA: Sage, 2005:383-9.
[17] Fachini A, Aliane PP, Martinez EZ, Furtado EF. Efficacy of brief alcohol screening intervention for college students (basics): a meta-analysis of randomized controlled trials. Subst Abuse Treat Prev Policy 2012;7:40.
[18] Centers for Disease Control and Prevention. Behavioral risk factor surveillance system survey data. Atlanta, GA: US Department Health Human Services CfDCaP, 2008.
[19] Berg CJ, Ling PM, Hayes RB, Berg EN, Nehl E, Choi WS, et al. Smoking frequency among current college student smokers: distinguishing characteristics and factors related to readiness to quit smoking. Health Educ Res 2012;27(1):141-50.
[20] Schane RE, Glantz SA, Ling PM. Nondaily and social smoking: and increasingly prevalent pattern. Arch Intern Med 2009;169:1742-44.
[21] Primack BA, Sidani JE, Agarwal AA, Donny EC, Shadel WG, Eissenberg TE. Prevalence of and associations with water-pipe smoking among US university students. Ann Behav Med 2008;36:81-6.
[22] Sepetdjian E, Shihadeh A, Saliba NA. Measurement of 16 polycyclic aromatic hydrocarbons in narghile waterpipe tobacco smoke. Food Chem Toxicol 2008;46:1582-90.
[23] Tsuang MT, Francis T, Minor K, Thomas A, Stone WS. Genetics of smoking and depression. Hum Genet 2012;131:905-15.
[24] Lasser K, Boyd JW, Woolhandler S, Himmelstein DU, McCormick D, Bor DH. Smoking and mental illness: a population-based prevalence study. JAMA 2000;284:2606–10.
[25] McClernon FJ, Kollins SH. ADHD and smoking: From genes to brain to behavior. Ann NY Acad Sci 2008;1141:131-47.
[26] Issa JS, Abe TO, Moura S, Santos PCJL, Pereira AC. Effectiveness of coadministration of varenicline, bupropion, and serotonin reuptake inhibitors in a smoking cessation program in the real-life setting. Nicotine Tob Res 2012 Nov 05. [Epub ahead of print]
[27] Harrison ELR, Desai RA, McKee SA. Nondaily smoking and alcohol use, hazardous drinking, and alcohol diagnoses among young adults: Findings from the NESARC. Alcohol Clin Exp Res 2008;32(12):2081-7.

[28] Winhusen T, Somoza E, Brigham GS, Liu, D, Green CA, Covey LS, et al. Does treatment of attention deficit hyperactivity disorder (ADHD) enhance response to smoking cessation intervention in ADHD smokers? A randomized trial. J Clin Psychiatry 2010;71(12):1680-8.

[29] Covey LS, Hu MC, Winhusen T, Weissman J, Berlin I, Nunes EV. OROS-methylphenidate or placebo for adult smokers with attention deficit hyperactivity disorder: Racial/ethnic differences. Drug Alcohol Depend 2010;110:156-9.

[30] American College Health Association. American College Health Association-National College Health Assessment II: Reference Group Executive Summary Spring 2012. Hanover, MD: American College Health Association, 2012.

[31] Caldeira KM, Arria AM, O'Grady KE, Vincent KB, Wish ED. The occurrence of cannabis use disorders and other cannabis-related problems among first-year college students. Addict Behav 2008;33:397-411.

[32] Elliot JC, Carey KB. Correcting exaggerated marijuana use norms among college abstainers: A preliminary test of a preventive intervention. J Stud Alcohol Drugs 2012;73:976-80.

[33] Kalant H. Adverse effects of cannabis on health: An update of the literature since 1996. Progr Neuro-psychopharmacol Biol Psychiatr 2004;28(5):849-63.

[34] Primack BA, Kim KH, Shensa A, Sidani JE, Barnett TE, Switzer GE. Tobacco, Marijuana, and alcohol use in university students: A cluster analysis. J Am Coll Health 2012;60:5:374-86.

[35] Danovitch I, Gorelick DA. State of the art treatments for cannabis dependence. Psychiatr Clin North Am 2012;35(2):309-26.

[36] Gray KM, Carpenter MJ, Baker NL, DeSantis SM, Kryway E, Hartwell KJ, et al. A double-blind randomized controlled trial of N-Acetylcysteine in cannabis-dependent adolescents. Am J Psychiatry 2012;169(8):805-12.

[37] Moussawi K, Pacchioni A, Moran M, Olive MF, Gass JT, Lavin A, et al. N-Acetylcysteine reverses cocaine-induced metaplasticity. Nat Neurosci 2009;12:182-9.

[38] Substance Abuse and Mental Health Services Administration. Results from the 2007 National Survey on Drug Use and Health: National findings. Rockville, MD: Office of Applied Studies, DHHS Publication No SMA 08-4343, 2008.

[39] Johnston LD, O'Malley PM, Bachman JG, Schulenberg JE. Monitoring the future national survey results on drug use, 1975–2006: Volume II, college students and adults ages 19–45 years. Bethesda, MD: National Institute Drug Abuse, NIH Publication No 07-6206, 2007.

[40] Kasperski SJ, Vincent KB, Caldeira KM, Garnier-Dykstra LM, O'Grady KE, Arria AM. College students' use of cocaine: Results from a longitudinal study. Addict Behav 2011;36:408-11.

[41] Weyandt LL, DuPaul G. ADHD in college students. J Attent Disord 2006;10(1):9-19.

[42] McCabe SE, Knight JR, Teter CJ, Wechsler H. Non-medical use of prescription stimulants among US college students: prevalence and correlates from a national survey. Addiction 2005;99:96-106.

[43] Sepulveda DR, Thomas LM, McCabe SE, Cranford JA, Boyd CJ, Teter CJ. Misuse of prescribed stimulant medication for ADHD and associated patterns of substance use: Preliminary analysis among college students. J Pharm Pract 2011;24(6):551-60.

[44] Teter CJ, McCabe SE, LaGrange K, Cranford JA, Boyd CJ. Illicit use of specific prescription stimulants among college students: Prevalence, motives, and routes of administration. Pharmacotherapy 2006;26(10):1501-10.

[45] Musso MW, Gouvier WD. "Why is this so hard?" A review of detection of malingered ADHD in college students. J Attention Disord 2012;5:1-16.

[46] Upadhyaya HP, Rose K, Wang W, O'Rourke K, Sullivan B, Deas D, et al. Attention-deficit/hyperactivity disorder, medication treatment, and substance use patterns among adolescents and young adults. J Child Adolesc Psychopharmacol 2005;15(5):799-809.

[47] Kollins SH, McClernon J, Fuemmeler BF. Association between smoking and attention-deficit/hyperactivity disorder symptoms in a population-based sample of young adults. Arch Gen Psychiatry 2005;62:1142-7.

[48] Alder LA, Wilens T, Zhang S, Dittmann RW, D'Souza DN, Schuh L, et al. Atomoxetine treatment outcomes in adolescents and young adults with attention-deficit/hyperactivity disorder: results from a post hoc, pooled analysis. Clin Ther 2012;34(2):363-73.

[49] Solhkhah R, Wilens TE, Daly J, Prince JB, Van Patten SL, Biederman J. Bupropion SR for the treatment of substance-abusing outpatient adolescents with attention-deficit/hyperactivity disorder and mood disorders. J Child Adolesc Psychopharmacol 2005;15(5):777-86.
[50] Wilens TE, Prince JB, Waxmonsky J, Doyle R, Spencer T, Martelon M, et al. An open trial of sustained release bupropion for attention-deficit/hyperactivity disorder in adults with ADHD plus substance use disorders. J ADHD Relat Disord 2010;1(3):25-35.
[51] Sallee FR, McGough J, Wigal T, Donahue J, Lyne A, Biederman J. Guanfacine extended release in children and adolescents with attention-deficit/hyperactivity disorder: a placebo controlled trial. J Am Acad Child Adolesc Psychiatry 2009;48(2):155-65.
[52] Solanto MV, Marks DJ, Wasserstein J, Mitchell K, Abikoff H, Alvir JM, et al. Efficacy of meta-cognitive therapy for adult ADHD. Am J Psychiatry 2010;167(8):958-68.
[53] Safren SA. Cognitive-behavioral approaches to ADHD treatment in adulthood. J Clin Psychiatry 2006;67(8):46-50.
[54] Conners CK, Erhardt D, Epstein JN, Parker JDA, Sitarenios G, Sparrow E. Self-ratings of ADHD symptoms in adults I: Factor structure and normative data. J Attention Disord 1999;3(3):141-51.

Submitted: August 05, 2013. *Revised:* October 01, 2013. *Accepted:* October 10, 2013.

Chapter 19

ADOLESCENT ATHLETES AND SPORTS DOPING

Dilip R Patel[*], MD,
and Donald E Greydanus, MD, Dr, HC (ATHENS)

Department of Pediatric and Adolescent Medicine,
Western Michigan University School of Medicine,
Kalamazoo, Michigan, United States of America

ABSTRACT

Use of drugs and nutritional supplements is widespread at collegiate, professional and elite level sports. Although, less is known about use of drugs and supplements to enhance sports performance in high school age athletes, such use does occur and is a reason for grave concerns.

Research on these products remains limited and athletes rely on word of mouth from fellow sports enthusiasts, coaches, nutrition store personnel, advertisements, and other unscientific sources for information on what drugs, herbs, or other available agents will help them improve their athletic performance or their lives in general. This paper reviews the use by athletes of anabolic agents, human growth hormone, clenbuterol, creatine, stimulants, and erythropoietin.

Keywords: substance abuse, sports, doping, adolescence

INTRODUCTION

For thousands of years, humans have sought the use of medicines, herbs, and other chemicals to improve their lives in various ways. Some scholars have interpreted the story of Adam and Eve in Genesis (see introduction) as a story of the original humans seeking to be strong (wise) like God (1). Extensive pharmacopoeias have been developed in China and India over the

---

[*] Correspondence Professor Dilip R Patel, MD, Department of Pediatric and Adolescent Medicine, Western Michigan University School of Medicine 1000 Oakland Drive, D48G, Kalamazoo, MI 49008-1284 United States. Dilip.patel@med.wmich.edu.

past eons (2). The first classifier of medicinal herbs is noted by historians as the Chinese emperor Shen-Nung 2737 BC, and there is a classic recorded painting of him holding leaves of Ephedra (machuang) leaves (3). An early historical record of medical treatments is the Ebers Papyrus (1500 BC), which lists more than 700 medicines of various origins (mineral, vegetable, and animal) (2, 4).

In recorded history, competitive athletes have used various mixtures of animal and plant origins, taken from known and unknown products, in attempts to improve their athletic performance and gain the perceived benefits of victory (5). For example, athletes during the Greek and Roman Games used wines, mushrooms, and opioids; stimulants (i.e., strychnine) were popular at the beginning of the twentieth century. Galen, the famous Greek who became the physician to the gladiators of ancient Rome, observed the belief of athletes of his time (180 AD) that consuming mushrooms and herbal teas was beneficial to their overall performance (3). In 1886, a cyclist died during a race in France because of a stimulant overdose (3). Such sports doping practices have continued in advocates of sport and others to the present age, even though such practices have been banned by sports officials. For example, the death of a British athlete at the Tour de France in 1967 was attributed to the use of amphetamines complicated by a state of dehydration, and 9 riders were ruled ineligible for the Tour de France in 2006 because of suspected sports doping (6).

Athletes of the past and of today have been willing to take various chemicals even without any proof of their benefit, in hope of improving their general health or their sports performance (7). Over thousands of years, athletes have consulted experts from the ancient days of sorcery and alchemy to modern-day biochemistry and pharmacology to find effective yet safe performance-enhancing drugs (5). The milieu of "victory at any cost" that existed millennia ago continues to the present. In 1982, Goldman and colleagues asked 198 world-class athletes if they would take a chemical that would guarantee them success but would lead to their death in 5 years; in this survey, 52% reported they would take this chemical and this report remained at this level in repeat surveys between 1982 and 1995 (8, 9). Connor and Mazanov posed this Faustian bargain to members of the general public in Australia; they noted that only 2 of the 250 individuals surveyed agreed to take such a chemical. These sagacious members of the general public were not obsessed with victory at any cost (9). As we enter a new millennium and century, it is sobering to realize that only a handful of the thousands of available herbal remedies of old or of modern chemistry have been shown to actually work as prescribed to better one's health (2, 4, 10). Proof of improving sports performance with various chemicals (including herbs) is even more limited. Yet, today's athletes are taking various products (see Table 1) in ever-increasing numbers because they are driven to succeed to obtain the perceived glories of winning in contemporary society (11–21). The teenage athlete should be carefully counseled that there are few substances (if any) that consistently and safely improve the performance of a well-trained individual. Also, the use of these agents has considerable potential to cause physical and psychological damage. Misuse of drugs in this manner should be discouraged. Our sports youth live in a modern-day Faustian dilemma often with the encouragement of coaches, trainers, parents, the media, and other members of society obsessed with success at any price.

Table 1. Partial list of drugs and supplements misused by athletes as ergogenic products

Alpha-lipoic acid	Chrysin	Niacin
Anabolic steroids	Chromium	Nicotine
Androsteindione	Clenbuterol	Nonsteroidal anti-
Antioxidants	Coenzyme Q10	inflammatory drugs (ibuprofen,
(vitamin C, vitamin E,	Creatine	mefenamic acid, naproxen,
beta-carotene)	Diuretics (furosemide,	others)
Amphetamines	spironolactone,	Omega-3 fatty acids
Bee pollen	hydrochlorothiazide)	Oxygen
Beta-blockers	Dihyhroepiandrostenedione	Pantothenic acid
(i.e., propranolol)	Engineered dietary supplements	Phosphorus
Beta-hydroxy-beta-	Ephedrine	Pyridoxine (vitamin B6)
methylbutyrate	Erythropoietin	Selenium
Blood	Folic acid	Vanadium
Boron	Ginkgo biloba	Zinc
Caffeine	Ginseng	
Calcium	Glycerol	
Carnitine	Human-growth hormone	
Choline	Inosine	
	Insulin-like growth factor-I	
	Iron	

PROTECTION FOR CONSUMERS

Some progress was made in the twentieth century to help consumers understand whether or not the medications or chemical agents they take are beneficial and safe. In 1906, the Pure Food and Drug Act required foods and drugs, which were sent between various states, to be provided with accurate labels. It was not required that medications be tested for safety until the 1938 Federal Food, Drug and Cosmetic Act (FFDCA). It was also not required that these drugs be proven effective for their intended use until the 1962 Harris-Kefauver Amendment of the FFDCA. However, the 1994 Dietary Supplement Health and Education Act (DSHEA) reversed some of these gains acquired over the previous 88 years. DSHEA allowed products classified as dietary supplements to avoid the scrutiny applied to drugs or medications. Thus, manufacturers of dietary supplements (defined as a vitamin, mineral, herb, other botanic, amino acid, metabolites of these products, related metabolites, related concentrations, or extracts or combinations) do not need to prove safety or efficacy of their products. All that is needed is to note that their products "maintain health or normal structure and function" (10).

This opened up the commercial floodgates to various agents used by athletes in the hope that the products they use are ergogenic (see Table 2) (22–24). It is important for physicians and medical educators to be aware of these various products and to be willing to provide education to society and their patients about what is known and not known about these products (18, 25, 26).

Research on these products remains limited and athletes rely on word of mouth from fellow sports enthusiasts, coaches, nutrition store personnel, advertisements, and other unscientific sources for information on what drugs, herbs, or other available agents will help them improve their athletic performance or their lives in general (24).

Table 2. Manufacturers' claims of ergogenic agents

Serve as an energy source
Decrease fatigue in sports events
Increase lean body mass and strength
Decrease adipose tissue
Alter weight in desirable directions
Improve aerobic capacity
Enhance motor capacity
Improve appearance
Enhance overall sports performance

Most research has been done on adult men, who are involved in competitive athletics and not on teenage athletes. The potency and purity of nutritional agents are not known and the long-term effects of these various substances are also unknown at present. However, the use of ergogenic agents remains popular, and more than 30,000 individual commercial products are available throughout the world (20, 27, 28). Unproven claims (see Table 1) remain while the hope of victory burns strong in athletes of all ages whether competing at the high school (or below) level or at the Olympic level of competition (29, 30).

DEFINITIONS

The term doping is derived from the Dutch word "dop" in reference to the practice of providing race horses with an opium mixture to act as a stimulant and enhance victory of the competing animal (17). Sports doping refers to the attempt of improvement or stimulation of sports performance in Homo sapiens in the eternal quest for victory at any cost. The promise of having a drug that is a true sports doping chemical often belies an eternal quest for the product having an ergogenic quality, and this term is derived from the Greek words ergon (to work) and gennan (to produce). The International Olympic Committee defines doping as "…use of an expedient (substance or method) which is potentially harmful to athletes' health and/or capable of enhancing their performance, or the presence in athletes' body of a prohibited substance or evidence of the use thereof or evidence of the use of prohibited method" (26).

The American Academy of Pediatrics defines performance enhancing agents as "…any substance when taken in nonpharmacological doses specifically for the purposes of improving sports performance. A substance should be considered performance enhancing if it benefits sports performance by increasing strength, power, speed or endurance (ergogenic) or by altering body weight or body composition" (22).

ANABOLIC AGENTS

Anabolic steroids or anabolic-androgenic steroids (AAS) are a class of chemicals that are synthetic derivatives of testosterone and represent a drug class often abused by adolescent and adult athletes (31). The roots of their use can be traced over 6 millennia ago when ancient farmers noted the quieting or passive effects that castration had on animals (32). Testosterone was isolated in 1935 and developed to improve metabolism; it was used by athletes to gain strength as early as the 1940s. Concern over the use of anabolic steroids by athletes led to an inaugural definition of sports doping by the International Olympic Committee (IOC) in 1964, the banning of these drugs by the IOC, the start of antidoping programs by the IOC in 1967, and the first official testing for these chemicals at the 1976 Montreal Olympic Games (5).

The term anabolic refers to the stimulation of protein synthesis, whereas androgenic implies the stimulation of male secondary sex characteristics. The terms steroids or steroid hormones refer to chemicals that are derived from cholesterol and include corticosteroids and sex hormones (i.e., testosterone, estrogen, and progesterone). Anabolic steroids stimulate several receptors: androgen, estrogen, progestin, and glucocorticoid. Some examples of oral and injectable anabolic steroids are listed in Table 3. The US Food and Drug Administration (FDA) has classified these chemicals as Schedule II drugs since 1990. Adequate training and protein intake are necessary for maximal effect on protein synthesis in muscle tissue and the individual response is variable. Anabolic steroids have become the sine qua non of the Faustian bargain awaiting our youth.

Table 3. Examples of anabolic steroids

ORAL	INJECTABLE	TOPICAL
Oxandronolone	Testosterone cypionate	Testosterone gel
Oxymetholone	Testosterone enanthate	Testosterone transdermal
Stanozolol	Nandrolone phenpropionate	
	Nandrolone decanoate	

Epidemiology

According to the Monitoring the Future Study, AAS are used predominantly by males. In 2011, annual prevalence rates were 1.0%, 1.4%, and 1.8% for boys in grades 8, 10, and 12, compared with 0.4%, 0.4%, and 0.5% for girls. It is clear that many youth try anabolic steroids including one-third who are not athletes (31–35). Various studies over the past few decades confirm that 5% to 11% of high school boys and 0.5 to 2.5% of high school girls in the United States have tried anabolic steroids; of these, 50% used these chemicals before 16 years of age and 33% of these youth were not athletes (31, 33, 36–50).

These youth have limited knowledge of the dangers of these drugs (41, 51-53). Abuse of these chemicals may be increased in the nonathletic population versus the athletic adolescent population (52). Adolescents who take anabolic steroids may also be involved in other high-risk behaviors, including illicit drug use such as cocaine, alcohol, cigarettes, marijuana, smokeless tobacco, and various injectable drugs (43, 47–55). Adolescents obtain these drugs from many sources, even from veterinary suppliers. Although abuse of anabolic steroids by American professional athletes has decreased somewhat in recent years, the use of these and other drugs by famous athletes has long encouraged teenagers to try these substances (56–58). Youth often believe that these chemicals are natural hormones and are endorsed by their sports heroes (54). Many teenagers are convinced that these drugs are valuable and worth any risk, even in very high doses.

Oral anabolic steroids are 17 alpha-alkylation chemicals that slow liver inactivation and cause much of the liver side effects of these drugs. The injectable forms are from 19 beta-esterification processes and pose infectious disease risks, including hepatitis (B and C) and human immunodeficiency virus (HIV)/AIDS. The therapeutic doses of such drugs as used for treatment of various medical disorders are 8 to 30 mg depending on the particular drug being used. Because teenage athletes are often not afraid (nor informed) of risks, they may use prolonged and heavy (supraphysiologic) doses. They may use these drugs in various combinations in a method called stacking, that is, cycles of 6 to 12 weeks on and then off (47, 53, 59). Increasing a drug dose in a cycle is called pyramiding, and doses may be 10 to more than 40 times the usual therapeutic doses (59). While taking several drugs together (i.e., stacking), some athletes use up to 200 mg per day. These athletes may not have any fear of side effects in their quest for ergogenic qualities or even in attempts to simply improve appearance.

Effects

Numerous studies have established that anabolic androgenic steroid use results in increased muscle mass, muscle size and maximal voluntary strength, especially when used in combination with proper training and adequate protein intake (60). Because the gains from AAS use in aerobic capacity are minimal at best, their popularity among endurance athletes is difficult to understand.

Athletes use anabolic steroids in the hope of increasing lean body mass, strength, and/or aggressiveness; as noted, some only wish to improve appearance (33, 61). Athletes at particular risk for the use of anabolic steroids include those engaged in sports such as weight lifting, shot putting, discus throwing, bodybuilding, sprinting, football, and wrestling.

Whether or not athletes get a significant increase in athletic performance remains controversial, and individualized results are the norm.

Adverse effects

Side effects of anabolic steroids are legion and reviewed in Table 4 (33, 45, 46, 62-74).

Use of additional or concomitant doping agents with AAS

Users of AAS may use other drugs as well (48). For example, they may use human growth hormone (hGH), methamphetamine, or clenbuterol (see later discussion) to augment the anabolic effects of AAS. Human chorionic gonadotropin (HCG) may be added to raise testosterone synthesis and counter the anabolic steroid-induced effect of testicular atrophy. Diuretics (e.g., furosemide, spironolactone, hydrochlorothiazide) may be used to reduce fluid retention, produce the desired rippled look, or dilute urine to subvert a drug-screening regimen. The use of diuretics to lose weight quickly is not an unusual plan of wrestlers. The use of such medications can result in increased weakness such that a wrestler can be injured by competing against a stronger opponent. Electrolyte dysfunction and other side effects of diuretics may complicate the picture. Pulmonary embolism has been reported in a high school wrestler using such a regimen (74).

Table 4. Side effects of anabolic steroids

Behavioral	Aggressiveness, irritability, depression, addiction
Cardiovascular	Lower high density lipoprotein, increased low density lipoprotein, cardiac hypertrophy, sudden cardiac death
Endocrine and Metabolic	Suppression of hypothalamic-pituitary-testicular axis, hyperglycemia, decreased follicle stimulating hormone, decreased luteinizing hormone, hepatic dysfunction, liver tumors, peliosis hepatitis, gynecomastia, acne
Unique to Female	Hirsutism, cliteromegaly, menstrual irregularity, amenorrhea, deep voice, coarsening of skin
Unique to Male	Decreased spermatozoa, decreased testosterone levels, reduced testicular size, prostatic enlargement
Unique to Children	Acceleration of maturation, premature fusion of growth plates, virilization in boys, masculinization in girls
Related to Injections	Systemic infections, local infections
Musculo-Tendinous	Increased risk for tendon ruptures

Stimulants may be taken along with AAS to increase the drive for exercise and competition, whereas anti-acne medications are used to deal with the anabolic steroid-induced acne. Antiestrogens (as tamoxifen or clomiphene) may be used to prevent male feminization effects (i.e., gynecomastia) of anabolic steroids. These athletes may use other drugs as well in the course of their training, such as antibiotics, corticosteroids (i.e., prednisone), and analgesics (e.g., morphine, propoxyphene, meperidine, oxycodone, and others). Narcotics and other illicit drugs are abused for their pleasure-granting effects as well. Corticotrophin (ACTH) is used to raise levels of internally produced corticosteroids and to produce a sense of euphoria.

Prevention

Anabolic have been banned by the (IOC), the National Collegiate Athletic Association (NCAA), the National Football League (NFL), and many other sporting associations. However, it is often difficult for the adolescent user to stop because many young people have difficulty understanding the consequences of their actions (concrete thinking) and have difficulty avoiding the win-at-all-cost attitude prevalent in the global sports milieu (29, 30, 41, 56, 57, 75-78). It is important to educate youth about these sports doping agents (59). Parents and coaches must be taught about these chemicals and they should not encourage the use of such potentially dangerous chemicals under the guise of "Winning is Everything!"

Although there may be some medical indications for these drugs (i.e., treatment of HIV-associated wasting or chronic renal failure), seeking to improve sports performance should not be one of the medical indications to use these drugs (11, 44, 79). The effort to ban anabolic steroids has now been complicated with the appearance of designer steroids, the first of which was norbolethone that was initially detected by a laboratory in Los Angeles in 2002 (5). Other identified designer steroids include madol (desoxy-methyl testosterone) and tetrahydrogestrinone. Unfortunately, experts and amateurs in the biochemistry industry continue to produce such drugs and the cat and mouse game between sports dopers and sports officials will continue in perpetuum.

Dihyroepiandrostenedione (DHEA)

DHEA is a mildly androgenic hormone naturally produced in the adrenal glands and testes. It is the precursor to testosterone (as well as dihydrotestosterone) and estrogen. Although DHEA is banned by the FDA and has no proven ergogenic effects, it is used by athletic teens and adults as an alternative to anabolic steroids (31, 48, 80). The ergogenic attempt is based on a hope and hype that DHEA will increase testosterone and an anabolic insulin-like growth factor (IGF-I). Despite animal studies having shown some DHEA-induced liver toxicity, it is marketed to adults (middle-aged and older) as an over-the-counter alternative to anabolic steroids with additional unproven claims of promoting euphoria, enhancing libido, delaying cardiovascular disease, preventing cancer, and boosting one's immunity (17). Research is limited on DHEA (65). One study evaluated men (average age 24 years) who used 1600 mg per day for 4 weeks; serum testosterone levels were not altered (81). Another study called the Andro Project also noted no ergogenic qualities of DHEA (82).

DHEA is given at a dose of 50 to 100 mg per day for 6 to 12 months in oral or injectable forms, up to 1600 mg. Side effects may occur as with ingestion of sex hormones. At doses of more than 100 mg/day, gynecomastia (irreversible) in men and hirsutism in women can occur; cancer (prostate or endometrial) may be worsened (83). DHEA should be considered as an anabolic steroid and teenagers should be advised not to use it. The FDA has ruled it has no medical usage, and it has been banned from the National Hockey League, the IOC, the NFL, among others.

Androstenedione

Androstenedione is another androgen produced by the adrenal gland and testes; it is a precursor of estrogen and testosterone (as well as dihydrotestosterone) and is found in Scotch pine tree pollen (84–86). It is used as a T-booster in hope of increasing testosterone; serum testosterone/estrogen ratios are normalized within 1 day of stopping this drug. High doses (as 100–300 mg per day and 60 minutes before an event) may increase lean muscle mass and strength. Studies note that 300 mg of androstenedione increases testosterone, estrone, and estradiol levels by more than 100 mg (26). It is often used in combination with different anabolic steroids in various cycling methods (80).

Androstenedione is a banned chemical with unknown long-term safety. Side effects are the same as noted with anabolic steroids; the potency and safety of available products are unknown. It should be avoided with growing athletes and for those at risk for prostate or breast cancer. Androstenedione and other steroidal supplements may be packaged with various other chemicals, such as ephedrine, caffeine, saw palmetto, and others (65).

HUMAN GROWTH HORMONE (hGH)

hGH has been used especially by power and speed athletes in attempts to increase lean muscle mass and strength, often in combination with anabolic steroids (11, 31). However, ergogenic effects have not been proven, even when using supraphysiologic doses (87). Although tests are available, it is difficult to detect all users and the user runs the risk of having an impure product obtained illegally (88, 89). Recombinant DNA technology has provided recombinant hGH (rhGH) to those able to pay the high cost of this agent (more than US$3000 per month) (89). A survey of more than 200 high school male athletes noted that 5% were on hGH (48). The question of hGH purity as a natural product was previously raised with the development of Creutzfeld-Jacobs disease. Side effects of hGH supplementation may include jaw enlargement, gigantism, hypertension, hyperglycemia, fluid retention, carpal tunnel syndrome, slipped capital femoral epiphysis, and pseudotumor cerebri (18, 89). Although several amino acids (arginine, ornithine, lysine, and tryptophan) are used to induce release of hGh, doses usually used do not significantly raise hGH in the body.

GAMA-HYDROXYBUTYRATE

Gama-hydroxybutyrate (GHB, Liquid Ecstasy, G, Georgia home boy) is a central nervous system depressant that leads to euphoria and lowering of inhibition (90, 91). GHB is popular with body builders with the hype and hope of increasing growth hormone release during sleep and enhancing muscle growth. GHB can be made at home with recipes found on the Internet and with ingredients easily purchased. It is made as a clear liquid or white powder; tablets or capsules are available. It is also used as a date-rape pill to enhance sexual assault; as a colorless, odorless and tasteless liquid, it is easily slipped into party drinks to produce sedation and amnesia; effects are noted in 10 to 20 minutes and last for 4 hours. It is quickly cleared from the body and is hard to detect. Thus, it has become a popular date-rape drug. An overdose can lead to profound respiratory depression, coma, and death.

Because the United States government is cracking down on GHB use, some are taking GHB metabolites or precursors, such as gama-butyrolactone (GBL) and even the industrial solvent, 1,4-butanediol (BD). After ingestion of GBH, it becomes GHB. Some companies are substituting BD for GHB, even though BD has been declared a potentially life-threatening drug by the FDA. It is marketed as a dietary supplement in various sleep aid and muscle builder products. Although it is promoted to enhance sexual performance, BD slows breathing and can lead to unconsciousness, emesis, seizures, and death.

CLENBUTEROL

Clenbuterol is a beta-2 agonist bronchodilator (substituted phenylethanolamine) that is used with anabolic steroids in attempts to improve lean body mass and decrease adipose tissue (11, 44, 54, 92–94). It is available in Europe, Central America, and South America. Clenbuterol can be given orally with full absorption, whereas aerosol and injection forms are also available. If used therapeutically for asthma, the dose is 0.02 to 0.04 mg per day; if used ergogenically, a dose of 0.02 to 0.16 mg per day is tried. Clenbuterol can be used in a 2-day on and 2-day off cycle for several weeks and then stopped before the athletic event, because it can be detected for 2 to 4 days after the last dose.

However, it is not proven that it increases muscle mass and reduces adipose tissue, certainly not to the extent attributed to anabolic steroids. Several side effects are observed, including tachycardia, headaches, anxiety, dizziness, nausea, tremor, and insomnia. Concern is raised that it may lead to arrhythmias, myocardial infarction, cardiac muscle hypertrophy, and cerebrovascular accidents. It is banned by many sport agencies, including the IOC, United States Olympic Committee, NCAA, and others.

Table 5. Substances and methods prohibited by sport governing bodies

PROHIBITED AT ALL TIMES	
Main categories of prohibited substances	Anabolic agents
	Peptide hormones, growth hormones and related substances
	Beta-2 agonists
	Hormone agonists and metabolic modulators
	Diuretics and other masking agents
Main categories of prohibited methods	Enhancement of oxygen transfer
	Chemical and physical manipulation
	Gene doping
PROHIBITED IN-COMPETITION	
Main categories of prohibited substances	Stimulants
	Narcotics
	Cannabinoids
	Glucocorticoids

Source www.usada.org/prohibited-list accessed 12/20/2012.

To avoid sanctions for using a medication (even with a prescription) at Olympic competition levels, rules of the World Anti-Doping Code must be followed in which the International Standard for Therapeutic Use Exemptions are used (95). Sports doping has been viewed by authorities as being an unfair and unethical advantage in sports competition. The IOC developed a medical commission in 1967 and they have produced a list of substances that are prohibited (Table 5) for athletes to use as well as various antidoping regulations (96). Specific screening for prohibited drugs was initiated at the 1972 Munich Olympic Games. In 1999, the World Anti-Doping Agency (WADA) was developed and this agency organized a worldwide effort to standardize and enforce antidoping regulations (31). Athletes must be careful even with prescription drugs that are prescribed for them or misuse of medications that are being prescribed for someone else (97).

CREATINE

Creatine is an essential amino acid synthesized from arginine, glycine, and methionine, mainly in the kidneys, and to a lesser extent in the liver and pancreas. It is available in milk, meat, fish, and other foods, although meat and fish are the main food sources and supply more than half of the daily requirement (27, 28, 31, 80, 90, 98). The usual diet provides 1 to 2 g of creatine per day. It is a tasteless crystalline powder that is readily dissolved in liquids and is usually marketed as creatine monohydrate or with phosphorus (990. At all levels of competition (from high school to professional), creatine is the most popular nutritional supplement sold today as an ergogenic Agent (27, 28, 31, 90, 98, 100–104).

All but 5% of creatine is stored in skeletal muscle (especially the fast twitch, type II muscle), two-thirds as a phosphorylated form, and one-third as free creatine. This substance serves as an energy substrate for the contraction of skeletal muscle in the body. Cells with high-energy requirements use creatine in the form of phosphocreatine, which functions as a donor of phosphate to produce adenosine triphosphate from adenosine diphosphate. Cells in the skeletal muscles store enough phosphocreatine and adenosine triphosphate (ATP) for about 10 seconds of high-intensity action (80, 100). The purpose of creatine supplementation is to increase resting phosphocreatine levels in muscles and free creatine to briefly postpone fatigue, with potential ergogenic results (99, 100). Phosphocreatine maintains high energy ATP levels, acts as a proton buffer, and can lead to reduced glycolysis. When the phosphocreatine levels decrease, glycolysis increases. Maximal exercise eventually stops because of muscle fatigue, probably because of accumulation of lactate and hydrogen ions in addition to a decrease in ATP.

Studies in adult athletes suggest that with creatine supplementation there may be a 5%to 15% improvement in short-term (less than 30 seconds), repetitive/intermittent, high-intensity exercise (18, 27, 28, 102, 105–107). Creatine is beneficial for those in power sports (i.e., football, sprinters), but not for those in endurance sports (e.g., swimming). Some athletes may have a low intracellular concentration of creatine and thus may respond to it, whereas those with a higher level do not respond. Most in vivo studies show no improvement in sports performance (80). Also, no studies report any improvement with long-term endurance activities.

Athletes use different dosage regimens for creatine supplementation (108-115). The work of Harris and colleagues has led to the current practice of many athletes using a loading dose of 20 g per day (5 g four times a day) for 5 to 7 days followed by 2 to 5 g per day for maintenance (113, 114). Other loading and maintenance doses are also used. For example, research suggests an equally beneficial effect may be seen with 3 g a day versus a loading dose of 20 g a day (115). The loading routine may maximize the amount of phosphocreatine in muscles, whereas a maintenance dose may keep muscles filled. Positive results are best with an active exercise program, although there is no need to take creatine specifically before or during exercise. Increased weight may result because of fluid (water) retention and not increased protein synthesis (114). An increase of 0.7 to 3 kg. in 1 month has been reported; weight gain can be maintained on 5 g per day of creatine during a 10-week period of detraining and maintained 4 weeks after its use is stopped.

Although creatine is generally regarded as safe, there may be side effects and risks, especially when consuming more than 20 g per day. The best-known effect is weight gain because of fluid (water) retention. Other adverse effects that are often cited but not proven include anecdotal reports of muscle cramps, strains, dehydration in hot/humid weather, renal function deterioration, suppression of endogenous synthesis, and possible cardiac muscle hypertrophy. Other anecdotal concerns include abdominal pain, dyspnea, nausea, emesis, diarrhea, anxiety, fatigue, migraine headaches, seizures, myopathy, and atrial fibrillation (17,

80). Supplementation does reduce endogenous creatine production, with unknown results on the body. Although it is not banned by any major sports groups, the American College of Sports Medicine recommends that those less than 18 years of age should not use creatine (115). Recommendations of the International Society of Sports Nutrition for use of creatine use in children are listed in Table 6.

Table 6. Recommendations of International Society of Sports Nutrition for use of creatine

The athlete is past puberty.
Athletes is involved in competitive training in which creatine supplementation may be beneficial.
Athletes is consuming well-balanced, performance enhancing diet.
The athlete and athlete's parents understand effects of creatine supplementation.
Athlete's parents approve of creating supplementation.
Athlete takes supplementation under proper professional supervision.
Quality creatine supplements are used.
That athlete does not exceed recommended dosages.

Source: http://www.jissn.com/content/4/1/6 accessed 12/18/2012.

STIMULANTS

Ephedrine

Ephedrine is a medication that can have beneficial effects in disease states (e.g., asthma), but which is not acceptable to various sports medicine committees because of potential harmful effects (18, 20, 116, 117). It is an example of using a stimulant drug to seek improvement in one's performance in training or competition. Although not proven to be ergogenic, it has been used by various athletes in this regard. Other stimulants include amphetamine and caffeine. They are used to reduce the sense of being tired, lessen the feeling of pain, and heighten aggressiveness (45). As noted earlier, stimulants have been used by athletes over the eons as performance-enhancing chemicals. The Incas in South America chewed coca leaves to help them run long distances (1).

In the case of ephedrine, many believe its sympathomimetic action gives the user an unfair advantage and is thus banned. However, such beta-2 agonists such as terbutaline and salbuterol are accepted in the Olympics if the athlete has documented asthma and informs the Olympic Committee of their use. The purpose is to allow the athlete proper treatment of a verified disorder (i.e., asthma), but not to allow him or her to gain an unfair advantage over the competitors (i.e., using stimulants).

Ephedrine alkaloids are derived from ephedra herbs (also called ma huang). Athletes use dietary supplement products that contain ma huang to improve muscle tone and energy levels, although there is no proof of these claims (10, 17). Numerous adverse event reports have been investigated by the FDA. These incidents involved otherwise healthy young to middle-aged adults who developed various complications while on these products; these included hypertension, arrhythmias, anxiety, tremors, insomnia, seizures, paranoid psychoses, cerebrovascular accidents, myocardial infarctions, and death (118). In 2004 the FDA banned sale of all dietary supplements containing ephedra.

Caffeine

Caffeine is a xanthine derivative that is used by many athletes (31, 119). In a study of 520 British athletes in which 36.1% reported use of creatine, while caffeine use as a sports doping agent was reported by 23.8% (104). It may improve performance in steady state endurance activities that rely on fat for fuel, because this chemical increases lipid metabolism. It increases the release of free fatty acids from adipocytes and stimulates catecholamine activity (44, 120). Studies have noted that ingestion of 2 to 3 cups of coffee (100–150 mg of caffeine per cup) increases the endurance of individuals cycling to exhaustion on bicycle ergometers. Coffee seems to reduce the perception of fatigue and allow further performance. However, an excessive amount increases sympathomimetic stimulation, which can interfere with overall athletic performance. Its diuretic effect can also interfere with such performance. Excessive amounts are banned from competition and is defined by NCAA as more than 15 mg/mL in the urine; this usually results from ingestion of 6 to 8 cups of coffee. Other sources of caffeine include tea, over-the-counter pills for sleepiness, and some analgesic pills that contain caffeine.

BLOOD DOPING AND ERYHROPROTEIN (EPO)

Blood doping (bloodboosting or blood packing), in which athletes receive transfusions of their own blood, is an attempt to increase aerobic performance (31, 121, 122). Hemoglobin levels may reach 19 to 20 g/dL, especially during intense competition (e.g., cycling competition at high altitudes), which leads to dehydration (44).

EPO is a renal glycoprotein that stimulates red cell production (31, 121, 122). Recombinant EPO (rEPO) is used to increase aerobic capacity and thus has become popular with endurance athletes (e.g., runners and cyclists) (44). rEPO is difficult to detect and has a half-life of 20 hours. As noted with blood doping, several side effects are reported, including increased blood viscosity, hypertension, coronary artery occlusion, cerebrovascular accidents, seizures, and sudden death. Dehydration from intense sports activity may trigger some of these complications. It is as effective in increasing aerobic capacity as blood doping and its use is banned (121, 122).

MISCELLANEOUS SPORTS DOPING AGENTS

Beta-blockers (i.e., propranolol, clinetrol, metoprolol) have been used to reduce anxiety, lessen hand tremor, control tachycardia, and reduce hypertension. Hand control is important in sports such as archery and riflery; these athletes may also use benzodiazepines and barbiturates for relief of anxiety and insomnia (44). Potential side effects of beta-blockers include various well-known cardiovascular, hematologic, central nervous system, and gastrointestinal symptomatology (5).

Ergolytic illicit drugs include alcohol (also used in small amounts for hand control), marijuana, nicotine, cocaine, amphetamines, and others (55). Nicotine may improve central nervous system attention span in some, but may also worsen hand steadiness. Insulin has been misused in sports by some because of its anabolic and anticatabolic effects. Drug testing has been developed to detect this practice (123). Selective androgen receptor moderators are a class of drugs with the potential for use and abuse as sports doping agents and drug testing technology is being developed to detect SARMs (124). A selective progesterone receptor modulator is an agent that works on the progesterone receptor with an agonist action on some tissues and an antagonist action in others. Sodium bicarbonate is an alkaline salt that has been used to delay fatigue during bouts of exercise that are limited by acidosis; this may be helpful in cases where the blood flow can increase to accommodate an increase in the by-products of increased muscles at work (17, 44). Nonsteroidal anti-inflammatory agents have been used to relieve pain and allow athletes to increase their performance despite painful injuries; this can lead to greater, more permanent injuries (44). Such medications have erroneously been used to quicken healing of muscle soreness after exercise. Side effects of such medications include gastrointestinal bleeding, reduced platelet aggregation, reduced renal perfusion, increased salt/water retention, and thermal regulation dysfunction with resultant heat illness. Another agent falsely used as an anti-inflammatory agent by athletes is dimethyl sulfoxide (DMSO). This chemical has been available in over-the-counter preparations and is rubbed onto sore or injured areas. Its effectiveness as an anti-inflammatory agent has never been proved by research and its production does not occur under standards acceptable for human use.

There are many other substances sold as ergogenic agents, such as ginkgo biloba, ginseng, yohimbine (yohimbe), coenzyme Q10, and others as listed in Table 1 (17, 125). The purity and safety of these products are not guaranteed but this does not prevent youth and other athletes from using them in high amounts. Clinicians providing sports medicine care to youth, whether through anticipatory guidance or direct sports medicine management, should educate their young patients about the never-ending hype and hyperbole of these ergogenic products (11, 17, 25, 126).

Conclusion

The ancient Olympic Games took place from 776 BCE to 393 AD and sports doping was quite common among athletes of ancient societies (5). The modern Olympic Games began in 1886 in Athens, Greece, under the influence of Baron Pierre de Coubertin who emphasized the need for sports to honor competition over winning (3). Unfortunately, the milieu of winning is everything persists and athletes will accept the Goldman challenge in their pursuit of performance-enhancing drugs. Most consumed agents do not improve performance, and risks of severe adverse effects continue to complicate the Faustian dilemma that athletes at all levels face in the early twenty-first century. Sports doping is also a part of the greater issue of illicit drug use that is so prevalent in youth and adults of the world (52, 56, 57). Our children and youth must be educated about proper exercise and nutrition. They are curious about using potential sports doping chemicals of all types (127). We must teach our children and adolescents that sports doping is neither a safe nor effective way to succeed in the game of life on or off the field (128). We need to reinstate Baron Pierre de Coubertin's view of competition over victory as the raison d'être for sports participation among our children and youth. Sports doping is an important cause of hors de combat in contemporary twenty first century sports society.

ACKNOWLEDGMENT

Adapted with permission from Greydanus DE, Patel DR. Sports doping in the adolescent: the Faustian conundrum of Hors de combat. Pediatr Clin North Am 2010;57:729-50.

REFERENCES

[1] Csaky TZ. Doping. J Sports Med Phys Fitness 1972;12(2):117–23.
[2] Grollman AP. Alternative medicine: the importance of evidence in medicine and medical evidence. Foreword: is there wheat among the chaff? Acad Med 2001;76:221–3.
[3] De Rose EH. Doping in athletes: an update. Clin Sports Med 2008;27:107–30.
[4] Porter R. The greatest benefit to mankind: a medical history of humanity. New York: WW Norton, 1998.
[5] Botre' F, Pavan A. Enhancement drugs and the athlete. Neurol Clin 2008;26:149–67.
[6] Lippi G, Franchini M, Guidi GC. Switch off the light on cycling, switch off the light on doping. Br J Sports Med 2007. Accessed 2013 Jan 02. URL: http://dopingjournal.org/noteworthy/achive/2007_11_01<archive.html.
[7] Gregory AJ, Fitch RW. Sports medicine: performance-enhancing drugs. Pediatr Clin North Am 2007;54(4):797–806.
[8] Goldman B, Bush PJ, Klatz R. Death in the locker room. London: Century; 1984:32.
[9] Connor JM, Mazanov J. Would you dope? A general population test of the Goldman dilemma. Br J Sports Med 2009;43:871–2.
[10] Talalay P, Talalay P. The importance of using scientific principles in the development of medicinal agents from plants. Acad Med 2001;76:175–84.
[11] Greydanus DE. Use and abuse of drugs and supplements. In: Bhave S, Patel DR, Greydanus DE, eds. Sports medicine. New Delhi: Jaypee Brothers Medical Publishers, 2008:122–33.
[12] Greydanus DE, Patel DR. Sports doping in the adolescent athlete. Asian J Paediatr Prac 2000;4(1):9–14.
[13] Fragakis S, Thompson C. Popular dietary supplements, 3rd ed. Chicago: American Dietetic Association, 2007.
[14] Catlin DH, Fitch KD, Ljungqvist A. Medicine and science in the fight against doping in sport. J Intern Med 2008;264(2):99–114.
[15] Rogol AD. Sports, hormones and doping in children and adolescents. In: Ghigo E, Lanfranco F, Strasburger CH, eds. Hormone use and abuse by athletes. New York: Springer, 2011;51-62.
[16] Castillo EM, Comstock RD. Prevalence of use of performance-enhancing substances among United States adolescents. Pediatr Clin North Am 2007;54(4):663–75.
[17] Greydanus DE. Performance enhancing drugs and supplements. In: Patel DR, Greydanus DE, Baker R, eds. Pediatric practice: Sports medicine. New York: McGraw-Hill Medical Publishers, 2009:63–77.
[18] Wang D. Understanding performance-enhancing drug use. Conn Med 2012;76(8):487-91.
[19] Fitch K. Proscribed drugs at the Olympic Games: permitted use and misuse (doping) by athletes. Clin Med 2012;12(3):257-60.
[20] Petroczi A, Naughton DP. Supplement use in sport. J Occup Med Toxicol 2007;2:4.

[21] Petroczi A, Naughton DP. The age-gender-status profile of high performing athletes taking nutritional supplements: lessons for the future. J Int Soc Sports Nutr 2008;5:2.
[22] American Academy of Pediatrics Policy statement: Use of performance enhancing substances. Pediatrics 2005;116:1103-6.
[23] Catlin DH, Murray TH. Performance enhancing drugs, fair competition and Olympic sport. JAMA 1996;276:231.
[24] Clarkson PM, Thompson HS. Drugs and sport: research findings and limitations. Sports Med 1997;24:366.
[25] Sampson W. The need for educational reform in teaching about alternative therapies. Acad Med 2001;76:248–50.
[26] International Olympic Committee. Accessed 2013 Jan 02. URL: www.ioc.org.
[27] Volek JS, Kraemer WJ. Creatine supplementation: its effect on human muscular performance and body composition. J Strength Cond Res 1996;10:200–10.
[28] Williams MH, Branch JD. Creatine supplementation and exercise performance: an update. J Am Coll Nutr 1998;17:216–34.
[29] Patel DR, Greydanus DE, Pratt HD. Youth sports: more than sprains and strains. Contemp Pediatr 2001;18:45.
[30] Pratt HD, Patel DR, Greydanus DE. Sports and the neurodevelopment of the child and adolescent. In: DeLee JC, Drez DD, Miller MD, eds. Orthopaedics sports medicine. Philadelphia, PA: WB Saunders, 2003:624–42.
[31] Greydanus DE, Patel DR. Sports doping: use of drugs and supplements to enhance performance. Int Public Health J 2009;1(4):1–7.
[32] Dotson JL, Brown RT. The history of the development of anabolic-androgenic steroids. Pediatr Clin North Am 2007;54(4):761–9.
[33] Kerr JM, Congeni A. Anabolic-androgenic steroids: use and abuse in pediatric patients. Pediatr Clin North Am 2007;54(4):771–85.
[34] Graham MR, Davies B, Grace FM, et al. Anabolic steroid use: patterns of use and detection of doping. Sports Med 2008;38(6):505–25.
[35] Sjö̈qvist F, Garle M, Rane A. Use of doping agents, particularly anabolic steroids, in sports and society. Lancet 2008;371(9627):1872–82.
[36] Buckley WE, Yesalis CE III, Friedl KE, et al. Estimated prevalence of anabolic steroid use among male high school seniors. JAMA 1988;260:3441–6.
[37] Faigenbaum AD, Zaichkowsky LD, Gardner DE, et al. Anabolic steroid use by male and female middle school students. Pediatrics 1998;101:E6.
[38] Foley JD, Schydlower M. Anabolic steroid and ergogenic drugs use by adolescents. Adolesc Med State Art Rev 1993;4(2):341–52.
[39] Johnson MD, Jay MS, Shoup B, et al. Anabolic steroid use by male adolescents. Pediatrics 1989;83:921–4.
[40] Kindlundh AM, Isacson DG, Berglund L, et al. Doping among high school students in Uppsala, Sweden: a presentation of the attitudes distribution, side effects, and extent of use. Scand J Soc Med 1998;26:71.
[41] Komoroski EM, Rickert VI. Adolescent body image and attitudes to anabolic steroid use. Am J Dis Child 1992;146:823–8.
[42] Massad SJ, Shier NW, Koceja DM, et al. High school athletes and nutritional supplements: a study of knowledge and use. Int J Sport Nutr 1995;5:232.
[43] Middleman AB, Faulkner AH, Woods ER, et al. High-risk behaviors among high school students in Massachusetts who use anabolic steroids. Pediatrics 1995;96:268–72.
[44] Patel DR, Greydanus DE. The adolescent athlete. In: Hofmann AD, Greydanus DE, eds. Adolescent medicine, 3rd ed. Stamford, CT: Appleton Lange, 1997:607–38.
[45] Pope HC Jr, Katz DL. Psychiatric and medical effects of anabolic-androgenic steroid use. Arch Gen Psychiatry 1994;51:375–82.
[46] Tanner SM, Miller DW, Aongi C. Anabolic steroid use by adolescents: prevalence, motives, and knowledge of risks. Clin J Sport Med 1995;5:109–15.

[47] Rogal AD, Yesalis CE III. Anabolic-androgenic steroids and the adolescent. Pediatr Ann 1992;21:175–88.
[48] Sturmi JE, Diorio DJ. Anabolic agents. Clin Sports Med 1998;17:261–82.
[49] Yesalis CE, Kennedy NJ, Kopstein AN, et al. Anabolic-androgenic steroid use in the United States. JAMA 1993;270:1217–21.
[50] DuRant RH, Rickert VI, Ashworth CS, et al. Use of multiple drugs among adolescents who use anabolic steroids. N Engl J Med 1993;328:922–6.
[51] Monitoring the future. Accessed 2013 Jan 02. URL: www.Monitoring the future.org.
[52] Harmer PA. Anabolic-androgenic steroid use among young male and female athletes: is the game to blame? Br J Sports Med 2010;44:26–31.
[53] DuRant RH, Escobodo LG, Heath GW. Anabolic steroid use, strength training and multiple drug use among adolescents in the United States. Pediatrics 1995;96:23–6.
[54] Heischober BS, Hofmann AD. Substance abuse. In: Hofmann AD, Greydanus DE, eds. Adolescent medicine, 3rd ed. Stamford, CT: Appleton Lange; 1997:703–39.
[55] Schydlower M, Rogers PD. Adolescent substance abuse and addictions. Adolesc Med State Art Rev 1993;4:227–477.
[56] Greydanus DE, Patel DR. Substance abuse in adolescents: current concepts. Curr Probl Pediatr Adolesc Health Care 2005;35(3):78–98.
[57] Greydanus DE, Patel DR. Substance abuse in adolescents: current concepts. Disease-a-Month 2005;51(7):392–431.
[58] Josefson D. Concern raised about performance enhancing drugs in the United States. BMJ 1998;317:702.
[59] American Academy of Pediatrics. Adolescents and anabolic steroids: a subject review. Committee on sports medicine and fitness. Pediatrics 1997;99:1–7.
[60] Brower KJ. Anabolic steroids. Psychiatr Clin North Am 1993;16:97–102.
[61] Casavant MJ, Blake K, Griffith J, et al. Consequences of use of anabolic androgenic steroids. Pediatr Clin North Am 2007;54(4):677–90.
[62] Bhasin S, Storer TW, Berman N, et al. The effects of supraphysiologic doses of testosterone on muscle size and strength in normal men. N Engl J Med 1996;335:1–7.
[63] Kanayama G, Hudson JI, Pope HG Jr. Long-term psychiatric and medical consequences of anabolic-androgenic steroid abuse: a looming public health concern? Drug Alcohol Depend 2008;98(1–2):1–12.
[64] Blue JG, Lombardo JA. Steroids and steroid-like compounds. Clin Sports Med 1999;18:667–89.
[65] Kashkin KB, Kleber HD. Hooked on hormones? An anabolic steroid addiction hypothesis. JAMA 1989;262:3166–70.
[66] Yesalis CE III, Streit AL, Vicary JR, et al. Anabolic sterid use: indications of habituation among adolescents. J Drug Educ 1989;19:103–16.
[67] Duclos M. Use, abuse, and biomedical detection of anabolic steroids and glucocorticoids in sports. Ann Endocrinol (Paris) 2007;68(4):308–14.
[68] Malone DA, Dimeff RJ, Lombardo JA, et al. Psychiatric effects and psychoactive substance use in anabolic-androgenic steroid users. Clin J Sport Med 1995;5:25–31.
[69] Cohen JC. Hypercholesterolemia in male power lifters using anabolic-androgenic steroids. Phys Sportsmed 1988;16:49–59.
[70] Dickerman RD, Schaller F, Prather I, et al. Sudden cardiac death in a 20-year old bodybuilder using anabolic steroids. Cardiology 1995;86:172–3.
[71] Ferenchick GS. Are androgenic steroids thrombogenic? N Engl J Med 1990;322:476.
[72] Fisher M, Applyby M, Rittoo D, et al. Myocardial infarction with extensive intracoronary thrombus induced by anabolic steroids. Br J Clin Pract 1996;50:222–3.
[73] Kennedy MC, Lawrence C. Anabolic steroid abuse and cardiac death. Med J Aust 1993;158:346–8.
[74] Luckstead EF, Greydanus DE. Use and abuse of drugs. In: Medical care of the athlete. Los Angeles: Practice Management Information, 1993:195–205.
[75] Greydanus DE, Pratt HD. Psychosocial considerations for the adolescent athlete: lessons learned from the United States experience. Asian J Paediatr Prac 2000;3:19–29.

[76] Patel DR, Pratt HD, Greydanus DE. Adolescent growth, development and psychosocial aspects of sports participation: an overview. Adolesc Med State Art Rev 1998;9:425–40.
[77] Mulcahey MK, Schiller JR, Hulstyn MJ. Anabolic steroid use in adolescents: identification of those at risk and strategies for prevention. Phys Sportsmed 2010;38(3):105-13.
[78] Wood RI, Stanton SJ. Testosterone and sport: current perspectives. Horm Behav 2012;61(1):147-55.
[79] Dobs AS. Is there a role for androgenic anabolic steroids in medical practice? JAMA 1999;281:1326–7.
[80] Creatine and androstenedione—two "dietary supplements." Med Lett Drugs Ther 1998;40:105–6.
[81] Nestler JE, Barlascini CO, Clore JN, et al. Dehydroepiandrosterone reduces serum low density lipoprotein levels and body fat, but does not alter insulin sensitivity in normal men. J Clin Endocrinol Metab 1988;66:57–61.
[82] Broeder CE, Quindry J, Brittingham K, et al. The Andro Project. Arch Intern Med 2000;160:3093–104.
[83] Shelby MK, Crouch DJ, Black DL, Robert TA, Heltsley R. Screening indicators of dehydroepiandrosterone, androstenedione, and dihydrotestosterone use: a literature review. J Anal Toxicol 2011;35(9):635-55.
[84] Di Luigi L. Supplements and the endocrine system in athletes. Clin Sports Med 2008;27:131–51.
[85] Smurawa TM, Congeni JA. Tesosterone precursors: use and abuse in pediatric athletes. Pediatr Clin North Am 2007;54(4):787–96.
[86] Johnson M. Anabolic steroid use in adolescent athletes. Pediatr Clin North Am 1990;37:111.
[87] Buzzini S. Abuse of growth hormone among young athletes. Pediatr Clin North Am 2007;54:823–43.
[88] Erotokritou-Mulligan I, Bassett EE, Kniess A, et al. Validation of the growth hormone (GH)-dependent marker method of detecting GH abuse in sport through the use of independent data sets. Growth Horm IGF Res 2007;17(5):416–23.
[89] Kamboj M, Patel DR. Abuse of growth hormone by athletes. Int Public Health J 2009;3:10–8.
[90] Lattavo A, Kopperud A, Rogers PD. Creatine and other supplements. Pediatr Clin North Am 2007;54(4):735–60.
[91] Denham BE. Association between narcotic use and anabolic-androgenic steroid use among American adolescents. Subst Use Misuse 2009;44(14):2043–61.
[92] Parr MK, Koehler K, Geyer H, et al. Clenbuterol marketed as dietary supplement. Biomed Chromatogr 2008;22(3):298–300.
[93] Beckett AH. Clenbuterol and sport. Lancet 1992;340:1165.
[94] Roberts CA. The impact of long-term clenbuterol on athletic performance in horses. Vet J 2009;182(3):377.
[95] Hilderbrand RL. The world anti-doping program and the primary care physician. Pediatr Clin North Am 2007;54(4):701–11.
[96] Barroso O, Mazzoni I, Rabin O. Hormone abuse in sports: the antidoping perspective. Asian J Androl 2008;10(3):391–402.
[97] Alaranta A, Alaranta H, Helenius I. Use of prescription drugs in athletes. Sports med 2008;38(6):449–63.
[98] Rogol AD. Drugs of abuse and adolescent athlete. Ital J Pediatr 2010;36:19.
[99] Stricker PR. Other ergogenic agents. Clin Sports Med 1998;17:283–97.
[100] Clark JF. Creatine and phosphocreatine: a review of their use in exercise and sport. J Athletic Train 1997;32:45–51.
[101] Engelhardt M, Neumann G, Berbalk A, et al. Creatine supplementation in endurance sports. Med Sci Sports Exerc 1998;30:1123–9.
[102] Greenhaff P. Creatine and its application as an ergogenic aid. Int J Sport Nutr 1995;5:S100–10.
[103] Grindstaff PD. Effects of creatine supplementation on repetitive sprint performance and body composition in competitive swimmers. Int J Sport Nutr 1997;7:330–46.
[104] Petroczi A, Naughton DP, Mazanov J, et al. Performance enhancement with supplements: incongruence between rationale and practice. J Int Soc Sports Nutr 2007;4(1):19.

[105] Brannon TA, Adams GR, Conniff C, et al. Effects of creatine loading and training on running performance and biochemical properties of rat skeletal muscle. Med Sci Sports Exerc 1997;29:489–95.
[106] Greenhaff PL, Casey A, Short AH, et al. Influence of oral creatine supplementation on muscle torque during repeated bouts of maximal voluntary exercise for men. Clin Sci 1993;84:565–71.
[107] Williams M. Nutritional ergogenics and sports performance. President's Council Phys Fitness Sports Res Digest 1998;3:1–8.
[108] Burke LM, Pyne DB, Telford RD. Effect of oral creatine supplementation on single effort sprint performance in elite runners. Int J Sport Nutr 1996;6:222–33.
[109] Cooke WH, Grandjean PW, Barnes WS. Effect of oral creatine supplementation on power output and fatigue during bicycle ergometry. J Appl Physiol 1995;78:670–3.
[110] Mujika I, Chatard JC, Lacoste L, et al. Creatine supplementation does not improve sprint performance in competitive swimmers. Med Sci Sports Exerc 1996;28:1435–41.
[111] Buford TW, Kreider RB, Stout JR, Greenwood M, Campbell B, Spano M, et al. International Society of Sports Nutrition position stand: creatine supplementation and exercise. J Int Soc Sports Nutr 2007;4:2-8.
[112] Cristani A, Romagnoli E, Boldrini E. Sport's medicalization. Recenti Prog Med 2007;98(9):433–6.
[113] Harris R, Sderlund K, Hultman E. Elevation of creatine in resting and exercise muscles of normal subjects by creatine supplementation. Clin Sci 1992;83:367–74.
[114] Hultman E, Sderlund K, Timmons JA, et al. Muscle creatine loading in men. J Appl Physiol 1996;81:232–7.
[115] Terjung RL, Clarkson P, Eichner ER, et al. American College of Sports Medicine roundtable. Physiological and health effects of oral creatine supplementation. Med Sci Sports Exerc 2000;32:706–17.
[116] Keisler B, Hosey R. Ergogenic aids: an update on ephedra. Curr Sports Med Rep 2005;4:231–5.
[117] Bent S, Tiedt TN, Odden MC, et al. The relative safety of ephedra compared to other herbal products. Ann Intern Med 2003;138:468–71.
[118] www.fda.org accessed December 20, 2010.
[119] Burke LM. Caffeine and sports performance. Appl Physiol Nutr Metabol 2008;33(6):1319–34.
[120] Duchan E, Patel ND, Feucht C. Energy drinks: a review of use and safety for athletes. Physician Sportsmedicine 2010;38:1-9.
[121] Pommering TL. Erythropoietin and other blood-boosting methods. Pediatr Clin North Am 2007;54(4):691–9.
[122] Jelkmann W, Lundby C. Blood doping and its detection. Blood 2011;118(9):2395-404.
[123] Thevis M, Thomas A, Schanzer W. Mass spectrometric determination of insulins and their degradation products in sports drug testing. Mass SpectromRev 2007. Accessed 2013 Jan 02. URL: http://dopingjournal.org/noteworthy/achive/2007_11_01<archive.html.
[124] Thevis M, Kohler M, Maurer J, et al. Screening for 2-quinolinone-derived selective androgen receptor agonists in doping control analysis. Rapid Commun Mass Spectrom 2007;21(21):3477–86.
[125] Powers SK, Hamilton K. Antioxidants and exercise. Clin Sports Med 1999;18:525–36.
[126] Patel DR, Luckstead EF. Sport participation, risk taking and health risk behaviors. Adolesc Med State Art Rev 2000;11:78.
[127] Petroczi A, Naughton DP. Popular drugs in sports: descriptive analysis of the enquiries made via the Drug Information Database (DID). Br J Sports Med 2009;43:811–7.
[128] Martinsen M, Bratland-Sanda S, Eriksson AK, et al. Dieting to win to be thin? A study of dieting and disordered eating among adolescent elite athletes and non-athlete controls. Br J Sports Med 2010;44:70–6.

Submitted: August 05, 2013. *Revised:* October 01, 2013. *Accepted:* October 10, 2013.

In: Public Health Yearbook 2015
Editor: Joav Merrick

ISBN: 978-1-63484-514-4
© 2016 Nova Science Publishers, Inc.

Chapter 20

TEENAGE PREGNANCY: PRENATAL DRUG EXPOSURE

Colleen Dodich[*], MD, Shalin Patel, MD, and Amanda Williams, MD

Department of Pediatric and Adolescent Medicine,
Western Michigan University School of Medicine, Kalamazoo, Michigan,
United States of America

ABSTRACT

Although teenage pregnancy has been on the decline, substance abuse in the pregnant adolescent population is still a problem that needs to be addressed. The rate of illicit drug use in pregnant teenagers was 20.9% for ages 15-17 and 8.2% for ages 18-25 years for the combined 2010-2011 time frame. It is important to screen all women, particularly teenagers, for substance abuse during their initial obstetrical visit, as substance abuse can encompass all ages and socioeconomic groups. This paper reviews the recommended screening tools that are available to the practitioner along with parameters used to determine the need for laboratory testing. Substance use, abuse, tolerance and dependence are all defined, as well. Also discussed are the main substances that are abused by this population of adolescents and the management and follow-up that is needed for each substance. The maternal, fetal and neonatal complications caused from these substances are also addressed. The substances described in this paper include alcohol, nicotine, marijuana, opioids, cocaine, amphetamines/methamphetamines, benzodiazepines and inhalants.

Keywords: substance abuse, adolescence, pregnancy, teenage pregnancy

---

[*] Correspondence: Colleen Dodich MD, Assistant Professor, Department of Pediatric and Adolescent Medicine, Western Michigan University School of Medicine, 1000 Oakland Drive, D48G, Kalamazoo, MI, 49008-1284, United States. E-mail: colleen.dodich@med.wmich.edu.

INTRODUCTION

Teenage pregnancy has been on the decline for many years with a record low in 2010, yet the teen birth rate in the United States is still higher than most of its industrialized counterparts. The birth rate in 2010 for adolescents aged 15-19 was 34%. This is a nearly 10% drop from 2009 and the lowest number of teenage births reported in more than 60 years (1, 2). Unfortunately, although teenage pregnancy is on the decline, teenage drug use during pregnancy is still a problem. The rate of illicit drug use in pregnant teenagers was 20.9% for ages 15-17 and 8.2% for ages 18-25 years for the combined 2010-2011 time frame. For the younger teenagers, the rate of illicit drug use is similar between those who are pregnant and those who are not (1).

It is important to screen all women, particularly teenagers, for substance abuse during their initial obstetrical visit, as substance abuse can encompass all ages and socioeconomic groups. This screening should then be repeated throughout the pregnancy, such as every trimester. The youngest women report the greatest substance abuse while pregnant. The American College of Obstetricians and Gynecologists (ACOG) promotes screening for substance abuse as a part of complete obstetric care and recommends asking all pregnant women about their use of alcohol, tobacco and illicit drugs. Early screening and diagnosis of substance abuse or dependence can lead to earlier intervention and management, which can thus lead to improved maternal and neonatal outcomes (3).

There can be barriers to this screening process, though. First, substance abusers, particularly teenagers, may not present for prenatal care for a host of different reasons. They may not know they are pregnant, or be in denial, and they may also have a sense of guilt, shame and/or fear surrounding the pregnancy. If substance abuse is also part of the picture, that shame, guilt and fear can be increased. When the adolescent does present for obstetrical care, they may not initially be upfront in regards to substance abuse, as they may feel that they will be reprimanded, subjected to legal consequences, have their child taken away from them or further ostracized. They may also be in denial that their substance use is a big deal or that it will harm themselves or their unborn child. It is important for the provider to cultivate a trusting environment with the patient so that a truthful history can be obtained.

Although all illicit substance abuse is potentially harmful to both the mother and the fetus, it is important to determine the pattern of drug use for correct diagnosis, management and monitoring of adverse effects to both the mother and baby. *Substance use* is considered to be sporadic consumption of a drug with no adverse effects from that usage. In some countries, sporadic alcohol use during pregnancy is not considered harmful. Per defined criteria based on the DSM-IV guide, Substance Abuse is consumption of a drug that causes adverse effects leading to clinically significant impairment or distress to the user. It is further defined as a manifestation of one of the following criteria within a 12 month period: recurrent use resulting in failure in work, school or home obligations, recurrent use in hazardous situations; recurrent substance-related legal problems or recurrent social or interpersonal problems due to the substance. The frequency of use may vary depending on the substance being abused and the individual abuser's needs and wants.

Substance dependence, as defined by the DSM-IV criteria, includes a pattern of use that leads to impairment or distress with the manifestation of at least three of the following criteria in the past 12 months: tolerance, withdrawal symptoms, increase or more frequent usage than intended, inability to cut down when desiring to do so, exorbitant amounts of time spent in substance related activities, decrease or cessation of important social or work-related activities due to substance use or continued use of the substance despite knowledge of harm (both to the mother and to the fetus). *Substance tolerance* is defined as the need to increase the amount of drug taken to achieve the same effect (3, 4).

There are numerous risk factors that should alert providers to an increased risk of substance abuse. A young age at conception is a risk factor on its own, thus all pregnant teenagers should be screened. In addition to age, a late start to prenatal care, inconsistent prenatal care, an unstable home environment, concomitant STIs, relational problems, and problems with school or work may signal a substance abuse problem. Also, changes in behavior during appointments, depression symptoms, weight loss or other health concerns may point to substance abuse. If the pregnant adolescent has had other children who are no longer under her care, has a partner with an abuse problem, a family history of substance abuse, a personal history of drug abuse, a history of legal problems or a diagnosis of a mental health condition, the risk of substance abuse is increased (4).

SCREENING AND DIAGNOSIS

When screening for substance abuse in pregnant teens, validated screening tools are recommended. Some of the usual substance abuse questionnaires may not be appropriate, as it is important to know if *any* substances are being used during the pregnancy. The 4P's Plus Screen© is a screening tool used in pregnancy to determine past or current substance use (5). If this screening tool elicits a positive response, further assessment should be done. A limitation of this screening tool is that it is copyrighted and may not be reproduced. Another screening tool is the CRAFFT Substance Abuse screen and this is available to be used without restriction. Some research has been done on this tool and it has been found to have a better response than the medical record and the T-ACE alcohol screen (6). This is also a preliminary screening tool and if there are two or more positive responses, further investigation should be performed. Other screening tests that have been used in this population with varying results are the T-ACE, TWEAK and AUDIT-C screening tools (7). It is important that with any screening tool, there is a question regarding any substance use.

When asking pregnant teenagers about substance use, it is best to ask questions about legal substances, such cigarettes and alcohol first, though depending on the age of the adolescent, these may be illegal as well. The questioning can then progress to use/misuse of over-the-counter, prescription and herbal drugs and finally to the use of illegal substances. The questions should be asked in a neutral, respectful tone and the provider should be sensitive in the wording of these questions. The patient may also be asked if she has any history of participation in substance abuse programs, such as Alcoholics Anonymous or Narcotics Anonymous or participation in rehabilitation programs. If the history is positive for substance use, it is then important to find out all the substances used, the frequency of the usage, the duration of the usage and the last time the substance(s) was used. It is also important to find out the quantity of the substance used.

Laboratory testing for drug use can be used following a positive screen, but laboratory tests have their limitations. Universal laboratory screening of pregnant adolescents is not recommended and random testing in which the adolescent did not give consent is unethical. Although there is no consensus as to who should undergo laboratory testing, there are some clinical situations that would indicate testing. These situations would include a previous positive drug test, late prenatal care or frequently missed prenatal appointments, an unstable social environment, monitoring for methadone use or previous involvement with Child Protective Services.

Additional medical complications that would potentially indicate a need for testing include placental abruption, idiopathic preterm labor, idiopathic IUGR or an unexplained fetal demise. It is important to receive consent from the pregnant adolescent before performing this testing, and it is important to follow the state's requirements for testing and reporting of the test results. The adolescent should be made aware of the legal and economic implications of the testing. Consent is not needed when a pregnant adolescent presents unconscious or under the influence of a substance and that substance needs to be identified for further medical management (4).

The most common mode of testing is via the mother's urine. Blood, hair and saliva may also be used for drug testing. Screening can be performed for a single substance or for multiple substances. The common substances tested are opiates, marijuana, amphetamines and cocaine, although other specific substances can be tested for, based on history. Maternal urine drug testing does have limitations, most notably that it can only be used to detect recent drug use. Amphetamines and cocaine can be detected for 2-3 days, opiates can be detected for 1-3 days, PCP can be detected for 7-14 days and marijuana can be detected 1-7 days for light use and up to one month for chronic moderate to heavy use (4). Alcohol is hard to screen for in a urine or blood test due to its short half-life.

In addition, there are other medications and foods that can create a false positive drug screen. If drug testing does come back positive for a specific substance, it may be worthwhile to look for concomitant drug use at that time. Studies show that half of mothers who use illicit drugs are also using tobacco and/or alcohol (8). Drug testing can also be performed on the infant after birth. A neonatal urine drug screen can be easily obtained and, unlike maternal testing, most times consent is not needed to test the neonate. Both hair and meconium can provide information on longer-term substance use during pregnancy.

ALCOHOL

Alcohol is one of the leading preventable causes of birth defects. Women who may be pregnant or may become pregnant are urged to abstain from alcohol for this reason. The CDC reports that 7.6% of pregnant women have used alcohol during pregnancy and 1.4% admitted to binge drinking during pregnancy. This is based on 2006–2010 Behavioral Risk Factor Surveillance System (BRFSS) data (9).

There is no known safe level of alcohol use in pregnancy; therefore women should not drink any alcohol while pregnant. Yet, binge drinking while pregnant appears to have a greater negative effect than comparable consumption of smaller amounts more frequently (9, 10). A good history during the first prenatal visit that includes the use of alcohol is important. Screening tools are available to investigate the mother's level of alcohol use, as described above. Screening tools assess for such things as mother's alcohol tolerance, if she feels the need to cut back on drinking, how many drinks are consumed and how often drinks are consumed. If a mother's initial screen comes back positive, intervention will be needed. Intervention includes counseling on the risks of alcohol intake during pregnancy, increasing the amount of prenatal visits, informing the pediatrician of the risk for neonatal withdrawal (11).

Alcohol crosses the placenta and is known to be damaging to the fetus. The damage ranges from short term withdrawal symptoms to long term chronic disorders. Withdrawal typically begins within the first 3-12 hours after delivery. Initially, the symptoms include hyperactivity, irritability, tremors, sleep disturbances and seizures. These initial symptoms can last approximately 72 hours. During this time the pediatrician must also watch for hypoglycemia and acidosis. After the initial 72 hours the infant may experience up to 48 hours of a lethargic phase. Soon after, the infant may return back to normal. Treatment during this time includes symptomatic care. Infants benefit from low stimulation including dim lights, swaddling and keeping the room quiet. Good nutrition is also important as the infant's metabolic needs are increased. Also, monitor for and correct any metabolic derangements. Benzodiazepines may be needed for treatment of seizures (11).

The long-term effects of alcohol are placed into a spectrum, termed fetal alcohol spectrum disorder, with fetal alcohol syndrome (FAS) being the most severe end of the spectrum. FAS is the most common identifiable cause of mental retardation (11) (see chapter 14). It is estimated that FAS affects anywhere from 0.2-2.0 cases per 1,000 live births (12). Abnormalities in several areas are required for diagnosis of FAS: poor growth, central nervous system abnormalities and dysmorphic facies. The infant may face poor growth starting in utero and continuing into childhood. CNS abnormalities include irritability, jitteriness and increase response to noise, as well as permanent brain damage with resulting adverse effects to the child's neurodevelopmental outcome. The characteristic facial features include a smooth philtrum, thin vermillion boarder, and small palpebral fissures (11). The effects even extend into adolescence with significant cognitive impairment, ADHD symptoms (hyperactivity, impulsivity, and poor concentration), poor memory and reasoning. Prenatal exposure to alcohol does not have to be confirmed for a diagnosis of FAS to be diagnosed.

Other less severe forms of the fetal alcohol spectrum disorder exist as well. Like FAS the following syndromes and defects have been confirmed with prenatal alcohol exposure. Infants with partial fetal alcohol syndrome have the same facial dysmorphisms and either poor growth or CNS disturbances. Alcohol-related birth defects include the abnormal facies with structural anomalies in other organs (renal and cardiac involvement) without poor growth or CNS abnormalities. Alcohol-related neurodevelopmental disorders occur in patients without the facial abnormalities and normal growth. They do however show behavioral and cognitive impairment with risk for diminished memory skills and lower IQ (12). One study showed that consuming two or more drinks per day during pregnancy resulted in a seven point decrease in IQ at seven years of age (13).

Per the American Academy of Pediatrics (AAP), alcohol is compatible with breastfeeding yet adverse effects (such as drowsiness, diaphoresis, weakness, a decrease in linear growth and abnormal weight gain) may occur in infants of mothers with a high alcohol intake (14). In addition, with ingestions larger than 1g/kg/day, the milk ejection reflex is decreased and may cause a decrease in breast milk supply (15). Yet, there are some studies suggesting that beer ingestion can increase milk production due to an increase in serum prolactin (16, 17).

TOBACCO

It is reported by the CDC that 13% of pregnant women reported smoking during the last three months of pregnancy. Of those who try to quit smoking during pregnancy, about half will relapse by the time the infant is 6 months of age (18). Screening the mother for cigarette smoking in addition to other drug use is an important part of the first prenatal visit. Cigarette smoking has been proven over time to be detrimental to the fetus. Smoking increases the risk of placental abnormalities (abruption and previa), premature rupture of membranes, preterm labor resulting in preterm delivery, low birth weight infants, and sudden infant death syndrome (SIDS). These complications are of concern as they increase the risk of neonatal mortality (18). In addition, studies have shown that infants exposed to tobacco in utero show increased signs of stress, hypertonicity, excitability and irritability (19). It is uncertain if these effects are from nicotine toxicity or withdrawal.

Maternal smoking also increases the infant's risk of type II diabetes later in life (20). Prenatal exposure to nicotine has also been linked to an increased risk of psychiatric problems later in life including substance abuse (21). Cognitive ability has been suspected to be affected by cigarette smoke as well but when studies adjusted for maternal IQ and education levels there was no significant effect on IQ. Behavioral issues increased when children were exposed to tobacco in utero and there is an increased incidence of ADHD and conduct disorder in males. It has also been shown that the female offspring are at a greater risk of smoking later in life (22).

It has been noted that prenatal smoking is associated with other drug use. Second hand smoke is a problem as well, in utero and after birth. It has been shown that pregnant women exposed to second hand smoke were at greater risk of delivering a low birth weight infant. After the mother has delivered it is important to encourage her to continue to abstain from smoking and to decrease the infant's exposure to smoking. Second hand smoke exposure after delivery increases the infant's risk of Sudden Infant Death Syndrome (SIDS), upper respiratory infections, ear infections, and asthma attacks (18). In order to preserve the health of the child, as well as the mother, it is important encourage smoking cessation.

Per the American Academy of Pediatrics (AAP), breastfeeding while smoking is recommended although under consideration. Nicotine is present in breast milk in concentrations between 1.5 and 3.0 times the simultaneous maternal blood concentration and its elimination half-life is 60 to 90 minutes in both milk and plasma. There is no evidence to document whether this amount of nicotine presents a health risk to the nursing infant (15). Mothers who smoke have a lower breast milk supply, a lower milk fat content and tend to supplement with formula and wean sooner (16). A mother who wants to breastfeed is an excellent opportunity to discuss smoking cessation.

MARIJUANA

Marijuana is a commonly used substance worldwide with about 4% of the world's population reporting use of cannabis at least once in 2004 (23). It is also the most common illegal substance used during pregnancy in the United States (4). Even though it is a commonly used substance in pregnancy the outcomes to the neonates are not clear. Research has shown associations but no strong evidence of adverse effects related to marijuana use in utero. One confounding factor is that there are not many people using cannabis alone (4). The Avon Longitudinal Study of Pregnancy and Childhood surveyed mothers asking about cannabis use and neonatal outcomes including late fetal and perinatal death, special care admission of the newborn infant, birth weight, birth length, and head circumference.

Results suggested that the use of cannabis during pregnancy was not associated with a greater risk of neonatal morbidity or mortality (24). Yet, infants of mothers who abused marijuana while pregnant can have neurobehavioral effects such as a decreased ability to self soothe, increased fine tremors, increased startle reflex, sleep disturbances and increased hand to mouth activity (3). In addition, mothers who use marijuana may sleep heavily after use and may not be unresponsive to her infant's needs. Second hand smoke, or passive smoke is a significant issue to the infants, though (17).

Per the American Academy of Pediatrics (AAP), breastfeeding is contraindicated with marijuana use (15). A case-control study looking at maternal marijuana use and breastfeeding found that infants exposed to marijuana in breast milk during the first month postpartum appeared to have a decrease in motor development at one year of age (25). An article published in the Journal of Reproductive Medicine looked at the transition of THC through pregnancy and breast milk in rhesus monkeys. It was found that THC readily crossed the placenta and was also transferred in the breast milk. The infant receives 0.8% of the mother's dose per kg from one joint (26). Significant depressant effects were seen in the mother and the neonates if THC was ingested one hour prior to either birth or breastfeeding (27), although data is limited.

OPIOIDS

Opioids are a class of natural, endogenous and synthetic compounds that activate μ-opioid receptors in the CNS (see chapter 9). The term opiate refers to a subclass of alkaloid opioids. Morphine is one of the natural opioids while, endorphins, enkephalins and endomorphone are endogenous opioids. Synthetic opioids include codeine, heroin, hydromorphone (Dilaudid), fentanyl and methadone (28).

Opioids acutely inhibit the release of noradrenaline at synaptic terminals. Tolerance develops with chronic opioid exposure as the rate of noradrenaline release over time increases toward normal. Abrupt discontinuation of exogenous opioids results in supranormal release of noradrenaline and causes withdrawal (28).

Opioid abuse during pregnancy results in high obstetrical complications and increased perinatal morbidity and mortality. Heroin and methadone are the two most commonly abused opioids in pregnancy. Fluctuations in daily opioid use due to voluntary abstinence or lack of access to the drug during pregnancy can affect the fetus, as well. Abrupt blood drug level changes can result in fetal abstinence syndrome, fetal demise, premature delivery, stillbirth and low birth weight (28, 29). If a mother is abusing certain opioids, such as heroin, it is important that this is not stopped abruptly.

Prenatal opioid exposure has been associated with low birth weight and length, low head circumference at birth and sudden infant death syndrome (SIDS). Opioid use during pregnancy has been associated with obstetrical complications including toxemia of pregnancy and antepartum hemorrhage. It also increases risk of postpartum hemorrhage (3, 29). It has been shown that 55 to 94 percent neonates exposed to opioids in utero can suffer from opioid withdrawal syndrome (28). The constellation of clinical findings associated with opioid withdrawal has been termed the neonatal abstinence syndrome (NAS). These clinical findings are mentioned in detail Figure 1 (28).

The clinical presentation of NAS varies with the type of opioids, the maternal drug history including last use of the drug, maternal metabolism, infant metabolism and placental metabolism. It also depends on the use of concomitant substances such as cocaine, barbiturates, sedatives and nicotine. NAS is more common and severe with methadone exposure in comparison to those exposed to heroin or buprenorphine (28). The onset of withdrawal symptoms depends on half-life of the drug. Withdrawal from heroin usually begins within 24 hour of birth, while withdrawal from methadone usually begins around 24 to 72 hours of age. Sometimes, withdrawal effects may be delayed up to 5 to 7 days with both opioids (28).

Pregnant women addicted to heroin specifically benefit from opioid agonist therapy such as methadone maintenance treatment (MMT). It should be the standard of care for all opioid-dependent women during pregnancy (3). MMT can sustain a stable serum opioid concentration in the mother and fetus in ranges that minimizes fetal abstinence and decreases perinatal mortality. MMT also provides several additional benefits including reduction in use of illegal heroin, optimization of prenatal care and maternal health (3, 28, 29). But, there are few disadvantages to MMT. NAS is more severe and prolonged after methadone exposure in comparison to heroin exposure and it is extremely unlikely to achieve successful detoxification after delivery (28).

Other slow-release opioid preparations like bupronorphine may be considered if methadone is not available. Antenatal planning for intrapartum and postpartum analgesia may be offered for all women in consultation with appropriate health care providers. Opioid detoxification should be reserved for selected women because of the high risk of relapse to opioids. Few studies have showed that opioid detoxification in the second and third trimester of pregnancy is not linked to increased adverse perinatal events if done under close observation (3, 30). Thus, due to high relapse rate to opioids, detoxification is not advisable during pregnancy (3).

It is also critical to provide psychosocial support and treat co-morbid medical problems including STI's and mental disorders for better pregnancy outcomes (26). Opioid-dependent women should be informed that neonates exposed to heroin, prescription opioids, methadone, or buprenorphine during pregnancy are monitored closely for symptoms and signs of neonatal withdrawal after birth.

Newborns exposed to opioids prenatally should be observed closely for withdrawal symptoms and scored based on their clinical pictures. The modified Finnegan Neonatal Abstinence Scoring System is commonly used in the United States. Neonates consistently scoring high on that scale benefit from pharmacotherapy. Morphine and methadone are first line treatments for moderate to severe NAS followed by second line treatment of phenobarbital in unresponsive neonates. Mild NAS can be managed by non-pharmacological interventions. Supportive care includes an environment with low stimulation such as being placed in a dark and quiet room and swaddled carefully to avoid any auto-stimulation (28).

NEONATAL ABSTINENCE SCORING SYSTEM

SYSTEM	SIGNS AND SYMPTOMS	SCORE	AM	PM	COMMENTS
CENTRAL NERVOUS SYSTEM DISTURBANCES	Continuous High Pitched (or other) Cry	2			Daily Weight:
	Continuous High Pitched (or other) Cry	3			
	Sleeps <1 Hour After Feeding	3			
	Sleeps <2 Hours After Feeding	2			
	Sleeps <3 Hours After Feeding	1			
	Hyperactive Moro Reflex	2			
	Markedly Hyperactive Moro Reflex	3			
	Mild Tremors Disturbed	1			
	Moderate-Severe Tremors Disturbed	2			
	Mild Tremors Undisturbed	3			
	Moderate-Severe Tremors Undisturbed	4			
	Increased Muscle Tone	2			
	Excoriation (Specific Area)	1			
	Myoclonic Jerks	3			
	Generalized Convulsions	5			
METABOLIC/VASOMOTOR/RESPIRATORY DISTURBANCES	Sweating	1			
	Fever 100.4°-101°F (38°-38.3°C)	1			
	Fever > 101°F (38.3C)	2			
	Frequent Yawning (>3-4 times/interval)	1			
	Mottling	1			
	Nasal Stuffiness	1			
	Sneezing (>3-4 times/interval)	1			
	Nasal Flaring	2			
	Respiratory Rate >60/min	1			
	Respiratory Rate > 60/min with Retractions	2			
GASTRO-INTESTINAL DISTURBANCES	Excessive Sucking	1			
	Poor Feeding	2			
	Regurgitation	2			
	Projectile Vomiting	3			
	Loose Stools	2			
	Watery Stools	3			
	TOTAL SCORE				
	INITIALS OF SCORER				

Figure 1. Modified Finnegan's neonatal abstinence scoring tool (Hudak ML et al., Pediatrics 2012;129:e540-60).

The risks and benefits of breastfeeding should be weighed on an individual basis. Per the AAP, methadone is compatible with breastfeeding, but heroin is contraindicated (15). Heroin is excreted in breast milk in quantities sufficient to cause addiction. All opiates have been documented in breast milk in small amounts and some clinical effects that may be seen include tremors, restlessness, vomiting and poor feeding (31). Lactating mothers should use codeine with caution as some women have a genetic predisposition to convert codeine to morphine at a faster rate (3). Mothers who are enrolled in a supervised methadone maintenance program should be encouraged to breastfeed, as long as their HIV status is negative. They should abstain from breastfeeding 2-4 hours after their methadone dose (32). Women on methadone maintenance should only breast feed for up to 5 months, after which the volume of milk consumed by the baby is large enough to supply a sedating dose of methadone to the baby and may produce NAS when breastfeeding is ceased. Chaotic substance use by a breastfeeding mother may result in the infant receiving fluctuating doses of opioids. Fluctuating levels may mean that breastfeeding is not reliable enough to be used as a method for preventing withdrawal.

COCAINE

Cocaine is an addictive central nervous system (CNS) stimulant that prevents uptake of extracellular dopamine into the pre-synaptic cell by blocking its transporter, resulting in excess stimulation of dopamine receptors in the synaptic cleft (33). It is also known as "coke," "C," "snow," "flake," or "blow." A combination of cocaine and heroin is known as a "speedball" (34).

There are several research studies showing that cocaine abuse during pregnancy can increase the risk of intrauterine growth restriction (IUGR), placental abruption, premature rupture of membrane and premature deliveries.

It also increases the risk of spontaneous abortion and precipitous delivery. Due to its vasoconstrictive effects, its abuse can increase the risk of pregnancy-induced hypertension (3, 29). Cocaine abuse during pregnancy has also been associated with genitourinary malformations, fetal demise and intracranial bleeding in neonatal period. In addition, it has associated with low birth weight and length and microcephaly (3, 29, 35).

An abstinence syndrome after intrauterine exposure to CNS stimulants like cocaine and amphetamine has not been clearly defined. Several studies have showed that cocaine-exposed infants had no clinically significant withdrawal signs (28).

Cocaine abuse is a complex problem like any other substance abuse. Management of cocaine abuse should be systematic and should be focused on medical management as well as psychosocial aspects. There are two main phases to the management for cocaine abuse during pregnancy. The first phase includes treatment of withdrawal symptoms with the cessation of the drug. Sometimes, women may benefit from a supportive admission to a non-medical withdrawal management center (3).

The second phase focuses on prevention of a relapse by providing psychosocial support for abstinence in addition to treating co-morbid medical problems including STI's and mental disorders (3). Currently, there are no FDA approved pharmacological treatment options available to treat cocaine abuse and to help with cessation and withdrawal symptoms. A few medications including vigabatrin, tiagabine, topiramate, modafinil and disulfiram have shown reduction in cocaine use in controlled clinical trials (34).

Behavioral interventions are the main stay of management for cocaine abuse. Contingency management or motivational incentives have proven to be an effective treatment for cocaine dependence, especially during the achievement of initial abstinence. Cognitive behavior therapy (CBT) is also a very effective approach to prevent relapse (34).

Per the AAP, cocaine is contraindicated in breastfeeding due to its vasoconstrictive effects (15). Cocaine is excreted into breast milk in fairly high concentrations and his been detected in the serum of breastfed babies. Effects on the infant include irritability, vomiting, diarrhea, tremors and seizures (31). Mothers should be advised that it is best to abstain from cocaine use while nursing (3).

METHAMPHETAMINE/AMPHETAMINES

Amphetamines are also CNS stimulants (see chapters 9 and 10). They are different from cocaine in terms of mechanism and have a prolonged half-life up to 12 hours. They reverse the actions of monoamine transporters and enhance the release of dopamine, norepinephrine and serotonin into the synaptic cleft, increasing their availability to act upon post-synaptic receptors. Amphetamines can also block the re-uptake and degradation of these neurotransmitters, further increasing their concentrations in the synaptic cleft (33). Methamphetamine is commonly known as "speed," "meth," "chalk," "ice," "crystal," "crank," and "glass." (36)

There are very few studies showing the consequences of prenatal methamphetamine abuse. However, methamphetamine abuse during pregnancy has been associated IUGR, fetal demise and placental abruption at same rate as cocaine abuse (28). Due to its vasoconstrictive effects, its abuse can increase the risk of pregnancy-induced hypertension. Methamphetamine abuse during pregnancy has been associated with several congenital anomalies involving the CNS and cardiovascular systems, oral clefts and limb anomalies (3, 29). Prescription amphetamines should also be avoided during pregnancy due the pregnancy related complications and the risk of perinatal mortalities (29).

Behavioral therapies like CBT and contingency management are also very effective for the management for amphetamine abuse. Currently, there are no specific pharmacological options available that help to reduce abuse and prevent relapse. Bupropion has shown some effectiveness in clinical trials by reducing methamphetamine-induced "high" and drug cravings (36).

An abstinence syndrome after intrauterine exposure to CNS stimulants like cocaine and amphetamines has not been clearly defined. One study showed that only four percent of infants exposed to methamphetamine in utero were treated for drug withdrawal but concomitant abuse of other drugs could not be excluded (28). Breastfeeding should be evaluated on an individual basis, as amphetamines have been shown to cross through breast milk (37). Effects on the infant from the contaminated breast milk include irritability and a poor sleeping pattern (31). Breastfeeding is contraindicated when the mother is taking in high doses of the drug, due to the vasoconstrictive properties (15).

BENZODIAZEPINES

Benzodiazepines are one of the most common classes of anxiolytic drugs used in the United States and are commonly prescribed to women of reproductive age and to pregnant women (see chapter 9). When benzodiazepines are used in pregnancy and lactation, the benefits to the mother have to be weighed against the risks to the fetus and neonate. These drugs are classified into three different groups: long acting, intermediate acting and short acting. The effects of these drugs, although not fully described physiologically, appear to be mediated through the inhibitory neurotransmitter gamma-aminobutyric acid (GABA). The drugs appear to act on the central nervous system to produce sedative and hypnotic effects, reduction of anxiety, anticonvulsant effects, and skeletal muscle relaxation (38).

All benzodiazepines diffuse readily through the placenta and pass through breast milk. The amount that passes through depends on the specific drug. Among the whole drug class, the most studied drug is diazepam. Several studies have shown an increased risk of oral clefts in fetuses of mothers who used diazepam in the first trimester of their pregnancy, although the results of this connection are not universally accepted. Studies also have shown an increased risk of low birth weight and microcephaly (38, 39). A neonatal withdrawal syndrome has been reported among infants exposed to diazepam during labor for preeclampsia, eclampsia, and sedation in the mother and has also been seen with more prolonged use of the lower dosages that are commonly prescribed for anxiety disorders. This syndrome can present a few days to a few weeks after birth and can last up to several months. Symptoms of neonatal withdrawal include hypertonia, hyperreflexia, restlessness, irritability, abnormal sleep patterns, inconsolable crying, tremors or jerking of the extremities, bradycardia, cyanosis, suckling difficulties, apnea, risk of aspiration of feeds, diarrhea and vomiting, and growth retardation (39).

In addition, acute use of diazepam during labor and delivery can lead to "floppy baby syndrome" which includes hypothermia, lethargy, respiratory problems, and feeding difficulties; in addition to other withdrawal symptoms.

Per the AAP, the risk of breastfeeding while taking benzodiazepines is unknown and it may be of concern (15). Published data regarding these drugs is highly variable. Neonatal withdrawal symptoms have been noted after exposure to alprazolam (Xanax) during breastfeeding but the drug has a relatively short half-life. Long-acting benzodiazepines such as diazepam and its metabolites can accumulate in infants, and have the potential to cause lethargy, sedation, and weight loss in infants. If an infant is abruptly weaned or the mother has rapid cessation of long-term treatment/use this may cause infant withdrawal symptoms. If breastfeeding is going to be accomplished while a mother is taking a benzodiazepine, it is best to wait 6-8 hours after a single dose of the drug before nursing.

INHALANTS

Inhalant abuse is prevalent in the adolescent population, particularly in younger adolescents. Nearly 20% of middle school and high school students have experimented with inhalants. Abused substances include fuels, solvents, propellants, glues, adhesives, and paint thinners (40). Inhalant abuse can produce a wide variety of physical and psychiatric side effects and when used during pregnancy, can lead to fetal abnormalities. There is an increased risk of spontaneous abortion in pregnant adolescents who abuse inhalants. In addition, it can cause fetal solvent syndrome, which includes symptoms of low birth weight, microcephaly, abnormal brain development, dysmorphic facies and muscle tone abnormalities (41). These symptoms are similar to those seen in fetal alcohol syndrome. Studies have also shown long term residual deficits in speech, motor and cognitive delays (42).

Management of inhalant abuse includes strict abstinence from the substance and supportive care. Counseling and support groups can also be offered. It is important to screen for other substance use, as inhalants are often a gateway to other illicit drugs. Withdrawal symptoms in the neonate are still being studied but tremors, malaise and gastrointestinal symptoms have been documented (3). It is important for these infants to be closely monitored for alcohol-like withdrawal symptoms.

The AAP has not thoroughly reviewed inhalants and breastfeeding, but many solvents that are used as inhalants will readily cross over into the breast milk and they do have short half-lives. An infant's nervous system continues to develop after birth and nursing infants may be more sensitive to the neurotoxic effects of solvents (43).

Conclusion

It is important to thoroughly screen all pregnant adolescents for substance use and abuse. It is also important to develop a trusting relationship with the adolescent so that an honest and complete history can be obtained. Depending on the substance that is being abused, the effects on the mother, fetus and neonate can vary widely. Substance-using women need additional support from their health care providers during the postpartum period to address their complex medical and psychosocial needs. They need support with breast-feeding; follow-up of medical problems including mental problems and sexually transmitted infections; support with child protective services involvement and assessment of substance use and encouragement to continue attending drug treatment program.

Acknowledgments

This paper is a revised and adapted version of an earlier publication in the book "Substance abuse in adolescents and young adults. A manual for pediatric and primary care clinicians" edited by Donald E Greydanus, Gabriel Kaplan, Dilip R Patel and Joav Merrick with Walter de Gruyter in Berlin, 2013.

References

[1] Hamilton BE, Ventura SJ. Birth rates for U.S. teenagers reach historic lows for all age and ethnic groups. NCHS data brief, no 89. Hyattsville, MD: National Center Health Statistics, 2012.

[2] Substance Abuse and Mental Health Services Administration, Results from the 2011 National Survey on Drug Use and Health: Summary of national findings. Rockville, MD: Substance Abuse Mental Health Services Administration, NSDUH Series H-44, HHS Publication No (SMA) 12-4713, 2012.

[3] Chasnoff IJ, et al. The 4P's Plus screen for substance use in pregnancy: clinical application and outcomes. J Perinatol 2005;25(6):368-74.
[4] Chang G, Orav EJ, Jones JA, et al. Self-reported alcohol and drug use in pregnant young women: a pilot study of associated factors and identification. J Addict Med 2011;5:221.
[5] Burns E, Gray R, Smith LA. Brief screening questionnaires to identify problem drinking during pregnancy: a systemic review. Addiction 2010;105:601.
[6] CDC. Alcohol use and binge drinking among women of childbearing age. United States, 2006-2010. MMWR 2012;61(28):534-8.
[7] Sielski LA. Infants of mothers with substance abuse. In: Basow DS, ed. UpToDate. Waltham, MA: UpToDate, 2012.
[8] CDC. Fetal alcohol spectrum disorder. Accessed 2013 Jan 02. URL: http://www.cdc.gov/ncbddd/fasd/index.html.
[9] Streissguth AP, Barr HM, Sampson PD. Moderate prenatal alcohol exposure: Effects on child IQ and learning problems at age 7 1/2 Years. Alcohol Clin Exp Res 1990;14(5):662-9.
[10] Ebrahim SH, Gfroerer J. Pregnancy-related substance use in the United States during 1996-1998. Obstet Gynecol 2003;101:374.
[11] CDC. PRAMS and smoking. Accessed 2013 Jan 02. URL: http://www.cdc.gov/prams/Tobaccoand Prams.htm.
[12] Montgomery SM, Ekbom A. Smoking during pregnancy and diabetes mellitus in a British longitudinal birth cohort. BMJ 2002;324(7328):26–7.
[13] Ernst M, Moolchan E, Robinson M. Behavioral and Neural Consequences of Prenatal Exposure to Nicotine. J Am Acad Child Adolesc Psychiatry 2001;40(6):630-41.
[14] Chang G. Overview of illicit drug use in pregnant women. In: Basow DS, ed. UpToDate. Waltham, MA: UpToDate, 2012.
[15] Bailey JA, DuPont RL, Teitelbaum SA. Cannibis use disorders: Epidemiology, comorbidity and pathogenesis. In: Basow DS, ed. UpToDate. Waltham, MA: UpToDate, 2012.
[16] Fergusson DM, Horwood LJ, Northstone K, et al. Maternal use of cannabis and pregnancy outcome. BLOG 2002;109(1):21.
[17] Astley SJ, Little RE. Maternal Marijuana use during lactation and infant development at one year. Neurotoxicol Teratol 1990;12(2):160-8.
[18] Asch RH, Smith CG. Effects of delta 9-THC, the principal psychoactive component of marijuana, during pregnancy in the rhesus monkey. J Reprod Med 1986;31(12):1071-81.
[19] Hudak ML, Tan RC. Neonatal drug withdrawal. Am Acad Pediatrics 2012;101(6):540-60.
[20] Luty J, Nikolaou V, Bearn J. Is opiate detoxification unsafe in pregnancy? J Subst Abuse Treat 2003;24(4):363-7.
[21] Minnes S, Lang A, Singer L. Prenatal tobacco, marijuana, stimulant, and opiate exposure: Outcomes and practice implications. J Natl Inst Drug Abuse 2011;6(1):57-70.
[22] National Institute on Drug Abuse. Cocaine: Abuse and addiction. National Institute on Drug Abuse Research Report Series, 10(4166). Accessed 2013 Jan 02. URL: http://www.drugabuse.gov/publications/research-reports/cocaine-abuse-addiction.
[23] National Institute on Drug Abuse. Methamphetamine abuse and addiction. National Institute on Drug Abuse Research Report Series, 06(4210). Accessed 2013 Jan 02. URL: http://www.drugabuse.gov/publications/research-reports/methamphetamine-abuse-addiction.
[24] Slutsker L. Risks associated with cocaine use during pregnancy. Obstet Gynecol 1992;79(5(Pt 1)):778-89.
[25] Thompson BL, Levitt P, Stanwood GD. Prenatal exposure to drugs: Effects on brain development and implications for policy and education. Nat Rev Neurosci 2009;10:303–12.
[26] Wong S, Ordean A, Kahan M. Substance use in pregnancy. J Obstet Gynaecol Can 2011;33(4): 367-84.
[27] Steiner E, Villen T, Hallberg M, Rane A. Amphetamine secretion in breastmilk. Eur J Clin Pharmacol 1984;27:123–4.
[28] Shor S, Nulman I, Kulaga V, Koren G. Heavy in utero ethanol exposure is associated with the use of other drugs of abuse in a high-risk population. Alcohol 2010;44:623.

[29] American Academy of Pediatrics Committee on Drugs. Transfer of drugs and other chemicals into human milk. Pediatrics 2001;108:776.
[30] Section of Breastfeeding. Breastfeeding and the use of human milk. Pediatrics 2012;129:e827.
[31] Law KL, Stroud LR, LaGasse LL, et al. Smoking during pregnancy and newborn neurobehavior. Pediatrics 2003;111:1318.
[32] Maier SE, West JR. Drinking patterns and alcohol-related birth defects. Alcohol Res Health 2001;25:168.
[33] Anderson CE, Loomis GA. Recognition and Prevention of Inhalant Abuse. Am Fam Physician 2003;68(5):869-74.
[34] Jones HE, Balster RL. Inhalant abuse in pregnancy. Obstet Gynecol Clin North Am 1998;25:153–67.
[35] Howard MO, Bowen SE, Garland LE, et al. Inhalant use and inhalant use disorders in the United States. Addict Sci Clin Pract 2011;6(1):18–31.
[36] American Academy of Pediatrics Committee on Drugs. Transfer of drugs and other chemicals into human milk. Pediatrics 2001;108(3):776-89.
[37] Ho E, Collantes A, Kapur BM, Moretti M, Koren G. Alcohol and breast feeding: calculation of time to zero level in milk. Biol Neonate 2001;80(3):219-22.
[38] Hale TW. Medications and mother's milk: A manual of lactational pharmacology, 11th ed. Amarillo, TX: Pharmasoft Medical, 2004.
[39] Royal Women's Hospital Drug Information Centre. Misuse of drugs in pregnancy and breastfeeding. Carlton, Vic: Royal Women's Hospital, 2003.
[40] Anderson PO. Drugs and breastfeeding. In: Anderson PO, Knoben JE, Troutman WG, eds. Handbook of clinical drug data, 10th ed. New York: McGraw-Hill, 2002.
[41] Liston J. Breastfeeding and the use of recreational drugs-alcohol, caffeine, nicotine and marijuana. Breastfeed Rev 1998;6(2):27-30.
[42] McElhatton PR. The effects of benzodiazepine use in pregnancy and lactation. Reprod Toxicol 1994;8(5):461-75.
[43] Iqbal MM, Sobhan T, Ryals T. Effects of commonly used benzodiazepines on the fetus, the neonate, and the nursing infant. Psychiatr Serv 2002;53(1):39-49.

Submitted. August 05, 2013. *Revised:* October 01, 2013. *Accepted:* October 10, 2013.

Section Three - Public health issues

In: Public Health Yearbook 2015
Editor: Joav Merrick

ISBN: 978-1-63484-514-4
© 2016 Nova Science Publishers, Inc.

Chapter 21

MEASUREMENTS OF SOCIAL ISOLATION AND SOCIAL SUPPORT FOR RARE LUNG DISEASE PATIENTS: AN INTEGRATIVE REVIEW

Susan K Flavin[*], MSN, RN

College of Nursing, Medical University of South Carolina,
Charleston, South Carolina, United States of America

ABSTRACT

Social support is an integral component of health. The risk of social isolation and perceptions of minimal support are high for persons living with rare chronic lung diseases such as sarcoidosis or alpha-1 antitrypsin deficiency. The study of social support and isolation requires validated, reliable instruments to quantify their influence. Objectives: The objective of this integrative review is to identify and critically appraise validated, reliable instrumentation to measure social isolation and related concepts in persons with rare lung diseases such as sarcoidosis or alpha-1 antitrypsin deficiency. Design: Integrative review. Methods: A review of the literature was conducted using PubMed, Medline, CINAHL and PsycINFO databases between 1970-2013. Eleven studies were included which encompassed eight instruments. Results: The Friendship Scale and the UCLA Loneliness Scale demonstrate past psychometric performance suggesting future suitability for use in persons with sarcoidosis or alpha-1 antitrypsin deficiency. Conclusion: Existing instruments would be suitable for an initial assessment of social isolation and social support in rare lung disease patients. Relevance to clinical practice: As the era of genomics and genetics continues to evolve, it is likely that conditions that were unrecognized previously may be identified as disease conditions. Moreover, simplification of testing for rare genetic conditions is becoming more commonplace, and clinicians may be faced with managing such patients. Knowledge of the potential or actual social impact of such conditions is necessary in order to provide for holistic management of such patients, and simple, existing tools can be useful.

Keywords: social isolation, loneliness, rare disease, chronic disease

---

[*] Correspondence: Susan K Flavin, MSN, RN, 132 Barton Drive, Spring City, PA 19475, United States. E-mail: sflavin622@comcast.net.

INTRODUCTION

An estimated 30 million Americans live with a diagnosis of one of the 6,000 to 8,000 known rare diseases (1) and such conditions affect approximately 30 million individuals in the EU (2). EURORDIS (Rare Diseases Europe) has identified the need to address the social aspects of the rare diseases as one component of living well within the context of a rare condition (3). Such social aspects include, but are not limited to, social support, extent of social network, and perceptions of loneliness and social isolation. Social isolation has been anecdotally reported in individuals suffering from various rare diseases (4, 5). Few studies have identified how social isolation affects people with rare diseases, despite the National Research Council's call for investigations into the linkages between social isolation and health (6). The impact of social isolation and social support has been explored in other populations. In their seminal work, House, Landis and Umberson (7) reviewed prospective epidemiological studies of social isolation in humans, and found that that social isolation was a significant risk factor for broad-based morbidity and mortality.

Operationally, social isolation is defined as the perception of a stigmatized environment, societal indifference, a personal-societal disconnection, or personal powerlessness (8). It is characterized by a lack of support system or a small/nonexistent social network. Few published studies have explored the experiences of living with a rare disease; no studies identified have investigated social isolation in rare lung diseases such as AATD or sarcoidosis.

Sarcoidosis is a rare, complex, granulomatous disease of unknown etiology. The incidence of sarcoidosis varies throughout the world, with 10-40 per 100,000 persons in the US and northern Europe developing this condition (9). Many organ systems can be affected, although lung involvement is most common, occurring in greater than 75% of all patients (10). Depression has been documented in these individuals (11), and more recently, social isolation has been identified as a concern (12). However, no published studies of social isolation have been identified to date.

Alpha-1 antitrypsin deficiency (AATD) is an uncommon genetic disease which that affects approximately 1 in 2,000 to 1 in 5,000 individuals and predisposes to liver disease and early-onset emphysema (13). Previous studies have confirmed adverse psychosocial effects related to an AATD diagnosis (14). Social isolation has been explored in individuals with COPD (15, 16) but no published studies were identified that investigated social isolation in AATD patients specifically.

Recognition of the importance of research into rare lung diseases is growing (17). Many studies have adopted a population-based approach to rare diseases, but the patients' viewpoint on having such a disorder has remained unattended (18). Despite the number of people affected by rare diseases, resources are lacking. Patients often feel isolated, unable to get the information and support they need (19). Delays in diagnosis and/or misdiagnosis may promote distrust of health care providers and counselors. Information on the psychosocial burden of these diseases is needed, of which social isolation is one component of the continuum.

SOCIAL ISOLATION AS A CONCEPT

The term "social isolation" has multiple meanings. Carpenito-Moyet succinctly defined social isolation as 'the state in which the individual or group expresses a need or desire for contact with others but is unable to make that contact' (20). Individuals at risk for such states include ethnic/cultural minorities, persons with chronic physiological and psychological illnesses or deformities, and elderly persons (8), such as individuals grappling with living with rare conditions.

In his concept analysis of social isolation in older adults, Nicholson (21) suggested that determinants of isolation include 'number of contacts, feelings of belonging, fulfilling relationships, engagement with others, and quality of network members' (p. 1349). Killeen suggests that isolation with choice is aloneness, while social isolation without choice equates to loneliness (22). This may be why some scales designed to measure loneliness also measure perceived social isolation or some measure of social network (e.g., the UCLA Loneliness Scale) (23).

This overview outlined the defining characteristics of social isolation and demonstrates that the term is not uniformly defined and consensus is elusive. This challenges measurement of the concept in this patient population. An integrative review of established instruments tested in diverse populations can inform studies that need to measure social isolation in populations living with rare disease such as sarcoidosis or alpha-1 antitrypsin deficiency.

For the purposes of this integrated review, instruments purporting to measure one or more constructs as delineated by Nicholson (21) (number of contacts, feelings of belonging, fulfilling relationships, engagement with others, and quality of network members) or Warren (stigmatized environment, societal indifference, personal-societal disconnection, or personal powerlessness) were included (8).

Objectives

The purpose of this paper is to present the findings of an integrative review of a number of instruments that were explicitly designed and tested to measure social isolation and concepts related to social isolation (such as loneliness or social support or network), and to review their relevance and appropriateness for the pilot measurement of social isolation in populations with sarcoidosis or alpha-1 antitrypsin deficiency.

METHODS

The integrated review methodology publicized by Whittemore and Knafl (24) was utilized to examine studies related to the concept to fully comprehend the depth and breadth of information related to social isolation. This particular approach allows for the inclusion of diverse methodologies (i.e., experimental and non-experimental research) to provide for a more holistic assimilation of information.

Literature search

An extensive review of the literature was conducted using PubMed, Medline, CINAHL and PsycINFO databases encompassing a range of years, as indicated in the attached table, but in general, between 1970-2013. This range was chosen in order to capture any seminal works that may have been published. GoogleScholar was also utilized to refine reviews. The search terms entered were "sarcoidosis," "alpha-1" "social isolation," "social support," "instrument," "questionnaire," "loneliness," "chronic disease," "lung disease" "pulmonary disease, "respiratory disease" and "social support" and combinations of these terms. In addition, the following three questionnaires were also used in the initial search, under the assumption that these could lead to other instruments measuring the same or similar constructs: "Social Support Questionnaire (SSQ)," "Lubben Social Network Questionnaire," and "Friendship Scale." The initial search captured over 500,000 articles; after multiple refinements, a total of 11 studies were included which encompassed eight instruments (see Figure 1).

Inclusion criteria

The inclusion criteria included published material with one of the search terms as the subject heading, and published in English. Literature relevant to instruments for measuring perceived social isolation or social support or loneliness was extracted from peer-reviewed journals. The initial search included the broader terms in order to assess for items within scales that might be similar to one another. Following this electronic search for articles, a hand-search of the references of the selected articles was conducted.

Exclusion criteria

Literature focusing on animal studies was excluded. Studies were excluded if they evaluated populations other than adults. Dissertation, theses, or websites were excluded.

Summary of the literature

As shown in Table 1, a total of 8 scales were reviewed from 11 studies. The theoretical frameworks ranged from Weiss' theory of social support used in the development of the Personal Resource Questionnaire-85 (PRQ85) (25) and Sarason's Social Support Questionnaire (26), the use of Kahn's social support theory in the development of the Norbeck Questionnaire (27) and various references to other social support theorists such as Cassel, Cobb and Bowlby in the Friendship Scale (28) and the Sarason Social Support Questionnaire.

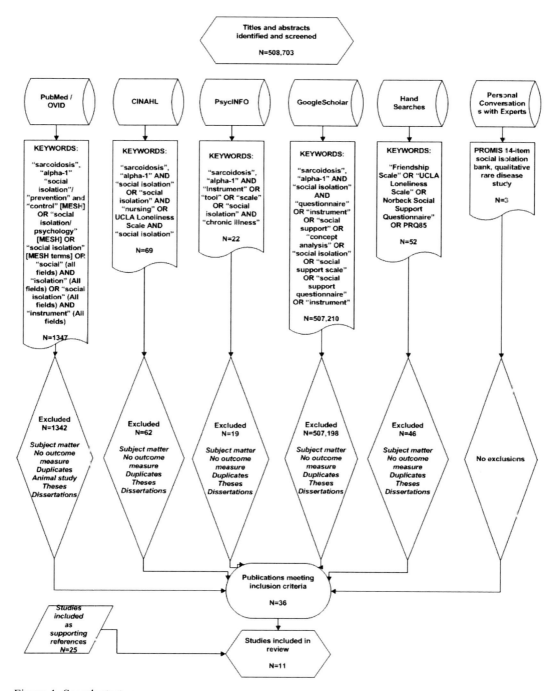

Figure 1. Search strategy.

Table 1.

Instrument/Reference	Theoretical Framework	Sample/Subjects/Disease/Condition	Instrument Description	Scoring	Method of Measurement	Reliability	Validity	Feasibility	Level of Evidence	Outcomes
Friendship Scale Hawthorne, G. (2006). Measuring Social Isolation in Older Adults: Development and Initial Validation of the Friendship Scale. *Social Indicators Research, 77,* 521-548.	Based upon three theories of social support (Cassel, Cobb, Bowlby)	(N=829). Four older adult cohorts, defined as those over 60 years, were recruited. Four cohorts were (1) older adults living in supported housing or nursing homes; (2) hospital outpatients with chronic disability; (3) older veterans; (4) healthy subjects from the community.	The six items measure six of the seven important dimensions that contribute to *social isolation* and its opposite, *social connection*.	Scoring involves reversal of items 1, 3 and 4 followed by summation across all items. The score range is 0–24. A high score represents social connectedness and a score of "0" complete social isolation.	Quantitative Questionnaire Self-administered	Cronbach α = 0.83	Correlates well with SF12 MCS, WHOQOL-Bref Psychological scale, AQoL Social relationships scale – Correlates *less well* with SF12 PCS, WHOQOL-Bref Physical scale, AQoL Physical senses scale	Short, 6 item questionnaire	1b	Initial paper outlining the development of the friendship scales. The psychometric properties suggest that it has excellent internal structures and that it possesses reliability and discrimination.
Functional Social Support Questionnaire	None specified	(N=401). Family medicine clinic patients selected from randomized time-frame sampling blocks during office hours.	8 item, 5 point Likert scale; contains questions in four content areas defined as *quantity of support, confidant support, affective support and instrumental support*	The item response options are on a 5-point scale ranging from 1 (much less than I would like) to 5 (as much as I would like). Higher scores reflect higher perceived social support.	Interviewer or self-administered	Test-retest reliability evaluated over a 2-week time period.	Construct validity demonstrated by significant correlations of individual items with measures of symptom status and emotional function.	Takes ~ 5 minutes to complete	1b	Reliability and validity for this scale was supported by the testing done as detailed in this study.

Instrument/ Reference	Theoretical Framework	Sample/Subjects/ Disease/Condition	Instrument Description	Scoring	Method of Measurement	Reliability	Validity	Feasibility	Level of Evidence	Outcomes
Broadhead, W. E., Gehlbach, S. H., de Gruy, F. V., & Kaplan, B. H. (1988). The Duke-UNC Functional Social Support Questionnaire: Measurement of social support in family medicine patients. *Med Care, 26*(7), 709-723.		No specific disease or conditions noted.				Correlation coefficient of .66. Item-remainder correlations were used to assess internal consistency and ranged from .50 for useful advice, to .85 for help around the house. To improve instrument reliability the original 14-item scale was reduced to eight items.	These measures have been shown to relate to social support. Concurrent validity was supported by significant correlations with 3 out of 4 activities measures.			The authors stated that the use of the scale in black, elderly, and male populations may be limited, and suggested further testing. They also suggested that the small number of items and the relative ease of completion should support its use as a cost-effective measurement tool.
Lubben Social Network Scale-6	None specified	(N=7,432). Take from three populations	6-item scale. It has been translated into many languages and applied to older adult populations of diverse ethnic backgrounds.	Score is an equally weighted sum of the 6 items.	Quantitative Questionnaire	Internal consistency for the LSNS-6 was consistent across sites (a=0.83).	The validity for LSNS-6 was established using EFA and criterion validity	6 item scale. Also available in 18 and 12-item versions. Available for free via the developer's website.	1b	Across all samples, the LSNS-6 showed high internal consistency and a consistent factor structure,

Table 1. (Continued)

Instrument/ Reference	Theoretical Framework	Sample/Subjects/ Disease/Condition	Instrument Description	Scoring	Method of Measurement	Reliability	Validity	Feasibility	Level of Evidence	Outcomes
Lubben, J...Stuck, A. E. (2006). Performance of an Abbrev. Version of the Lubben Social Network Scale Among Three European Community-Dwelling Older Adult Populations. *The Gerontologist, 46*(4), 503-513.		Samples comprised of patients seen by family medicine clinic for a variety of conditions; no specific diseases or conditions noted.	Designed to gauge *social isolation* in older adults by measuring *perceived social support* received by family, friends and mutual supports (e.g., neighbors), including confidant relationships. It consists of 6 items which measure size, closeness and frequency of contacts of a respondent's social network.	Scores range from 0 to 30 with higher scores indicating a greater level of social support and low risk for isolation. Scores for each question range from zero to five, with 0 = minimal social integration and 5= substantial social integration. A score < 20 may indicate a person with an extremely limited social network and high risk for isolation.	Self-administered questionnaire with health professionals as informants					even though there were relevant differences among the three samples in terms of demographic and health characteristics

Instrument/Reference	Theoretical Framework	Sample/Subjects/Disease/Condition	Instrument Description	Scoring	Method of Measurement	Reliability	Validity	Feasibility	Level of Evidence	Outcomes
Norbeck Social Support Questionnaire

Norbeck, J. S., Lindsey, A. M., & Carrieri, V. L. (1981). The development of an instrument to measure social support. *Nurs Res*, 30(5), 264-269. | Kahn's Social Support | (N=135). This initial testing of the NSSQ was done with 75 master's students in nursing and 60 senior nursing students.

None of the subjects were presented as having a chronic disease or condition. | Total of 9 items. Participants list and rate the amount of Affect, Affirmation and Aid they perceive is available to them from up to 24 network members of their choosing. After completing the network list, they are instructed to successively turn the half pages and rate each listed network member (0-4) on six functional support questions measuring three types of support: affect, affirmation, and aid (see Table 1). Network members' support scores are then summed. | Because support ratings for each network member are summed, support scores (range = 0-576) vary greatly due to network size alone. Average scores have been suggested to eliminate the bias for subjects with multiple network members. | Quantitative Questionnaire

Self-administered

However, in part due to the 'free text' entry, Because of this self-report feature, the NSSQ requires a unique layout (available from Prof. Norbeck at no cost). | Pearson correlations among the items and subscales were calculated.
• Each of the two items for each subscale, were highly correlated: Affect, .97; Affirmation, .96; and Aid, .89.
• The correlations among the four items measuring Affect and Affirmation ranged from .95 to .98, suggesting that these two functions might not be distinct. | Affect, Affirmation, and Aid correlated with the C&L Emotional Support component at .51, .56, and .44, respectively. Affirmation correlated at .33 with the C&L Informational Support, but the correlation between Aid and the C&L Tangible | Free from author on UCSF College of Nursing Website

Takes' 10 minutes to complete | 1b | The Norbeck Social Support Questionnaire is a valid and reliable measure of total network support, as well as three functional types of social support. The three functional types of social support should be calculated |

Table 1. (Continued)

Instrument/ Reference	Theoretical Framework	Sample/Subjects/ Disease/Condition	Instrument Description	Scoring	Method of Measurement	Reliability	Validity	Feasibility	Level of Evidence	Outcomes
						The correlations between the Aid items and the Affect and Affirmation items ranged from .72 to .78. • The correlations among the three network properties (Number in Network, Duration of Relationships, and Frequency of Contact) ranged from .88 to .96; and these network properties correlated highly with Affect and Affirmation (.88 to .97) and moderately with Aid (.69 to .80).	Support was -.03; however, the C&L Tangible Support scale was a weak construct with a Coefficient Alpha of .31.			

Instrument/ Reference	Theoretical Framework	Sample/Subjects/ Disease/Condition	Instrument Description	Scoring	Method of Measurement	Reliability	Validity	Feasibility	Level of Evidence	Outcomes
						Test-Retest Reliability. The test-retest correlations were Affect, .89; Affirmation, .88; and Aid, .86. Similar high correlations were found for the three network properties, which were each .92				
Norbeck SSQ Gigliotti, E., & Samuels, W. E. (2011). Use of averaged Norbeck social support questionnaire scores. *ISRN Nurs*, 2011	Kahn's definition of social support	(N=609). A secondary analysis was conducted on data from three different samples of women who were mothers attending college for their first postsecondary school degree (n = 157, n = 263, n = 189).	Using a unique layout, participants are first asked to list from 1 to 24 network members "who provide personal support for you or who are important to you.	Because support ratings for each network member are summed, support scores (range = 0–576) vary greatly due to network size alone.	Quantitative questionnaire Subject completed	Not purpose of this paper	Not purpose of this paper	Not purpose of this paper	2a	In all three samples, there are no statistically significant decreases in averaged total functional support scores, affect or affirmation as network size increases.

Table 1. (Continued)

Instrument/ Reference	Theoretical Framework	Sample/Subjects/ Disease/Condition	Instrument Description	Scoring	Method of Measurement	Reliability	Validity	Feasibility	Level of Evidence	Outcomes
		None of the subjects were presented as having a chronic disease or condition	After completing the network list, they are instructed to successively turn the half pages and rate each listed network member (0–4) on six functional support questions measuring three types of support: affect, affirmation, and aid. Network members' support scores are then summed.							
				In fact, in the three samples [9–11] used in the present study, network size was very highly correlated with affect scores (.95, .94, and .95, resp.) and affirmation scores (.92, .90, and .92, resp.)						Thus, averaged total functional support scores and averaged affect and affirmation scores do not lower scores as one's network size increases.

Instrument/ Reference	Theoretical Framework	Sample/Subjects/ Disease/Condition	Instrument Description	Scoring	Method of Measurement	Reliability	Validity	Feasibility	Level of Evidence	Outcomes
				and a bit less with aid scores (.81, .82, and .82, resp.). As network size increased, support scores increased.						This is not true for averaged aid scores. In all three samples, there are stat. sig. decreases in averaged aid support scores as network size increases. Averaged Norbeck Social Support Questionnaire (NSSQ) support scores remove the influence of network size variability but may unduly lower scores for participants with large networks.

Table 1. (Continued)

Instrument/Reference	Theoretical Framework	Sample/Subjects/Disease/Condition	Instrument Description	Scoring	Method of Measurement	Reliability	Validity	Feasibility	Level of Evidence	Outcomes
Norbeck SSQ Norbeck, J. S., Lindsey, A. M., & Carrieri, V. L. (1983). Further development of the Norbeck Social Support Questionnaire: normative data and validity testing. *Nurs Res, 32*(1), 4-9.	Kahn's social support	This was considered the second phase of testing the NSSQ. Involved three studies with sample sizes of 136, 75 and 55.	Participants are first asked to list from 1 to 24 network members "who provide personal support for you or who are important to you. After completing the network list, they are instructed to turn the half pages and rate each listed network member (0–4) on six functional support questions measuring three types of support: affect, affirmation, and aid. Network members' support scores are then summed.	Because support ratings for each network member are summed, support scores (range = 0–576) vary greatly due to network size alone.	Quantitative questionnaire Subject self-report		Construct validity of the instrument was established by comparing convergent and discriminant constructs to the NSSQ. Concurrent validity with another social support questionnaire was demonstrated. Predictive validity was tested in a sample of 53 graduate students through assessing the buffering effect of social support on measures of negative mood following life stress.		1b	In the second and third studies, the instrument was found to be very stable over a seven-month interval and sensitive to changes within the social support networks of a group of graduate students during their first year of study.

Instrument/ Reference	Theoretical Framework	Sample/Subjects/ Disease/Condition	Instrument Description	Scoring	Method of Measurement	Reliability	Validity	Feasibility	Level of Evidence	Outcomes
PROMIS Item Bank Hahn, E. A., Devellis, R. F., Bode, R. K., Garcia, S. F., Castel, L. D., Eisen, S. V., ... Group, P. C. (2010). Measuring social health in the patient-reported outcomes measurement information system (PROMIS): item bank development and testing. *Qual Life Res*, 19(7), 1035-1044.	None specified	(N=956) general population respondents who answered Ability to Participate and Satisfaction with Participation items.	These were items that were evaluated, and not a defined scale. The authors identified and reviewed 1,781 Social Function items; 112 items were retained and edited. New items were written to fill content gaps. This process produced 56 items for Ability to Participate and 56 for Satisfaction with Participation within four contexts (family, friends, work and leisure). All items were written as statements, using a 7-day reporting period.	The Ability items used a 5-point frequency rating scale (Never, Rarely, Sometimes, Often and Always) and the Satisfaction items used a 5-point intensity rating scale (Not at all, A little bit, Somewhat, Quite a bit and Very much).	Quantitative items	N/A	Content validity was sought by examining previous models and by collecting patient experiences about their social well-being and limitations [20, 21]. Sub-domain structures emerged from qualitative data, expert consensus and quantitative results of extensive field tests. Although Ability to Participate and its three subdomains were essentially unidimensional (based on EFA and CFA),	N/A	1b	After extensive item preparation and review, EFA, CFA and IRT-guided item banks help provide increased measurement precision and flexibility. Two Satisfaction short forms are available for use in research and clinical practice.

Table 1. (Continued)

Instrument/ Reference	Theoretical Framework	Sample/Subjects/ Disease/Condition	Instrument Description	Scoring	Method of Measurement	Reliability	Validity	Feasibility	Level of Evidence	Outcomes
							they did not fit the item response theory model, when examined either separately or together			This initial validation study resulted in revised item pools that are currently undergoing testing in new clinical samples and populations.
PRQ-85 Weinert, C. (1987). A social support measure: PRQ85. *Nurs Res, 36*(5), 273-277.	Weiss' model of relational functions	Three studies: sample of 132 older adults, 100 and 132 middle-aged adults. None of the samples were presented as having a chronic disease or condition.	Measures *situational and perceived social support*. Two part questionnaire: Part 1: 10 life situations where an individual might be expected to need assistance- provides information concerning the person's resources and satisfaction with the help received from those resources. Part 2: 25 item, 7-point Likert scale that measures the person's perceived level of social support	Scale scores range from 25-175; higher scores indicate higher levels of social support	Quantitative questionnaire Self-administered	Established in 3 separate samples of 132 and 100 subjects. Cronbach's alpha ranged from .87 (132 subjects) to .90 (100 subjects). Third sample (132 subjects) demonstrated alpha of .90.	Content validity was established by 2 nurse researchers not familiar with the instrument. Construct discriminate validity established using the BDI and Trait Anxiety Scale. Moderate correlations were obtained between Part 2 of the tool and the BDI (r=.33) and the Trait Anxiety Scale (r=-.39).	Takes ~15 minutes to complete	1b	The findings from this initial use of the PRQ-85, combined with ~5 years of psychometrics on previous version of the tool (PRQ82) support validity and reliability of the instrument.

Instrument/ Reference	Theoretical Framework	Sample/Subjects/ Disease/Condition	Instrument Description	Scoring	Method of Measurement	Reliability	Validity	Feasibility	Level of Evidence	Outcomes
PRQ-85 Weinert, C., & Tilden, V. P. (1990). Measures of social support: assessment of validity. *Nurs Res, 39*(4), 212-216.	Weiss' model of relational functions	Two samples of adults N=333 who were part of a large health project and N=99 who participated in a methodological study.	The PRQ-85 Measures situational and perceived social support. Two part questionnaire: Part 1: 10 life situations where an individual might be expected to need assistance provides information concerning the person's resources and satisfaction with the help received from those resources. Part 2: 25 item, 7-point Likert scale that measures the person's perceived level of social support. The CRI is a self-report questionnaire which consists of 38 Likert type items purported to measure four subscales of social support: social support, reciprocity, cost and conflict	The PRQ-85 Scale scores range from 25-175; higher scores indicate higher levels of social support.	Quantitative questionnaire Self-administered	Internal consistency reliability was found to be .90 for the ORQ85 and for the CRI subscales: .93 for support, .95 for conflict, .81 for reciprocity and .92 for cost.	Convergence was evaluated and confirmed. Construct validity of the PRQ85 and CRI behave similarly. Discriminant validity was also assessed and found to be lacking across some of the subscales.	Both questionnaire are self-administered and take ~15 minutes to complete.	1b	Both of the instruments each measure social support. Each of the measures taps somewhat different aspects of social support and CRI scores may be more global and measure a larger and more tightly focused aspect of social networks.

Table 1. (Continued)

Instrument/ Reference	Theoretical Framework	Sample/Subjects/ Disease/Condition	Instrument Description	Scoring	Method of Measurement	Reliability	Validity	Feasibility	Level of Evidence	Outcomes
Social Support Questionnaire (Sarason) Sarason, I. G., Levine, H. M., Basham, R. B., & Sarason, B. R. (1983). Assessing social support: The Social Support Questionnaire	Not based on one specific framework, although Weiss' theory of social support was cited, as well as Kelly and Caplan	Four studies included. Samples of college students: N=602, N=227, N=295 and N=40 in each study, respectively.	The SSQ is a 27-item scale which investigates (1) the *number of perceived social support events* in a person's life and (2) the degree to which they are personally satisfying.	Satisfaction rating for each situational circumstance is the same regardless of the situation given. A six point rating scale (from "very satisfied" to "very dissatisfied") is used to rate the individual's satisfaction with his or her support available. A support score for each item is calculated by the number of individuals the participant listed (number score)..	Quantitative Questionnaire Self-administered questionnaire	The number scores yielded an inter-item correlation ranging from 0.35 to 0.71 (m=0.54). The Cronbach's alpha for internal reliability was 0.97.	Criterion validity tests show a significant negative correlation between the SSQ and a depression scale (ranging from -0.22 to -0.43), and correlations of 0.57 and 0.34 were obtained between an optimism scale and the satisfaction score and the number score, respectively (Sarason et al., 1983).	5 minutes to administer	1b	The paper describes the development of the SSQ to measure social support. The reliability of the tool is quite high and correlates with other measures

Instrument/ Reference	Theoretical Framework	Sample/Subjects/ Disease/Condition	Instrument Description	Scoring	Method of Measurement	Reliability	Validity	Feasibility	Level of Evidence	Outcomes
Journal of *Personality and Social Psychology*, 44(1), 127-139.				The overall support score (SSQN) is calculated by the mean of this scores across the items. The overall satisfaction score is calculated by the means of the 27 satisfaction scores (McDowell & Newell, 1996		The inter-item correlations for the satisfaction scores ranged from 0.21 to 0.74, and the coefficient alpha was 0.94. Test-retest correlations of 0.90 for overall number scores and satisfaction scores of 0.83 were obtained (Sarason et al., 1983).				The SSQ does not seem to be highly biased by the social desirability response set. The SSQ investigates two aspects of social support: (a) the number of perceived social supports in a person's life and (b) the degree to which they are personally satisfying.
UCLA Loneliness Scale (v3)	Not stated	Data from four previous studies using the scale was used to assess the psychometrics of version three of the scale. Study 1 consisted of 489 college students;	Developed to assess subjective feelings of loneliness or social isolation. It is a 20 item scale; 10 positively worded and 10 negatively worded items.	Choices range from 1 ("never") to 4 ("often"). Each person's responses to the questions are summed, with higher scores indicating greater loneliness.	Quantitative self-administered	Coefficient alpha ranges from .89-.94; test-test reliability over 1 year (r=0.73)	Convergent and construct validity supported by analyses of previous studies.	Takes about 5 minutes to complete	1b	The data support the reliability and validity of the version 3 of the UCLA

Table 1. (Continued)

Instrument/Reference	Theoretical Framework	Sample/Subjects/Disease/Condition	Instrument Description	Scoring	Method of Measurement	Reliability	Validity	Feasibility	Level of Evidence	Outcomes
Russell, D. W. (1996). UCLA Loneliness Scale (Version 3): Reliability, Validity, and Factor Structure. Journal of Personality Assessment, 66(1), 20.		Study 2 consisted of 310 nurses; study 3 consisted of 316 teachers; 301 elderly comprised study 4	The Scale has become the most widely used measure of loneliness, with over 500 citations in the Social Science Citation Index of the 1980 publication on the measure. Scores on the loneliness scale have been found to predict a wide variety of mental (i.e., depression) and physical (i.e., immunocompetence, nursing home admission, mortality) health outcomes in our research and the research of others				CFA of multiple studies provided support for viewing the scale as a unidimensional measure.			Loneliness Scale in a variety of populations, ranging from college students to the elderly. Psychometric data from version 3 are comparable to values reported for the first two versions.

Three of the instruments (the Functional Social Support Questionnaire, the Lubben Social Network Scale, the UCLA Loneliness Scale) as well as the PROMIS Social Isolation Item bank have unspecified theoretical foundations (29-31). The sample sizes for psychometric testing scores ranged from 55 subjects in the second phase of testing of the Norbeck Social Support Questionnaire (32) to 7,432 subjects for the Lubben Social Network Scale, distributed across three sites in Europe, with each site having greater than 1,900 participants at each (33).

None of the instruments reviewed were tested in rare disease populations. The Lubben Social Network Scale has been utilized in studies of patients with chronic obstructive pulmonary disease (34), a lung disease which can be caused, in rare instances, by alpha-1 antitrypsin deficiency. COPD and these rare lung diseases share symptoms of breathing and mobility challenges, so that prior testing in those populations with strong psychometric performance helps support content validity in choosing to adapt them to study social isolation in sarcoidosis or alpha-1 antitrypsin deficiency patients.

RESULTS

The search criteria included only studies of adults. In addition, the search was broadened to include studies of all disease populations, as no studies were identified that specifically explore social phenomena in sarcoidosis or alpha-1.

Evaluation of instruments

Seven instruments that assess adult perceptions of social support, measure social isolation or loneliness were identified: 1) the Friendship Scale, 2) the Lubben Social Network Scale, 3) the Norbeck Social Support Questionnaire, 4) the Personal Resource Questionnaire-85 [PRQ85], 5), the Social Support Questionnaire, 6) the UCLA Loneliness Scale – Revised and 7) the Functional Social Support Questionnaire, In addition, an eighth tool, an item bank derived from PROMIS [Patient-Reported Outcomes Measurement Information System] was included in this review. This 14 item bank of questions is referred to as the "Social Isolation Item Bank," and contains items purported to measure various facets of social isolation.

Instrument description

Instruments ranged from 6 items to 27 items comprising a scale. All instruments had the ability to be self-administered and all utilized at minimum, a Likert scale. The Friendship Scale, the PROMIS Social Isolation Item Bank, the UCLA Loneliness Scale and the Duke-UNC Functional Social Support Questionnaire gathered responses via only a Likert scale. The Lubben Social Network Scale is a composite instrument which utilizes a Likert scale as well as an ordinal ranking scale to confirm number of support persons available.

Two of the questionnaires required free text entry. Both the Sarason Social Support Questionnaire and the Norbeck Social Support Questionnaire asked the patient to list individual persons that they can count on for support. The Personal Resource Questionnaire-85 (PRQ-85) presented a listing of individuals (parent, spouse, friend, neighbor, etc) that the individual was asked to confirm as being available in times of help. The Duke-UNC Functional Social Support Questionnaire was reputed to be either self- or interviewer-administered. However, the instrument is presented to the patient as a Likert-scale, so it could easily be completed via patient self-administration.

Consistent with the lack of consensus definition of what constitutes social isolation is the variety of different constructs that the instruments measure. Although all of the constructs measured are linked to social isolation, the most common construct found in the review of instruments is perceived social support. The Personal Resource Questionnaire-85 (PRQ85), the Social Support Questionnaire and the Lubben Social Network Scale have all been found to measure this construct (25, 26, 33).

Method of perceptions and scoring

Four to 6 point Likert scales were most commonly used, with a summed lower Likert number generally indicating less social support (25, 29, 33, 35, 36) or greater social isolation (31, 33, 37, 38). The (Sarason) Social Support Questionnaire provides two scores: an overall support score (SSQN) is calculated by the mean of scores across various situational circumstances. The overall satisfaction score is calculated by the means of the 27 satisfaction scores (26).

Method of administration

All instruments are completed via pencil and paper.

Reliability

In general, all of the studies spoke to reliability of the instrument on various levels. Of the eight instruments that were evaluated, all instruments with the exception of the Norbeck Social Support Questionnaire demonstrated acceptable internal consistency as supported by Cronbach's alpha scores >.70 (25, 26, 28, 29, 31, 33, 39). Since the Norbeck SSQ is not a summative scale, the reliability of this instrument was demonstrated using Pearson product-moment correlation calculations (27). Each of the two items for each subscale, were highly correlated: Affect, .97; Affirmation, 96; and Aid, .89. The correlations among the four items measuring Affect and Affirmation ranged from .95 to .98, suggesting that these two functions might not be distinct. The correlations between the Aid items and the Affect and Affirmation items ranged from .72 to .78. The correlations among the three network properties (Number in Network, Duration of Relationships, and Frequency of Contact) ranged from .88 to .96; and these network properties correlated highly with Affect and Affirmation (.88 to .97) and moderately with Aid (.69 to .80) (27).

Of the eight instruments evaluated, test-test reliability was reported for four of the instruments - the Duke UNC Functional Social Support Questionnaire, the Norbeck Social Support Questionnaire, the UCLA Loneliness Questionnaire, and the Sarason Social Support

Questionnaire (26, 29, 31, 32) - and found to be acceptable (greater than .7). Four of the instruments - the PRQ85, the Friendship Scale, the Lubben Social Network Scale, and the PROMIS item bank - did not report this statistic (28, 33, 37, 39). The PROMIS item bank for social isolation is not a validated scale in and of itself. As such, reliability and validity estimates are not reported for this bank. Rather, researchers are free to access the various item banks from the PROMIS repository for use in testing.

Validity

Presentation of validity findings was inconsistent across the various studies. Concurrent validity was reported for three of the instruments, the Norbeck SSQ, the Friendship Scale and the Duke UNC Functional Social Support Questionnaire (27-29, 32). Convergent validity was noted for two of the eight tools, the UCLA Loneliness Scale and the Lubben Social Network Scale (31, 33), and criterion validity was reported only for the Sarason SSQ (26).

Construct validity was noted for five of eight instruments, the Friendship Scale, the Lubben Social Network Scale, the UCLA Loneliness Scale, the Norbeck SSQ and and the Duke UNC Functional Social Support Questionnaire (28, 29, 31, 33, 35). These five instruments presented findings on factor analyses, demonstrating additional scientific rigor in validity testing. Factor analyses are used as an additional technique to assess the construct validity of an instrument, by statistically evaluating the internal structure of a scale and the various dimension(s) within that scale (40). Hawthorne performed a principal component analysis to evaluate construct validity for the Friendship Scale, and found that for six of the seven intended items, PCA results showed formed a unidimensional scale with mean loadings between 0.63 and 0.84 (28), and which is considered acceptable, since in general, a cut-off of .40 would be considered reasonable to retain the item (40). Lubben also reported on the factor analysis for the Social Network Scale, which incorporated an arbitrary cut-off of 0.5 (33). They found that the factor structure for the LSNS-6 was acceptable among the six items, and also reported eigenvalues of >1, suggesting a strong principle component. Broadhead performed factor analyses for the Duke UNC Functional Social Support Questionnaire which resulted in all of the items being retained, with r-values between .52 and .72 (29).

The validity of the PROMIS social isolation item bank was not reported.

Feasibility of instrument use

Feasibility is the ease and cost of instrument use, as well as time necessary for completion. Some questionnaires specifically requested that the user report back the results of any studies done using the instrument to the developer as per the developers' websites. The majority of the instruments require between 5 and 15 minutes to complete. It is not clear if all of the instruments are available in multiple languages, which is a desirable option.

RESULTS

There are no validated instruments that measure social isolation (or social support, loneliness, or social networking) in these suffering from sarcoidosis or alpha-1 antitrypsin deficiency. No instruments were identified that measure any of these constructs in chronic interstitial lung disease.

In this particular review (as illustrated in Table 1) a number of the studies reviewed did specify a theoretical framework that either guided the development of the instrument or the study overall. The findings of this review suggest that instruments proven to be valid and reliable in measuring social isolation do exist, albeit tested in other populations. The instruments reviewed have been tested in adult populations, in ages ranging from college-aged to older adults, and included a variety of races and ethnicities. This is encouraging when considering the instruments for use in the sarcoidosis or alpha-1 population and the fact that these patients are generally middle-aged to older adults. Somewhat discouraging is the fact that when demographics of the instruments were presented, the majority of the sample subjects were Caucasian. Of the eight instruments reviewed, five - the PRQ85, the Sarason Social Support Questionnaire, the Friendship Scale, the Lubben Social Network Scale and the UCLA Loneliness Scale- were lacking any information regarding race in the original psychometrics (23, 25, 26, 28, 33) and three - the Norbeck Social Support Questionnaire, the Duke-UNC Functional Social Support Questionnaire, and the PROMIS item bank - were evaluated in largely Caucasian populations (27, 29, 37). Thus, the utility of these instruments in culturally diverse and in rare disease populations warrants further exploration.

As shown in Table 1, eight instruments were reviewed that measured social isolation, loneliness, social networking, social support or a combination thereof. It is important to note that some of the items overlapped between questionnaires. Of the eight instruments surveyed, two have published psychometric results that suggest potential generalizability in content validity, construct validity and cultural sensitivity: The Friendship Scale (28) and the UCLA Loneliness Scale (31). These two instruments contain items which closely link to the characteristics of social isolation as described by Nicholson (21) and Warren (8). The PROMIS Social Isolation item bank also could be considered for pretesting psychometric performance as a tool to assess social isolation. The tool has no psychometric testing results in any population to date but are available for consideration at: http://www.nihpromis.org. Pilot testing of the bank as a secondary measure would be appropriate in a one of these populations using another instrument as a primary assessment tool.

One of the major limitations of this review was the ability to conduct an equivalent comparison of the various tools. This was due in part to the inconsistency in the reporting of the psychometric properties of the tools, as well as the variety of different populations tested. As illustrated in the descriptions of the psychometrics of the instruments, in general, reliability and validity of these tools was acceptable in the populations studied.

DISCUSSION

The experience of sarcoidosis or alpha-1 antitrypsin deficiency, as with other rare diseases, can be physically as well as emotionally devastating. In addition to the medical management of symptoms, there are numerous potential social consequences of living with a rare disease, including goal setting and life objectives. Equally as important, it may lead to stigmatization, isolation and exclusion from one's social community. Sarcoidosis and/or alpha-1 may currently be considered "orphan" or rare diseases at the moment, but better, more refined medical diagnostics combined with tools to assist the clinician in screening for and managing psychosocial issues could provide for a more holistic overall approach to patient care.

The lack of a consensus definition of what constitutes social isolation, and how to measure it remains one of the main challenges for researchers interested in this phenomenon. Throughout the literature, the idea of perceived social support being an important component of the subjective perception of social isolation appeared frequently, and was in fact, the most common construct found in the review of instruments.

Conclusion

The experience of living with sarcoidosis or alpha-1 antitrypsin deficiency as with other rare diseases, has largely been understudied and poorly documented. Although the psychosocial issues associated with rare disease sufferers are many and varied, one common characteristic that many of these individuals share is the feeling of isolation. As a first step in exploring this phenomenon, the use of existing instruments would be of use in measuring the magnitude of social isolation in this population. The relatively small number of items on these questionnaires might lend themselves to web-based distribution (after consultation with the developers) for interested and consenting participants from a broad demographic area. Since populations in rare diseases are small and geographically dispersed, creative recruitment strategies would be beneficial, and consideration of web-based recruitment and/or test administration is warranted.

One construct not captured by any of the instruments identified in this search, or which was discovered in any literature search, is perceptions of public support for the care or cure of the disease. Public empathy for rare disease support is an important component of the reported experience of many rare diseases. Exploration among rare disease populations, by qualitative methods such as cognitive interviewing and focus groups, to learn whether these perceptions are a quantifiable construct in social isolation will inform content and construct validation of social isolation instrumentation in the study of persons with rare diseases.

Relevance to clinical practice

As the era of genomics and genetics continues to evolve and expand, it is likely that conditions that were unrecognized previously may be identified as disease conditions. Moreover, simplification and enhancement of testing for rare and/or genetic conditions is becoming more commonplace, and more clinicians may be faced with managing such patients. Knowledge of the potential or actual social impact of such conditions is necessary in order to provide for holistic management of such patients, and simple, existing tools can be useful. This review provides for a summary review of tools available to clinicians to screen for perceived social isolation in rare lung disease patients, a valuable asset to any clinician.

REFERENCES

[1] Griggs RC, Batshaw M, Dunkle M, Gopal-Srivastava R, Kaye E, Krischer J, et al. Clinical research for rare disease: opportunities, challenges, and solutions. Mol Genet Metab 2009;96(1):20-6.
[2] Joppi R, Bertele' V, Garattini S. Orphan drugs, orphan diseases. The first decade of orphan drug legislation in the EU. Eur J Clin Pharmacol 2013;69(4):1009-24.
[3] EURORDIS. Position paper on rare disease research EURORDIS: The voice of rare disease patients in Europe, 2012. URL: http://www.eurordis.org/sites/default/files/EURORDIS_Rapport_Research_2012.pdf2012.
[4] Esmann S, Jemec GB. Psychosocial impact of hidradenitis suppurativa: a qualitative study. Acta Derm Venereol 2011;91(3):328-32.
[5] Henderson SL, Packman W, Packman S. Psychosocial aspects of patients with Niemann-Pick disease, type B. Am J Med Genet A 2009;149a(11):2430-6.
[6] National Research Council. New horizons in health: An integrative approach. Washington, DC: National Academy Press, 2001.
[7] House JS, Landis KR, Umberson D. Social relationships and health. Science 1988;241(4865):540-5.
[8] Warren BJ. Explaining social isolation through concept analysis. Arch Psychiatr Nurs 1993;7(5):270-6.
[9] Chen ES, Moller DR. Sarcoidosis: scientific progress and clinical challenges. Nat Rev Rheumatol 2011;7(8):457-67.
[10] Patterson KC, Hogarth K, Husain AN, Sperling AI, Niewold TB. The clinical and immunologic features of pulmonary fibrosis in sarcoidosis. Transl Res 2012;160 (5): 321–31.
[11] Chang B, Steimel J, Moller DR, Baughman RP, Judson MA, Yeager H, Jr, et al. Depression in sarcoidosis. Am J Respir Crit Care Med 2001;163(2):329-34.
[12] Victorson DE, Cella D, Grund H, Judson MA. A conceptual model of health-related quality of life in sarcoidosis. Qual Life Res 2014;23(1):89-101.
[13] Stoller JK, Aboussouan LS. A review of α1-antitrypsin deficiency. Am J Respir Crit Care Med 2012;185(3):246-59.
[14] Stoller JK, Smith P, Yang P, Spray J. Physical and social impact of alpha 1-antitrypsin deficiency: results of a survey. Cleveland Clin J Med 1994;61(6):461-37.
[15] Ellison L, Gask L, Bakerly ND, Roberts J. Meeting the mental health needs of people with chronic obstructive pulmonary disease: a qualitative study. Chronic Illn 2012;8(4):308-20.
[16] Seamark DA, Blake SD, Seamark CJ, Halpin DM. Living with severe chronic obstructive pulmonary disease (COPD): perceptions of patients and their carers: An interpretative phenomenological analysis. Palliat Med 2004;18(7):619-25.
[17] Gupta S, Bayoumi AM, Faughnan ME. Rare lung disease research: strategies for improving identification and recruitment of research participants. Chest 2011;140(5): 1123-9.
[18] Huyard C. What, if anything, is specific about having a rare disorder? Patients' judgements on being ill and being rare. Health Expect 2009;12(4):361-70.
[19] Colledge V, Solly J. The rare disease challenge and how to promote a productive rare disease community: Case study of Birt-Hogg-Dube Symposia. Orphanet J Rare Dis 2012;7(1):63.
[20] Carpenito-Moyet JL. Handbook of nursing diagnosis, 11 ed. Philadelphia, PA: Lippincott Williams Wilkins, 2006.
[21] Nicholson NR, Jr. Social isolation in older adults: an evolutionary concept analysis. J Adv Nurs 2009;65 (6): 342-52.
[22] Killeen C. Loneliness: an epidemic in modern society. J Adv Nurs 1998; 28(4):762-70.
[23] Russell D, Peplau LA, Cutrona CE. The revised UCLA Loneliness Scale: concurrent and discriminant validity evidence. J Pers Soc Psychol 1980;39(3):472-80.
[24] Whittemore R, Knafl K. The integrative review: updated methodology. J Adv Nurs 2005;52(5):546-53.
[25] Weinert C. A social support measure: PRQ85. Nurs Res 1987;36(5):273-7.
[26] Sarason IG, Levine HM, Basham RB, Sarason BR. Assessing social support: The Social Support Questionnaire. J Pers Soc Psychol 1983;44(1):127-39.

[27] Norbeck JS, Lindsey AM, Carrieri VL. The development of an instrument to measure social support. Nurs Res 1981;30(5):264-9.
[28] Hawthorne G. Measuring Social Isolation in Older Adults: Development and Initial Validation of the Friendship Scale. Soc Indicat Res 2006;77:521-48.
[29] Broadhead WE, Gehlbach SH, de Gruy FV, Kaplan BH. The Duke-UNC Functional Social Support Questionnaire. Measurement of social support in family medicine patients. Med Care 1988;26(7):709-23.
[30] Lubben J, Blozik E, Gillmann G, Iliffe S, von Renteln Kruse W, Beck JC, et al. Performance of an abbreviated version of the Lubben Social Network Scale among three European community-dwelling older adult populations. Gerontologist 2006;46(4):503-13.
[31] Russell DW. UCLA Loneliness Scale (Version 3): Reliability, Validity, and Factor Structure J Pers Assess 1996;66(1):20-40.
[32] Norbeck JS, Lindsey AM, Carrieri VL. Further development of the Norbeck Social Support Questionnaire: normative data and validity testing. Nurs Res 1983;32(1):4-9.
[33] Lubben J, Blozik E, Gillmann G, Iliffe S, von Renteln Kruse W, Beck JC, et al. Performance of an Abbreviated Version of the Lubben Social Network Scale Among Three European Community-Dwelling Older Adult Populations. Gerontologist 2006;46(4):503-13.
[34] Keele-Card G, Foxall MJ, Barron CR. Loneliness, depression, and social support of patients with COPD and their spouses. Public Health Nurs 1993;10(4):245-51.
[35] Gigliotti E, Samuels WE. Use of averaged norbeck social support questionnaire scores. ISRN Nurs 2011;2011:567280.
[36] Tilden VP, Weinert C. Social support and the chronically ill individual. Nurs Clin North Am 1987;22(3):613-20.
[37] Hahn EA, Devellis RF, Bode RK, Garcia SF, Castel LD, Eisen SV, et al. Measuring social health in the patient-reported outcomes measurement information system (PROMIS): item bank development and testing. Qual Life Res 2010;19(7):1035-44.
[38] Hawthorne G. Perceived social isolation in a community sample: Its prevalence and correlates with aspects of peoples' lives. Soc Psychiatry Psychiatr Epidemiol 2008;43(2):140-50.
[39] Weinert C, Tilden VP. Measures of social support: assessment of validity. Nurs Res 1990;39(4):212-6.
[40] Di Lorio CK. Measurement in Health Behavior. San Francisco, CA: Jossey-Bass, 2005.

Submitted: April 14, 2014. *Revised:* June 01, 2014. *Accepted:* June 17, 2014.

In: Public Health Yearbook 2015
Editor: Joav Merrick

ISBN: 978-1-63484-514-4
© 2016 Nova Science Publishers, Inc.

Chapter 22

ALCOHOL CONSUMPTION IN RUSSIA DURING THE PAST 50 YEARS

Sergei V Jargin[*]

People's Friendship University of Russia, Moscow, Russia

ABSTRACT

There is abundant literature about alcohol consumption and alcoholism in Russia. The problem is immense; but nonetheless there is a tendency to exaggerate it, which is visible for inside observers. Such exaggeration tends to veil shortcomings of the health care system, with responsibility for the low life expectancy especially among men shifted onto the patients, that is, self-inflicted diseases caused by excessive alcohol consumption. The purpose of this review is to draw attention to this and other problems related to the alcohol consumption, such as the instable quality of alcoholic beverages, which have sometimes caused poisonings even after consumption in moderate doses, and offences against alcoholics and people with alcohol-related dementia aimed at appropriation of their immobile or other properly.

Keywords: alcohol, alcoholism, public health, Russia

INTRODUCTION

Alcohol consumption in the former Soviet Union (SU) has been a theme of extensive research despite the difficulties of obtaining valid statistics. The fact that the state, at various times, encouraged alcohol sales is known to the international community (1). Veiled propaganda of alcohol consumption was recognizable during the 1960-1980s (before the start of the anti-alcohol campaign in 1985) and took place also earlier (2, 3). Some editions such as the extremely popular "Book about delicious and healthy food" re-edited several times during the period 1939-64 (4), praised gustatory and medicinal properties of some alcoholic beverages,

---

[*] Correspondence: Sergei V Jargin, People's Friendship University of Russia, Clementovski per 6-82, 115184 Moscow, Russia. E-mail: sjargin@mail.ru.

which was accompanied by appetizing illustrations with bottles standing on a richly covered table, admired by many children.

The most efficient tool of the alcohol propaganda was creation by certain mass media and films of an attractive image of a drunkard, suitable for self-identification: carefree, cheerful and manly. The carrier of this notion was, for example, the popular magazine 'Crocodile,' whose feuilletons and caricatures were formally directed against alcohol but, in fact, romanticized alcohol consumption and the reckless drunken atmosphere. The 'Crocodile' and other mass media created and poetized alcoholic stereotypes: vodka-i-seliodka (consumption of vodka with salty herring), butylka-na-troikh (a bottle for three) etc. Association of harmless pastimes such as fishing trips or domino play with alcohol consumption was maintained by numerous pictures and cartoons. In the same way acted the most popular Soviet-time films with participation of the famous actor Yuri Nikulin, who personified the image of a charismatic drunkard; more details are in (2). Alcohol consumption at workplaces was not only tolerated but also visibly encouraged among workers, students and intelligentsia. Some Soviet festivals were associated with drinking, the best example being the New Year: eating and drinking started well before midnight; then, at midnight, sparkling wine was consumed, and then followed a continuation, until the daybreak in many cases. Other festivals associated with alcohol consumption were the Women's Day on March 8 and professional holidays such as the Builder's Day on the second Sunday of August, when many people related to a corresponding profession became inebriated. Birthdays and other personal events were regularly celebrated in many working teams. Parties at workplaces were often initiated or indirectly inspired by the management, which was common also in medical, educational and scientific institutions. In such institutions, technical or medicinal alcohol was consumed, which was knowingly tolerated by the management. It was known and seen that the management purloined alcohol themselves. Moreover, in workers,' students' and other companies, the ringleaders could be observed, who manipulated others towards drinking in excess. Non-drinkers were sometimes stigmatized.

Treatment and prevention of alcoholism was inefficient, while placebos and persuasion were the usual methods (5). Aversion (emetic) therapy and repeatedly induced teturam-alcohol reactions were applied (6). Correctional centers, the so-called work-and-treatment prophylactoriums, were in fact a form of detainment for 1-2 years (http://ru.wikipedia.org/wiki/Лечебно-трудовой_профилакторий) for chronic alcoholics evading treatment, violating community order or working discipline (according to an official definition); while loopholes were left for the inhabitants to obtain alcohol. The prophylactoriums were criticized as contradictory to human rights (6). There was business with teturam preparations for the implantation, having a placebo effect at best (7, 8): patients or their relatives were persuaded about efficiency and paid considerable amounts of money for the implantation. Finally, the so-called ultra-rapid psychotherapy or stress-therapy of alcoholism, known in the former SU as the 'coding,' should be mentioned. The method was started during the anti-alcohol campaign; it was criticized as unethical (9) because of intimidating verbal suggestion and unpleasant manipulations: spraying the throat with ethyl chloride, massage of the trigeminal nerve branches, backwards movements of the patient's head by the therapist's hands (9-11). Certain modifications of the method included general anesthesia (12). The method is used in the former SU for treatment of alcohol and drug addiction now as before (13).

ANTI-ALCOHOL MEASURES AND THEIR IMPACT

The anti-alcohol campaign (1985-88) was initially successful but ended with a failure. It was accompanied, along with a temporary decrease in the alcohol-related mortality (1), by numerous fatal cases because of the increased consumption of alcohol-containing surrogates and technical fluids. The quality of alcoholic beverages deteriorated during that period (14). After the campaign, the alcohol consumption increased again, with vodka forming a larger share in the total (15), having partly replaced wine (16).

As mentioned in the preceding section, veiled propaganda of alcohol consumption was recognizable from 1970 to 1985 but took place also earlier (3); more details are in (2). Retrospectively, it becomes clear that the anti-alcohol campaign (1985-88) was used for the same purpose: its failure and the recoil-effect was predictable and occurred when it was required. Massive alcohol consumption after the anti-alcohol campaign facilitated the economic reforms of early 1990s. It is known that alcohol abusers can experience emotions of shame, guilt and have a low self-esteem (17), therefore being probably easier to manipulate and to command. Workers did not oppose privatizations of state-owned enterprises partly due to their drunkenness, involvement in workplace theft and other illegal activities, e.g., use of the factories' equipment for private purposes, which was often tolerated by the management at that time.

Similarly, the impact of earlier anti-alcohol measures was sometimes quite different from the proclaimed goals. In 1972, the sale of vodka and other spirits on Sundays, and between 7 p.m. and 11 a.m. on all other days, was prohibited. However, after 7 p.m. till the closing of shops at 8-10 p.m., and on Sundays, fortified wines with the alcohol concentration 17-19% were sold. Some cheaper fortified wines were poor quality, being noticed to induce more severe intoxication and hangover than vodka. In practice, workers who finished work at around 5 p.m., considering that there were usually queues at the shops, started drinking vodka (often at the workplace) but continued with fortified wines or consumed the latter only. It was generally known by drinkers that it is not advisable to consume fortified wine after vodka: it often brought about more severe intoxications, vomiting, sleeping down in public places etc. At the same time, 0.25l vodka bottles disappeared almost completely, replaced by 0.5l bottles. On the rare occasions when the 0.25l bottles were on sale, it induced a visibly positive emotional reaction. For aged alcoholics in particular, it was preferable to purchase a 0.25l bottle of vodka after work and to go home: after that he or she would wake up next morning in a better condition for the next workday. Instead, they often continued with poor quality fortified wines, which caused deeper intoxications, being associated with higher health-related and social risks. This was a foreseeable consequence of the anti-alcohol measures of 1972.

During the Soviet time, even beyond the anti-alcohol campaigns, alcoholic beverages were not as easily available as in many other countries: number of bottle stores was limited, queues were usual. It was difficult to buy a bottle of beer in case of an occasional demand such as stress. After standing a queue, larger amounts of alcohol were usually purchased and consumed. Analogously, people rarely came to a beerhouse just for one drink: after standing a queue, companies or couples usually stayed there for hours. In the author's opinion, technically complicated availability of alcohol is one of the factors contributing to deeper alcohol intoxications.

After the anti-alcohol campaign (1985-88), the quality of alcoholic beverages deteriorated (14), but they have become easily available. However, recent governmental measures in Russia, limiting availability of alcohol, in particular, a prohibition of small (0.33l) beer cans, contribute even today to alcohol consumption in higher doses: one cannot take for an occasional stress just a small can of beer. Another recent "anti-alcohol" measure – prohibition from the 1 January 2013 of beer selling between 23 p.m. and 8 a.m. (18) apparently results in purchasing by some people larger amounts in advance with subsequent consumption. Prohibition of beer sales at small kiosks (18) will probably have a similar effect in the places with no shops near at hand. There is an opinion that the latter measure would have no impact on the volume of beer sales (19). The pro forma anti-alcohol measures of this kind and accompanying rhetoric are in fact distracting public attention from the problems, which the government does not tackle, among them the insufficient public health and social security systems (20, 21).

CHANGING PATTERN OF ALCOHOL CONSUMPTION

According to the author's observations, the pattern of alcohol consumption in Russia has been changing since approximately the year 2000, with the average amounts of consumed alcohol tending to decrease. The decrease was mentioned in some publications (22, 23); but for an inside observer this tendency seems to be more pronounced, especially in the large cities such as Moscow. During the Soviet time and the 1990s, many inebriated individuals could be seen in public places: drinking, sleeping, making noise, etc. In contrast with the past, there are almost no heavily drunk people in the streets today; even the marginalized are rarely seen drunk in public.

Concomitantly, the pattern of alcohol consumption has changed: less heavy binge drinking of vodka, partly replaced by the moderate consumption of beer (16). A similar tendency is also generally noticed in smaller towns and rural areas, favored by the ongoing immigration from the regions with less widespread alcohol consumption, such as Middle Asia and the Caucasus, or explained by the fact that local alcoholics have "died out" with fewer successors. Other reasons for these changes have been discussed previously: the more responsible way of life under the conditions of the market economy, intimidation and crime against alcoholics and people with alcohol-related dementia, including appropriation of their residences and other property (24-26). Conversely, some alcohol abusers, particularly those facing economic difficulties, are involved in illegal activities.

A discussion of the changing pattern of alcohol consumption in Russia would be incomplete without an overview of social transformations during the two last decades, including the dissolution of the social strata containing the majority of alcohol consumers in urban areas - workers and intelligentsia. Their carefree lifestyle, often accompanied by alcohol consumption, was largely lost after the economic reforms of the early 1990s: many factories and scientific institutions were closed or restructured; and personnel faced unemployment in conditions of an underdeveloped social security system with by far insufficient unemployment benefits. Many people, in order to preserve a current or to find a new job, had to discontinue or reduce their alcohol consumption. In addition, the ongoing replacement of ethnic Russian workers by immigrants from less drinking regions has further contributed to the per capita decrease in alcohol consumption by workers.

ALCOHOL CONSUMPTION AND LIFE EXPECTANCY

It was discussed in the preceding sections that certain governmental measures, purportedly aimed at reducing of mass alcohol abuse, have in fact contributed to deeper intoxications and increased mortality due to the widespread consumption of surrogates. After the anti-alcohol campaign (1985-88), average life expectancy at birth decreased sharply, especially in men: by 1993 it had slumped to about 59 years (15), today being estimated to be 64 years (20). According to a widespread opinion, many Russian alcohol abusers do not live long enough to die of liver cirrhosis or its complications. Among the most frequent causes of death of alcoholics are bronchopulmonary diseases including chronic bronchitis, bronchopneumonia, pleural empyema, and tuberculosis (28-31). This is probably partly caused by the cold climate coupled with the limited availability of warm public houses for the people with low incomes, so that they often drink and loiter outdoors and can fall asleep in a cold place. Smoking of poor-quality cigarettes is also likely to be a contributing factor, although the quality of cigarettes has improved in recent decades, cheap cigarettes without filter having largely disappeared.

Another cause of the relatively high mortality has been the poor quality of alcoholic beverages, in particular, consumption of counterfeit products and surrogates sold also in legally operating shops (14). During the anti-alcohol campaign, many poisonings were caused by alcohol-containing technical fluids. The quality of legally sold alcoholic beverages deteriorated during that period; after the campaign, poor-quality alcoholic beverages were produced and sold en masse (Figure 1) (32). Numerous cases of death after the ingestion of moderate amounts (33), with a relatively low blood alcohol level (32) were reported, obviously caused by the substances other than ethanol contained in the consumed products. However, according to the author's observations, there has been a gradual improvement in the average quality of alcoholic beverages over the last decade.

Furthermore, a relatively high mortality rate from cardiovascular diseases in Russia has been reported (34, 35). A cause of the high registered cardiovascular mortality in the former SU is evident for anatomic pathologists. Since the Soviet time, autopsy has remained obligatory for all patients dying in hospitals; but the attitude towards post-mortem examinations has become less rigorous. Autopsies were often performed incompletely (36). Two examples: in the late 1990s, a young pathologist in a central clinical hospital in Moscow performed an autopsy and wrote as a post mortem diagnosis "cancer of oral mucosa" without looking into the oral cavity, on the basis of a preceding cytological report mentioning "atypical cells" in a smear from the oral cavity.

Another example from the same institution: aplastic anemia was diagnosed post mortem referring to clinical data in an elderly patient with red bone marrow in the femoral diaphysis without its histological examination and iron stain. Both diagnoses were approved by a professor and head of pathology services. If a cause of death is not entirely clear, it is usual to write on a death certificate: 'Ischemic heart disease with cardiac insufficiency' or a similar formulation.

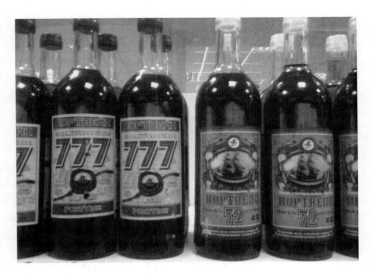

Figure 1. Beverage named 'Portwein' tasted like a flavored sweetened solution of poor quality alcohol. Portwein 72 was inexpensive red fortified wine of acceptable quality during the Soviet time. It has disappeared; and the popular name is used for selling of the surrogates. "Port wine" 777 appeared later in the 1980s and has been of poor quality from the beginning.

A tendency to overdiagnose cardiovascular diseases also exists for people dying at home and not undergoing autopsy. This is likely to be one of the causes of the considerable increase in cardiovascular mortality since the 1970s, especially among men (37). It can be indirectly confirmed by the following statement: 'Increases and decreases in mortality [have been] related to cardiovascular diseases (CVD), particularly to 'other forms of acute and chronic ischemia' and 'atherosclerotic heart disease,' but not to myocardial infarction, the proportion of which in Russian CVD-related mortality is extremely low.' (38) The explanation for this discrepancy is evident: the diagnosis of myocardial infarction is usually based on clear clinical and/or pathological criteria, while entities such as 'acute and chronic ischemia' or 'atherosclerotic heart disease' can be used post mortem without strong evidence; more details are in (21). It also indicates that many patients with myocardial infarction remain undiagnosed and untreated.

The following typical statement should be commented upon: 'Numerous epidemiological studies led to the consensus that vodka binge drinking is a key reason for these observed changes,' i.e., for premature mortality (34). It is difficult to generalize without reliable statistics, but heavy binge drinking is visibly in decline in today's Russia, especially in large cities such as Moscow (14). The role of alcohol as a cause of premature death cannot be denied, but this role was obviously more significant during the 1990s, when alcohol consumption increased as a recoil effect after the anti-alcohol campaign (1985-88). The causative role of alcohol in Russian mortality rates was obviously exaggerated in some publications, e.g., (39), where "the enormous scale of alcohol-related mortality" was reiterated without mentioning the insufficient availability and quality of health care as another cause of premature death. There is a tendency in the Russian-language literature to exaggerate the topic alcohol abuse and its cause-effect relationship with mortality, especially from cardiovascular diseases, e.g., (28, 29, 32, 39, 40). In this way, responsibility for higher mortality rates, partly caused by the shortages of the health care system, is in a sense shifted onto the patients themselves: they allegedly suffered from self-inflicted diseases due to their excessive alcohol consumption. In fact, statements such like 'Alcohol accounts for most of the large fluctuations in Russian mortality, and alcohol and tobacco account for the large difference in adult mortality between Russia and Western Europe.' (41) tend to veil another significant cause of such difference: insufficient availability of modern health care.

For example, it was stated on the basis of a large autopsy study that all studied 654 deceased individuals classified as hard drinkers were diagnosed post mortem with cardiomyopathy; while in the majority of the patients classified as chronic alcoholics (172 cases) the cardiomyopathy was graded as pronounced (29). According to the monograph (28), clinically significant cardiomyopathy was diagnosed in approximately 50% of habitual alcohol consumers. Accordingly, cardiomyopathy has been used to explain for sudden death cases amongst alcohol consumers (29), while the real cause could have been unnatural, including poisonings by alcohol-containing fluids (38). The tendency to exaggerate the cause-effect relationship between alcohol and the cardiovascular morbidity/mortality is relatively new in the Russian-language literature. An earlier epidemiological study reported that rates of cardiovascular diseases including hypertension were not significantly higher among excessively drinking men compared to the general male population (30); a lesser prevalence of atherosclerosis in alcoholics older than 40 years compared to the controls was reported in (31).

Finally, it should be mentioned that evaluating results of surveys (42-44), it should be taken into account that surveys and questionnaires have been largely discredited in Russia by means of obtrusive solicitations to partake in different surveys, often asking for private information: in the streets, per telephone, and previously also by agents coming to private homes. Answers to the questionnaires can be biased, especially with regard to such a delicate topic as alcohol use and misuse.

CONCLUSION

Societies should care for vulnerable members, including aged citizens suffering of alcoholism and alcohol-related dementia (45). This is feasible today in view of the economic growth in Russia. Furthermore, apart from excessive alcohol consumption, the following causes of the relatively low life expectancy in Russia, not clearly perceptible from the literature, should be pointed out: insufficient quality and availability of the health care, particularly for middle-aged and elderly men, including those prone to the alcohol consumption; low quality and toxicity of some alcoholic beverages, acknowledging however that there have been improvements over approximately the last decade.

REFERENCES

[1] McKee M. Alcohol in Russia. Alcohol Alcohol 1999;34(6):824-9.
[2] Jargin SV. On the causes of alcoholism in the former Soviet Union. Alcohol Alcohol 2010;45(1):104-5.
[3] Pelipas VE, Miroshnichenko LD. Problems of the alcohol policy. In: Ivanets NN, Vinnikova MA. (Editors) Alcoholism. Moscow: MIA, 2011:817-51. [Russian].

[4]   Sivolap IK, ed. Book about delicious and healthy food. Moscow: Pishchepromizdat, 1964. [Russian].
[5]   Fleming PM, Meyroyan A, Klimova I. Alcohol treatment services in Russia: a worsening crisis. Alcohol Alcohol 1994;29(4):357-62.
[6]   Altshuler VB. Alcoholism. Moscow: GEOTAR-Media, 2010. [Russian].
[7]   Johnsen J, Mørland J. Depot preparations of disulfiram: experimental and clinical results. Acta Psychiatr Scand Suppl 1992;369:27-30.
[8]   Wilson A, Blanchard R, Davidson W, McRae L, Maini K. Disulfiram implantation: a dose response trial. J Clin Psychiatry 1984;45(6):242-7.
[9]   Voskresenskii VA. Critical evaluation of ultra-rapid psychotherapy of alcoholism (concerning the article by A.R. Dovzhenko et al. "Ambulatory stress psychotherapy of alcoholics"). Zh Nevropatol Psikhiatr Im S S Korsakova 1990;90(9):130-2. [Russian].
[10] Dovzhenko AR, Artemchuk AF, Bolotova ZN, Vorob'eva TM, Manuilenko IuA. Outpatient stress psychotherapy of patients with alcoholism. Zh Nevropatol Psikhiatr Im S S Korsakova 1988;88(2):94-7. [Russian].
[11] Lipgart NK, Goloburda AV, Ivanov VV. Once more about A.R. Dobzhenko's method of stress psychotherapy in alcoholism. Zh Nevropatol Psikhiatr Im S S Korsakova 1991;91(6):133-4.
[12] Belokrylov IV, Agibalova TV, Rovenskikh IN. Psychotherapy of alcoholism technology. In: Ivanets NN, Vinnikova MA, eds. Alcoholism. Moscow: MIA, 2011:396-438 [Russian].
[13] Torban M, Heimer R, Ilyuk RD, Krupitsky EM. Practices and attitudes of addiction treatment providers in the Russian Federation. J Addict Res Ther 2011;2:104.
[14] Jargin SV. Letter from Russia: minimal price for vodka established in Russia from 1 January 2010. Alcohol Alcohol 2010;45(6):586-8.
[15] Ryan M. Alcoholism and rising mortality in the Russian Federation. BMJ 1995;310(6980):646-8.
[16] WHO. Russian Federation. Global Information System on Alcohol and Health (GISAH), Geneva: World Health Organization, 2011.
[17] Scherer M, Worthington EL, Hook JN, Campana KL. Forgiveness and the bottle: promoting self-forgiveness in individuals who abuse alcohol. J Addict Dis 2011;30(4):382-95.
[18] News. Sales of beer in kiosks prohibited. Food Industry (Moscow) 2013;(2):5-6. [Russian].
[19] MacFarlane S. Regulation of brewing in RF – one of the most strict. Beer Beverages (Moscow) 2013;(1):48-9.
[20] Jargin SV. Barriers to the importation of medical products to Russia: in search of solutions. Healthcare Low-resource Settings 2013;1:e13.
[21] Jargin SV. Health care and life expectancy: a letter from Russia. Public Health 2013;127(2):189-90.
[22] Koshkina EA, Kirzhanova VV. Prevalence of alcoholism and alcoholic psychoses in Russia. In: Ivanets NN, Vinnikova MA, eds. Alcoholism. Moscow: MIA, 2011:32-39. [Russian].
[23] Seregin SN. Structure policy in Russian food independence problem solving. Food Processing Industry (Moscow) 2008;(6):38-44. [Russian].
[24] Jargin SV. Changing pattern of alcohol consumption in Russia. Adicciones 2013;25(4):356-7.
[25] Jargin SV. Social vulnerability of alcoholics and patients with alcohol-related dementia: a view from Russia. Alcohol Alcohol 2010;45(3):293-4.
[26] Jargin S. Alcohol consumption in Russia 1970-2014. Saarbrücken: LAP Lambert Academic Publishing, 2014.
[27] Rehm J. Russia: lessons for alcohol epidemiology and alcohol policy. Lancet 2014;383(9927):1440-2.
[28] Vertkin AL, Zairat'iants OV, Vovk EI. Final diagnosis. Moscow: Geotar-Media, 2009. [Russian].
[29] Paukov VS, Erokhin IuA. Pathologic anatomy of hard drinking and alcoholism. Arkh Patol 2004;66(4):3-9.
[30] Kopyt NIa, Gudzhabidze VV. Effect of alcohol abuse on the health indices of the population. Zdravookhr Ross Fed 1977;(6):25-8.
[31] Gukasian AG. Chronic alcoholism and condition of internal organs. Moscow: Meditsina, 1968. (Russian).
[32] Nuzhnyi VP, Kharchenko VI, Akopian AS. Alcohol abuse in Russia is an essential risk factor of cardiovascular diseases development and high population mortality (review). Ter Arkh 1998;70(10):57-64.

[33] Govorin NV, Sakharov AV. Alkohol-related mortality. Tomsk: Ivan Fedorov, 2012. [Russian].
[34] Zatonski WA, Bhala N. Changing trends of diseases in Eastern Europe: closing the gap. Public Health 2012;126(3):248-52.
[35] Razvodovsky YE. Beverage-specific alcohol sale and cardiovascular mortality in Russia. J Environ Public Health 2010;2010:253853.
[36] Jargin SV. The practice of pathology in Russia: On the eve of modernization. Basic Appl Pathol 2010;3:70-3.
[37] Zatonski W. The East-West Health Gap in Europe - what are the causes? Eur J Public Health 2007;17(2):121.
[38] Davydov MI, Zaridze D G, Lazarev AF, Maksimovich DM, Igitov VI, Boroda AM, Khvastik MG. Analysis of mortality in Russian population. Vestn Ross Akad Med Nauk 2007;(7):17-27.
[39] Nemtsov AV. Alcohol-related human losses in Russia in the 1980s and 1990s. Addiction 2002;97(11):1413-25.
[40] Razvodovsky YE. Estimation of alcohol attributable fraction of mortality in Russia. Adicciones 2012;24(3):247-52.
[41] Zaridze D, Brennan P, Boreham J, Boroda A, Karpov R, Lazarev A, Konobeevskaya I, Igitov V, Terechova T, Boffetta P, Peto R. Alcohol and cause-specific mortality in Russia: a retrospective case-control study of 48,557 adult deaths. Lancet 2009;373(9682):2201-14.
[42] Cook S. De Stavola B, Saburova L, Kiryanov N, Vasiljev M, McCambridge J, McKee M, Polikina O, Gil A, Leon DA. Socio-demographic predictors of dimensions of the AUDIT score in a population sample of working-age men in Izhevsk, Russia. Alcohol Alcohol 2011;46(6):702-8.
[43] Pomerleau J, McKee M, Rose R, Haerpfer CW, Rotman D, Tumanov S. Hazardous alcohol drinking in the former Soviet Union: a cross-sectional study of eight countries. Alcohol Alcohol 2008;43(3):351-9.
[44] Zaridze D, Lewington S, Boroda A, Scélo G, Karpov R, Lazarev A, Konobeevskaya I, Igitov V, Terechova T, Boffetta P, Sherliker P, Kong X, Whitlock G, Boreham J, Brennan P, Peto R. Alcohol and mortality in Russia: prospective observational study of 151,000 adults. Lancet 2014;383(9927):1465-73.

Submitted: April 14, 2014. *Revised:* May 26, 2014. *Accepted:* June 06, 2014.

In: Public Health Yearbook 2015
Editor: Joav Merrick

ISBN: 978-1-63484-514-4
© 2016 Nova Science Publishers, Inc.

Chapter 23

EXERCISE CULTURE AMONG IMMIGRANTS LIVING IN THE MIDWESTERN UNITED STATES

Goodwill Apiyo, MA, MDA, and Cecilia S Obeng, PhD*

Department of Applied Health Science, School of Public Health,
Indiana University, Bloomington, Indiana, United States of America

ABSTRACT

The purpose of this study was to explore shared lived exercise experiences among new African immigrants residing in the Midwest of the United States. Participants (n=32) were recruited through non-probability purposive and snowball sampling procedures. Open-ended probing interviews were administered in the study. The interview transcripts were analyzed thematically in a stepwise procedure as outlined by Collaizi. (1) Themes emerging from participant narratives included: a) culture which included the wearing of veils by women in the presence of men and modes on dress; b) family commitments and commitments to schoolwork; and c) personal grooming dealing with cultural expectations on taking care of one's body and hair. Because of the central role of culture on immigrant exercise behavior, the study recommends that resources on women-only gyms, childcare assisting social support groups, and education debunking hair care myths be made available to this population.

Keywords: fitness, exercise, immigrants, public health, education

INTRODUCTION

Physical inactivity/exercise is a priority health risk behavior and a leading contributor to morbidity and mortality in the United States (US). It has been mentioned as a risk factor for cardiovascular disease (2), obesity (3) and other chronic conditions that reduce individuals' quality of life and place huge financial burden on families (3). Healthy People 2020 lists

---

[*] Correspondence: Cecilia S Obeng, PhD, Associate Professor, Indiana University, School of Public Health, 1025 E. 7th Street, SPH 116, Bloomington, IN 47405, United States. E-mail: cobeng@indiana.edu.

increasing the proportion of children, adolescents, and adults participating in physical activity as one of its four overarching goals (4).

Few physical activity/exercising research studies have been done on immigrants from Africa residing in the US. Existing research mainly focuses on socioeconomic facilitators and barriers to physical activity in a segment of African immigrants in the US (5-8), but is mostly silent on salient cultural issues surrounding exercising in the population. Our study explores the role of culture in influencing exercise behavior among recent immigrants from Africa who reside in the US Midwest. Such an investigation, we believe, is important given Kreuter et al. (9) argument that culture is a shared group characteristic (seen in its norms, values, practices, and other social regularities) that has passed on to future generations and directly or indirectly influences a group's health-related behavior. Secondly, immigrants are the fastest growing segment of the U.S. population (10) and immigrants from Africa represent one of the fastest growing groups resettling in the US (5). The population's health status therefore impacts the overall health standing of the country.

New immigrants tend to present better health indicators in general and weigh less than native-born individuals in the US. With increasing duration of residence in the country, however, exhibited health and weight advantages diminish (10-12). Several studies (13-15) indicate that migration to Western countries is significantly associated with weight gain among immigrants from some parts of the world; with obesity being more prevalent among Africans who migrate to Western countries than among their counterparts in Africa (16, 17). Studies also find significantly elevated risks of developing obesity among children from communities with a high proportion of immigrants (14). These changes in health and weight among immigrants are attributed in-part to a combination of dietary and exercise factors. In a process referred to as diet acculturation, migration often makes individuals change their food habits (14). Empirical evidence indicates that migrants from Africa to Western countries usually change their dietary habits from a consumption of traditional staple foods low in fat and rich in fiber to processed and refined foods high in saturated fats and sugar (14, 15). Additionally, consistent with studies on adult immigrants from other Western countries, (18) foreign-born individuals in the US have been found to be more often sedentary than the host population (10). According to the Center for Disease Control and Prevention (CDC) (19), physical activity levels and dietary behaviors among immigrants and refugees to high income nations are usually less healthy than the non-immigrant majority populations.

Little is known about exercise culture among African immigrants in the US. Qualitative studies among segments of African men (6), women (7) and youth (8) originally from Somalia suggests inadequate levels of physical activity after resettlement in the US. It is also not clear if the population's cultural perceptions concerning obesity/overweight changes when they settle in the US, and whether that is reflected in the population's exercise culture. In several parts of Africa, attitudes toward overweight and obesity are positive (20) and people generally associate fatness with good health and beauty. (21-23) CDC guidelines recommend obesity prevention through exercise and diet (24).

The purpose of this study was therefore to explore shared lived exercise experiences of immigrants by investigating the phenomena as described by recent immigrants from Africa living in the US Midwest. Identification of salient cultural barriers that influence exercising behavior in this sub-population will help to elucidate why the population loses health and weight advantages that it enjoys over the host population when it first arrives in the US; and subsequently help inform culturally sensitive programs that promotes public health.

METHODS

Phenomenology was used to explore this topic. Phenomenology is seen as both a research method and a philosophy striving to elucidate a phenomenon as it really is (25, 26). Sokolowski (26) asserts that as a methodology, phenomenology involves the use of thick description and close analysis of lived experiences with the aim of deepening an understanding of the range of immediate experiences. Starks and Trinidad (25) further posit that the methodology pursues the uncovering of essential invariant features of those unique experiences.

Phenomenology fits well with this study because it allows participants to focus on their individual lived exercise experiences, and to describe how their cultures influence their exercising behavior. The methodology thus helps facilitate our understanding of common features of exercise experiences among recent immigrants from Africa who reside in Indiana (Indianapolis and Bloomington).

The study conducted open-ended probing interviews with thirty-two immigrants. Recruitment for the study was done through non-probability purposive and snowball-sampling procedures in which recruited participants' recommended additional useful potential candidates. Potential participants were contacted either in person or by email and phone. Participants were informed that the study was voluntary and had to give their informed consent before participating in the study. The study protocol was approved by Indiana University's Institutional Review Board. The inclusion criteria were as follows: adult (18+ years old); originally from Africa (living in the US for less than 10 years); living in Indiana (Bloomington, or Indianapolis) at the time of the study; ability to speak and write English; and ability to give informed consent. The study excluded children (< 18 years) and people who were unable to give informed consent.

Because qualitative studies scholars are usually more interested in understanding complex human issues (e.g., the exercise culture of the immigrants) rather than the generalizability of the results (27) and because the literature on qualitative research is not categorical on sample size (28), this study settled on a sample of 50 possible informants who had recently immigrated from Africa and were living in Bloomington and Indianapolis at the time of the study.

From the 50 participants contacted, 32 gave their consent to take part in the study and 18 declined. The researchers' local knowledge of the study population ensured that the participants' were purposefully recruited to represent a range of religious, geographic, and demographic influences and to also provide a variety of expressions.

To diminish disruption of the participant's daily routine, interviews took place either within the participants' home or at a university library easily accessible by public transportation. Open-ended questionnaires were used to allow probing for detail and clarity on individual participant's lived exercise experiences (29). The interviewer (GA) asked and completed questionnaires based on responses from study participants. Questionnaires took 20-25 minutes to complete and were all in English.

Questionnaires were first pilot tested with eight foreign students from Africa studying at Indiana University in Bloomington, Indiana, and revised based on feedback to enable capture key concepts. Individual interview questions solicited demographic information on age, marital status, occupation, gender, and country of origin. The questions further solicited information on physical activity/exercise that increases one's heart rate and makes one breathe hard some of the time. These were classified into regular, moderate and mild depending on duration and intensity of the physical activity/exercise. To capture the shared group (cultural) characteristics that influenced exercising, a specific question was also asked on group values, norms, practices, beliefs, and other social regularities that influenced the type, duration, seasonality, place, and frequency of physical activity/exercise.

Immigrants were defined as people originally from Africa who had resettled in the US as green card holders, as well as refugees and those on student visas. Exercise was used interchangeably with physical activity and was defined as any form of physical activity that increases one's heart rate and makes one breathe hard some of the time (19). The Center for Disease Control and Prevention (CDC) classifies exercise into i) vigorous: 10+ minutes, causes heavy sweating or large increases in breathing or heart rate; and ii) moderate: 10+ minutes, causes light sweating or slight to moderate increase in breathing or heart rate.

Data analysis

Interview transcripts (texts) were analyzed thematically in a stepwise procedure (30) as outlined by Colaizzi (1). Each completed interview text was first read several times to gain a good grasp of the whole picture. After several readings of the text, significant statements were extracted and key words relating to the phenomenon under study identified. We then formulated meanings for each of these significant statements and repeated the process across participants' narratives. This enabled us to cluster experiences into recurrent meaningful themes based on shared patterns among the participants (25, 31).

All judgments on coding and categorizing were done by a research team that consisted of the first author (interviewer) and the second author (a senior faculty with advanced qualitative research skills). Themes were identified and confirmed after wide consultations in which discrepancies and contradictory issues were clarified. As recommended (26) for phenomenological analysis, both researchers (with intimate knowledge of the study population) recognized and set aside their prior knowledge and assumptions and had an open mind about the study participants' accounts. To be sure that study findings reflected the essence of the immigrant's lived exercise experiences, the interviewer returned to seven informants chosen at random to validate emerging themes.

RESULTS

A total of 32 immigrants from Africa living in the US Midwest participated in the study. They ranged in age from 21 to 49 years (mean age 31 years) and their duration of stay in the US ranged from 3 months to 7 years. A majority of them (62.5%) were students and their countries of origin were Kenya, Uganda, Tanzania, Ghana, South Africa, Nigeria, and Sudan. Additional details of study participants are indicated in Table 1.

Table 1. Characteristics of the study participants (n = 32)

Characteristics	N	%
Gender		
Female	20	62.5
Male	12	37.5
Marital Status		
Single	19	59.4
Married	13	40.6
Country of Origin		
Kenya	5	15.6
Uganda	3	9.4
Tanzania	4	12.5
Ghana	5	15.6
Nigeria	7	21.9
Sudan	3	9.4
South Africa	5	15.6
Age Range		
20-29 years	10	31.3
30-39 years	17	53.1
40 - 49 years	5	15.6
Duration of Stay in the USA		
<1 year	9	28.1
1-4 years	18	56.3
-7 years	5	15.6
Place of Residence in the USA		
Bloomington, IN	14	43.8
Indianapolis, IN	18	56.3
Religion		
Christian	17	53.1
Muslim	11	34.4
Others	4	12.5

Religion

For religious reasons, some female participants could not exercise around men. They also stated that no fitness centers in their neighborhoods were appropriate for their culture and that they preferred gender based fitness clubs serving women only.
Two participants stated:

> Muslim women from my country cover their head if there are men around. Therefore, we do not like to exercise just anywhere (Tanzanian woman, age 27).

> …We prefer closed clubs just for women ….which means we can take our head cover off and wear swimming suits and exercise clothes…… in the United States gyms have men around so Muslim women from my culture don't feel comfortable (Nigerian woman, age 31).

Dressing

Perceptions about the type of exercise that the community deemed appropriate or the kind of clothing that the society viewed as decent for women of a certain age emerged as a barrier to exercising. A participant stated:

> There are certain exercises that are not acceptable for women, especially elderly women from my culture. It is also difficult to dress lightly for sports because in my culture such dressing is seen as inappropriate and indecent (Kenyan woman, age 49).

Personal grooming

A participant described how he could not exercise because sweating was not good for his hair as a hair stylist had advised him that it would make his dreadlocks, part of his cultural heritage, to untangle. He noted:

> I can't afford to sweat. I just started making dreadlocks and my hair stylist advised me against getting my hair wet...

> .... If I exercise I will sweat and this bad for dreadlocks as wet hair will not lock. ...It also become very itchy. ....sweating may force me to start this process all over again. I don't want to do that. ... it will take 6-12 months before the twists form locks that cannot untangle.... This is part of my heritage and religion so if I have to wait 6-12 months to exercise, so be it... absolutely (a man from South Africa, age 41).

Societal attitudes toward weight gain and exercise

Some participants perceived that their community had a favorable attitude toward weight gain; while others believed that loss of weight as a result of exercising could result in stigmatization in the community:

> If I run I will lose weight you know, everyone I call in Africa asks me how much weight I have gained............It's a sign of living good, you know,... fat people are admired in my country (Ugandan woman, age 20).

> You don't want to lose weight from exercising.... people talk.... they may talk behind your back saying you have HIV (South African woman, age 33).

Beside these, some participants in this study held the view that studying and working to uplift living standards of relatives still left in Africa was more important than exercising, and that exercising took away valuable time that could be used for study and work.

Other factors

Finally, additional barriers to exercising that emerged included cold temperatures; commitment to work, study, and parenting; and inconvenience (i.e., no transportation to the gym or no childcare for their offspring while they are at the gym). A participant observed:

> I do not have time. I am a mother studying fulltime. When my daughter comes home from school, she has to find food ready and I also have to assist her with homework. When we are finished, I then have to start with my school work and by the time I finish, I would be very tired (Ghanaian woman, age 33).

DISCUSSION

The aim of this study was to gain an insight into the exercise culture among new immigrants from Africa living in the US. The group's norms, practices, beliefs, and other social regularities appear to play a central role in their exercise behavior. For religious reasons, some females could not exercise around men and were of the opinion that no fitness centers in their neighborhoods were appropriate for their culture. Similar findings have been recorded in a study by Rothe et al. (8), where the Somali community limited interaction with the opposite sex beyond a certain age; and by Devlin et al. (7), who found that clothing was a barrier to exercising among Somali women.

Some elderly female participants in our study stated that they could not dress lightly to exercise because their culture considered it inappropriate or indecent. This finding complements results of a study looking at barriers to exercising among male immigrants from Africa, which noted that old Somali men were embarrassed to wear standard exercising attire in the United States for fear of what female counterparts from their community would say (6). Other participants in our study described how their community viewed work and studies positively, to assist relatives still in Africa, and considered time spent exercising as one that could be wisely spent working to make money. Similar findings have previously been noted by other scholars (6).

Other participants in our study expressed reservations about exercising because of positive communal attitudes toward being overweight. A study (15) conducted in Africa (where the immigrants hail from) confirms this finding as it notes that unlike in the West where obesity is viewed negatively, the perception of obesity in Africa is largely positive. Our study also found that some participants expressed reservations toward exercising for fear of being stigmatized. They perceived that any resultant weight loss, stemming from exercising, could be associated with HIV status by their community members. Previous studies in five African countries have reported HIV/AIDS stigmatizing behavior resulting from symptoms such as loss of weight (32). It is interesting that the view is still held by some people who have already migrated from the continent.

Research conducted among African American women has identified hair as one of the barriers preventing women from being physically active (33-35). To our knowledge, no study has reported similar findings among immigrants from Africa living in the US. Our study therefore adds to the literature by finding that even among recent immigrants from Africa, sweaty hair (especially among participants with dreadlocks) was also a factor preventing people from adopting exercising behavior. The study further highlights the potential influence of hair stylists on some participants' exercise behavior in that our study finds that some study participants were not exercising because they were in the process of locking their hair and were merely following the advice given to them by their hair stylists not to make their hair wet.

This study further adds to the literature by identifying the central role that culture plays in the exercise behavior of recent migrants from Africa. In trying to understand why immigrants arriving in the US with superior health indicators than the host population lose these advantages with longer duration of stay in the country, many reasons have been advanced (10, 14) including acculturation, where immigrants adopt dietary habits low on fibers and high on sugars and acquire more sedentary lifestyles.

Our study adds to the literature through findings that immigrants from Africa also retain elements of their culture that may also contribute to diminished health indicators in the group, with longer duration of stay in the country. For example, the study finds that even after migrating from Africa, some participants still harbor positive attitudes towards weight gain (prevalent in the source continent where people generally associate fatness with beauty, good health, and affluence) (15). Other immigrants also retain beliefs about appropriate clothing and types of exercising for the females/elderly that is inhibitive to adopting exercising behavior. A combination of practices acquired in the host country (i.e., through acculturation) and retained from the source continent (such as positive attitudes on weight gain) potentially explains the diminishing health of this population with increased duration of stay in the US.

The study additionally finds cold temperature, commitments with work, study, and parenting, as well as inconvenience of exercise facilities being inaccessible (i.e., either too expensive or far from one's place of residence) as being barriers to exercising behavior. Similar results have been noted elsewhere by studies investigating barriers to physical activity (6-8, 12, 34).

There are several limitations to the study. First, interviews were conducted only in English. Important information on the lived exercise experiences of the group could therefore have been lost because English is not the first language of the participants. Second, generalizability to all immigrants from Africa may be limited because Africa is a heterogeneous continent with many subgroups and subcultures. The sample of 32 participants drawn from seven countries could therefore hardly be a true representation of the continent. In qualitative approaches, however, improved understanding of complex human issues is usually more important than the generalizability of results (27).

Recommendations

Among our sample of recent immigrants from Africa to the US, we found that culture played a significant role in determining their exercise behavior. The study therefore recommends culturally sensitive education programs to: a) address misconceptions associating being overweight with good living; myths that sweating makes dreadlocks to untangle; and attitudes that exercising is a waste of time that could otherwise be well spent on studies or work; b) provide resources on where to find gender based exercise facilities; c) link single mothers with social support groups that can help with childcare and school-work duties and subsequently allow them time to exercise; and d) recommend walking/exercise buddies for outdoor walking, and indoor exercises during winter.

Previous research indicates that many black churches are effective channels for delivering health programs to African Americans in the US (36). Given our finding of religion as playing a central role in determining exercise behavior of the study participants, we recommend that mosques provide gender based exercise facilities for their congregants; and if exercise facilities exist within the establishments, then they should allocate exclusive times for females to exercise freely without worrying about the presence of men around. We further recommend that information be made available to this population about women-only gyms that exist in their communities. Lastly, given the dearth of studies on physical activity on immigrants from Africa to the US, we also recommend further scholarship investigating the cultural facilitators of exercising behavior in this population.

REFERENCES

[1] Colaizzi PF. Psychological research as the phenomenologist views it. Existential phenomen-ological alternatives for psychology. New York: Oxford University Press, 1978.
[2] Dassanayake J, Dharmage SC, Gurrin L, Sundararajan V, Payne WR. Are Australian immigrants at a risk of being physically inactive. Int J Behav Nutr Phys Act 2011;8:53.
[3] Haskell WL, Lee I-M, Pate RR, Powell KE, Blair SN, Franklin BA, et al. Physical activity and public health: updated recommendation for adults from the American College of Sports Medicine and the American Heart Association. Circulation 2007;116(9):1081.
[4] Healthy people 2020, 2011. URL: http://www.healthy people.gov/2020/default.aspx.
[5] Carroll J, Epstein R, Fiscella K, Volpe E, Diaz K, Omar S. Knowledge and beliefs about health promotion and preventive health care among Somali women in the United States. Health Care Women Int 2007.28(4):360-80.
[6] Mohamed AA, Hassan AM, Weis JA, Sia IG, Wieland ML. Physical activity among Somali men in Minnesota. Barriers, facilitators, and recommendations. Am J Men's Health 2014;8(1):35-44.
[7] Devlin JT, Dhalac D, Suldan AA, Jacobs A, Guled K, Bankole KA. Determinants of physical activity among Somali women living in Maine. J Immigr Minor Health 2012;14(2):300-6.
[8] Rothe E, Holt C, Kuhn C, McAteer T, Askari I, O'Meara M, et al. Barriers to outdoor physical activity in wintertime among Somali youth. J Immigr Minor Health 2010;12(5):726-36.
[9] Kreuter MW, Lukwago SN, Bucholtz DC, Clark EM, Sanders-Thompson V. Achieving cultural appropriateness in health promotion programs: targeted and tailored approaches. Health Educ Behav 2003;30 (2):133-46.
[10] Goel MS, McCarthy EP, Phillips RS, Wee CC. Obesity among US immigrant subgroups by duration of residence. JAMA 2004;292(23):2860-7.
[11] Barcenas CH, Wilkinson AV, Strom SS, Cao Y, Saunders KC, Mahabir S, et al. Birthplace, years of residence in the United States, and obesity among Mexican-American adults. Obesity 2007;15(4):1043-52.
[12] Park Y, Neckerman KM, Quinn J, Weiss C, Rundle A. Place of birth, duration of residence, neighborhood immigrant composition and body mass index in New York City. Int J Behav Nutr Phys Activity 2008;5(1):19.
[13] Oza-Frank R, Cunningham SA. The weight of US residence among immigrants: a systematic review. Obes Rev 2010;11(4):271-80.
[14] Magnusson MB, Hulthen L, Kjellgren KI. Obesity, dietary pattern and physical activity among children in a suburb with a high proportion of immigrants. J Hum Nutr Dietetics 2005;18(3):187-94.
[15] Adeboye B, Bermano G, Rolland C. Obesity and its health impact in Africa: a systematic review: review article. Cardiovasc J Afr 2012;23(9):512-21.

[16] Agyemang C, Owusu-Dabo E, de Jonge A, Martins D, Ogedegbe G, Stronks K. Overweight and obesity among Ghanaian residents in The Netherlands: how do they weigh against their urban and rural counterparts in Ghana? Public Health Nutr 2009;12(07):909-16.

[17] Jackson M, Walker S, Cruickshank J, Sharma S, Cade J, Mbanya J, et al. Diet and overweight and obesity in populations of African origin: Cameroon, Jamaica and the UK. Public Health Nutr 2007;10(02):122-30.

[18] Fischbacher C, Hunt S, Alexander L. How physically active are South Asians in the United Kingdom? A literature review. J Public Health 2004;26(3):250-8.

[19] Control CfD, Prevention. Prevalence of fruit and vegetable consumption and physical activity by race/ethnicity--United States, 2005. MMWR 2007;56(13):301.

[20] Walker A, Adam F, Walker B. World pandemic of obesity: the situation in Southern African populations. Public Health 2001;115(6):368-72.

[21] Siervo M, Grey P, Nyan O, Prentice A. Urbanization and obesity in The Gambia: a country in the early stages of the demographic transition. Eur J Clin Nutr 2006;60(4):455-63.

[22] Amoah AG. Sociodemographic variations in obesity among Ghanaian adults. Public Health Nutr 2003;6(08):751-7.

[23] Holdsworth M, Gartner A, Landais E, Maire B, Delpeuch F. Perceptions of healthy and desirable body size in urban Senegalese women. Int J Obes 2004;28(12):1561-8.

[24] Khan LK, Sobush K, Keener D, Goodman K, Lowry A, Kakietek J, et al. Recommended community strategies and measurements to prevent obesity in the United States. MMWR Recomm Rep 2009;58(RR-7):1-26.

[25] Starks H, Trinidad SB. Choose your method: A comparison of phenomenology, discourse analysis, and grounded theory. Qual Health Res 2007;17(10):1372-80.

[26] Sokolowski R. Introduction to phenomenology. Cambridge: Cambridge University Press, 2000.

[27] Marshall MN. Sampling for qualitative research. Fam Pract 1996;13(6):522-6.

[28] Holloway I, Wheeler S. Qualitative research in nursing and healthcare, 3rd ed. Bognor Regis, UK: Wiley-Blackwell Science, 2009.

[29] Creswell JW, Hanson WE, Plano VLC, Morales A. Qualitative research designs selection and implementation. Couns Psychol 2007;35(2):236-64.

[30] Patton MQ. Qualitative evaluation and research methods. Thosand Oaks, CA: Sage, 1990.

[31] Goulding C. Grounded theory, ethnography and phenomenology: A comparative analysis of three qualitative strategies for marketing research. Eur J Marketing 2005;39(3/4):294-308.

[32] Holzemer WL, Uys L, Makoae L, Stewart A, Phetlhu R, Dlamini PS, et al. A conceptual model of HIV/AIDS stigma from five African countries. J Adv Nurs 2007;58(6):541-51.

[33] Henderson KA, Ainsworth BE. A synthesis of perceptions about physical activity among older African American and American Indian women. Am J Public Health 2003;93(2):313-7.

[34] Im E-O, Ko Y, Hwang H, Yoo KH, Chee W, Stuifbergen A, et al. Physical activity as a luxury. African American women's attitudes toward physical activity. West J Nurs Res 2012;34(3):317-39.

[35] Hall RR, Francis S, Whitt-Glover M, Loftin-Bell K, Swett K, McMichael AJ. Hair care practices as a barrier to physical activity in African American women. JAMA Dermatol 2013;149(3):310-4.

[36] Resnicow K, Jackson A, Braithwaite R, DiIorio C, Blisset D, Rahotep S, et al. Healthy Body/Healthy Spirit: a church-based nutrition and physical activity intervention. Health Educ Res 2002;17(5):562-73.

Submitted: March 14, 2014. *Revised:* May 10, 2014. *Accepted:* June 05, 2014.

Chapter 24

HEALTHCARE WORKERS' BREASTFEEDING PRACTICES AND BELIEFS IN GHANA

Cecilia S Obeng[*], PhD, and Donisha Reed, MPH

Department of Applied Health Science, School of Public Health,
Indiana University, Bloomington, Indiana, United States of America

ABSTRACT

Scholarship on breastfeeding indicates that breastfeeding knowledge and skills increase mothers' chances of nursing a baby. This paper uses an interpretative phenomenological perspective to examine 31 Cape Coast (Ghana) healthcare workers' breastfeeding experiences in their work place. Also examined are their breastfeeding practice(s) and their beliefs about breastfeeding. The results indicate that majority of the healthcare workers had no training in breastfeeding practice. The participants reported that mothers who were sick did not want to breastfeed and this led to underfed and malnourished babies. Also, participants reported that parents' misconceptions about exclusive breastfeeding might lead to not doing exclusive breastfeeding. The study recommends intensive breastfeeding education for healthcare workers in Ghana.

Keywords: breastfeeding, health care workers, public health, Ghana

INTRODUCTION

According to a World Health Organization document, breastfeeding is the best source of nutrients for infants for the first six months of an infant's health (1). Majority of mothers with good information and good skills on breastfeeding will be able to nurse their babies for healthy development (1).

---

[*] Correspondence: Cecilia S Obeng, PhD, Associate Professor, Indiana University, School of Public Health, 1025 E. 7th Street, SPH 116, Bloomington, IN 47405, United States. E-mail: cobeng@indiana.edu.

Scholarships on Healthcare workers demonstrates that healthcare professionals' competence to help breastfeeding mothers depends on their breastfeeding skills, knowledge and attitudes towards breastfeeding and that some health care professionals have negative beliefs, and wrong information about human breast milk (2-4). Research has also shown that new mothers' attempt to breastfed their infants can be swayed by the information and skills they receive from their healthcare professionals (doctors and nurses), since they are the first people to be with the mother and the child (2-7).

Many scholars and mothers around the globe reported professional healthcare workers making mistakes that had impacted the breastfeeding efforts of mothers leading to frustration by a mother and her child (8-13).

Many scholars studied breastfeeding education on healthcare providers and came to the conclusion that breastfeeding education helped healthcare workers' clinical performance and positive health results for mothers and their children (14-16).

Concerning breastfeeding world-wide, according to the World Health Organization's Infant and Young Child Feeding, only 38% of babies receive breastfeeding for 6 months, and that about 800, 000 children's lives will be saved if they are exclusively breastfed (17).

In view of the above-mentioned research findings, this research aims to investigate the breastfeeding beliefs, knowledge and skills among healthcare workers in Ghana with the view to learning more about what influences this group of healthcare workers' knowledge and skill about breastfeeding practice.

METHODS

This study uses an interpretative phenomenological perspective to examine the breastfeeding experiences of healthcare workers in Cape Coast (Ghana). An interpretative phenomenological perspective was used in order to find out the ways in which participants make sense of their experiences. The study was conducted in the summer of 2013 by the lead author. Surveys were used to collect the data. The survey included open-ended questions that allowed the participants the opportunity to respond as they saw (it) fit. Open-ended questions were used since they require researchers to careful select words in order for the respondent to understand what is being asked (18). Also, open-ended questionnaires were used since they have the potential to gather information from a wider sample than can be reached by personal interviews. The questionnaire investigated participants' beliefs about breastfeeding and how such beliefs influence their profession. The questions also touched on problems that they could potentially come across as healthcare providers on breastfeeding, and their knowledge and opinion about skin-to-skin. Finally participants were asked about some ways that they believe will encourage mothers to breastfeed for at least 6 months or one year.

Participants

The target population was healthcare workers. This population was chosen because they are the first people to work with mothers if babies are born at the hospital and great target audience for giving breastfeeding information and skills. Knowing the beliefs and breastfeeding knowledge, and skills of health care workers in Ghana practices would provide information to tailor future educational training and interventions of this group.

Participants were recruited through a healthcare worker who assisted with the data collection. Criteria for participating included: being a healthcare worker and over 18 years old. Potential participants were encouraged to notify and refer other workers who fit the above criteria. Indiana University's Institutional Review Board approved this research project. Participants were provided with information about the purpose of the research project. Thirty-one participants participated in the study. The 31 participants sample was considered appropriate since they formed more than two-thirds of the people who worked at the hospital in the research area.

Analysis

Analysis of the data included a summary of their demographic data and using descriptive statistics to report their ages, educational background and their employment type. The survey data were put on a spreadsheet by the second author. Thematic analyses of the verbatim responses of the participants were made on the research questions. Entered survey reliability was checked by the lead author to make sure the information was recorded correctly. The lead author and a volunteer colleague coded transcripts. Each answered research question was put into theme(s).

We included verbatim quotations that emphasize what participants said within each theme. Participants' demographic information is presented in Table 1.

Table 1. Characteristics of participants

Age Demographics	Average Age:	32.96
	Age Range:	20 - 56
Relationship Status	Single, not married:	10
	Single, in a relationship:	11
	Married:	8
	Separated/Divorced:	1
	Did not provide response:	1
Employment Status	Full-Time:	25
	Part-Time:	3
	No response:	3

On the question of what problems could participants potentially come across as a healthcare provider on breastfeeding?

A majority of the participants reported that mothers who are sick do not want to breastfeed their children and even if they nursed their babies the babies are underfed and therefore become malnourished. Poor positioning and attachment of baby-to-breast were also reported by the healthcare providers as a problem in their hospitals. Others problems reported by the participants were: breast engorgement, breast abscess, crack nipples, infected nipples, mastitis, babies with no sucking reflexes, mothers who do not know how to breastfeed, mothers with small/little amount of breast milk and mothers with bilateral breast infections.

Some participants reported that some mothers had beliefs about exclusive breastfeeding that prevented them from nursing their children. Verbatim parents' beliefs about exclusive breastfeeding as reported are given below:

> Many mothers especially in the villages do not belief the 6 month exclusive breastfeeding because they thought it is some kind of punishment to the child

> Most mothers are not able to do exclusive breastfeeding due to the nature of their work and some wrong perception that children who are exclusively breastfed do not like food

> Doubt about breastfeeding and its importance

> Engorged breast, inverted nipples, no knowledge on breastfeeding, breast infection

> Mothers not adhering to proper breastfeeding, mothers sometimes listen to their mothers about how to breastfeed babies and not the instructions given to them from health care providers

> The problem is in a situation where the mothers refuse to give only breast milk for the babies in the first 6 months of birth. Just because they lack the knowledge about the importance of breastfeeding or breast milk to the child

> One breast contain water and the other breast contain milk

Concerning the healthcare workers' knowledge on skin–to– skin, a majority of the healthcare workers had not heard about skin-to-skin. Only twelve out of the thirty-one healthcare workers indicated that they had some knowledge about it.

Regarding what participants believe will encourage breastfeeding for at least six months or one year, this is what the participants wrote: teaching health education on the importance of breast milk to mothers and periodically teaching it to the public by emphasizing the fact that breast milk is the best food for infants. The healthcare providers also said it should be taught to families, that it is not expensive, it saves time, it could be used as a family planning method, and it protects the child and improves child growth. Also, participants wrote that demonstrating to mothers the positioning and attachment of the baby during breastfeeding will help both the mothers and babies. Participants also noted that using successful mothers to campaign on the importance of breast-milk to the family, the community and the nation as a whole, and having a national policy on breastfeeding, increasing duration of maternity leave to at least 6 months, adding breastfeeding to the secondary school curriculum and giving awards for successful breastfeeding families will all help increase exclusive breastfeeding in Ghana. Finally, a majority of the participants wrote that clarifying misconceptions about exclusive breastfeeding would help the country increase exclusive breastfeeding.

DISCUSSION

This paper makes contribution to breastfeeding practice and policy that are needed to increase exclusive breastfeeding in Ghana. The fact that majority of the healthcare workers had no knowledge on such an important terminology concept as skin–to -skin which contributes to successful initiation of breastfeeding had implication for practice. Specifically, it points to the fact that educators of healthcare providers will need to emphasize breastfeeding in child health courses. Also, since breast-milk is known as the best food for infant health (1) because it is tailored specifically for a particular child and it is known to cut down many childhood diseases (19), effort should be made to allocate resources to educate healthcare providers to assist in their efforts to help mothers. Assistance provided by healthcare workers will help mothers and their children to begin a quality of life free from malnourishment.

Concerning mothers' knowledge and misconceptions on breastfeeding, improved education as indicated by the healthcare workers and access to lactation educators should be used to help mothers improve their breastfeeding knowledge and hence improve their children's development and health.

It is important to note that this research surveyed mostly women healthcare workers from Cape Coast. Also it is important to say that this data are rich but lack generalization since the data were collected from one town and generalizations cannot be made for the whole country based on information acquired from just one town. Although we asked questions that were straight forward and carefully constructed in order for the respondents to understand what was being asked (18) and the questions were designed to encourage respondents to provide accurate, unbiased and complete information, we believe some participants may have misinterpreted some of the questions since we were not around when they filled the survey. Also, since it was self-reported, some participants may have had biases toward breastfeeding and may have overly reported or underreported their beliefs about breastfeeding; these might affect our results on participants' practice and beliefs about breastfeeding in Ghana.

In conclusion, this paper has revealed what healthcare workers believe will increase exclusive breastfeeding for children in the research area. The recommendations such as breastfeeding education to mothers, including breastfeeding in secondary school curriculum, giving incentives to families, and expelling misconceptions on breastfeeding will help mothers and their infants' health. Finally, if the above suggestions are implemented by all stakeholders of child-health this will help improve children's health and their quality of life in Ghana.

REFERENCES

[1] World Health Organization. Health topics: Breastfeeding, 2014. URL: http://www.who.int/topics/breastfeeding/en/.
[2] Bernaix LW. Nurses' attitudes, subjective norms, and behavioral intentions toward support of breastfeeding mothers. J Hum Lact 2000;16:201-9.
[3] Register N, Eren M, Lowdermilk D, Hammond R, Tully M. Knowledge and attitudes of pediatric office nursing staff about breastfeeding. J Hum Lact 2000;16(3):210-5.
[4] Spear HJ. Nurses' attitudes, knowledge, and beliefs related to the promotion of breastfeeding among women who bear children during adolescence. J Pediatr Nurs 2004;19(3):176-83.
[5] Obeng CS, Shiver A. Mothers shared their experiences on breastfeeding. Int J Child Health Hum Dev 2013; 6(3), in press.
[6] Oluwatosin AO. Nurses' knowledge of and attitudes to exclusive breastfeeding in South West Nigeria. Afr J Nurs Midwifery 2007; 9(1):73-81.

[7] Lu MC, Lange L, Slusser W, Hamilton J, Halfon N. Provider encouragement of breast-feeding: Evidence from a national survey. Obstet Gynecol 2001; 97:290–5.
[8] Bramhagen A, Axelsson I, Hallstrom I. Mothers' experiences of feeding situations – an interview study. J Clin Nurs 2006;15:29–34.
[9] Cox SG, Turnbull CJ. Breastfeeding – a gradual return to mother's autonomy. Breastfeed Rev 2000;8(2):5–8.
[10] Bentley ME, Dee DL, Jensen JL. Breastfeeding among low income, African-American women: Power, beliefs and decision making. J Nutr 2003;133(1):S305-9.
[11] Hannon PR, Willis SK, Bishop-Townsend V, Martinez IM, Scrimshaw SC. African-American and latina adolescent mothers' infant feeding decisions and breastfeeding practices: A qualitative study. J Adolesc Health 2000;26(6):399-407.
[12] Dykes F, Moran VH, Burt S, Edwards J. Adolescent mothers and breastfeeding: experiences and support needs- an exploratory study. J Hum Lact 2003;19(4):391–401.
[13] Hailes JF, Wellard SJ. Support for breastfeeding in the first postpartum month: perceptions of breastfeeding women. Breastfeed Rev 2000;8(3): 5–9.
[14] Humenick SS, Hill PD, Spiegelberg PL. Breastfeeding and health professional encouragement. J Hum Lact 1998;14(4):305–10.
[15] Hillenbrand KM, Larsen PG. Effect of an educational intervention about breastfeeding on the knowledge, confidence, and behaviors of pediatric resident physicians. Pediatrics 2002;110(5):e59.
[16] Kronborg H, Væth M, Olsen J, Harder I. Health visitors and breastfeeding support: influence of knowledge and self-efficacy. Eur J Public Health 2008;18(3):283-8.
[17] World Health Organization. Infant and young child feeding, 2014. URL: http://www.who.int/mediacentre/factsheets/fs342/en/.
[18] Crawford IM. QuestionnairedDesign. In: Crawford IM, ed. Marketing research and information wystems. Rome: Food Agriculture Organization United Nations, 1997. URL: http://www.fao.org/docrep/W3241E/w3241e05.htm.
[19] Bartick M, Reinhold A. The burden of sub-optimal breastfeeding in the United States: A pediatric cost analysis. Pediatrics 2010;125(5). doi: 10.1542/peds.2009-1616.

Submitted: March 20, 2014. *Revised:* May 22, 2014. *Accepted:* June 05, 2014.

In: Public Health Yearbook 2015
Editor: Joav Merrick
ISBN: 978-1-63484-514-4
© 2016 Nova Science Publishers, Inc.

Chapter 25

PRIAPISM IN SICKLE CELL DISEASE: NEED FOR IMPARTING SEX EDUCATION IN RURAL INDIA

Ranbir S Balgir*, MSc(Hons), PhD

Department of Biochemistry, Regional Medical Research Centre for Tribals (Indian Council of Medical Research), Jabalpur, Madhya Pradesh, Central India

ABSTRACT

The sickle cell hemoglobinopathy is a common disabling disease profoundly affects human morbidity, mortality and quality of life. Priapism in sickle cell disease is a condition that cause sustained, painful, and unwanted erection of the penis in boys or men without any sexual stimulation. Sickled cells are short lived and can cause vaso-occlusive crisis in affected persons. A few case reports from India have shown the rare occurrence of priapism in sickle cell disease in India. The present cross-sectional and hospital based study showed around 3% (2.97%) prevalence of priapism in cases suffering from sickle cell disease in a tertiary hospital at Jabalpur in Madhya Pradesh of Central India. It is a common practice in India that any problem related to sex or sex organs is intentionally not disclosed (kept secret) to elderly family members because of shyness or psycho-social implications or due to a stigma attached to it. It is never brought to the notice of a medical doctor. This is due to utter lack of sex education in rural areas, resulting in deteriorated sexual health and related complications. Priapism in sickle cell disease is a pathological condition of penile erection and recovery of the erectile function is dependent on prompt counseling and urgent intervention. Priapism in sickle cell disease should be considered as a medical and surgical emergency and should not be taken as lightly or ignored.

Keywords: priapism, sickle cell disease, ischemic priapism, stuttering, prevalence, rural India

---

* Correspondence: Ranbir S Balgir, PhD, Scientist F/Deputy Director (Senior Grade) & Head, Department of Biochemistry, Regional Medical Research Centre for Tribals (Indian Council of Medical Research), Near NSCB Medical College & Hospital, P.O: Garha, Nagpur Road, Jabalpur-482 003, Madhya Pradesh, Central India. E-mail: balgirrs@yahoo.co.in.

INTRODUCTION

Sickle cell anemia is a common hereditary disabling disorder profoundly affecting human morbidity, mortality and quality of life. The sickle cell disease (SCD) is an autosomal recessively inherited condition caused by a point mutation in the β-globin gene, resulting in substitution of the valine for glutamic acid at 6th position of the β-globin chain (Glu^6Val). This mutation results in abnormal sickle hemoglobin (Hb S) which is when deoxygenated, polymerizes damaging the sickle erythrocyte. Sickling is dependent on multiple variables including hemoglobin concentration, hydration status, pH and degree of deoxygenation. Sickling is more common in vascular beds with low-flow states including the splenic sinusoids, bone marrow, and the penile corpora during an erection, or in any inflamed tissue. The combined influence of these factors can result in a vicious cycle of inflammation, hypoxia, and acidosis resulting in increased sickling, vessel occlusion, and ischemia. Priapism is a patho-physiologically sustained, painful, and unwanted erection of the penis due to either increased arterial inflow (i.e., high flow) or more commonly, the failure of venous outflow (i.e., low flow or veno-occlusive flow) resulting in blood trapping within the erectile bodies. Although uncommon in the general population, priapism was recognized as a serious complication of the SCD as early as 1934 (1). Since then, many researchers have estimated its incidence and prevalence including various treatment strategies and choices in different populations.

Considering the embarrassing nature of the problem and the dire consequences to erectile function, it is important to inform patients, parents, and health providers about the relationship of SCD to prolonged painful erections. Ideally, patients at high risk for the development of such episodes should be identified early to increase the education of risks of prolonged priapism and to institute potential prophylactic strategies. Increased awareness of the signs of priapism and educational needs for early treatment may be the best way to prevent long term sequelae.

The occurrence of priapism since time immemorial is not uncommon in India. It is widely encountered in length and breadth of the country. It is a common practice in India that any problem related to sex or sex organs is intentionally kept hidden because of shyness or psycho-social implications or due to a stigma attached to it. It is never brought to the notice of elderly members of the family or to a medical doctor. Further, there is utter lack of sex education in India, resulting in deterioration of health related complications. The case of priapism especially its occurrence in sickle cell disease is one of such examples.

This article emphasizes the need of imparting sex education to rural masses especially associated with the sickle cell disease in India.

METHODS

This study was a part of our major ongoing research project undertaken on 'Reproductive Outcome in Carrier Couples of Hemoglobinopathies in a Tertiary Hospital in Central India.' Ethical approval of this project was obtained from the Human Ethical Committee, Regional Medical Research Centre for Tribals (ICMR), Jabalpur. A total of 1,279 subjects suspected to be suffering from anemia/hemoglobinopathies referred from a tertiary hospital, Netaji

Subhash Chandra Bose Medical College & Hospital, Jabalpur in Central India were screened for different hemoglobinopathies during the cross-section period from March 2010 to December 2012.

About 2-3ml. of blood was intravenously taken under aseptic conditions with disposable syringes and needles using disodium salt of ethylene diamine tetra acetic acid (EDTA) as anticoagulant after taking informed/written consent from each individual who was free of blood transfusion at least one month prior to screening for hemoglobinopathies. Blood so collected was transported to laboratory at RMRCT, Jabalpur under wet-cold conditions for analysis. All the adopted procedures and techniques standardized in the laboratory were followed for diagnosis as described elsewhere (2-4). Hematological indices were measured using MS_59 Hematological Analyzer (Melet and Schloesing Laboratories, Cergy-Pontoise Cedex, France).

Laboratory investigations were carried out following standard procedures. Some blood samples of doubtful cases were further subjected to confirmation by hemoglobin variant analysis (Bio-Rad Diagnostics Group, Hercules, California, USA). For quality control, results were cross-checked periodically. Family studies were carried out to confirm the diagnosis, wherever it was felt necessary.

RESULTS AND DISCUSSION

It is a matter of great concern for the Indian physicians that priapism in Indian sickle cell patients is prevalent, although its frequency is reported to be low because of several confounding factors. The present study does support this contention that priapism in the Indian sickle cell disease patients is not absent but prevalent in low frequency (3%) in India.

The penile erection normally occurs in response to physical or psychological stimulation. This stimulation causes certain blood vessels to relax and expand, increasing blood flow to spongy tissues in the penis. Blood vessels, that control the flow of blood out of the penis, contract and result in trapping of blood. Consequently, the blood-filled penis becomes erect. After stimulation ends, the blood flows out, and the penis returns to its non-rigid (flaccid) state or detumescence. Priapism probably results from abnormalities of the blood vessels and nerves that cause blood to become trapped in the erectile tissue (corpora cavernosa) of the penis. Thus, priapism occurs when some part of this system — the blood, blood vessels or nerves — changes normal blood flow. Subsequently, an unwanted erection persists. There are several factors that can contribute to priapism or to erectile dysfunction or impotence.

Priapism is a full or partial erection that persists for more than 4 hours. There are three kinds of priapism: ischemic priapism (veno-occlusive, low flow), stuttering priapism (recurrent ischemic priapism), and non-ischemic priapism (arterial, high flow). Ischemic priapism is a pathologic phenotype of SCD. Ischemic priapism is a urologic emergency when untreated priapism results in corporal fibrosis and erectile dysfunction.

The type and severity of complications vary significantly between individuals. Common manifestations include vaso-occlusive crises, the result of hypoxic injury or infarction, which may affect the brain, pulmonary vessels, spleen, bone marrow, kidney, retina, penis or other tissues resulting in sequelae such as acute chest syndrome with pulmonary infarction, stroke or splenic infarction. Splenic infarction and subsequent fibrosis ultimately contribute to increased susceptibility to infections from encapsulated bacteria leading to increased risk of septicemia and meningitis, the most common causes of death in children with SCD. Leg ulcers are another common manifestation of vaso-occlusion.

The average allele frequency of the sickle cell hemoglobinopathy has been observed to be 4.3% in India (5). The prevalence of the disease has been recorded to be high among some scheduled tribes, scheduled castes, other backward castes as well as among some general castes of central India (2). Sickle cell anemia is one of the most common causes of priapism, and is an inherited disorder characterized by abnormally shaped red blood cells. These abnormally shaped red cells can block the flow of blood and cause priapism.

The first reported case of priapism in patient with homozygous sickle cell disease was presented to the New York Society for Clinical Psychiatry as a 'castration fear complex' in 1932 (1), although Diggs and Ching (6) were the first to recognize this association with sickle cell disease. Subsequently, the priapism was recognized as a complication of sickle cell disease in various reports and reviews (7). Among the precipitating factors of priapism, may follow a sexual intercourse (8), masturbation (9), and alcohol ingestion (10), and other drugs (11). Other causes may be spontaneous nocturnal erections, night dreaming, night stuttering attacks, which cease during painful crises, but resume after resolution of the pains.

In the present cross-sectional and hospital based study, out of a total of 1279 subjects screened, 101 had homozygous sickle cell disease, and out of 101 patients (7.9%), 3 patients who were belonging to adjoining rural areas of Jabalpur town in Central India, and were affected with priapism, giving a prevalence rate of 2.97%. A summary of salient hematological findings and other features of three cases of priapism are presented in Table 1.

Sickle cell anemia is the most common cause of priapism in boys. There is a wide age range of onset of priapism but involvement in childhood under the age of 18 years has been reported common in sickle cell disease (13). Priapism appears rare among Indian and Eastern Province of Saudi Arabians even when they are directly asked (14-16). Priapism is most common in boys between ages 5 and 10 years old and in men from ages 20 to 50 years (17). In our series, the age of patients was 22, 23 and 24 years.

Priapism is an uncommon condition that needs immediate medical attention. Prompt treatment for priapism is usually needed to prevent tissue damage that results in the inability of the penis to become or stay erect with sexual arousal (erectile dysfunction). Ischemic priapism — the result of blood not being able to exit the penis — is an emergency situation that requires immediate treatment. The occlusion of the outflow vessels from the corpora cavernosa is most likely by sickled cells. The aspiration of the static reservoirs of the corpora yields a thick, dark-red, viscous fluid (18, 19) consisting of sickled cells (20). Priapism in homozygous sickle cell disease is of low-flow ischemic type, although high-flow priapism occurs and one case was treated by selective embolization of the cavernous and dorsal penile arteries (21). The mechanism of high-flow priapism in sickle cell disease is still unclear.

Among the characteristics of priapism in sickle cell disease is that it typically affects only the corpora cavernosa and spares the corpus spongiosum. In literature, two different patterns are observed: stuttering and major attacks (22, 23). Stuttering attacks are typically brief (< 3 h), nocturnal, recurrent, and are associated with normal intervening sexual function. They may act as a prodrome and are found to proceed to major attacks. Stuttering attacks may cause a loss of sleep and daytime sleepiness. Relief from stuttering episodes is most commonly sought by gentle exercise such as walking or cycling, ice or cold water directly applied to the penis, drinking cold water, passing urine, or by taking cold showers (22, 23).

Table 1. A comparative study of hematological parameters and other features in cases with priapism in sickle cell disease in Madhya Pradesh, India

Salient Features	Normal Range	Patient-1	Patient -2	Patient -3	Patient*	Patient*
Caste	-	Katiya (Scheduled Caste)	Goud (Scheduled Tribe)	Jharia (Scheduled Caste)	-	-
District	-	Balaghat	Jabalpur	Narsinghpur	-	-
Sex	Male	Male	Male	Male	Male	Male
Age (in years)	-	24	22	23	24	23
Hb (g/dl)	12-18	9.7	9.9	6.9	7.8	12.2
RBC(m/mm3)	4-5.9	4.5	3.9	2.1	-	-
MCV (fl)	83-98	76.9	78.2	100.5	80	82
HCT (%)	35-54	34.7	30.5	20.3	-	-
MCH (pg)	25-33	21.5	25.3	34.1	-	-
MCHC (g/dl)	28-40	28.0	32.4	33.9	31	30
RDW (%)	8-15.5	14.0	13.8	13.8	-	-
WBC(m/mm3)	3-14	5.1	11.7	4.6	-	-
PLT (m/mm3)	150-450	309	391	355	-	-
Hb F (%)	<2.0	16.4	6.3	2.7	5.8	22.8
Reticulocytes (%)	3-5	6.9	9.5	9.7	26	11.5
T. Serum Bilirubin	1-2.5mg/dl	5.4mg/dl	3.5mg/dl	4.2mg/dl	3.4mg/dl	2.5mg/dl
Type of Priapism	-	Ischemic	Stuttering	Ischemic	-	-
Treatment	-	Penis Blood Aspiration	Phenylephrine (Medication)	Glucose drip and Hydration	-	-
Red cell Morphology	-	Lymphocytosis, Hypochromia	Microcytosis, Normo-chromia	Lmphocytosis, Macrocytemia, Hemolytic Anemia	-	-

Table 1. (Continued)

Salient Features	Normal Range	Patient-1	Patient -2	Patient -3	Patient*	Patient*
Clinical Features	-	Pallor, Abdominal & Joint pains, H/o jaundice, Hepatomegaly (3-4cm), Splenomegaly (5-6 cm), Occasional epistaxis, Retarded growth and development, Premature cataract, H/o Blood trans-fusion, Painful priapism, Pains during urination, Bended Penis.	Pallor, Abdominal pains, Body ache, Bony or joint pains	Fatigue, Pallor H/o Jaundice, Joint pains, Splenomegaly (3-5cm)	Asymptomatic with fever, Abdominal pains, Severe painful erection	Enlarged swollen & soft Penis

*Data from reference No. 12.

It has been reported that major attacks usually exceed 24 h, do not recur, and are generally followed by impotence, although the prognosis is better in patients aged less than 15 years (22, 24, 25). Prompt recognition and appropriate treatment of a priapism episode in males with sickle cell disease is critical as the end result of prolonged and/or repeated episodes of priapism can be ischemia and fibrosis in the corpus cavernosa of the penis, potentially leading to impaired sexual function and impotence. They are characterized by extremely severe pain in the penis which may persist for several days. Pain may also occur in the lower abdomen and perianal region, and may be associated with dysuria (23, 26), acute urinary retention (27-30), penile and/or scrotal edema (31, 32) and a large, boggy, tender prostate (33). After a major attack, further episodes of either stuttering or major forms are mostly unusual.

Stuttering or recurring priapism is a form of ischemic priapism that occurs off and on. A stuttering erection is usually painful but generally lasts fewer than three hours.

A comparison of hematological characteristic features in patients (Table 1) with and without a history of priapism revealed that the priapism group has lower fetal hemoglobin levels and higher platelet counts (22). Other studies have also shown associated risk for priapism in hemolytic diseases. Lactate dehydrogenase (LDH), bilirubin and reticulocyte count were all elevated in men with SCD who experienced priapism compared with men with SCD who had never experienced an episode of priapism (33). The hematological findings of the present study are more or less consistent with the previous studies on the subject of priapism in sickle cell disease (22).

Thus, the priapism in sickle cell disease is under reported in India due to several confounding factors including the lack of sex education, although it is an emergency condition and needs immediate attention for medication, treatment, and the relief.

Conclusion

Priapism in sickle cell disease is a pathological condition of penile erection that persists beyond four hours or is unrelated to sexual stimulation. Clinically and pathologically, two subtypes are seen—the high flow (non-ischemic) variety and the low flow (ischemic) priapism. The low flow type is more dangerous as these patients are susceptible to greater complications and the long term recovery of erectile function is dependent on prompt and urgent intervention. As such, priapism should be considered as a medical and surgical emergency. Moreover, the priapism in sickle cell disease is not uncommon India but under reported due to poverty, ignorance, shyness, and psycho-social factors.

Acknowledgments

Author is grateful to Dr. V. M. Katoch, Secretary, Department of Health Research, Government of India, and Director General, Indian Council of Medical Research, New Delhi for the permission and providing the necessary research facilities.

Conflict of interest: Author declares no conflict of interest.

REFERENCES

[1] Obendorf CP. Priapism of psychogenic origin. Arch Neurol Psychiatr 1934;31:1292-96.
[2] Balgir RS. Public health challenges of sickle cell disorders, β-thalassemia syndrome and G6PD deficiency in scheduled caste and scheduled tribe communities of central
[3] India. Intl Public Health J 2011;3:307-18.
[4] Balgir RS. Hematological profile of pregnant women with carrier status of hemoglobin disorders in coastal Odisha, India. Int J Child Health Hum Dev 2011;4:325-32.
[5] Dacie JV, Lewis SM. Practical Hematology. 7th Edn. Edinburgh: Churchill Livingstone. 1991;227-58.
[6] Balgir RS. Genetic epidemiology of the three predominant abnormal hemoglobins in India. JAPI 1996;44:25-28.
[7] Diggs LW, Ching RE. Pathology of sickle cell anemia. Southern Med J 1934;27:839- 45.
[8] Hasen HB, Raines SL. Priapism associated with sickle cell disease. J Urol 1962;88:71- 76.
[9] Krauss L, Fitzpatrick T. The treatment of priapism by penile aspiration under controlled hypotension. J Urol 1961;85:595-98.
[10] Karayalcin G, Imran M, Rosner F. Priapism in sickle cell disease: report of five cases. Am J Med Sci 1972;264:289-93.
[11] Conrad ME, Perrine GM, Barton JC, Durant JR. Provoked priapism in sickle cell anemia. Am J Hemat 1980;9:121-22.
[12] Kassim AA, Fabry ME, Nagel RL. Acute priapism associated with the use of sildenafil in a patient with sickle cell trait. Blood 2000; 95:1878-79.
[13] Dash BP, Kar BC. Priapism is rare in sickle cell disease in India. JAPI 2000;48:255.
[14] Winter CC, McDowell G. Experience with 105 patients with priapism: update review of all aspects. J Urol 1988;140:980-83.
[15] Al-Awamy B, Taha SA, Naeem MA. Priapism in association with sickle cell anemia. Acta Haematol 1985;73:181-82.
[16] Kar BC, Satapathy RK, Kulozik AE, Kulozik M, Sirr S, Serjeant BE, Serjeant GR. Sickle cell disease in Orissa State, India. Lancet 1986; ii:1198-201.
[17] Padmos MA, Roberts GT, Sackey K, Kulozik A, Bail S, Morris JS, Serjeant BE, Serjeant GR. Two different forms of homozygous sickle cell disease occur in Saudi Arabia. Br J Haematol 1991;79:93-98.
[18] Serjeant GR, Serjeant BE. Sickle Cell Disease. 3rd Edn. Oxford: Oxford University. 2001; 326-30.
[19] Rosokoff J, Brodie EL. Priapism complicating sickle cell anemia: a case report. J Urol 1946;56:544-46.
[20] Gillenwater JY, Burros HM, Kornblith PL. Priapism as the first and terminal manifestation of sickle cell disease. Southern Med J 1968; 61:133-38.
[21] Diggs LW. Sickle cell crises. Am J Clin Pathol 1965;44:1-19.
[22] Ramos CE, Park JS, Ritchey ML, Benson GS. High flow priapism associated with sickle cell disease. J Urol 1995;153:1619-21.
[23] Emond AM, Holman R, Hayes RJ, Serjeant GR. Priapism and impotence in homozygous sickle cell disease. Arch Intern Med 1980;140:1434-37.
[24] Fowler JE, Koshy M, Strub M, Chinn SK. Priapism associated with the sickle cell hemoglobinopathies: prevalence, natural history and sequelae. J Urol 1991;145:65-68.
[25] Sharpsteen JR, Powars D, Johnson C, Rogers ZR, Williams WD, Posch RJ. Multisystem damage associated with tricorporal priapism in sickle cell disease. Am J Med 1993;94: 289-95.
[26] Chakrabarty A, Upadhyay J, Dhabuwala CB, Sarnaik S, Perlmutter AD, Connor JP. Priapism associated with sickle cell hemoglobinopathy in children: long-term effects on potency. J Urol 1996;155:1419-23.

[27] Erman S, Bloomberg HH. Priapism in sickle cell anemia: treatment by estrogenic hormone. J Urol 1960;84:345-46.
[28] Grace DA, Winter CC. Priapism: an appraisal of management of twenty three patients. J Urol 1968; 99:301-10.
[29] Seeler RA. Intensive transfusion therapy for priapism in boys with sickle cell anemia. J Urol 1973;110:360-61.
[30] Noe HN, Wilimas J, Jerkins GR. Surgical management of priapism in children with sickle cell anemia. J Urol 1981;126:770-71.
[31] Sawan E, Cawley RD. Priapism due to thrombosis in sickle cell anemia. Clin Proc Child Hospital Washington DC 1947;3:241-43.
[32] Baron M, Leiter E. The management of priapism in sickle cell anemia. J Urol 1978;119: 610-11
[33] Arduinc LJ. Urological complications of sickle cell disease. Am Surg 1954;29:1213-18.
[34] Nolan VG, Wyszynski DF, Farrer LA, Steinberg MH. Hemolysis-associated priapism in sickle cell disease. Blood. 2005;106:3264–67.

Submitted. April 02, 2014. *Revised:* May 28, 2014. *Accepted:* June 06, 2014.

In: Public Health Yearbook 2015
Editor: Joav Merrick

ISBN: 978-1-63484-514-4
© 2016 Nova Science Publishers, Inc.

Chapter 26

WHO DO SMOKERS FEEL OUGHT TO BE RESPONSIBLE FOR INFORMING PEOPLE ABOUT THE DANGERS ASSOCIATED WITH SMOKING AND REGULATING SMOKING BEHAVIORS?

Claire E Sterk[1], PhD, Hugh Klein[1,2], PhD, and Kirk W Elifson[1], PhD

[1]Rollins School of Public Health, Emory University, Atlanta, Georgia, United States of America
[2]Kensington Research Institute, Silver Spring, Maryland, United States of America

ABSTRACT

Purpose: The focus of this paper is to examine the extent to which a community-based sample of current cigarette smokers believes it to be the responsibility of outside persons and agencies to inform the public about the dangers of smoking and/or to regulate smoking behaviors (herein termed REGULATE). Also investigated is how REGULATE relates to smokers' attitudes toward cigarette smoking and actual smoking practices, and whether REGULATE matters when the influence of other key variables is taken into account.
Method: Questionnaire-based interviews were conducted with a community-based sample of 485 adult current cigarette smokers recruited from the Atlanta, Georgia metropolitan area. Active and passive recruiting approaches were used, along with a targeted sampling strategy.
Results: Participants were divided in their beliefs pertaining to REGULATE. Their beliefs were related consistently to smoking-related attitudes but much less to actual smoking behaviors. Four factors (greater religiosity, older age of first purchasing a cigarette, lower levels of depression, and sexual abuse history) were found to underlie REGULATE. Structural equation analysis revealed that REGULATE is an influential measure to consider when trying to understand overall attitudes toward smoking and actual smoking behaviors.

Conclusion: REGULATE is an important variable to consider when aiming to understand the factors associated with how people feel about their smoking practices, including actual cigarette use. It may be construed as a proxy measure for locus of control; and the implications of this are discussed.

Keywords: cigarette smoking, tobacco regulation, locus of control

INTRODUCTION

Locus of control is defined as the extent to which people perceive themselves as having the ability or "agency" to determine what happens to them versus believing that outside forces and/or other persons are, to a greater extent, responsible for their experiences and actions. When discussing locus of control, researchers typically conceptualize people falling onto a continuum that is bounded, on one side, by those who are internally oriented (believing in their own ability to determine their own fate and experiences) and, on the other side, those who are externally oriented (believing that what happens to them is the result of outside forces that are beyond their personal control). Locus of control has been linked to a variety of health practices, such as cigarette smoking and tobacco cessation (1–3), smoking during pregnancy (4), substance use and abuse (5), healthy eating practices (1), and risky sexual behaviors (5), among others. This had led researchers to coin the term "health locus of control" to apply the underlying principles of locus of control to the scientific study and understanding of people's health practices (6–8). Typically, research has found that people who are more internally oriented when it comes to locus of control tend to engage in lower rates of risky behaviors and higher rates of behavioral practices that can be considered to be beneficial or health protective in nature (2, 6, 9).

Closely related to the notions of locus of control and health locus of control is the construct of "powerful others" (10). Powerful others are people or institutions that are perceived as being dominant, persuasive, influential, and/or controlling in terms of determining how events in one's life unfold. For persons who score higher on the external rather than the internal end of the locus of control continuum, powerful others are construed as being the principal source and the main underlying force of their experiences and actions, to the point where the individuals themselves believe that they have limited, if any, responsibility or agency for their life events. Research has demonstrated that people whose locus of control orientation supports the belief in powerful others are more apt to have adverse substance use/abuse outcomes than their peers who are not oriented toward believing in the importance of powerful others (1, 11).

In the present paper, the focus is on one specific measure that, conceptually, may be construed as a proxy for internal/external locus of control–namely, the extent to which people believe that outside persons, organizations, and agencies (such as public health agencies and tobacco companies) ought to be responsible for informing the public about the potential health hazards of smoking and for regulating the public's access to and usage of cigarettes. In this article, we examine the following research questions: 1) To what extent do adult smokers believe that it should be the responsibility of these "powerful others" to inform the public about the dangers of smoking and to regulate tobacco use in the United States? 2) How, if at all, does adhering to the external orientation locus of control-related belief in other persons and agencies being responsible for informing the public and regulating tobacco use relate to actual smoking practices and to smokers' attitudes toward smoking? 3) What factors underlie greater versus lesser adherence to the belief that outside persons and agencies should be responsible for providing the public with information about the dangers of smoking and with regulating cigarette use/policy? 4) When we try to understand the factors that affect people's smoking behaviors, does the extent to which they believe that outside persons and agencies should be responsible for providing the public with information about the dangers of smoking and with regulating cigarette use/policy matter when the effects of other relevant variables are taken into account?

As part of addressing the latter three questions, we employ a conceptual model (see Figure 1) that owes its origins to syndemics theory (12). One of the principal tenets of syndemics theory is that certain types of influences may co-occur in such a manner so as to heighten the effects of one another and thereby make adverse health outcomes even more severe than they would have been had these measures not co-occurred. In the model used in the present research, four types of measures are hypothesized to interact syndemically with one another in the way that they influence one another, the main smoking-related outcome measure, *and* the REGULATE endogenous measure. These are 1) demographic characteristics, 2) lifetime maltreatment experiences, 3) early-life/initial smoking practices and 4) psychological/psychosocial functioning. In other published studies (13-17), syndemics theory has been used to study a wide array of populations and health behaviors, almost always including substance use/abuse measures as part of the analyses.

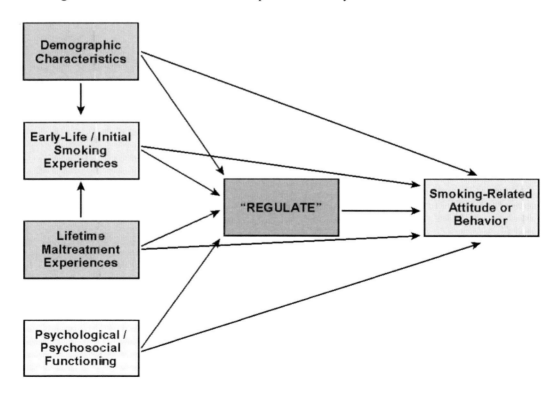

Figure 1. Conceptual Model.

Worth noting is the fact that only a few published studies have specifically included measures of smoking behaviors in their syndemic-focused models (18, 19). Interestingly, to the present authors' knowledge, no other published study has utilized syndemics theory to examine smoking behaviors as an outcome measure, thus enabling the present study to make an important and unique contribution to the scientific literature.

METHODS

The data presented in this paper are part of the *Persistent Smokers Project (PSP)* in Atlanta, Georgia. The community-based sample of 485 current smokers is distinct from those reported in many other studies, which have been based on younger, school-based research populations or those recruited at clinics or other institutional settings. Data were collected between September 2004 and July 2007. To be eligible, the participants had to be aged 18 years or older and reside in the Atlanta metropolitan area. Study participants had to have smoked at least 100 cigarettes during their lifetime (which is consistent with the National Health Interview Survey (NHIS) classification (20) as "ever smoked") and have smoked in the last week (which is consistent with the NHIS classification (20) as "current smoker").

Participant recruitment involved purposive sampling, including a combination of active and passive recruitment techniques. Using a short screening form, potential study participants were screened in the setting where they were recruited, such as near office buildings or other work locations, at restaurants, in social entertainment settings, in parks, and in other public settings. Passive recruitment involved posting flyers in local venues such as stores, restaurants, and community centers. Interested individuals, who called the project phone line listed on the flyers, initially were screened over the phone using the same short form used in the active recruitment. Two-thirds of the respondents ($n = 325$) were brought into the study via active recruitment, with the remaining one-third being identified through passive recruitment ($n = 160$). We did not identify any significant difference in the sample characteristics or in the outcome variables based on the recruitment strategy.

Once a person was identified as eligible, the staff member described the study and time required to participate. The most common reason for ineligibility was having smoked an insufficient number of cigarettes to qualify, either during the person's lifetime or during the preceding week. The interviews took place at a mutually-convenient location, such as one of the project offices, the respondent's home, a local restaurant or coffee shop, or at community centers. Additional information was provided on the nature of the study, the time required, and the informed consent and other confidentiality procedures. The questionnaire contained items covering the respondent's social background characteristics, smoking behaviors, attitudes, and opinions, as well as items about alcohol and other drugs, a health inventory, and self and identity items. The average length of the interview as 90 minutes and respondents received $20 as compensation for their time and participation. Prior to implementation in the field, all study protocols were reviewed and approved by the institutional review boards at Emory University and Georgia State University.

Measures used

The principal variable of interest in this paper is a 15-item scale (Cronbach's alpha = 0.78) that was created specifically for use in this study, based on formative research conducted by the study's investigators. Throughout the remainder of this paper, in an effort to keep verbiage to a minimum and to keep the writing simpler and easier to read/follow, this scale measure will be referred to as REGULATE. Taken as a group, the items comprising REGULATE assess the extent to which study participants believe that it ought to be the responsibility of outside persons and agencies to regulate smoking, to inform the public about the dangers associated with smoking, and to put into place various laws to regulate when and where smoking can occur legally.

Table 1. Perceptions of the Responsibilities of Outside Persons and Agencies to Inform the Public about the Potential Dangers of Smoking and/or to Regulate Smoking Behaviors

REGULATE Measure	% Agree	% Disagree
Cigarette companies should be required to provide more information about how to stop smoking.	54.3	45.7
Cigarette companies should be required to provide more information about the health risks of smoking.	64.1	35.9
Cigarette companies should be required to provide more information about how to get screened for the diseases caused by smoking.	63.4	36.6
Cigarette companies should be required to provide more information about chemicals in cigarette smoke.	77.5	22.5
Public health agencies should be required to provide more information about how to stop smoking.	72.7	27.3
Public health agencies should be required to provide more information about the health risks of smoking.	73.8	26.2
Public health agencies should be required to provide more information about how to get screened for the diseases caused by smoking.	74.6	25.4
Public health agencies should be required to provide more information about chemicals in cigarette smoke.	76.7	23.3
Regulation of smoking in public spaces is a good thing.	69.2	19.8
Smoking should be permitted in bars.	11.6	79.6
Smoking on television or in movies should be prohibited.	25.0	64.1
Taxes on cigarettes should be increased.	14.7	76.9
Smoking should not be permitted in restaurants.	55.0	30.2
Smoking bans should be unconstitutional.	49.1	29.3
I have a right to smoke anywhere I want.	72.2	19.2

NOTE: In some instances, the percentages do not add up to 100% due to the exclusion of "neutral" or "don't know: responses from this table.

Table 1 shows the items comprising this scale measure. Individual items used in the construction of REGULATE were scored on a five-point Likert scale with responses ranging from "strongly disagree" to "strongly agree." As appropriate, individual items have been recorded so that higher scores on the scale indicate a greater belief or perception that outside persons or agencies ought to be more responsible for informing the public and/or for regulating smoking behaviors.

To examine Research Question #2, 13 behavioral and 11 attitudinal/psychosocial measures were used. Regarding the former, *number of cigarettes smoked* was assessed based on the number of cigarettes smoked per week (continuous measure). This was computed from the number of days respondents reported having smoked during the preceding month, the average number of cigarettes smoked on a typical weekday, and the average number of cigarettes smoked over the course of a typical weekend. *Needing a cigarette to function* was derived from the question "How often do you feel that you need a cigarette to help you function?" Response choices were: "never" (coded as 0), "less than once a month" (1), "about once a month" (2), "a few times a month" (3), "about once a week" (4), "several times a week" (5), "daily" (6), and "every 2-3 hours or more often" (7). *Making a special trip to get cigarettes* involved the question "How often do you make special trips to get cigarettes?" *Chain smoking frequency* was assessed by asking "How often do you chain-smoke, that is, smoke one cigarette right after another?" *Smoking more than intended* was derived from the question "How often do you smoke more cigarettes than you intend to smoke?" Response choices for these last three measures were "never" (coded as 0), "less than once a month" (1), "about once a month" (2), "a few times a month" (3), "about once a week" (4), "several times a week" (5), and "daily" (6). *Trying to get the most out of one's smoking* was an eight-item scale (all items coded yes/no) measuring the number of different things (e.g., smoking a cigarette to a shorter length, inhaling more deeply, removed a cigarette's filter, holding cigarette smoke inside one's lungs longer prior to exhaling) that smokers did in an effort to maximize the effects of their cigarette use (Kuder-Richardson$_{20}$ = 0.68). *The number of times trying to quit smoking* and *the number of times trying to cut down on smoking without actively trying to quit* were both continuous measures. Twenty-one yes/no items were used to develop a scale to assess *the number of different ways that the person tried to quit smoking* (e.g., used medication to help stop smoking, stopped buying cigarettes from the store, used gum or candy to help stop smoking, used a nicotine lozenge). This scale assessed the variety of strategies that people employed to try to quit smoking (Kuder-Richardson$_{20}$ = 0.78). Among persons who had previously tried to quit smoking, the final scale assessed *the number of negative effects the person experienced* the last time he/she tried to quit smoking. Sixteen yes/no items (e.g., became irritable, felt impatient, inability to think clearly, felt frustrated) comprised this scale (Kuder-Richardson$_{20}$ = 0.90). *Smoking more cigarettes on weekends* was assessed with a single yes/no item, as were *lying to friends and relatives about one's smoking practices* and *whether or not people had ever tried to quit smoking at any point in the past*.

The perceived benefits of smoking (the first of the attitudinal/psychosocial measures) was assessed via 16 items scored in a five-point Likert fashion, with responses ranging from "strongly disagree" to "strongly agree" (Cronbach's alpha = 0.81). Examples of items comprising this scale include "Smoking energizes me" and "Smoking calms me down when I feel nervous" and "Cigarettes can really make me feel good." *The perceived negative consequences of smoking* was assessed via four items scored in similar fashion to the previous scale (Cronbach's alpha = 0.82), with examples including such measures as "Smoking is hazardous to my health" and "By smoking, I risk heart disease and lung cancer." *The number of reasons for continuing to smoke* was assessed via a nine-item scale (Cronbach's alpha = 0.69), with all items again scored using a five-point Likert fashion, with responses ranging from "strongly disagree" to "strongly agree." Constituent items included such measures as continuing to smoke due to physical dependence, as a form of weight control, to help in social situations, and coping with negative feelings. *The perceived level of safety of light cigarettes* is another scale (Cronbach's alpha = 0.85), assessed by eight items scored on a five-point Likert scale with responses ranging from "definitely not true" to "definitely true." It included statements such as "Light cigarettes are healthier" and "Light cigarettes give you less tar." *Perceived extent of cigarette industry efforts to make smoking safer* is a scale measure comprised by six yes/no items, asking respondents whether they believed that Big Tobacco had been taking steps such as adding filters to make cigarettes less dangerous, reducing the amount of tar in cigarettes, and removing additives to cigarettes (Kuder-Richardson$_{20}$ = 0.84). *Having a negative self-view as a result of smoking* is a 32-item scale measure (Cronbach's alpha = 0.87), comprised by items scored on a five-point Likert scale with responses ranging from "strongly disagree" to "strongly agree." It included such items as hating the way one smells after smoking, feeling looked down upon because of one's smoking, and perceiving oneself to be viewed as a criminal by others as a result of one's smoking. *Having friends and relatives complain about one's smoking* was a scale comprised by seven yes/no items (Kuder-Richardson$_{20}$ = 0.74) that addressed such issues as friends complaining about the residual odor resulting from smoking, the amount of money that the person has spent on cigarettes, and how smoking has affected their health. Two separate scales assessed *the number of reasons the person had for wanting to quit smoking* (14 yes/no items; Kuder-Richardson$_{20}$ = 0.81) and *the number of reasons the person had for wanting to reduce his/her cigarette use without quitting* (12 yes/no items; Kuder-Richardson$_{20}$ = 0.84). People's *overall attitudes toward quitting smoking* were assessed via an 18-item scale (Cronbach's alpha = 0.71) comprised by five-point Likert-scored items with responses ranging from "strongly disagree" to "strongly agree." Examples of items in this scale include: "I would quit if I knew I would not gain weight" and "I need to be ready before I will even try to quit smoking" and "I need to have a good reason to quit." Higher scores on this scale indicate a greater overall willingness to consider quitting smoking. *Perceived riskiness of smoking* was another scale measure (Cronbach's alpha = 0.71), assessed in a similar fashion, utilizing six items such as "Cigarettes still have not been proven to cause cancer" and "Lung cancer has more to do with genetics than with actual smoking" and "Pollution causes more lung cancer than does cigarette smoking."

To examine Research Question #3, which examined the factors underlying higher/lower scores on REGULATE, items from four domains–demographic characteristics, earlier-life or initial smoking practices, lifetime maltreatment experiences, and psychological/psychosocial functioning–were used. *Demographic characteristics* included in this part of the analysis were: gender (male versus female), age (continuous measure), race (coded as African American versus all others), employment status (unemployed versus employed), educational attainment (continuous measure), marital/relationship status ("involved" versus not "involved"), and religiosity (a three-item scale measure; Cronbach's alpha = 0.79). Two *earlier-life or initial smoking practices* measures were examined: age of first time smoking a cigarette (continuous measure) and age of first time purchasing a cigarette (continuous measure). *Lifetime maltreatment experiences* were assessed with three measures asking people the number of times during their lifetime that they had experienced emotional abuse, physical abuse, or sexual abuse. For analytical purposes, in this paper, each item was dichotomized into "ever experienced" and "never experienced" each type of maltreatment. Six scales measuring various aspects of *psychological or psychosocial functioning* were utilized in this part of the analysis. They were: sociability (derived from Watson and Friend's (21) *Social Avoidance and Distress Scale*) (11 items; Cronbach's alpha = 0.89), social isolation (11 items; Cronbach's alpha = 0.87), depression (the *Center for Epidemiologic Studies Depression (CES-D)* scale (22)) (20 items; Cronbach's alpha = 0.90), perceived predictability/randomness of events in one's life (derived from Schuessler's (23) *Doubt about Self-Determination Scale*) (12 items; Cronbach's alpha = 0.75), impulsiveness (derived from Zuckerman et al. (24) *Zuckerman-Kuhlman Personality Questionnaire*) (12 items; Cronbach's alpha = 0.81), and self-esteem (Rosenberg's (25) *Self-Esteem Scale*) (10 items; Cronbach's alpha = 0.86).

Analysis

Research Question #1–pertaining to how study participants feel about the prospect of having outside persons and agencies provide information about and regulate smoking practices–is analyzed with the use of descriptive statistics. In most instances, because the attitudinal and behavioral outcome measures in question are continuous variables (as is the REGULATE measure that serves as the focal point for this study), Research Question #2–examining how REGULATE relates to smoking-related attitudes and smoking practices–was analyzed via the computation of zero-order correlation coefficients (Pearson's r). The only exceptions to this were the three yes/no behavioral outcomes items (smoking more on weekends, lying to friends/relatives about smoking, ever tried to quit smoking), for which logistic regression was deemed to be the more appropriate analytical approach.

For Research Question #3–identifying the factors underlying higher/lower scores on REGULATE–the analysis was undertaken in two steps. Initially, bivariate analyses were conducted to learn which items were found to be related to REGULATE. Whenever the independent variable was dichotomous in nature (e.g., gender, race, any lifetime physical abuse), Student's t tests were performed to ascertain whether the comparison groups differed from one another on the dimension in question. Whenever the independent variable was continuous in nature (e.g., religiosity, age, self-esteem), the bivariate analyses entailed the use of correlation coefficients. Subsequently, items found to be associated with REGULATE in the bivariate analyses either significantly (i.e., $p < .05$) or marginally (i.e., $.10 > p > .05$) were entered into a multiple regression equation, to determine which ones contributed to the REGULATE scale scores when the effects of the other measures were taken into account. Items that were nonsignificant were removed from the equation in stepwise fashion, until a final "best fit" model containing only statistically-significant measures was derived.

For Research Question #4–determining whether REGULATE remains influential in the prediction of attitudes toward smoking and/or actual smoking behaviors when the effects of other relevant measures were taken into account–the analysis entailed a three-step process. The first two steps were similar to those described for Research Question #3, but using REGULATE as one of the independent variables instead of using it as the dependent variable in question. In these analyses, a smoking-related attitudinal measure or a smoking behavioral outcome measure served as the dependent variable; and separate multivariate analyses were performed for each outcome measure in question. The third step in this part of the analysis entailed subjecting the multivariate findings to structural equation analysis, to determine whether or not the relationships identified in the multivariate analyses "hold up" when considered as a totality. Separate structural equation analyses were undertaken for each of the different outcome measures. SAS's PROC CALIS procedure was used to assess the overall fit of each model to the data. When we use this type of structural equation analysis, we look for several specific outcomes, including 1) an appropriate goodness-of-fit index, 2) an acceptable Bentler-Bonett normed fit index value, 3) an overall chi-square value for the model that is statistically *non*significant, and 4) a root mean square error approximation value close to zero. If these conditions are met, then the relationships depicted are considered to indicate a good fit with the data. Throughout the analyses, results are reported as statistically significant whenever $p < .05$.

RESULTS

Slightly more than one-half of the study participants (56.8%) were male. Most respondents were either Caucasian (54.6%) or African American (39.0%). The median age was 34 (range = 18–70, mean = 36.4, $s.d.$ = 12.3). This is a fairly well-educated sample, with 34.2% of the respondents having completed college and an additional 40.6% having attended college without completing it. Although most (55.1%) of the study participants were employed on a full-time basis, substantial proportions of them were working on a part-time basis (32.9%) or unemployed (12.0%). Respondents were relatively evenly split between those who were single (42.7%) or involved in a marital-type relationship (44.5%). Approximately one person in six (16.5%) self-identified as gay, lesbian, or bisexual.

Research Question #1 – How do people feel about the regulation of smoking-related behaviors?

Overall, summed across all items comprising the REGULATE scale, approximately one-half of the study participants (51.3%) scored in the moderate range in terms of their beliefs about the extent to which outside agencies ought to be responsible for informing the public about the potential dangers of smoking and/or to regulate cigarette smoking practices (see Table 1).

Very few people gave responses indicating that they did not feel that these duties were important and incumbent upon outside agencies and regulators (2.5%) or, alternatively, that they felt strongly that outside agencies and persons should be responsible for informing the public about the potential dangers of smoking and/or to regulate cigarette smoking practices (1.0%). Respondents were about equally likely to score in the lower-moderate part of the range versus in the moderately-high part of the range on the REGULATE scale (25.4% versus 19.8%, respectively).

As Table 1 shows, there were large differences from item to item in terms of respondents' likelihood of endorsing a particular measure. For example, approximately three-quarters of the study participants believed that cigarette companies and public health agencies should be required to provide more information about the chemicals in cigarette smoke (77.5% and 76.7%, respectively), public health agencies should be required to provide more information about how to get screened for the diseases caused by smoking (74.6%), public health agencies should be required to provide more information about the health risks of smoking (73.8%), and public health agencies should be required to provide more information about how people can stop smoking (72.7%). In contrast, most study participants believed that: smoking portrayals should not be prohibited on television or in movies (64.1%) or that taxes on cigarettes should not be increased (76.9%).

Table 1 shows that participants in this study believed that it was incumbent upon public health agencies (and to a slightly lesser extent, cigarette companies) to provide more information to the public about how to control smoking behaviors, while these same people were less inclined to agree with measures that would implement and enforce tobacco/smoking control policies.

Research Question #2 – How do people's views regarding smoking regulation relate to their actual smoking behaviors and to their actual attitudes toward smoking?

Although not all measures demonstrated a relationship between REGULATE and people's actual smoking-related perceptions and behaviors, most did (see Table 2). This was true for the perception and behavioral items alike.

Regarding the former (i.e., smoking-related perceptions), as Table 2 demonstrates, endorsement of REGULATE was associated with: adhering to a greater overall perception that smoking yields a variety of benefits for the smoker ($r = .19$, $p < .001$), adhering to a greater overall perception that smoking causes a variety of adverse consequences for the smoker ($r = .19$, $p < .001$), having a larger number of reasons for continuing to smoke cigarettes ($r = .17$, $p < .001$), perceiving so-called light cigarettes not to be safer to smoke than regular cigarettes ($r = -.11$, $p = .013$), having a more negative self-view as a result of one's smoking practices ($r = .21$, $p < .001$), adhering to a larger number of reasons for wanting to quit smoking ($r = .27$, $p < .001$), adhering to a larger number of reasons for wanting to cut down on one's tobacco use rather than quitting smoking altogether ($r = .28$, $p < .001$), having more-favorable attitudes toward quitting smoking ($r = .12$, $p = .011$), and a greater perception that smoking carries with it a variety of risks ($r = .31$, $p < .001$). Regarding the latter (i.e., behavioral outcomes), endorsement of REGULATE was found to be related to: smoking fewer cigarettes per week ($r = -.18$, $p < .001$), a greater number of previous times having tried to quit smoking ($r = .10$, $p = .028$), a greater number of different methods for having tried to quit smoking in the past ($r = .18$, $p < .001$), less frequent experiences of needing a cigarette in order to function properly ($r = -.11$, $p = .014$), and chain smoking less frequently ($r = -.14$, $p = .002$).

In addition to the preceding, logistic regression analysis revealed that REGULATE was not related to whether or not study participants smoked more cigarettes on weekends ($OR = 0.997$, $CI_{95} = 0.67–1.48$, n.s.) or to whether or not they lied to others about their smoking practices ($OR = 1.50$, $CI_{95} = 0.96–2.35$, $p = .074$). Conversely, the more that people endorsed the items comprising the REGULATE scale, the more likely they were to report having tried to quit smoking at least once before ($OR = 2.10$, $CI_{95} = 1.25–3.53$, $p = .005$).

Table 2. The Relationship between Perceptions Regarding the Regulation of Smoking and Actual Smoking Behaviors and Smoking-Related Attitudes

Smoking Behavior	Correlation Coefficient	Statistical Significance
Number of cigarettes smoked per week	−.18	<.001
Doing things to get the most out of smoking	.02	n.s.
Perceived positive benefits experienced by smoking	.19	<.001
Perceived negative consequences experienced by smoking	.19	<.001
Number of reasons for continuing to smoke	.17	<.001
Perceived level of safety of smoking light cigarettes	−.11	.013
Perceived extent of cigarette industry's efforts to make smoking safer over the years	−.08	.067
Extent of having negative self-view due to smoking	.21	<.001
Extent to which nonsmoking friends/relatives have commented negatively or complained about one's smoking	.06	n.s.
Number of times trying to cut down (but not quit) on smoking	.05	n.s.
Number of times trying to quit smoking	.10	.028
Number of reasons for wanting to quit smoking	.27	<.001
Number of reasons for wanting to cut down (not quit) smoking	.28	<.001
Number of different ways the person has tried to quit smoking	.18	<.001
Overall attitude toward quitting smoking	.12	.011
Number of negative effects experienced the last time the person attempted to quit smoking (among quit attempters only)	.05	n.s.
Extent to which person perceives smoking to be risky	.31	<.001
Frequency of needing a cigarette in order to function properly	−.11	.014
Frequency of making special trips in order to get cigarettes	−.05	n.s.
Frequency of chain smoking	−.14	.002
Frequency of smoking more than originally intended	.06	n.s.

Research Question #3 – What factors underlie people's views regarding the regulation of smoking practices?

Bivariate analyses revealed several variables that were related either significantly or marginally to REGULATE. In terms of the *demographic measures* examined, African Americans scored somewhat higher on REGULATE than members of other racial groups did (2.32 versus 2.25; $t = 1.66$, $p =.097$). There was a slight tendency for REGULATE to be endorsed more with advancing age ($r =.09$, $p =.060$). People who were unemployed at the time of their interview were somewhat less inclined to support REGULATE than their employed counterparts were (2.18 versus 2.29; $t = 1.76$, $p =.078$). The more religious people were, the more apt they were to endorse the REGULATE items ($r =.09$, $p =.043$).

Two *earlier-life or initial smoking practices* measures were examined, and were found to be related to people's responses to the REGULATE scale items. The older people were the first time they smoked a cigarette, the more likely they tended to endorse the REGULATE items ($r =.08$, $p =.093$). Similarly, the older they were the first time they purchased a cigarette, the more supportive of REGULATE they were ($r =.15$, $p =.001$).

Some of the *lifetime maltreatment experiences* measures were found to be related to REGULATE as well. People who had experienced emotional abuse at some point during their lifetimes tended to endorse the REGULATE items more than their never-emotionally-abused counterparts (2.30 versus 2.17; $t = 2.41$, $p = .016$). Persons who had been sexually abused were also more apt to support REGULATE than their counterparts who had not been subjected to such abuse (2.34 versus 2.25; $t = 1.86$, $p = .063$). Such a relationship was not found for physical abuse, however.

Similarly, some but not all of the *psychological/psychosocial functioning* measures were found to be related to REGULATE. Higher scores on REGULATE were found to be associated with: lower levels of social isolation ($r = -.11$, $p = .021$), greater belief in the randomness or unpredictability of events ($r = .09$, $p = .046$), lower levels of depression ($r = -.12$, $p = .011$), and lower levels of impulsiveness ($r = -.10$, $p = .036$) but not with sociability ($r = .05$, $p = .255$) or self-esteem ($r = .07$, $p = .132$).

When the appropriate items were entered into a multivariate equation to determine which ones mattered when the effects of the others were taken into account, four items were found to contribute uniquely and significantly to the prediction of REGULATE. These were: level of religiosity ($\beta = .09$, $p = .054$), age of first purchasing cigarettes ($\beta = .14$, $p = .002$), level of depression ($\beta = .14$, $p = .002$), and whether or not the person had been sexually abused during his/her lifetime ($\beta = 11$, $p = .012$). Together, these items explained 5.5% of the total variance in REGULATE. It should be noted that the religiosity measure was retained in this equation despite narrowly failing to maintain statistical significance because its removal reduced the model's overall explanatory power by a significant amount, therefore indicating the importance of its retention rather than its deletion.

Research Question #4 – When we try to understand the factors that affect people's smoking behaviors, does REGULATE matter when the effects of other relevant variables are taken into account?

As a general rule, the answer to the question posed here is "yes." Figures 2, 3, and 4 present three specific examples from the data to support this contention. In each instance, REGULATE is a key endogenous variable in the overall determination of the smoking-related outcome measure in question. This was true when the outcome measure in question was the frequency of chain smoking (see Figure 2), the number of cigarettes smoked per week (see Figure 3), and the number of perceived risks associated with smoking (see Figure 4). In each model, the structural equation analysis revealed that REGULATE contributed significantly to the determination of the smoking-related dependent variable in question, and that it was one of several variables (different from model to model, based on the specific outcome measure being examined) influencing the smoking measure in question.

As the information presented in the encircled portion of each figure shows, the structural equation analysis for all three of these models yielded strong statistical support for the applicability of each model. Further supporting its relevance and importance to the scientific understanding of smoking behaviors and smoking-related attitude/perception measures, we would like to point out that REGULATE was also retained as a multivariate predictor of several of the other smoking-related outcome measures that are listed in Table 2 but which, for brevity's sake, are not depicted in the figures presented in the current paper.

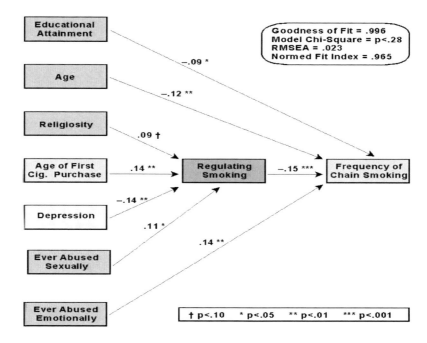

Figure 2. Beliefs about Regulating Smoking and the Frequency of Chain Smoking.

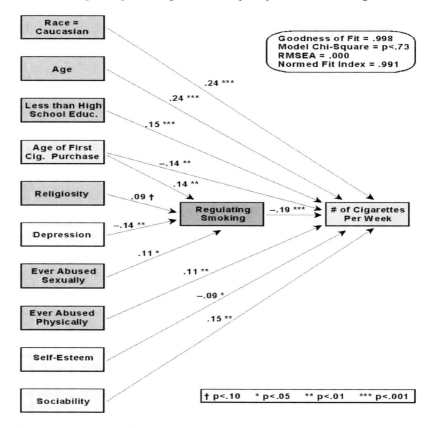

Figure 3. Beliefs about Regulating Smoking and the Number of Cigarettes Smoked per Week.

DISCUSSION

The analyses conducted in conjunction with this paper yielded several interesting and noteworthy findings with regard to REGULATE and its relevance to adult smokers' smoking behaviors. First, as a group, the smokers who participated in this study were quite mixed in their overall feelings about the extent to which they believed that outside agencies and persons should be responsible for informing the public about the dangers of smoking and/or for regulating smoking behaviors.

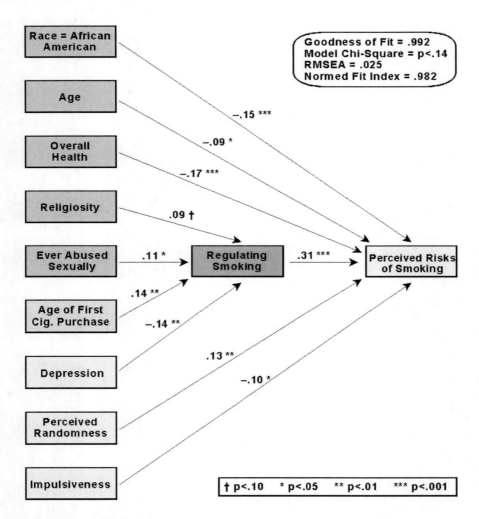

Figure 4. Beliefs about Regulating Smoking and the Perceived Risks of Smoking.

By approximately a 3:1 margin, they advocated a position indicative of a desire to hold public health agencies responsible for informing the public about the dangers of smoking. Interestingly and, to us, intriguingly, respondents were noticeably less inclined to assign this same responsibility to the cigarette companies that make the cigarettes that cause the smoking-related dangers in question available to the public. When it came to assessing the

REGULATE measures that pertained to individual liberties to smoke, our study participants were noticeably more divided in their responses, with many believing that it was acceptable to try to regulate or constrain smoking behaviors while many others adhered to beliefs standing in direct opposition to that mindset.

Our best professional judgment suggests that these findings might be interpreted as follows: It appears that the smokers who participated in this research construe it as a central responsibility of public health agencies to uphold the principles of public safety, thereby leading those agencies to be held most accountable by smokers for informing the public about the dangers associated with smoking. In contrast, while smokers generally believe that the cigarette companies ought to be responsible for telling the public about the dangers associated with smoking, their adherence to this position may be tempered somewhat by their recognition of the existence of the competing interests of the business-related profit motive that these companies also have. That is, the smokers understand that these companies exist for the purpose of making money, and in order for them to do that, they must sell their product. At the same time, however, there is a certain amount of responsibility to one's customers that comes with selling them a product that has known dangers associated with its use; and with that responsibility comes a perceived duty of protecting one's customers' safety, at least to some extent. When it comes to affecting individual liberties, however, smokers are far more reluctant to want outsiders to be able to exert influence over their smoking behaviors. It appears to us that the smokers feared the potential impact of too much regulation of smoking practices, perhaps out of a concomitant concern that such regulation could affect their ability to afford the cigarettes they intended to smoke and their ability to smoke wherever they wanted. Thus, when the items comprising the REGULATE construct are combined into the scale measure, people's scores are more disbursed, leaving them more mixed in their overall attitudes about the extent to which other persons and agencies ought to be responsible for informing the public about and for regulating smoking-related practices.

With respect to Research Question #2–whether or not REGULATE was related to people's smoking-related attitudes and/or to their actual smoking behaviors–the findings obtained were somewhat more complicated. REGULATE was related inconsistently to cigarette smoking practices. It was not related to such measures as taking steps to get more from one's smoking behaviors, the number of times people tried to cut down on (rather than quit) their smoking, the number of negative effects people experienced the last time they tried to quit smoking, smoking more than one intended, or making special trips to the store to ensure having cigarettes available. In contrast, greater endorsement of REGULATE was associated with smoking fewer cigarettes, a larger number of previous attempts to quit smoking, trying a larger number different ways to quit smoking, less frequent chain smoking, and experiencing less frequent urges to smoke in order to function properly. Overall, however, REGULATE was not found to be a strong, consistent predictor of the extent to which persistent adult smokers smoked cigarettes or of their smoking behavioral patterns. In contrast, however, REGULATE was related quite consistently with how people felt about their smoking behaviors. Generally speaking, the more that people believed that it ought to be the responsibility of other persons and agencies to inform the public about the dangers associated with smoking and for regulating smoking behaviors: the more they wanted to quit smoking, the more they wanted to cut down on their cigarette use, the more favorably disposed they were toward the notion of quitting smoking, the more they perceived smoking to be risky, the more they tended to perceive smoking to cause them problems, and the more they tended to view themselves negatively as a result of their smoking behaviors.

The greatest relevance of REGULATE, therefore, appears to be in the psychosocial/attitudinal domain rather than in the behavioral domain. Thus, REGULATE has its greatest impact upon smoking behaviors indirectly rather than directly, through its "behind the scenes" influence on the attitudes that underlie people's smoking practices rather than by impacting specifically and directly the smoking behaviors themselves. As the structural equation models presented in Figures 2, 3, and 4 clearly demonstrate, REGULATE matters greatly and centrally in the overall determination of a variety of smoking-related beliefs, attitudes, and behaviors; but it does so in the form of an endogenous variable.

As an endogenous variable, it becomes important to examine the findings obtained in conjunction with Research Question #3, which focused on identifying the factors associated with greater adherence to the belief that outside persons and/or agencies ought to be responsible for regulating smoking behaviors and/or informing the public about the dangers associated with smoking. Only by understanding more about the factors that underlie REGULATE can we determine which subgroups of smokers might be targeted for specific intervention and/or educational messages. In our analyses, four variables were identified as contributing uniquely and significantly to people's scores on the REGULATE scale: level of religiosity, age of first purchasing cigarettes, level of depression, and sexual abuse history. Each of these merits a brief discussion.

Regarding level of religiosity, our analysis showed that the more religious people tended to be, the more likely they were to endorse REGULATE. A few previous, recent studies have examined the relationship between religiosity and smoking behaviors in the United States, and the present research contributes to that small but evolving literature. Gillum (26), for example, reported that people who attended religious services more frequently were less likely to smoke cigarettes compared to their less-frequently-attending counterparts. Additionally, among current smokers, the frequency of religious service attendance was related inversely to the number of cigarettes that people smoked. In a study of older adult smokers in the American South (27), Roff and colleagues found that religiosity was related inversely to lifetime cigarette smoking. In their research on pregnant and post-partum women, Page, Ellison and Lee (28) found that the odds of smoking tobacco were significantly lower among people who attended worship services regularly or frequently when compared to their less-frequently-attending counterparts. Based on their study of Syracuse, New York residents, Masters and Knestel (29) found that religiosity was associated with whether or not people ever smoked cigarettes, being versus not being a current smoker, and the number of pack-years of cigarette use. Similar results were obtained by Hill and colleagues (30) based on their research on Texas adults, and by Salmoirago-Blotcher and colleagues (31) in their large study of post-menopausal women. As a result of the consistent nature of these studies' findings, Aldwin and colleagues (32, p. 16) concluded that "Both cross-sectional and longitudinal studies have demonstrated relationships between religious service attendance and less cigarette smoking." The current study's finding for the REGULATE scale contributes to this body of literature by demonstrating a slightly different way in which smoking practices are influenced by religiosity–namely, in the form of people's perceptions of the extent to which they believe that outside persons and/or agencies ought to be responsible for regulating smoking and informing the public about the dangers of cigarette use.

With respect to the age of first purchasing cigarettes, the older people were the first time they purchased a cigarette, the more likely they were to endorse REGULATE. A few studies have examined the age of onset of smoking behaviors, typically focusing on the age at which people begin using cigarettes regularly, and how age of onset relates to smoking practices later in life. In one study of early-onset cigarette smokers (defined as persons initiating use prior to age 12), about three-quarters of the young people (77.0%) became regular smokers by mid-adolescence (33). In their research on smoking initiation during the college years, Clarkin, Tisch, and Glicksman (34) found that about one out of nine (11.7%) students had their first cigarette while in college years and 10.8% of college students began smoking regularly at some point during their college years. Having a positive experience (e.g., experiencing relaxation) when first smoking a cigarette has been associated with an increased risk of current smoking, daily smoking, nicotine dependence, and cue-induced cravings for a cigarette (35). The present study's findings add to the literature on this subject by documenting one more way in which age of onset of smoking behaviors–in this specific instance, the age of making the decision to purchase one's first cigarette–is relevant to later-life tobacco use.

Regarding people's level of depression, the more depressed participants in the present study were, the less likely they were to endorse REGULATE. A substantial body of literature has been published on the topic of depression and smoking, with the large majority of studies reporting that depression tends to lead to increased cigarette smoking and/or that smokers have higher rates of depressive symptomatology when compared with their nonsmoking peers (36–38). The present study's finding regarding the relationship between depression and REGULATE is generally consistent with these other research reports; yet it focuses on an aspect of smoking–namely, the belief in who should be responsible for protecting and informing the public about smoking, and to what extent such persons/agencies should be expected to perform such duties–that has not been addressed in any other published reports that the present authors have identified.

With respect to sexual abuse history, the tendency was for people who had experienced sexual abuse to be more likely to endorse REGULATE. As with the preceding measures, previous research has documented a link between early-life sexual abuse experiences and later-life smoking behaviors, with the former generally shown to be a risk factor for the latter (39–41). Once again, the present study's findings are generally consistent with the scholarly literature and still able to extend this literature by virtue of focusing on a somewhat different smoking-related measure, in the form of REGULATE.

Finally, we would like to switch our focus and revisit the findings obtained in the present study as they apply to the notions of locus of control, health locus of control, and powerful others, as introduced earlier in this paper. As we discussed earlier, one way of conceptualizing REGULATE is to think of it as a proxy for locus of control (or at least, as a proxy for one aspect of locus of control). More specifically, people who score high on REGULATE may be construed as being more externally-oriented than those who score low on this scale, because of their belief in the responsibility of other persons and other agencies to determine social and regulatory policies regarding smoking practices. To the extent that REGULATE may be used as a substitute measure for locus of control, the present study's findings indicate that participants in the *Persistent Smokers Project* varied widely in their internal versus external locus of control when it came to their smoking behaviors. Previous researchers have found that people who are more internally oriented when it comes to locus of control tend to engage in lower rates of risky behaviors and higher rates of behavioral practices that can be considered to be beneficial or health protective in nature (2, 4, 6). In the present study, we found that people who scored higher on REGULATE–that is, those with a greater external locus of control orientation–generally had attitudes toward smoking that were aligned with a recognition of a need and/or a desire to stop smoking. This is the opposite of what we would have expected, based on the findings obtained by previous studies examining locus of control and health practices. It is possible that one reason for our finding is that REGULATE may not be a sufficiently precise measure of locus of control. It is also possible that locus of control operates differently with regard to attitudinal measures than it does with behavioral ones. Other interpretations of our finding may exist, too. Regardless of how one interprets our research findings, this is a subject worth exploring in future studies–namely, how, exactly, does locus of control affect smoking behaviors *and* the decision-making processes and attitudes that underlie smoking behaviors? This subject has been investigated only infrequently with regard to the behavioral outcomes in question and even less frequently with regard to the attitudinal/psychosocial measures that also pertain to smoking practices.

With regard to the construct of "powerful others" (also discussed in this paper's Introduction), the present study's findings suggest that participants in the *Persistent Smokers Project* adhered to beliefs that indicated both a respect for and a simultaneous fear of what these so-called powerful others could do with regard to smoking behaviors and smoking-related public policies. When "powerful others" is operationalized in terms of public health agencies, the smokers who participated in this study believed that these were the very individuals/agencies who should be responsible for informing people about the dangers of smoking and how to minimize these dangers. Even when "powerful others" is operationalized in terms of cigarette companies, most of the study participants still believed that these companies should be duty-bound to inform the public about the dangers of smoking.

When "powerful others" is operationalized in terms of lawmakers and policymakers, though, our study participants appeared to be more leery. Nearly 1 respondent in 3 did not agree that it was a good idea to regulate smoking in public places. More than 1 respondent in 3 said that smoking should be banned from television programs and/or movies. Nearly one-half of the *Persistent Smokers Project* study participants believed that smoking should not be banned in restaurants, and a comparably-large proportion of the people who took part in this study believed that smoking bans should be unconstitutional. Thus, when faced with the prospect of having "powerful others" help the public with regard to smoking information, our study participants believed that this was well within the purview of their "proper" domain; but when faced with the prospect of having "powerful others" use their power for regulatory purposes, they seemed to be more conflicted about the extent to which they wanted these "powerful others" to avail themselves of their authority. Little, if any, research has been conducted with a focus or an emphasis on "powerful others" and the role that they can play in promoting healthier behaviors, particularly in the realm of cigarette smoking. About the closest analog has been the multitude of studies that have been done with a "community gatekeepers" or a "key informants" approach; but those approaches typically have been used to gain access to difficult-to-find or difficult-to-recruit study participants rather than to help promote smoking cessation. Applying the construct of "powerful others" to the smoking cessation field might prove to be a fruitful endeavor for future intervention efforts, particularly (our findings suggest) if researchers/interventionists are able to tap into the respect-engendering aspects of what "powerful others" can do to bring about behavioral and attitudinal change while eschewing those other aspects of their powers and authority that are likely to instill fear into members of the target population.

Finally, we would like to touch upon the value of having used a syndemics theory approach to examining the topics at hand in this particular study. As the findings presented in Figures 2, 3, and 4 clearly demonstrate, elements from all of the domains that were included in the conceptual model shown in Figure 1 were relevant in these analyses. This indicates a strong level of support for the usefulness of syndemics theory for understanding the relationships amongst factors affecting smokers' attitudes toward smoking and their actual smoking behaviors. Thus, one additional contribution made by the present research is its ability to demonstrate the applicability of this theoretical model to the study of yet another health behavior–namely, cigarette smoking–thereby expanding its importance and relevance beyond such behavioral domains as obesity (42), HIV risk taking (15, 43, 44), health disparities (45, 46), criminal justice system involvement (47), and socioeconomic disadvantage (48) as other researchers have demonstrated in their own work.

Acknowledgments

This research was supported by a grant from the National Institute on Drug Abuse (R01 DA015707).

References

[1] Armitage CJ. The relationship between multidimensional health locus of control and perceived behavioural control: How are distal perceptions of control related to proximal perceptions of control? Psychol Health 2003;18:723-38.

[2] Sheffer C, MacKillop J, McGeary J, Landes R, Carter L, Yi R, et al. Delay discounting, locus of control, and cognitive impulsiveness independently predict tobacco dependence treatment outcomes in a highly dependent, lower socioeconomic group of smokers. Am J Addict 2012;21:221-32.

[3] Williams GC, McGregor HA, Sharp D, Levesque C, Kouides RW, Ryan RM, et al. Testing a self-determination theory intervention for motivating tobacco cessation: Supporting autonomy and competence in a clinical trial. Health Psychol 2006;25:91-101.

[4] Haslam C, Lawrence W. Health-related behavior and beliefs of pregnant smokers. Health Psychol 2004;23:486-91.

[5] Burnett AJ, Sabato TM, Walter KO, Kerr DL, Wagner L, Smith A. The influence of attributional style on substance use and risky sexual behavior among college students. Coll Stud J 2013;47:122-36.

[6] Reitzel LR, Lahoti S, Li Y, Cao Y, Wetter DW, Waters AJ, Vidrine JI. Neighborhood vigilance, health locus of control, and smoking abstinence. Am J Health Behav 2013;37:334-41.

[7] Wallston KA, Wallston BS, DeVellis R. Development of the Multidimensional Health Locus of Control (MHLC) scales. Health Educ Monogr 1978;6:160-70.

[8] Wallston BS, Wallston KA, Kaplan GD, Maides SA. The development and validation of the Health related Locus of Control (HLC) scale. J Consult Clin Psychol 1976;44:580-5.

[9] Haslam C, Lawrence W, Haefeli K. Intention to breastfeed and other important health-related behaviour and beliefs during pregnancy. Fam Pract 2003;20:1-5.

[10] Rotter JB. Some problems and misconceptions related to the construct of internal versus external control of reinforcement. J Consult Clin Psychol 1975;43:56-67.

[11] Dekel R, Benbenishty R, Amram Y. Therapeutic communities for drug addicts: Prediction of long-term outcomes. Addict Behav 2004;29:1833-7.

[12] Singer MC. Introduction to syndemics: A critical systems approach to public and community health. San Francisco, CA: John Wiley, 2009.
[13] Halkitis PN, Moeller RW, Siconolfi DE, Storholm ED, Solomon TM, Bub KL. Measurement model exploring a syndemic in emerging adult gay and bisexual men. AIDS Behav 2013;17:662-73.
[14] Illangasekare SL, Burke JG, McDonnell KA, Gielen AC. The impact of intimate partner violence, substance use, and HIV on depressive symptoms among abused low-income urban women. J Interpers Violence 2013;28:2831-48.
[15] Klein H. Using a syndemics theory approach to study HIV risk taking in a population of men who use the Internet to find partners for unprotected sex. Am J Men Health 2011;5:466-76.
[16] Meyer JP, Springer SA, Altice FL. Substance abuse, violence, and HIV in women: A literature review of the syndemic. J Women Health 2011:20:991-1006.
[17] Senn TE, Carey MP, Vanable PA. The intersection of violence, substance use, depression, and STDs: Testing of a syndemic pattern among patients attending an urban STD clinic. J Natl Med Assoc 2010;102:614-20.
[18] Greenwood GL, Paul JP, Pollack LM, Binson D, Catania JA, Chang J, et al. Tobacco use and cessation among a household-based sample of US urban men who have sex with men': Greenwood et al. respond. Am J Publ Health 2005;95:929-30.
[19] Yu F, Nehl EJ, Zheng T, He N, Berg CJ, Lemieux AF, et al. A syndemic including cigarette smoking and sexual risk behaviors among a sample of MSM in Shanghai, China. Drug Alcohol Depend 2013;132:265-70.
[20] Centers for Disease Control and Prevention. NHIS–Adult tobacco use information: Smoking status recodes. URL: www.cdc.gov/nchs/nhis/tobacco/tobacco_recodes.htm.
[21] Watson D, Friend R. Measurement of social-evaluative anxiety. J Consult Clin Psychol 1969;33:448-57.
[22] Radloff LS. The CES-D scale: A self-report depression scale for research in the general population. Appl Psychol Meas 1977;1:385-401.
[23] Schuessler K. Measuring social life feelings. San Francisco, CA: Jossey-Bass, 1982.
[24] Zuckerman M, Kuhlman DM, Joireman J, Teta P, Kraft M. A comparison of three strictiral models for personality: The Big Three, the Big Five, and the Alternative Five. J Pers Soc Psychol 1993;65:757-68.
[25] Rosenberg M. Society and the adolescent self-image. Princeton, NJ: Princeton University Press, 1965.
[26] Gillum RF. Frequency of attendance at religious services and cigarette smoking in American women and men: The Third National Health and Nutrition Examination Survey. Prev Med 2005;41:607-13.
[27] Roff LL, Klemmack DL, Parker M, Koenig HG, Sawyer-Baker P, Allman RM. Religiosity, smoking, exercise, and obesity among southern community-dwelling older adults. J Appl Gerontol 2005;24:337-54.
[28] Page RL, Ellison CG, Lee J. Does religiosity affect health risk behaviors in pregnant and postpartum women? Matern Child Health J 2009;13:621-32.
[29] Masters KS, Knestel A. Religious orientation among a random sample of community-dwelling adults: Relations with health status and health-relevant behaviors. Int J Psychol Relig 2011;21:63-76.
[30] Hill TD, Burdette AM, Ellison CG, Musick MA. Religious attendance and the health behaviors of Texas adults. Prev Med 2006;42:309-13.
[31] Salmoirago-Blotcher E, Fitchett G, Ockene JK, Schnall E, Crawford S, Granek I, et al. Religion and healthy lifestyle behaviors among postmenopausal women: The Women's Health Initiative. J Behav Med 2011;34:360-71.
[32] Aldwin CM, Park CL, Jeong YJ, Nath R. Differing pathways between religiousness, spirituality, and health: A self-regulation perspective. Psychol Relig Spiritual 2014;6:9-21.
[33] Vega WA, Gil AG. Revisiting drug progression: Long range effects of tobacco use. Addiction 2005;100:1358-69.
[34] Clarkin PF, Tisch LA, Glicksman AS. Socioeconomic correlates of current and regular smoking among college students in Rhode Island. J Am Coll Health 2008;57:183-90.
[35] Ursprung WWS, Savageau JA, DiFranza JR. What is the significance of experiencing relaxation in response to the first use of nicotine? Addict Res Theory 2011;19:14-21.

[36] Baek JH, Eisner LR, Nierenberg AA. Smoking and suicidality in subjects with major depressive disorder: Results from the National Epidemiologic Survey on Alcohol and Related Conditions (NESARC). J Affect Disord 2013;150:1158-66.
[37] Kenney BA, Holahan CJ, North RJ, Holahan CK. Depressive symptoms and cigarette smoking in American workers. Am J Health Promot 2006;20:179-82.
[38] Payne TJ, Ma JZ, Crews KM, Li MD. Depressive symptoms among heavy cigarette smokers: The influence of daily rate, gender, and race. Nicotine Tob Res 2013;15:1714-21.
[39] Choudhary E, Coben JH, Bossarte RM. Gender and time differences in the associations between sexual violence victimization, health outcomes, and risk behaviors. Am J Men Health 2008;2:254-9.
[40] Nichols HB, Harlow BL. Child abuse and risk of smoking onset. J Epidemiol Commun Health 2004;58:402-6.
[41] Smith PH, Homish GG, Saddleson ML, Kozlowski LT, Giovino GA. Nicotine withdrawal and dependence among smokers with a history of childhood abuse. Nicotone Tob Res 2013;15:2016-21.
[42] Candib LM. Obesity and diabetes in vulnerable populations: Reflection on proximal and distal causes. Ann Fam Med 2007;5:547-56.
[43] Lyons T, Johnson AK, Garofalo R. What could have been different: A qualitative study of syndemic theory and HIV prevention among young men who have sex with men. J HIV/AIDS Soc Serv 2013;12:368-83.
[44] Talman A, Bolton S, Walson JL. Interactions between HIV/AIDS and the environment: Toward a syndemic framework. Am J Public Health 2013;103:253-61.
[45] Bruce D, Harper GW. Operating without a safety net: Gay male adolescents and emerging adults' experiences of marginalization and migration, and implications for theory of syndemic production of health disparities. Health Educ Behav 2011;38:367-78.
[46] Egan JE, Frye V, Kurtz SP, Latkin C, Chen M, Tobin K, et al. Migration, neighborhoods, and networks: Approaches to understanding how urban environmental conditions affect syndemic adverse health outcomes among gay, bisexual and other men who have sex with men. AIDS Behav 2011;15:s35-s50.
[47] Kurtz SP. Arrest histories of high-risk gay and bisexual men in Miami: Unexpected additional evidence for syndemic theory. J Psychoactive Drugs 2008;40:513-21.
[48] Gonzalez-Guarda RM, McCabe BE, Florom-Smith A, Cianelli R, Peragallo N. Substance abuse, violence, HIV, and depression: An underlying syndemic factor among Latinas. Nurs Res 2011;60:182-9.

Submitted: June 02, 2014. *Revised:* July 15, 2014. *Accepted:* July 31, 2014.

In: Public Health Yearbook 2015
Editor: Joav Merrick

ISBN: 978-1-63484-514-4
© 2016 Nova Science Publishers, Inc.

Chapter 27

SERO-PREVALENCE OF RUBELLA-SPECIFIC IMMUNOGLOBULIN G ANTIBODIES AND ITS CORRELATES AMONG BLOOD DONORS IN ZAMBIA

Mazyanga L Mazaba-Liwewe [1],*, BSc, Mwaka Monze[2], MBChB, PhD, Olusegun O Babaniyi[1], MBBS, MPH, MSc, Seter Siziya[3], BA(Ed), MSc, PhD, Dia Phiri[4], BSc, Joseph Mulenga[4], MBChB, and Charles Michelo[5], BSc, MBChB, MPH, MBA, PhD

[1]World Health Organization, Lusaka, Zambia
[2]University Teaching Hospital, Lusaka, Zambia
[3]Copperbelt University, Ndola, Zambia/University of Lusaka, Lusaka, Zambia
[4]Zambia National Blood Transfusion Services, Lusaka, Zambia
[5]University of Zambia, Lusaka, Zambia

ABSTRACT

Rubella is a disease of public health importance in pregnant women causing major problems including abortions, miscarriages and Congenital Rubella Syndrome (CRS). The prevalence of rubella is not known in Zambia. The purpose of this study was to determine the rubella specific IgG antibody sero-prevalence and its correlates among blood donors. A cross sectional study was conducted in the nine provincial donor sites around Zambia. The rubella-specific IgG antibody levels were measured qualitatively by Enzyme-Linked Immuno-Absorbent Assay (ELISA) using Siemens Enzygnost® Anti-rubella-Virus/IgG. Proportions were compared using the Chi-squared test at the 5% significance level, and magnitudes of associations were determined using the odds ratio and its 95% confidence interval. A total of 331 blood donors aged 16-63 years

---

* Correspondence: Mazyanga L Mazaba-Liwewe, WHO, UN Annex, POBox 32346, Lusaka, Zambia. E-mail: mazmazli@yahoo.com.

participated in the survey. Overall, 203 (62.1%) of the participants were males, 48% were aged below 19 years, 66.7% had never been married and 46.2% attained primary level of education. Rubella sero-positivity was 94.8%. Compared to participants who had attained college or higher education level, participants who had no formal schooling were 2.73 (95% CI [1.05, 7.13]) times more likely to have rubella infection, while participants who had attained primary level of education were 69% (OR = 0.31, 95% CI [0.11, 0.83]) less likely to have the infection. Overall, 5.2% of the study population was still susceptible to rubella infection by age of 16 years. Measles vaccine should be replaced with measles-rubella vaccine in the under-five immunisation program to prevent continued circulation of the virus and a catch up campaign to include older children.

Keywords: rubella, IgG sero-prevalence, education, blood donors, Zambia

INTRODUCTION

Rubella is an acute, contagious viral infection caused by rubella virus, a member of the Togaviridae family. The virus is an enveloped single-stranded RNA genome (1). It is transmitted through the respiratory system, replicating in the nasopharynx and lymph nodes. The virus is found in the blood 5 to 7 days after infection and spreads throughout the body, and can be shed for even up to one year in children with CRS (2). Rubella disease affects both children and adult with common signs and symptoms including rash, low fever (<39°C), nausea and mild conjunctivitis and swollen lymph nodes that follow for up to three weeks after exposure to infection. In adults, more so women, arthritis and joint problems are common in the acute phase of the infection which can last up to 10 days (2). Rubella virus is the major cause of birth defects among the TORCH group of agents (Toxoplasma, Others, Rubella, Cytomegalo virus and Herpes virus) that cause congenital anomalies (3). Rubella infection in pregnancy can cause serious damage to unborn babies (4, 5), manifesting with severe teratogenic effects in the fetus where it stops or destroys cell development causing defects in organ development and sometimes foetal death a condition referred to as congenital rubella syndrome (CRS) (6-8) or other serious consequences including miscarriages. Despite a reduction in disease burden of several vaccine-preventable diseases through childhood immunization, CRS continues to account for preventable severe neurological damage, including microcephaly, cortical malformations, blindness, deafness, hydrocephalus and persistent seizures (6).

Rubella continues to be a disease of public health concern globally. In the Americas, rubella virus infection during pregnancy was estimated to have caused 30,000 still births and 20,000 children were born impaired or disabled as a result of CRS (9). The number of rubella cases reduced from the pre vaccine to vaccine era in the Americas and Europe where an elimination goal was set for 2010 and 2015, respectively. WHO estimates that in 1996, 22,000 children were born with CRS in Africa, 46,000 in Southeast Asia and almost 13,000 in the Western Pacific (10). Literature review by Goodson et al. (5) revealed 22 reports on studies conducted on rubella sero-prevalence between 1963 and 2009 from 14 out of the 46 countries in the Africa region. Seventeen of the 22 studies reported rubella sero-positivity of between 68 and 98%. Of the 22 studies, 17 reported sero-positivity results in the range of 71-99% and varied between study populations and age groups among persons aged older than 12 years or described as "women of reproductive age."

Socio-demographic factors such as age, sex and residency and socio-economic factors such as education and wealth have been associated with rubella infection (7, 11, 12). Factors associated with rubella vary among populations and it is important that they be determined in a population so that population-specific interventions may be tailored accordingly.

Rubella infections are prevented by active immunisation programs using live, disabled virus vaccines. Most countries in Africa have not introduced routine vaccination against rubella partly because studies on the burden of the disease, sero-prevalence of rubella or CRS have not been conducted (2, 13). The majority of studies that have been conducted to determine the sero-prevalence of rubella on populations or sub populations are in the developed world (7, 11, 12).

Mazaba-Liwewe et al. (14) confirmed the presence of rubella disease among suspected measles cases in persons aged below 5 years in Zambia. However, there is limited documentation on the burden of disease in older age groups in Zambia. A study by Watts (13) on sero-prevalence of rubella among mothers, though with a number of limitations including a small sample size of 100 respondents and limited geographical area (Lusaka) indicated at least 12% of this study population was vulnerable to rubella infection. Cutts et al. (15) using modelling method, estimated that in Zambia, the prevalence of infection by age 13 years was 75%, incidence of rubella infection per 100, 000 pregnancies between 15-44 years at 465 and incidence of CRS per 100,000 live births at 123 (15). Recently CRS was confirmed in four babies at the University teaching Hospital in Lusaka, Zambia indicating sero-negativity in the mothers to these babies at the time of pregnancy (16). This study however does not estimate the prevalence nor burden of rubella disease including CRS. The objective of the current study was to determine the rubella specific IgG antibodies sero-prevalence and its correlates among blood donors in all provincial centres of the Blood Bank in Zambia.

METHODS

A cross sectional study was carried out at the static blood donor sites in the 9 provincial headquarters. The study population included consecutively selected persons donating blood through the Zambia National Blood Transfusion Services (ZNBTS) centres. A 100% of blood donors in Zambia volunteer to donate blood. The volunteers included mostly students (70%) and persons in the community who met the criteria in the age range 16-65 years (17).

Considering a rubella IgM positive sero-prevalence rate of 76.9% (UTH Virology laboratory annual report 2011, unpublished), indicating these persons were not previously protected against rubella at the time of current infection, a population size of 108,296 (17) and using the Statcalc program in Epi Info version 3.5.4 for population surveys, the required sample size was 307 that was proportionally distributed among the provinces. All eligible persons were requested to participate in the survey.

The study included amongst its variables rubella IgG result (positive/negative IgG in ELISA test) as a dependent variable. The independent variables were socio-demographic factors including age, sex and residency, economic status including education and reported rubella infection or vaccination.

Blood samples were collected from consenting participants and sent to the provincial laboratory for serum separation and storage until transportation to the University Teaching

Hospital for testing. Generally it took an average of 5 days to collect data and samples per sample site except in Lusaka province where the sample size was larger.

Before data and specimen collection, the purpose of the study was explained to the participants (and members of staff in the case of school communities) at secondary schools and communities where blood donations were being sought. Participants who volunteered were assured of privacy, and confidentiality. Participants who consented to taking part in the study were interviewed privately by the researcher or research assistants who filled in the questionnaire. The research proposal was approved by the University of Zambia Biomedical Research Ethics Committee for approval. Permission to conduct the study was obtained from the ZNBTS and Ministry of Health.

Serum samples collected from consenting blood donors were analysed at the Virology laboratory, University Teaching Hospital in Lusaka. To determine the seroprevalence of rubella, the rubella Immunoglobulin G (IgG) antibodies were measured qualitatively (Figure 1) in blood sera using the Enzyme Linked Immunosorbent Assay (ELISA) manual method (18). The kit that was selected had high specificity and sensitivity of 98.5% and 100%, respectively (18), reducing any chance of "false positives" and ensuring at least sensitive enough to detect clinically important but very low levels of antibodies. Quality assurance was emphasized including the use of kit controls and standard operating procedures. All kits used were within expiry dates.

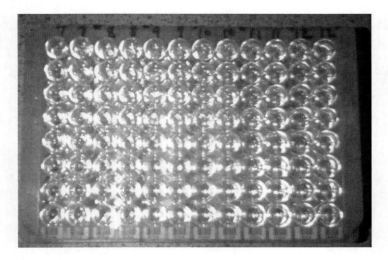

Figure 1. Final plate after addition of stop solution.

The difference in the optical densities (Absorbance), ΔA between the antigen and antigen control wells was calculated and results interpreted as follows:

Anti-Rubella-Virus/IgG negative $\Delta A < 0.100$
Anti-Rubella-Virus/IgG positive $\Delta A > 0.200$
Anti-Rubella-Virus/IgG equivocal $0.100 \leq \Delta A \leq 0.200$

Data was entered using Epi Data version 3.1. A unique identifier was used to link the questionnaire and laboratory data. Data were analyzed using SPSS version 16.0. Associations were determined using Pearson's Chi-squared test (higher tables than 2 by 2) and Yates corrected Chi-squared test (2 by 2 tables). Fisher's exact test was used when in 2 by 2 tables when expected frequency in any cell was less than 5. The cut off point for statistical significance was set at 5%. Odds ratio and its 95% confidence interval was used to measure the magnitude of association.

RESULTS

A total of 331 participants took part in the survey, 2 of whom refused to have samples drawn. Only those with the sample drawn were entered into the data base. Most of the participants were aged between 20-29 for males (31.7%) and less than 25 years for females (75.0%), as shown in Figure 2. Out of a total of 327 participants with known sex, 203 (62.1%) were males. Table 1 shows the distribution of the participants by socio-demographic factors and sex for 329 participants. Overall, 66.7% of the participants had never been married. Close to a third (37.7%) of the participants resided in rural areas of the country. Of the 266 participants with recorded highest level of education, 8.3% had no formal schooling, 6.8% attained college or higher level of education, and 46.2% attained primary level of education. Out of 112 participants with recorded current employment status, 42.0% were not working for pay. About 1 in 4 (24.0%) of the participants resided in Lusaka province. Only Lusaka and Copperbelt province were considered predominantly urban (Figure 3).

Of all persons who had knowledge of rubella, 20 (54.1%) had rubella vaccination and 7 (22.6) had previous rubella infection.

Table 1. Distribution of participants by socio-demographic and economic factors stratified by sex

FACTOR	Overall n (%)	Male n (%)	Female n (%)	p value
Marital status				
Never married	218 (66.7)	138 (68.0)	80 (64.5)	0.600
Currently or once married	109 (33.3)	65 (32.0)	44 (35.5)	
Residence				
Rural	124 (37.7)	77 (37.9)	47 (37.9)	1.000
Urban	205 (62.3)	126 (62.1)	77 (62.1)	
Education level				
No formal school	22 (8.3)	10 (6.6)	12 (10.5)	0.707
Up to secondary school	123 (46.2)	72 (47.4)	51 (44.7)	
Secondary school completed	103 (38.7)	60 (39.5)	43 (37.7)	
College/pre-university or higher	18 (6.8)	10 (6.6)	8 (7.0)	
Current employment				
Government/non-government	35 (31.2)	22 (31.9)	13 (30.2)	0.931
Self-employed/Employer	30 (26.8)	19 (27.5)	11 (25.6)	
Not working for pay	47 (42.0)	28 (40.6)	19 (44.2)	

*Total =327 [203 (62.1%) male, 124 female].

Table 2. Distribution of participants by vaccination, history of rubella infection and knowledge stratified by sex

FACTOR	Overall n (%)	Male* n (%)	Female* n (%)	p value
Rubella vaccination				
Yes	20 (54.1)	11 (45.8)	9 (69.2)	0.309
No	17 (45.9)	13 (54.2)	4 (30.8)	
History of rubella infection				
Yes	7 (22.6)	5 (26.3)	2 (16.7)	0.676
No	24 (77.4)	14 (73.7)	10 (83.3)	
Knowledge on symptoms of rubella				
Fever with rash				
Yes	26 (70.3)	16 (66.7)	10 (76.9)	0.711
No	11 (29.7)	8 (33.3)	3 (23.1)	
Diarrhoea				
Yes	3 (8.1)	1 (4.2)	2 (15.4)	0.278
No	34 (91.9)	23 (95.8)	11 (84.6)	
Knowledge on rubella prevention				
Vaccination	28 (75.7)	17 (70.8)	11 (84.6)	0.595
Drinking clean water or do not know	9 (24.3)	7 (29.2)	2 (15.4)	
Sources of knowledge				
Reading				
Yes	10 (27.0)	6 (25.0)	4 (30.8)	0.716
No	27 (73.0)	18 (75.0)	9 (69.2)	
Media				
Yes	12 (32.4)	8 (33.3)	4 (30.8)	1.000
No	25 (67.6)	16 (66.7)	9 (69.2)	
Friend				
Yes	7 (20.6)	4 (16.7)	3 (30.0)	0.394
No	27 (79.4)	20 (83.3)	7 (70.0)	
Health facility				
Yes	11 (29.7)	6 (25.0)	5 (38.5)	0.465
No	26 (70.3)	18 (75.0)	8 (61.5)	
Antenatal				
Yes	1 (2.7)	0 (0)	1 (7.7)	0.351
No	36 (97.3)	24 (100)	12 (92.3)	

Total = 37 (24 male, 13 female). Total for history of rubella infection is 31. *percents based on denominators <30.

Overall, 37 (11.5%) of the participants had ever heard of rubella. Sources of information included: reading (27.0%), Media (32.4%), Friends (88.7%), health facility (29.7%) and antenatal care (2.7%) as shown in Table 2.

Out of the 37 participants who had ever heard of rubella, 26 (70.3%) reported fever with rash as a symptom of rubella. Only 8.1% of the participants reported diarrhoea as a symptom of rubella. None of the participants reported cough as a symptom of rubella (Table 2).

Of the 37 participants who indicated that they had ever heard of rubella, 28 (75.7%) indicated that rubella can be prevented by vaccination, 2 (5.4%) said by drinking clean water and 7 (18.9%) reported that they did not know how rubella is prevented. Of the 37 participants who had heard of rubella, 54.1% had received rubella vaccination. Out of the 20 participants who reported to have received rubella vaccination, 4 were laboratory confirmed, one was not a laboratory confirmed case, and 2 did not know whether they were laboratory confirmed or not. Altogether, 22.6% of the participants had a history of rubella infection

(Table 2). All the persons who indicated exposure to rubella by vaccine (37) or infection (31) tested rubella IgG positive. A total of 310 (113 of whom were female, 195 males and 2 with no sex recorded) out of 327 participants were positive for rubella IgG giving a total positivity rate of 94.8%.

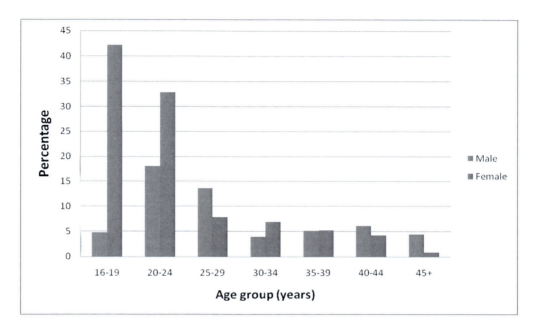

Figure 2. Age distribution by sex.

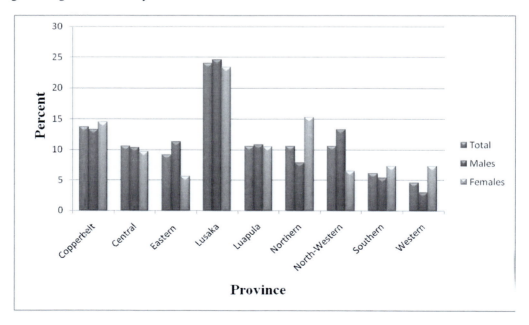

Figure 3. Distribution of participants by province stratified by sex.

Figure 4 shows the distribution of sero-positivity by province. All the participants from Eastern and Northern provinces were found to have rubella IgG antibodies.

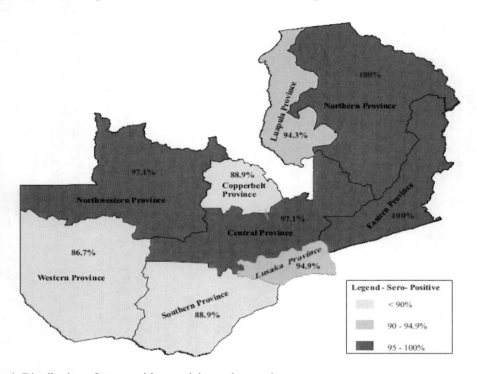

Figure 4. Distribution of sero-positive participants by province.

Table 3. Factors associated with rubella sero-positivity

FACTOR	IgG TOTAL	IgG POSITIVE (%)	OR (95% CI)
Age (years)			
<20	155	145 (93.5)	1.38 (0.71, 2.67)
20-24	75	72 (96.0)	0.83 (0.35, 1.97)
25+	95	91 (95.8)	1
Sex			
Male	202	195 (96.5)	0.64 (0.39, 1.05)
Female	123	113 (91.9)	1
Marital status			
Never married	216	201 (93.1)	2.00 (0.95, 4.22)
Currently or once married	96	94 (97.9)	1
Residence			
Urban	124	115 (37.1)	1.38 (0.85, 2.25)
Rural	203	195 (62.9)	1
Education level			
No formal school	22	18 (-)	2.73 (1.05, 7.13)
Up to secondary school	123	120 (97.6)	0.31 (0.11, 0.83)
Secondary school completed	101	95 (94.1)	0.77 (0.34, 1.76)
College/pre-university or higher	18	16 (-)	1
Current employment			
Government/non-government	35	33 (94.3)	1.16 (0.34, 3.95)
Self-employed/Employer	30	29 (96.7)	0.66 (0.15, 2.86)
Not working for pay	47	44 (93.6)	1

Of the factors considered in the analysis (Table 3), only education was significantly associated with the outcome. Compared to participants who had attained college or higher education level, participants who had no formal schooling were 2.73 (95% CI [1.05, 7.13]) times more likely to have a positive IgG result. Meanwhile, participants who had not completed secondary level of education were 69% (OR = 0.31, 95% CI [0.11, 0.83]) less likely to have a positive IgG result.

DISCUSSION

This study determined the rubella sero-prevalence and its correlates amongst blood donors in Zambia. The study population included blood donors from schools and the community between the ages 16 to 63 years, 37.9% of whom were female and almost half the participants belonging to the under 20 years age group. This study reveals a sero-prevalence of 94.8%, and this rate indicates a susceptible population (sero-negative) of 5.2% amongst blood donors in Zambia. Considering the presence of antibodies does not always assure immunity (19), we can assume that those at risk of rubella infection in this study population could be more than 5.2%.

The sero-prevalence in this study are close to those among a similar age group in other studies such as the study in Turkey, (though study population was only women) that found a sero-negativity of 4.5%. This study reveals a prevalence within the range described by Goodson and team who document that serological surveys throughout Africa estimated susceptibility to rubella virus among adults ranged from 1%–29% among the various study populations (5). It is also in agreement with that found in 22 African countries that have determined rubella sero-prevalence in various groups of their populations that indicate a range of sero-prevalence between 68 and 98% (5).

Our study participants were between 16 and 63 years of age including both males and females. All the participants who tested seronegative were between 16 and 33 years old which is within the child bearing age. Most studies indicate increasing sero-positivity with increased age while others showed advancing age to be associated with increased risk of rubella. This study reveals no significant association between age groups and sero-positivity. This could be due to the fact that the majority (71%) of the population in this study were below 25 years of age and hence the data skewed towards the younger age group. It has been documented that most children in the AFRO region would have gained a natural immunity (sero-positive) to rubella by 15 years of age. Most studies in Africa have looked at those above 12 years or "women of reproductive age." The females in this study had a sero-positivity of 91.9% indicating 8.1% of the female in this study population still susceptible to rubella infection. It is comparative to sero-prevalence in other studies in which sero-positivity was found to be 94.1% in women 14–18 years of age in Ethiopia, and 90.1% in women 15–45 years of age in Senegal, but higher than in in Côte d'Ivoire where sero-positivity was 84% in women 15–34 years of age (20, 21).

Though the rate in this study may not be a representative of the general population, it confirms that there is a part of the population that is still at risk of rubella infection. This implies continued rubella virus circulation and increased risk of CRS especially that Zambia has no deliberate policy with regards to control and prevention of rubella. If Zambia is to be in line with the WHO strategies to control and prevent rubella and CRS, a vaccination must be put in place. Our study agrees with conclusions by others whose epidemiological evidence has shown that while rubella virus continues to circulate among children, there is still a risk of infection in pregnant women, even though only 3% of them are non-immune, and there is little prospect of eliminating CRS (22, 23).

Rubella sero-prevalence and its association to various social, economic or demographic characteristics vary in different countries. Some studies have shown either one or more social, economic and demographic factors being associated with rubella sero-prevalence including age, residency (urban vs, rural), economic status among others (11, 12).

In this study education and employment status were used as a proxy measure to economic status. Though some schools of thought indicate a limitation in using education as a measure of social economic status (24), it is generally accepted that education is linked to income (25). This study reveals a significant association between education and the outcome with decreasing sero-negativity towards higher education. Participants who had no formal schooling were 2.73 times more likely to have a positive IgG result than those who had attained college or higher education. However, participants who had not completed secondary level of education were 69% less likely to have a positive IgG result. Low socio-economic status has also been seen to be associated with risk of rubella infection in some studies while others dispute having found no correlation was found between socioeconomic status and rubella sero-positivity (7, 11, 12). Our study reveals that those who did not complete secondary level of education were 31% less likely to be infected hence more susceptible than those who are in college or higher while those with no formal education were more than 2.7 times likely to be infected hence with lower sero-negativity. This could be due to the fact that the non-schooled and those schooling for a longer time socialize more in economic and school activities respectively hence more exposure to the disease (leading to natural immunity). The findings on those schooled in this study are in agreement with other studies including that by Cengiz et al. (26) who reported that rubella sero-negativity was 87.5% before school and decreased to 37.3% in primary school. Infection rates in susceptible populations is higher in closed quarters such as school and less in the home environment says Krugman et al. (27). Our findings are in dispute with those by Kombich et al. (12) who found that low socio-economic factors suggest an increased risk of infection in certain categories of society education which was also used as a proxy to measure of economic status was not significantly associated with risk to rubella infection. Karakoc et al. (7) also found no correlation was found between socioeconomic status and rubella sero-positivity.

The study though limited to the blood donor population is the first widespread sero-prevalence study in Zambia. It is an important step in generating baseline sero-prevalence data on rubella infection in Zambia. Findings from this study are useful in the development of rubella control programme in Zambia. This study identifies low socio-economic status (education) as a significant risk factor for rubella was identified. Though no significant association of age with outcome was found in this study it is noted that 5.2% of the study population was still susceptible to rubella infection by age of 16 years. We recommend the measles vaccine be replaced with measles-rubella vaccine in the under-five immunisation program to prevent continued circulation of the virus and a catch up campaign to include older children.

ACKNOWLEDGMENTS

I wish to thank the following for their contributions to the study. Dr William Moss (Johns Hopkins University, Baltimore, USA) for reagent support and technical advice, Southern Africa Consortium for Research Excellence (SACORE) for reagent support and financing sample and data collection, research assistants from Zambia National Blood Transfusion Services and the study participants for their cooperation.

REFERENCES

[1] Frey TK. Molecular biology of rubella virus. Adv Virus Res 1994;44:69–160.
[2] Reef SE, Strebel P, Dabbagh A, Gacic-Dobo M, Cochi S. Progress toward control of rubella and prevention of congenital rubella syndrome--worldwide, 2009. J Infect Dis 2011;204(Suppl 1):S24-7.
[3] Otaigbe BE, Brown T, Esu R. Confirmed congenital rubella syndrome. A case report. Niger J Med 2006;15(4):448-50.
[4] Freij BJ, South MA, Sever JL. Maternal rubella and the congenital rubella syndrome. Clin Perinatol 1988;15(2):247–57.
[5] Goodson JL, Masresha B, Dosseh A, Byabamazima C, Nshimirimana D, Cochi S, Reef S. Epidemiology of rubella in Africa in the prevaccine era, 2002-2009. J Infect Dis 2011;204(Suppl 1);S215-25.
[6] Dewan P, Gupta P. Burden of congenital rubella syndrome (CRS) in India: a systematic review. Indian pediatr 2012;49(5):377-99.
[7] Karakoc GB, Altintas DU, Kilinc B, Karabay A, Mungan NO, Yilmaz M, Evliyaoglu N., Seroprevalence of rubella in school girls and pregnant women. Eur J Epidemiol 2003;18(1):81-4.
[8] de Moraes JC, Toscano CM, de Barros EN, Kemp B, Lievano F, Jacobson S, Afonso AM, Strebel PM, Cairns KL; VigiFex Group. Etiologies of rash and fever illnesses in Campinas, Brazil. J Infect Dis 2011;204(Suppl 2):S627-36.
[9] Centers for Disease Control and Prevention. Achievements in public health: elimination of rubella and congenital rubella syndrome--United States, 1969-2004. MMWR 2005;54(11):279-82.
[10] GAVI Alliance. Measles-rubella vaccine support. Accessed 2014 July 01. URL: http://www.gavialliance.org/support/nvs/rubella/.
[11] Figueiredo CA, Afonso AM, Curti SP, Oliveira MI, Souza LT, Sato HK, Azevedo RS. Seroprevalence of rubella in urban and rural populations, Guaratinguetá. Rev Assoc Med Bras 2009;55(2):117-20.
[12] Kombich JJ, Muchai PC, Tukei P, Borus PK. Rubella seroprevalence among primary and pre-primary pupils at Moi's Bridge location, Uasin Gishu District, Kenya. BMC Public Health 2009;9:269.
[13] Watts T. Rubella antibodies in a sample of Lusaka mothers. Med J Zambia 1983;17(4):109-10.
[14] Mazaba Liwewe LM, Ndumba I, Chibumbya J, Msiska T, Mutambo H, Micheelo C, Babaniyi O, Monze M. Rubella amongst suspected measles cases under the EPI surveillance program in Zambia (2004-2011). 15th ICID. Bangkok, Thailand; June 13-16, 2012.
[15] Cutts FT, Vynnycky E. Modelling the incidence of rubella syndrome in developing countries. Int J Epidemiol 1999;28(6):1176-84.
[16] Mazaba-Liwewe ML, Mtaja A, Chabala C, Sinyangwe S, Babaniyi O, Monze M, Siziya S, Michelo C. Laboratory confirmed congenital rubella syndrome at the University Teaching Hospital in Lusaka, Zambia-case reports. Med J Zambia, in press.
[17] Ministry of Health. Highlights on national blood transfusion status and trends. Lusaka: Ministry Health, 2013.
[18] Siemens.Enzygnost®. Anti-Rubella Virus/IgG hand-book, July 2011.
[19] Kudesia G. Carrrington D. Subclinical rubella in pregnancy. Lancet 1985;1(8430)700.
[20] Cutts FT, Abebe A, Messele T, Dejene A, Enquselassie F, Nigatu W, Nokes DJ. Sero-epidemiology of rubella in the urban population of Addis Ababa, Ethiopia. Epidemiol Infect 2000;124(3):467-79.

[21] Gomwalk NE, Ahmad AA. Prevalence of rubella antibodies on the African continent. Rev Infect Dis 1989;11(1):116-21.
[22] Galazka A. Rubella in Europe. Epidemiol Infect 1991;107(1):43–54.
[23] Sadighi J Eftekhar H, Mohammad K. Congenital rubella syndrome in Iran. BMC Infect Dis 2005;5:44.
[24] Braveman PA, Cubbin C, Egerter S, Chideya S, Marchi KS, Metzler M, Posner S. Socioeconomic status in health research: one size does not fit all. JAMA 2005;294(22):2879-88.
[25] Montgomery MR, Gragnolati M, Burke KA, Paredes E. Measuring living standards with proxy variables. Demography 2000;37(2):155-74.
[26] Cengiz AT, Kıyan M, Dolapci GI, Aysev D, Tibet M. Serum rubella IgG and IgM antibodies with ELISA in different age groups. Turkish J Infect. 1996;10:249–52.
[27] Krugman S, Katz SL, Gershon AA, Wilfert CM. Infectious diseases of children, 9th ed. St Louis, MO: Mosby Year Book, 1992:381–401.

Submitted: June 10, 2014. *Revised:* August 01, 2014. *Accepted:* August 07, 2014.

Chapter 28

PARENTS OF CHILDREN WITH AUTISM: ISSUES SURROUNDING CHILDHOOD VACCINATION

April M Young, PhD, MPH[1,*], *Abigail Elliston*[2] *and Lisa A Ruble, PhD*[3]

[1]Department of Epidemiology, University of Kentucky College of Public Health, Lexington, Kentucky, United States of America
[2]Transylvania University, Lexington, Kentucky, United States of America
[3]Department of Educational, School, and Counseling Psychology, University of Kentucky College of Education, Lexington, Kentucky, United States of America

ABSTRACT

Parents of children with autism (PCA) are among those most affected by the controversy surrounding supposed links between vaccines and autism. In this chapter we describe the vaccine attitudes of PCA and their association with satisfaction with their child's healthcare provider. Fifty PCA completed questionnaires on vaccine attitudes, exposure to media discussing links between vaccines and autism ('vaccine-autism media'), and satisfaction with their child's healthcare. These characteristics, as well as autism severity and child cognitive functioning, were examined for their correlation with parents' belief that vaccines caused autism and desire to refuse future vaccination. The majority endorsed vaccines as effective and necessary, yet 56% believed they contributed to autism's cause and 16% would discourage others' vaccination. Nearly 80% discussed concerns with their child's provider and felt they were taken seriously. Attitudes were not associated with parents' demographic characteristics or satisfaction with healthcare, but were associated with trust in health institutions, vaccine safety, exposure to vaccine-autism media, and child's lower cognitive functioning. *Conclusions:* Although parents reported positive communication with providers, doubts about safety and exposure to vaccine-autism media were common. These findings underscore the importance for targeted campaigns addressing PCA's concerns and to mitigate mistrust.

---

[*] Correspondence: April M Young, Department of Epidemiology, University of Kentucky College of Public Health, 111 Washington Avenue, Lexington, KY 40536, United States. E-mail: april.young@uky.edu.

INTRODUCTION

Despite increasing evidence of genetic causes of autism spectrum disorder (ASD) (1-3) and an authoritative review rejecting a causal association between MMR vaccination and ASD (4), fear that childhood vaccines play a key role in the etiology of ASD persists (5). In fact, a review by Brown and colleagues (6) identified a significant association between parents' belief that vaccines cause autism and lower vaccine uptake. The controversy continues to attract media attention and many parents remain skeptical about the safety of childhood vaccines (7, 8). The issue is particularly salient for parents of children with autism (PCA) and, with an estimated ASD prevalence of one in 88 (9), vaccine uptake among this group could have a substantive impact on public health.

Online surveys of parents involved with autism organizations in the US and Canada revealed that 40% of parents believed that vaccines were among the most significant contributory factors involved in their child's autism (10). Many factors play a role in producing these beliefs, including the temporal proximity of childhood vaccination and the manifestation of autism, distrust of governmental agencies, perceptions of the risks posed by vaccine-preventable diseases (VPDs), and information from popular media sources (11). Several studies have suggested that the latter, especially web-based sources, may fuel distrust in childhood vaccinations (12-15); yet, given limitations in extant research, developing interventions to address these influences would be challenging (16).

Healthcare providers are on the frontlines in the debate about vaccines and autism, and can have a substantial influence on decisions about childhood vaccination (17-21). Therefore, it remains critical that healthcare providers offer information to caregivers, and to PCA, as early after diagnosis as possible (17). The purpose of this study was to examine attitudes toward childhood vaccination among PCA. The association between various dimensions of healthcare satisfaction, vaccine attitudes, and child autism severity and cognitive ability was explored, as was exposure to media sources portraying a link between vaccines and autism.

OUR STUDY

A convenience sample of PCA were recruited through their participation in randomized controlled trials of a parent-teacher consultation intervention in Kentucky and Indiana (22, 23). All children met the diagnostic and statistical manual IV-TR definition of autistic disorder (24) as confirmed by professionally-administered Autism Diagnostic Observation Schedule Modules 1 or 2 (25). Parents (n = 79) were mailed two self-administered surveys assessing their attitudes toward childhood vaccines and their satisfaction with their child's medical care. Fifty parents completed the Parent Satisfaction with Care Questionnaire and 49 completed the Vaccine Attitude Questionnaire (described below). Respondents were not significantly different than non-respondents in terms of child's age, parental education level, income, or race. All study procedures were approved by the University's Institutional Review Board.

Table 1. Bivariate analyses of parents' (n = 50) beliefs toward childhood vaccination and experiences with child's healthcare provider

Correlate	Total mean (SD)	Vaccines contributed to cause of child's autism. (n = 43) Disagree mean (SD)	Agree mean (SD)	p-value	Would refuse to vaccinate if there were no penalties. (n = 47) Disagree mean (SD)	Agree mean (SD)	p-value
Demographic and ASD-Related Characteristics							
White - n(%) (n = 47)	34 (68.0)	11 (57.9)	18 (81.8)	0.168	28 (71.8)	6 (85.7)	0.657
Mother attended college - n(%) (n = 41)[a]	27 (54.0)	10 (66.7)	13 (65.0)	1.000	21 (61.8)	5 (83.3)	0.399
Income greater than $25,000 - n(%) (n = 39)[b]	25 (50.0)	6 (46.2)	15 (75.0)	0.142	20 (62.5)	4 (66.7)	1.000
Child's gender (male) - n (%)	43 (86.0)	17 (89.5)	22 (91.7)	0.806	35 (85.4)	7 (87.5)	0.875
Child's age	5.8 (1.6)	5.4 (1.6)	6.2 (1.6)	0.115	5.8 (1.6)	5.8 (1.7)	0.991
Number of siblings (n = 47)	1.2 (1.1)	1.3 (1.3)	1.1 (1.1)	0.625	1.4 (1.1)	0.6 (1.2)	0.094
CARS Score (n = 48)	37.7 (8.5)	39.4 (8.4)	37.3 (9.1)	0.455	36.9 (9.0)	41.3 (6.0)	0.194
DAS Score	47.6 (21.2)	50.0 (24.4)	47.3 (20.5)	0.696	51.1 (21.2)	32.8 (13.9)	0.024*
Vaccine Attitudes							
Perception of vaccine safety/efficacy	2.0 (0.5)	2.5 (0.4)	1.8 (0.4)	<0.001[†]	2.2 (0.5)	1.7 (0.3)	0.002[†]
Negative consequences of non-vaccination	3.1 (0.5)	3.3 (0.5)	2.9 (0.5)	0.008[†]	3.2 (0.5)	2.8 (0.7)	0.102
Trust in health institutions	2.3 (0.7)	2.8 (0.6)	2.0 (0.5)	<0.001[†]	2.4 (0.6)	2.0 (0.7)	0.043*
Vaccine communication with PCP	3.0 (0.7)	3.1 (0.7)	3.0 (0.7)	0.860	3.0 (0.6)	3.0 (0.8)	0.373
Desired autonomy	2.5 (0.7)	2.3 (0.7)	2.8 (0.7)	0.036*	2.4 (0.6)	3.0 (0.6)	0.004[†]
Sense of responsibility to vaccinate	3.1 (0.6)	3.3 (0.6)	2.9 (0.6)	0.043*	3.2 (0.5)	2.9 (0.7)	0.058
Satisfaction with Medical Care							
Physician informativeness	2.9 (0.7)	2.9 (0.6)	2.9 (0.8)	0.788	2.9 (0.7)	2.9 (0.7)	0.927
Interpersonal sensitivity	3.2 (0.6)	3.3 (0.6)	3.3 (0.5)	0.864	3.2 (0.5)	3.3 (0.5)	0.875
Partnership building	2.9 (0.6)	3.0 (0.7)	3.1 (0.6)	0.691	3.0 (0.6)	3.0 (0.6)	0.846
Perceived competence	2.7 (0.7)	2.7 (0.7)	2.8 (0.7)	0.584	2.7 (0.7)	2.6 (0.7)	0.730
Accessibility of care	2.9 (0.5)	3.0 (0.5)	3.0 (0.6)	0.720	2.9 (0.5)	2.8 (0.6)	0.343
Affordability of care	2.8 (0.6)	3.1 (0.7)	2.7 (0.6)	0.065	3.0 (0.6)	2.6 (0.7)	0.126
Encountered information provoking fear about vaccine-autism link - n (%)	32 (65.3)	5 (27.8)	22 (91.7)	<0.001[†]	18 (54.5)	13 (92.9)	0.017*

SD: standard deviation, ASD: Autism Spectrum Disorder, CARS: Childhood Autism Rating Scale, DAS: Differential Ability Scales, PCP: Primary Care Provider. * $p < 0.05$, [†]$p < 0.01$.

[a] Response options for parents' education-level included, *"graduate/professional training," "college graduate," "some college," "high school/general equivalence degree," "some high school," "junior high school,"* and *"less than 7 years of education."* Data were dichotomized at the mean (1 = some college or greater, 0 = no college attendance). Given that 50% of respondents reported that father's education level was "not applicable," mother's educational attainment was used for analysis.

[b] Response options for household income included, *"Less than $10,000," "$10,000 - $24,999," "$25,000 - $49,999," "$50,000 - $100,000,"* and *"Greater than $100,000."* Data were dichotomized (1 = $25,000 or greater, 0 = Less than $25,000) at the mean and to closely correspond with the US Federal Poverty Level for a four person household (US Department of Health and Human Services, 2013).

Table 2. Description and internal consistency of subscales within the Parent Satisfaction with Care Scale

Scale	Items	Example Item	Coefficient α
Physician's informativeness	5	The doctor thoroughly explains everything to me.	0.87
Physician's interpersonal sensitivity	4	The doctor shows a genuine interest in my child's well-being.	0.81
Physician/caregiver partnership building	4	The doctor asks for my thoughts about autism.	0.80
Physician's Competence	3	The doctor's office has everything needed to provide complete medical care to a child with autism.	0.79
Accessibility of care	4	I can make doctors' appointments at a time that is convenient for my schedule.	0.51
Affordability of care	3	I have to pay for more of my child's medical care than I can afford.	0.71

Demographic information including child age, gender, race, household income, number of siblings, and parent education level was collected (described in Table 1). Measures assessing children's severity of autism (Childhood Autism Rating Scale; CARS) and cognitive ability (Differential Abilities Scale; DAS) were administered by the research team (23). The CARS is a valid and reliable, observational scale comprised of 15 items evaluating behaviors such as social relating, resistance to change, communication, and body use (26). The General Conceptual Ability subscore of the DAS, which has strong internal and test-retest reliability (27), was used to assess children's cognitive ability.

Participants also completed questionnaires assessing their satisfaction with their child's primary healthcare provider (PCP); Table 2 provides example items and coefficient alphas for subscales. The 24-item Parent Satisfaction with Care Questionnaire contained seven subscales and was based on a modification of two established measures for assessing individuals' satisfaction with medical care (28, 29). Five subscales examined parents' perceptions of their child's PCP, including his/her informativeness, interpersonal sensitivity, competence to care for a child with autism, and willingness to engage in partnership building with caregiver. Two additional subscales assessed parents' reported accessibility and affordability of healthcare for their child. Response options were arranged on a 4-point Likert scale ranging from strongly agree to strongly disagree.

Parents also completed a 43-item Vaccine Attitude Questionnaire, which was based in part on a study of MMR vaccine attitudes conducted in the United Kingdom (30).

The modified questionnaire contained six subscales examining parents' 1) perceived safety and efficacy of childhood vaccines, 2) perceived benefits of childhood vaccination, 3) trust in health institutions such as healthcare providers, the government, and pharmaceutical companies, 4) communication with the child's PCP about vaccination, 5) sense of responsibility to vaccinate their child for his/her welfare and the benefit to society and 6) desire for autonomy in making childhood vaccination decisions. Responses were arranged on a 4-point Likert scale ranging from strongly agree to strongly disagree. Table 3 provides items and coefficient alphas. Likert scale items on both the Parent Satisfaction with Care and Vaccine Attitude Questionnaires were recoded for analysis such that higher values indicated attitudes more positively associated with the subscale construct.

Caregivers were also queried about their exposure to information about links between vaccines and autism. Parents were asked the following three questions: 1) "Have you encountered information on/from [source] about links between vaccines and autism?"; 2) "Was the information useful?"; and 3) "Did the information increase your fears regarding vaccines and autism?" These questions were asked for six different sources (see Figure 1). From these data, a binary variable was created in which caregivers with an affirmative response on the third question for any source were assigned a 1 and their counterparts were assigned a 0

Table 3. Description and internal consistency of subscales within the Vaccine Attitude Questionnaire

Question	n (%)[a]	Coefficient α[b]
Vaccine safety and efficacy		0.85
Childhood vaccines are safe (n = 47)	18 (38.3)	
Childhood vaccines are very effective in preventing disease. (n = 47)	42 (89.4)	
More research is needed to fully investigate the effects of childhood vaccines. (n = 47)[c]	47 (100.0)	
Possible complications of vaccination can be very serious for children. (n = 47)[c]	45 (95.7)	
Scientific evidence has shown that vaccines do not cause autism. (n = 47)	14 (29.8)	
My child getting autism from vaccines is a major concern for me. (n = 49)[c]	35 (71.4)	
Consequences of non-vaccination		0.83
The diseases childhood vaccines prevent are serious. (n = 48)	44 (91.7)	
Without vaccines, my child would be at risk for getting the diseases they prevent. (n = 48)	42 (87.5)	
People who do not vaccinate their children put others at risk. (n = 47)	34 (72.3)	
More kids should be vaccinated so that outbreaks do not occur. (n = 48)	32 (66.7)	
Trust in health institutions involved with vaccination		0.80
I trust the opinion of my healthcare provider regarding safety of vaccines. (n = 47)	28 (59.6)	
I trust the companies producing my child's vaccines. (n = 47)	22 (46.8)	
The government would stop childhood vaccination programs if they were dangerous to children. (n = 49)	22 (44.9)	
The government is too defensive about childhood vaccines. (n = 48)[c]	35 (47.9)	
Communication about vaccination with healthcare provider		---[a]
I discuss my concerns about vaccination openly with my child's healthcare provider. (n = 47)	37 (78.7)	
My concerns about vaccination are taken seriously by my child's healthcare provider. (n = 47)	33 (70.2)	
Desired autonomy in vaccination decision		---[a]
Parents should make decisions regarding their child's vaccination rather than healthcare providers or the government. (n = 49)	35 (71.4)	
Vaccines should not be required to attend school. (n = 49)	11 (22.4)	
Sense of parental/societal responsibility to vaccinate		---[a]
I have a responsibility to vaccinate my children for the protection of all children. (n = 49)	41 (83.7)	
As a caregiver, I have a responsibility to vaccinate my child for his/her welfare. (n = 49)	45 (91.8)	

[a]Number and percent who indicated that they agreed or strongly agreed with the statement.
[b]Coefficient alpha not computed for scales comprised of fewer than three items.
[c]Items were reverse coded for computation of subscale score and coefficient alpha.

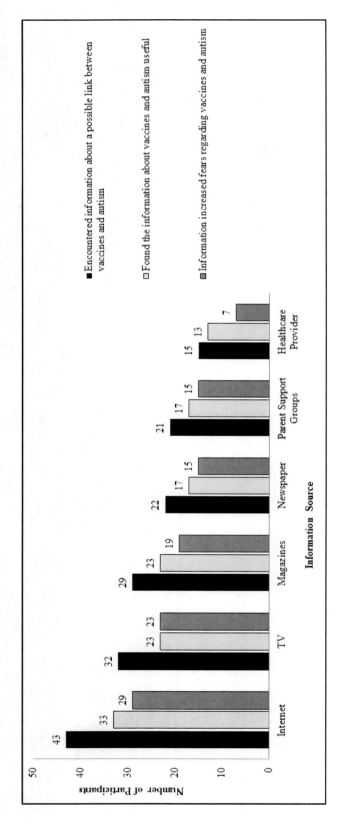

Figure 1. Caregivers' exposure to information regarding a link between vaccines and autism.

Three items on the Vaccine Attitude Questionnaire served as the outcome measures for analysis. Responses to the following three questions were dichotomized (1 = strongly agree/agree; 0 = strongly disagree/disagree): "Vaccines contributed to the cause of my child's autism," "I would recommend to others not to vaccinate their children," and "If there were no penalties for doing so, I would refuse to vaccinate my children."

Subscale scores were computed as an average of item ratings. Bivariate associations between the outcome variables and continuous and categorical correlates were assessed through a series of independent samples t-tests and chi-square tests, respectively.

OUR FINDINGS

Demographic characteristics of the sample are described in Table 1. The majority of the sample was white (68%), 50% reported a family income of greater than $25,000, and 54% of mothers had attended some college. The majority (86%) of children were male. The average age of children was 5.82 (range: 3 to 9); 22% were under the age of 5 years. Most children (70%) had at least one sibling.

Table 3 describes participants' attitudes toward childhood vaccination. Of note, only 38% believed that childhood vaccines were safe, 30% believed that scientific evidence had shown that vaccines do not cause autism, and 71% reported that they were concerned that their child could get autism from vaccines. However, the majority (89%) did believe that vaccines were effective in preventing disease. Most (92%) believed that VPDs were serious and 88% believed that their children would be at risk for those diseases without vaccination. The majority of parents (72%) also believed that people who do not vaccinate their children put others at risk. Similarly, 84% felt that they had a responsibility to vaccinate their children "for the protection of all children."

Parents' trust in regulatory and health-related institutions involved with vaccination was relatively low. For example, only 60% trusted the opinion of their child's PCP regarding the safety of vaccines, and 47% trusted the pharmaceutical companies producing vaccines. Fewer than half (45%) believed that the government would stop vaccination programs if they were found to be dangerous to children. Despite mistrust, most parents (79%) reported that they did discuss their concerns about vaccination openly with their child's PCP and 70% reported that their concerns were taken seriously. Most parents valued their autonomy in the vaccine decision process, with 71% reporting that vaccination should be a parental decision rather than one mandated by healthcare providers or the government. Moreover, nearly one-fourth (22%) reported that vaccines should not be mandatory for school attendance.

Figure 1 describes parents' exposure to information about the vaccine-autism controversy. The most common source was the internet (reported by 88%), followed by television, magazines, newspaper, parent support groups, and healthcare providers. The majority of parents reported that the information they obtained was useful, ranging from 65% of those receiving information from healthcare providers to 77% for that from parent support groups. Except for those who acquired information from a healthcare provider, the majority of parents reported that the information increased their fears about the association between vaccines and autism. Information obtained from parent support groups provoked fear among proportionally more parents (71%) than did television (70%), internet (67%), magazines

(63%), and newspapers (60%). Of note, among those encountering information from healthcare providers, comparatively fewer (37%) reported an increased fear of the links between vaccines and autism.

Over half (56%) of the parents believed that vaccines had contributed to the cause of their child's autism, 30% reported that they would refuse to vaccinate their children if there were no penalties for doing so, and 16% reported that they would recommend others not to vaccinate their children. Most parents (71%) believed that vaccines given later in childhood were less likely to cause autism than those given to children at a younger age and 60% believed that vaccines involving doses that were weeks or months apart were less likely to cause autism than vaccines given all that once.

Bivariate analyses

Table 1 presents results from bivariate analyses. Due to the low number (n = 8) of participants who reported that they would recommend others not to vaccinate their children, this variable was not included as an outcome in analyses.

Demographic characteristics and satisfaction with care. None of the demographic variables, including parent education level or child's autism severity, were associated with beliefs of vaccines as a cause of autism or refusal to vaccinate if no penalties existed. Of note, characteristics related to parents' perceptions of their child's PCP and accessibility/ affordability of medical care were not significantly associated with parents' belief that vaccines had contributed to their child's autism or to their desire to refuse vaccination.

Belief that vaccines contributed to child's autism. Parents who believed that vaccines had contributed to the cause of their child's autism were significantly more likely to report that they had encountered media that caused them to have fear about the possible links between vaccines and autism ($p < 0.001$). These parents had lower average ratings on subscales assessing perceived vaccine safety and efficacy ($p < 0.001$), negative consequences of non-vaccination ($p = 0.008$), trust in healthcare institutions ($p < 0.001$), and sense of responsibility to vaccinate for the welfare of their child and for other children ($p = 0.043$). Parents who believed vaccines had contributed to the cause of their child's autism also believed that parents should have more autonomy in childhood vaccination decisions ($p = 0.036$). Child autism severity nor child cognitive ability were significantly associated with parents' belief that vaccines had contributed to their child's autism.

Desire to refuse vaccination. Parents who reported that they would refuse to vaccinate their children if there were no penalties for doing so were significantly more likely to report that they had encountered media that caused them to have fear about the possible links between vaccines and autism ($p = 0.017$). These parents had a lower average ratings on subscales assessing perceived vaccine safety and efficacy ($p = 0.002$), lesser trust in healthcare institutions ($p = 0.043$), and believed that parents should have more autonomy in childhood vaccination decisions ($p = 0.004$). Parents who reported that they would refuse to vaccinate their children if there were no penalties for doing so had children with significantly lower DAS scores; however, autism severity was not significantly associated.

DISCUSSION

Among this sample of PCA, over half believed that vaccines had contributed to the cause of their child's autism, and over 70% reported that they were concerned that a child could get autism from vaccination. Nearly one-third reported that they would refuse to vaccinate their children if there were no penalties for doing so and nearly one in every six parents reported that they would discourage other parents from vaccinating their children. In this sample, nearly 90% believed that vaccines were effective in preventing disease and over 90% believed that the diseases vaccines prevent are serious. Moreover, nearly 88% of parents reported that, without vaccines, VPDs would pose a risk to their children. These findings are similar to those found in previous research (31). Many studies have reported that low perceived risk of VPDs and doubts about vaccine efficacy contribute to negative attitudes toward childhood vaccination (32-34), though there has been some evidence to the contrary (35).

Perceived safety of childhood vaccines was low, with fewer than 40% reporting that vaccines were safe. Parents who believed that vaccines had contributed to the cause of their child's autism and those who would refuse to vaccinate their children if there were no penalties for doing so reported significantly less confidence in vaccine safety and efficacy than did their counterparts. Distrust of health-related institutions responsible for ensuring safety was common, with fewer than half reporting that they trusted the companies producing vaccines and 45% believing that the government would stop an unsafe vaccination program. Parents who believed that vaccines had contributed to their child's autism and those who would refuse vaccination reported significantly less trust in health institutions. Previous research suggests that institutional trust and perceptions of safety are related. Parental trust in the institutions that develop and regulate vaccines may affect information-seeking behavior and how they receive, process, and react to risk communication from those sources, including material insisting upon vaccine safety (36). As such, vaccine promotion activities involving increased dissemination of information from sources perceived as having questionable credibility is likely to have a limited impact on vaccine attitudes, particularly when the material targets parents' risk:benefit calculus and fails to address underlying mistrust (36).

Of note, the majority of parents believed that alterations in the vaccine schedule would improve the safety of vaccines, specifically delaying vaccines until later in childhood and spacing the doses further apart. Similar attitudes have been identified in previous research (18) and national data suggest that delayed vaccination is not uncommon in the United States (37). These beliefs may be indicative of parents' attempt to educate themselves about vaccination and of their exposure to social discourses, advocated by vaccine-resistant groups and others, suggesting a moral imperative for parents to make empowered, informed, and educated decisions about vaccination to protect their children's health (38). Thus, in a sense, vaccine-resistant groups and public health authorities are promoting the same message: individuals should be informed and empowered to take personal responsibility for their health-related decisions. In this quest, however, individuals are exposed to various information sources and often to 'mixed messages' (38).

While the cross-sectional design precludes ability to draw conclusions about the origins of parents' attitudes, it is notable that 65% reported encountering information from popular media sources, parent support groups, and/or healthcare providers that increased their fear about the links between vaccines and autism. Parents who were exposed to information that provoked fears related to vaccines and autism were significantly more likely to report that vaccines had contributed to the cause of their child's autism and that they would refuse to vaccinate their children in the absence of penalties. Healthcare providers were described as the least frequent source eliciting fear, and the internet was the most common source of exposure to information about the controversy over vaccines and autism. These findings are consistent with those of Woo and colleagues (11) who found that information from magazines/newspapers, healthcare providers, and the internet played important roles in parents' suspicion about links between vaccination and their child's autism.

The implications of these findings for public health practice are complex. Parental mistrust in governmental and pharmaceutical institutions undermines these institutions' ability to discredit and/or counteract information from other sources. Moreover, mistrust may motivate parents to seek information from alternative sources, and circularly, information from alternative sources may contribute to further mistrust. Future longitudinal research is needed to unpack details about the temporality and directionality of these associations. Public health authorities' engagement in an 'information war' with other sources will likely be ineffective if content explicitly or implicitly communicates that vaccine resistance is an 'irrational' and/or ignorant miscalculation of risk without addressing trust, uncertainty, parent's personalized concepts of their children's vulnerability, and the social and political contexts in which scientific evidence is produced and vaccine decisions are made (36, 38, 39).

With the exception of information received from healthcare providers, information about autism and vaccination encountered from other sources provoked fear in the majority of those parents exposed to it. Interestingly, proportionally more parents who encountered information about autism and vaccines from parent support groups reported that it provoked fear than those who encountered the information from other sources. Previous research has shown that PCA perceive autism organizations to be an equally credible or more credible source of vaccine information than organizations such as the CDC, National Vaccine Information Center, and American Academy of Pediatrics (11). However, dimensions of trust and attitudes regarding credibility and authority are complex. For example, discourses of vaccine-resistant groups frame 'trusting blindly' in traditional scientific authority as symptomatic of disempowerment and entailing a substantive risk (38). Thus, vaccine promotion efforts aiming to improve public trust in traditional health-related institutions may be misguided if 'trust' is in itself seen by consumers as a risk (38). Of note, the present study did not inquire about the specific type of support groups with which parents were involved. Additional research about the types of organizations with which PCA typically affiliate, as well as informal and/or formal discourses about vaccination within these organizations is needed to more fully understand if and how parents' affiliation with these groups affects vaccination behavior. Furthermore, researchers and public health practitioners interested in working with and writing about these groups should be thoughtful in how they frame their language. Specifically, previous research cautions against the tendency to identify these groups with an anti-vaccine 'social movement,' as this attribution may inherently grant more social theoretic foundation to their claims by conflating it with broader political transformations focused on individual rights and resistance to authority (40).

Studies have highlighted the important role healthcare providers play in encouraging the uptake of childhood vaccination (17, 30). In fact, a literature review revealed that mistrust in healthcare systems and negative experience communicating healthcare providers about vaccination are often associated with lower vaccine uptake (6). In the present study, the vast majority of parents reported that they discussed their concerns about vaccination with their child's healthcare provider and that the provider took their concerns seriously. On average, parents had positive ratings of their healthcare providers' informativeness, sensitivity, competence, and partnership building. Nevertheless, only 60% reported that they trusted their provider's opinion regarding vaccine safety. This percentage is slightly less than that reported in a recent nationally representative survey of parents (41). Although somewhat low, the level of trust in healthcare providers exceeded that reported for other authorities associated with vaccination (pharmaceutical companies, government, etc.); thus, the patient-provider relationship may represent an opportunity for effective dialogue about childhood vaccination. Of note, however, none of the measures related to satisfaction with child's PCP or accessibility and affordability of medical care were significantly associated with vaccine attitude outcomes in this study. Given these findings and the logistical constraints faced by healthcare providers (12), immunization campaigns cannot rely solely on healthcare providers to promote vaccination, but must engage other mobilization activities and/or electronic, visual, and print media channels (41) directed at parents and support groups specifically.

Demographic and ASD-related characteristics were generally not associated with vaccine attitudes, with the exception that children of parents who reported they would refuse vaccination had lower cognitive functioning, as assessed by the DAS. Additional research is needed to investigate factors that mediate the association between childhood cognitive functioning and parents' attitudes toward childhood vaccination. For example, mediators may include differences in timing of diagnosis and appearance of symptoms of regression and/or variations in parents' information-seeking behavior according to child's level of cognitive functioning.

Most parents desired autonomy in vaccine decision-making, but the majority reported that they felt a personal obligation to vaccinate for the protection of others and the child. Parents who believed that vaccines contributed to the cause of their child's autism and those who would refuse vaccination desired significantly more decision-making autonomy than their counterparts. The former also felt significantly less responsibility to vaccinate. Interestingly, the concept of societal responsibility to vaccinate often has been ignored in vaccine promotion materials. Although the public health rationale for mitigating vaccine refusal is to maintain coverage levels necessary to achieve herd immunity, many promotional materials focus on presenting the individual-level risks and benefits of vaccination (36). In the present study, 84% of parents believed that they had a responsibility to vaccinate their children for the protection of all children, and parents' sense of societal responsibility to vaccinate was strongly associated with their vaccine attitudes; these findings highlight a pivotal point to target in vaccine promotion. Public health communications and efforts addressing vaccine uptake among PCA should leverage and include information addressing attitudes surrounding the societal implications of individual-level vaccine uptake.

Nevertheless, the tension between individual autonomy and government regulation in immunization has a long and contentious history in the United States and will be difficult to address (42). Nationally, parents are increasingly seeking nonmedical exemptions for vaccination (43), citing religious, ideological, and/or safety concerns (44, 45). As discussed above, in the public health arena, vaccine refusal is often assumed to be a matter of miscalculated of risk; however, autonomy in the context of social movements involving 'alternative' concepts of health and responsibility (36), empowered decision-making (38), and tendencies toward a more personalized approach to parenting and vaccine decision-making (39) also play a role. In the coming years, these and other significant health-related issues related to vaccine refusal (46-48) will force the public health community, policy makers, and the public to confront questions surrounding boundaries of personal autonomy and societal responsibility (44).

While this study provides important preliminary insights into the vaccine attitudes of PCA, the study is not without limitations. Though they were based on measures used in previous research in other settings, the questionnaires assessing parent satisfaction with care and vaccine attitudes were self-developed for this formative study and are in need of further evaluation and integration with validated measures developed since the commencement of this study (49). Additionally, although demographic differences between survey respondents and non-respondents were not observed, the response rate (63%) does raise concerns of participation bias. The study was based on a convenience sample of parents participating in a separate autism-related study; given that the vaccine attitudes of participating parents may differ from non-participants, the findings should be generalized with caution. The small sample size also resulted in limited statistical power to detect differences in some pairwise comparisons.

Conclusion

PCA are at the center of arguably one of the most heated debates surrounding vaccination in recent history (7, 8). The present study highlights the complexity of parents' beliefs about vaccination and underscores the failure of popular narratives dichotomizing attitudes as "pro-vaccine" and "anti-vaccine" to adequately portray nuances. In this study, most parents reported serious concerns about vaccine safety, but the majority viewed vaccines as necessary and effective. Concerns about safety are likely related, in part, to issues of trust, perceived credibility, and exposure to sources of information suggesting a link between vaccines and autism. From a public health perspective, the findings clearly point to a need to reestablish parents' trust in scientific evidence suggesting no link between vaccines and autism and in government-backed immunization programs more generally. This will be an ongoing and tenuous process that should involve transparent and truthful dialogue (50), engage trusted members of the community, and acknowledge the value of parent empowerment and information-seeking.

Acknowledgments

The authors would like to acknowledge Jennifer Woods for her contribution to the literature search and review, and would like to thank the reviewer for thoughtful suggestions that led to the improvement of this manuscript.

Funding source: No external funding was secured for this study.

Financial disclosure: The authors have no financial relationship relevant to this article to disclose.

Conflict of interest: The authors have no conflicts of interest to disclose.

REFERENCES

[1] Rosenberg RE, Law JK, Yenokyan G, McGready J, Kaufmann WE, Law PA. Characteristics and concordance of autism spectrum disorders among 277 twin pairs. Arch Pediatr Adolesc Med 2009;163(10):907-14.
[2] Hallmayer J, Cleveland S, Torres A, Phillips J, Cohen B, Torigoe T, et al. Genetic heritability and shared environmental factors among twin pairs with autism. Arch Gen Psychiatry 2011;68(11):1095-102.
[3] Ronald A, Happe F, Bolton P, Butcher LM, Price TS, Wheelwright S, et al. Genetic heterogeneity between the three components of the autism spectrum: a twin study. J Am Acad Child Adolesc Psychiatry 2006;45(6):691-9.
[4] National Research Council. Adverse effects of vaccines: Evidence and causality. Washington, DC: National Academies Press, 2012.
[5] Bazzano A, Zeldin A, Schuster E, Barrett C, Lehrer D. Vaccine-related beliefs and practices of parents of children with autism spectrum disorders. Am J Intellect Dev Dsabil 2012;117(3):233-42.
[6] Brown K, Kroll JS, Hudson MJ, Ramsay M, Green J, Long SJ, et al. Factors underlying parental decisions about combination childhood vaccinations including MMR: a systematic review. Vaccine 2010;28(26):4235-48.
[7] Offit PA. Vaccines and autism revisited -- the Hannah Poling case. N Engl J Med 2008;358(20):2089-91.
[8] Smith MJ, Ellenberg SS, Bell LM, Rubin DM. Media coverage of the measles-mumps-rubella vaccine and autism controversy and its relationship to MMR immunization rates in the United States. Pediatrics 2008;121(4):e836-43.
[9] Biao J. Prevalence of autism spectrum disorders. Autism and Developmental Disabilities Monitoring Network, 14 Sites, United States, 2008. MMWR 2012;61(SS03):1-19.
[10] Mercer L, Creighton S, Holden JJA, Lewis MES. Parental perspectives on the causes of an autism spectrum disorder in their children. J Genet Couns 2006;15(1):41-50.
[11] Woo E, Ball R, Bostrom A, Shadomy SV, Ball LK, Evans G, et al. Vaccine risk perception among reporters of autism after vaccination: Vaccine Adverse Event Reporting System 1990–2001. Am J Public Health 2004;94(6):990-5
[12] Pineda D, Myers MG. Finding reliable information about vaccines. Pediatrics 2011;127(Suppl 1):S134-S7.
[13] Kata A. A postmodern Pandora's box: Anti-vaccination misinformation on the Internet. Vaccine 2010;28(7):1709-16.
[14] Zimmerman RK, Wolfe RM, Fox DE, Fox JR, Nowalk MP, Troy JA, et al. Vaccine criticism on the world wide web. J Med Internet Res 2005;7(2):e17.
[15] Nicholson M, Leask J. Lessons from an online debate about measles-mumps-rubella (MMR) immunization. Vaccine 2012;30(25):3806-12.
[16] Brown K, Sevdalis N. Lay vaccination narratives on the web: are they worth worrying about? Med Decis Making 2011;31(5):707-9.
[17] Healy CM, Pickering LK. How to communicate with vaccine-hesitant parents. Pediatrics 2011;127(Suppl 1):S127-S33.
[18] Luthy KE, Beckstrand RL, Callister LC. Parental hesitation in immunizing children in Utah. Public Health Nurs 2010;27(1):25-31.
[19] Vannice KS, Salmon DA, Shui I, Omer SB, Kissner J, Edwards KM, et al. Attitudes and beliefs of parents concerned about vaccines: impact of timing of immunization information. Pediatrics 2011;127(Suppl 1):S120-S6.
[20] Carbone PS, Behl DD, Azor V, Murphy NA. The medical home for children with autism spectrum disorders: Parent and pediatrician perspectives. J Autism Dev Disord 2010;40(3):317-24.
[21] Kennedy A, Lavail K, Nowak G, Basket M, Landry S. Confidence about vaccines in the United States: understanding parents' perceptions. Health Affairs 2011;30(6):1151-9.

[22] Ruble LA, Dalrymple NJ, McGrew JH. The effects of consultation on Individualized Education Program outcomes for young children with autism: The collaborative model for promoting competence and success. J Early Intervent 2010;32(4):286-301.
[23] Ruble LA, McGrew JH, Toland M, Dalrymple NJ, Jung L. A randomized controlled trial of COMPASS web-based and face-to-face teacher coaching. J Consult Clin Psychol 2013;81(3):566-72.
[24] American Psychiatric Association. Diagnostic and statistical manual of mental disorders, 4th ed, text rev ed. Washington, DC: American Psychiatric Association, 2004.
[25] Lord C, Risi S, Lambrecht L, Cook EJ, Leventhal B, DiLavore P, et al. The autism diagnostic observation schedule-generic: a standard measure of social and communication deficits associated with the spectrum of autism. J Autism Dev Disord 2000;30(3):205-23.
[26] Schopler E, Reichler R, DeVellis R, Daly K. Toward objective classification of childhood autism: Childhood Autism Rating Scale (CARS). J Autism Dev Disord 1980;10(1):91-103.
[27] Elliott C. Differential Ability Scales. New York: Harcourt Brace Jovanovitch Psychological Corporation, 1990.
[28] Marshall GN, Hays RD. The patient satisfaction questionnaire short-form (PSQ-18). Santa Monica, CA: Rand, 1994.
[29] Street RL. Physicians' communication and parents' evaluations of pediatric consultations. Med Care 1991;29(11):1146-52.
[30] Casiday R, Cresswell T, Wilson D, Panter-Brick C. A survey of UK parental attitudes to the MMR vaccine and trust in medical authority. Vaccine 2006;24(2):177-84.
[31] Freed GL, Clark SJ, Butchart AT, Singer DC, Davis MM. Parental vaccine safety concerns in 2009. Pediatrics 2010;125(4):654-9.
[32] Salmon DA, Moulton LH, Omer SB, DeHart MP, Stokley S, Halsey NA. Factors associated with refusal of childhood vaccines among parents of school-aged children: a case-control study. Arch Pediatr Adolesc Med 2005;159(5):470-6.
[33] Fredrickson DD, Davis TC, Arnould CL, Kennen EM, Hurniston SG, Cross JT, et al. Childhood immunization refusal: provider and parent perceptions. Fam Med 2004;36(6):431-9.
[34] Allred N, Shaw K, Santibanez T, Rickert D, Santoli J. Parental vaccine safety concerns: results from the National Immunization Survey, 2001-2002. Am J Prev Med 2005;28(2):221-4.
[35] LaVail KH, Kennedy AM. The role of attitudes about vaccine safety, efficacy, and value in explaining parents' reported vaccination behavior. Health Educ Behav 2013;40(5):544-51.
[36] Hobson-West P. Understanding vaccination resistance: moving beyond risk. Health Risk Society 2003;5(3):273-83.
[37] Luman ET, Barker LE, Shaw KM, McCauley MM, Buehler JW, Pickering LK. Timeliness of childhood vaccinations in the United States. JAMA 2005;293 (10):1204-11.
[38] Hobson-West P. 'Trusting blindly can be the biggest risk of all': organised resistance to childhood vaccination in the UK. Sociol Health Illness 2007;29(2):198-215.
[39] Poltorak M, Leach M, Fairhead J, Cassell J. 'MMR talk'and vaccination choices: An ethnographic study in Brighton. Soc Sci Med 2005;61(3):709-19.
[40] Blume S. Anti-vaccination movements and their interpretations. Soc Sci Med 2006;62(3):628-42.
[41] Freed GL, Clark SJ, Butchart AT, Singer DC, Davis MM. Sources and perceived credibility of vaccine-safety information for parents. Pediatrics 2011;127(Suppl 1):S107-S12.
[42] Colgrove J. State of immunity: the politics of vacination in twentieth-century America. Berkeley, CA: University of California Press, 2006.
[43] Omer SB, Pan WKY, Halsey NA, Stokley S, Moulton LH, Navar AM, et al. Nonmedical exemptions to school immunization requirements: secular trends and association of state policies with pertussis incidence. JAMA 2006;296(14):1757-63.
[44] Salmon DA, Omer SB. Individual freedoms versus collective responsibility: immunization decision-making in the face of occasionally competing values. Emerg Themes Epidemiol 2006;3:13-3.
[45] Poland GA, Jacobson RM. Understanding those who do not understand: a brief review of the anti-vaccine movement. Vaccine 2001;19(17-19):2440-5.

[46] Salmon DA, Haber M, Gangarosa EJ, Phillips L, Smith NJ, Chen RT. Health consequences of religious and philosophical exemptions from immunization laws: individual and societal risk of measles. JAMA 1999;282(1):47-53.
[47] Omer SB, Enger KS, Moulton LH, Halsey NA, Stokley S, Salmon DA. Geographic clustering of nonmedical exemptions to school immunization requirements and associations with geographic clustering of pertussis. Am J Epidemiol 2008;168(12):1389-96.
[48] Feikin DR, Lezotte DC, Hamman RF, Salmon DA, Chen RT, Hoffman RE. Individual and community risks of measles and pertussis associated with personal exemptions to immunization. JAMA 2000;284(24):3145-50.
[49] Brown K, Shanley R, Cowley NA, van Wijgerden J, Toff P, Falconer M, et al. Attitudinal and demographic predictors of measles, mumps and rubella (MMR) vaccine acceptance: development and validation of an evidence-based measurement instrument. Vaccine 2011;29(8):1700-9.
[50] Poland GA, Spier R. Fear, misinformation, and innumerates: how the Wakefield paper, the press, and advocacy groups damaged the public health. Vaccine 2010;28(12):2361-2.

Section Four - Health and culture

Chapter 29

IMMIGRANT COLLEGE STUDENTS' EXPERIENCES WITH THEIR AMERICAN PHYSICIANS

Cecilia S Obeng*, PhD, Roberta E Emetu, MLS, and Sean Bowman, MA*

Department of Applied Health Science, School of Public Health,
Indiana University, Bloomington, Indiana, United States of America

ABSTRACT

Immigrant students face a myriad of problems in the United States. This study describes the experiences of immigrant college students with their American physicians. The study was conducted in the mid-west. One hundred and forty questionnaires were distributed to participants, and 86 answered the questionnaires giving a response rate of 61%. Aspects of qualitative methods—the Constant Comparative method and the Phenomenological approach—were used in this research. Findings indicated that the students were dissatisfied with some of the services received from their American physicians, but indicated that the American physicians were more helpful than physicians in their home countries. Recommendations include that American physicians take into consideration the culture of immigrants when providing services.

Keywords: immigrants, American physicians, college students, culture

INTRODUCTION

Preventative healthcare, which includes screening and regular check-ups, are an integral part of health. The Centers for Disease Control and Prevention (CDC) states that routine visits to the one's healthcare provider can extend life expectancy and decrease the cost of medical care (1). Immigrants in the United States (US) are from diverse backgrounds (2-5). Hispanic and

---

* Correspondence: Cecilia S Obeng, PhD, Associate Professor, Indiana University, School of Public Health, 1025 E 7th Street, SPH 116, Bloomington, IN 47405, United States. E-mail: cobeng@indiana.edu.

Asian Americans make up the fastest growing sector of the US population (6). Often times immigrants are unable to access, seek, or receive health care due to barriers. A study that examined responses of a nationally representative database of recent immigrants found that those who migrate to the US frequently experience a lack of access, high costs, and difficulty obtaining medical insurance along with barriers such as access to information, cultural or linguistic obstacles, and an inability to understand the US healthcare system (6). Gaining a better understanding of the experiences that immigrants undergo in the healthcare system is thus important.

The period when individuals enter college marks a period of transition from adolescence to adulthood. For many university students, college may be the first time away from home where they must independently make decisions. College students are regarded as a vulnerable population who are susceptible to many health problems. Research has illustrated that the period of adolescence is a stage when risky behavior is most common (7). Therefore, access to care is imperative for this subpopulation. The disposition of an international college student is vastly different from that of the traditional native college student. International students go through the federal process of applying and being granted a visa before entry into the country. Beyond this procedure, the acculturation process is expected immediately from international students. These students are expected to cross cultural, and at times, bilingual lines fairly quickly in addition to becoming accustomed to the policies at the higher educational institution.

Acculturation is defined as the process of incorporating and understanding behaviors, beliefs, and values of a culture; however, current research has focused on changes of a cultural group (8-10). Getting accustomed to the healthcare system is a form of acculturation for immigrants, including international college students. Therefore, information about healthcare access, utilization, and health informational sources is needed and should be available for incoming international studies. There is need for further investigation regarding acculturation of the healthcare system among international students, especially regarding the mental health concerns that may accompany it.

A meta-analysis revealed that international students face various stressors such as language barriers, educational stress, sociocultural difficulties, discrimination, practical stressors, and acculturative stress (11). Another study that sampled Asian International students' found that racial identity status, Asian values, ethnic identity affirmation and belonging were predictors of wellbeing (12). Even though international students tend to have a strong sense of identity, they are less likely to utilize medical facilities for healthcare and mental health services (13, 14). In a study that examined trends in health information utilization, in comparison to native students, international students reported a least likelihood of utilizing the medical center's health staff, health educators, faculty or coursework as a source of health information, but were more likely to utilize their parents as a health informational source (15).

Doctor-patient relationship is an important aspect to the adequate care. A qualitative study that interviewed 22 individuals (10 participates who saw their regular healthcare practitioner and 12 who saw an unfamiliar practitioner), found that patients preferred to create a personal relationship with their practitioner, and reported that it was difficult to change practitioner even if the care was poor (16). If care provided by a healthcare provider is perceived to be inadequate it could prompt the patient to not return to the practitioner. For international students, the inability to build a tangible relationship with a healthcare provider could have lasting effect on pursuing routine and preventative examinations.

Communication between a patient and their doctor is highly recognized as an integral part of patient care, particularly because it has implications for both successful treatment and adverse events. A study conducted at a hospital interviewed 84 patients about their general clarity of health information, responsiveness of concerns, explanation of problems, explanation of processes of care, explanation of self-care after discharge, empowerment, decision-making, and desire and ability to comply with recommendations (17). Results found that 44% of patents had health literacy inadequacy; in addition, patients rated the clarity of communication provided by their healthcare provider as the lowest (17). Adequate patient communication can be beneficial for assisting a patient with health literacy, procedures, and necessary treatment. It is imperative that adequate doctor-patient relationship and communication is addressed as an essential facet of healthcare as international student begin the process of becoming familiarized with the healthcare culture in the U.S. Therefore, the purpose of this study is to examine college students' experience with their American physicians while residing in the U.S.

METHODS

The study utilized purposeful sampling (18) to recruit college immigrant students living within a community containing a large university. All participants were born outside the U.S.

Instrument

The data collection instrument contained a list of 14 questions. The questionnaires consisted of both open- and closed- ended questions. The questionnaires were distributed to participants by hand as well as via email. Participants' responses to these questions formed the basis of the claims made in the research. The questionnaire also covered the research participants' level of education (undergraduate or graduate) and their utilization of clinics and hospitals in the US.

Procedure

Potential participants in this study were contacted through email, phone calls and, where possible, in person after the researchers were given approval by the University's Institutional Review Board Potential participants were notified that taking part in this study was voluntary. Consenting participants took approximately 20 minutes to independently complete the questionnaire at their convenience. Completed questionnaires were hand delivered to the researcher, where possible, or sent by email.

Data coding and analysis

Collected data from the questionnaire were coded and compared according to similar identified answers to the questionnaire, then grouped together and sorted into categories by theme. Constant Comparative Method was used, the data was coded inductively and then each segment of the data was taken in turn and compared to one or more categories to determine its relevance (19). As the coding of new segments of data were compared to the coding of existing data, "new analytic categories and new relationships between categories" were discovered (19). Moreover, phenomenological methods assisted the researcher in identifying commonalities within participants' personal experiences (19-22).

RESULTS AND DISCUSSION

The majority of participants were in their middle twenties, had 0-1 children, and also had health insurance. There were eighteen countries of origination identified among participants; however, the majority of participants' home country was either in China, S. Korea, or India.

Analysis of the results indicates that some of the immigrant students had problems communicating with their physicians. The excerpts below explicate and exemplify the above-mentioned claim:

> "the Physicians ask detailed questions that I did not understand"
> "I'm not sure whether my doctor would understand me.
> "I had no confidence in speaking English"
> "A participant noted "just hard to explain or express myself.""

As exemplified below, some participants indicated that American physicians could perform complicated procedures given the fact that they had sophisticated medical technology.

> "they have high tech equipment and facilities"
> "their technology is pretty advanced and help them take care of their patients efficiently."

Eleven participants believed that the physicians performed complicated procedures not because such procedures were necessary but because the physicians just wanted money. Note the following excerpts:

> "American Physicians are pretty well qualified compared to general standard. However my one complaint is that for e.g. even for a small stomach pain they would do all kinds of unnecessary test leading up to a large medical bill."
> "I think in Italy they care more about you. Here it is hard to meet a very good one, it's all about money."

Another participant indicated "they have long procedure of taking care of patients and too expensive comparing to other countries."

Some participants indicated that American physicians lacked compassion. For example, a participant noted:

"some issues that are important to me don't seem to be important to my doctor"

Another participant wrote:

"The physician in this country shows no affection to their patients. He rushed through exams since you are just a client. He does not care about you as a person."

Some participants noted that they were always given "pills" and that they could easily predict what they would be given by going to a doctor; which did not give them an incentive to go to the hospital. A participant opined: "I feel they always want to give me pills for everything even with small ailment that can go away by themselves."

Some participants said they had no confidence in American physicians. For instance, a participant noted: "I feel their service is mediocre and I have no confidence in them"

Although immigrant college students were dissatisfied with some of the services received from their American doctors, the students noted that American physicians are very helpful compared to the physicians in their home countries. Four participants wrote:

"they are professional and helpful compared to Physician back home"
"Does a good job understanding my illness"
"I just think that American Physicians understands specific health care much better than back home"
"They asked detailed information and very careful than doctors in my home country. Run through all the test before given medication."

A close attention to the data points to the fact that the study has uncovered both the positive as well as the negative experiences of international college students with their American physicians. Because majority of the participants were from different cultural backgrounds they indicated several times in the data that cultural differences were the biggest issue between them and their American doctors.

It is important to emphasize the necessity of adequate healthcare services, and the significance of differences with regards to culture and behavior. Being in the same environment or setting must not be seen as having identical behavior and culture. What international students considered lack of compassion may be considered doing one's work diligently in the American culture. Hence, emotional or behavioral patterns deemed appropriate in one culture may be seen as a taboo in another culture. Such opposite spectra can cause major problems between physicians and their patients. It is important to note that people from different cultures react to identical situations differently and how one reports the symptoms of his or her ailment or sickness depends on what is considered appropriate in one's culture and the community in which one were raised. Culture may determine how one reacts to a problem and the extent to which such a reaction influences one's health and in seeking help with illnesses. It is for this reason that cultural background and differences should be taken into consideration when discussing American physicians and their immigrant patients. Ignoring the cultural differences can result in one's inability to efficiently discuss and/or deal with this topic.

Also, participants' inability to tell their physicians their health problems because they had problems speaking English, contributed to their frustration with some of the services received from their American physicians. Majority of these college students had no confidence in speaking English, and they feared making mistakes linguistically. Also, some students were not sure whether people would understand them because of their accent. The participants in this study indicated that the above-mentioned issues contributed to their inability to communicate with their physicians.

This study has provided previously unavailable information on migration and utilization of healthcare services by immigrant college students. In particular, the findings of the study show that immigrants college students' country of origin or birth and their culture influence their health service utilization experiences in US.

RECOMMENDATIONS

Due to the above findings, this study recommends the need for American physicians to take the culture of immigrant college students into consideration when providing healthcare services, since ignoring culture could negatively impact the overall healthcare system and the healthcare access particular to immigrants.

REFERENCES

[1] Center of Disease Control and Prevention. Regular check-ups are important. URL: http://www.cdc.gov/family/checkup/#overview.
[2] Larsen LJ. The foreign-born population in the United States: 2003. Current population reports, US Census, 2004 Aug: 20-551.
[3] Bornstein MH, Cote LR. "Who Is sitting across from me?" Immigrant mothers' knowledge of parenting and children's development. Pediatrics 2004;114(5):e557-64.
[4] Hwang WC. The psychotherapy adaptation and modification framework: Application to Asian Americans. Am Psychol 2006;61(7): 702-15.
[5] Cruz GD, Chen Y, Salazar CR, Le Geros RZ. The association of immigration and acculturation attributes with oral health among immigrants in New York City. J Information 2009;99(S2): S474-80.
[6] Portes A, Fern?ndez-Kelly P, Light D. Life on the edge: immigrants confront the American health system. Ethnic Racial Stud 2012; 35(1): 3-22.
[7] Teese R, Bradley G. Predicting recklessness in emerging adults: A test of a psychosocial model. J Soc Psychol 2008;148(1):105-28.
[8] Berry JW. Acculturation as varieties of adaptation. In: Padilla AM, ed. Acculturation theory, models and some new findings. Boulder, CO: Westview Press, 1980: pp. 9–25.
[9] Berry JW. Immigration, acculturation, and adaptation. Appl Psychol 1997;46:5-68.
[10] Berry JW. A psychology of immigration. J Soc Issues 2001;57: 615-31.
[11] Smith RA, Khawaja NG. A review of the acculturation experiences of international students. Int J Intercult Relat 2011;35(6):699-713.
[12] Iwamoto DK, Liu WM. The impact of racial identity, ethnic identity, asian values and race-related stress on Asian Americans and Asian international college students' psychological well-being. J Couns Psychol 2010;57(1):79.

[13] Loya F, Reddy R, Hinshaw SP. Mental illness stigma as a mediator of differences in Caucasian and South Asian college students' attitudes toward psychological counseling. J Couns Psychol 2010;57(4):484-90.
[14] Kim J. Acculturation phenomena experienced by the spouses of Korean international students in the United States. Qual Health Res 2012;22(6):755-67.
[15] Vader AM, Walters ST, Roudsari B, Nguyen N. Where do college students get health information? Believability and use of health information sources. Health Promot Pract 2011;12(5):713-22.
[16] Thygeson M, Morrissey L, Ulstad V. Adaptive leadership and the practice of medicine: a complexity-based approach to reframing the doctor–patient relationship. J Eval Clin Pract 2010;16(5):1009-15.
[17] Kripalani S, Jacobson TA, Mugalla IC, Cawthon CR, Niesner KJ, Vaccarino V. Health literacy and the quality of physician-patient communication during hospitalization. J Hosp Med 2010;5(5):269-75.
[18] Patton MQ. Qualitative evaluation and research methods, 2nd ed. Newbury Park, CA: Sage, 1990.
[19] Schwandt TA. Dictionary of qualitative inquiry, 2nd ed. Thousand Oaks, CA: Sage, 2001.
[20] Smith JA, Osborn M. Interpretative phenomenological analysis. In: Smith JA, ed. Qualitative psychology: A practical guide to research methods. Thousand Oaks, CA: Sage, 2003.
[21] Moustakas C. Phenomenological research methods. Thousand Oaks, CA: Sage, 1994.
[22] Van Manen M. Researching lived experience. Ontario, Canada: Althouse, 1990.

Submitted: June 06, 2014. *Revised:* July 01, 2014. *Accepted:* July 12, 2014.

In: Public Health Yearbook 2015
Editor: Joav Merrick

ISBN: 978-1-63484-514-4
© 2016 Nova Science Publishers, Inc.

Chapter 30

FOOD CHOICES AND EATING PATTERNS OF INTERNATIONAL STUDENTS IN THE UNITED STATES: A PHENOMENOLOGICAL STUDY

*Bobbie H Saccone, MS, RD, and Cecilia S Obeng, PhD**

Department of Applied Health Science, School of Public Health, Indiana University, Bloomington, Indiana, United States of America

ABSTRACT

Despite extensive quantitative research on dietary changes of immigrants in the United States, only a handful of studies address the dietary changes international college students' face from their perspectives. This study examines the shifts in dietary patterns and health status of international students using a phenomenological approach. An open-ended survey was conducted with 25 participants at a public university. The results revealed three major themes: 1) changes in types of foods eaten; 2) factors affecting food choice decisions and eating patterns, and 3) health outcomes. The findings point to a resistance in accepting less indigenous foods and a protective negotiation when adopting foreign (US) foods or eating practices. The study will help international students in particular, and immigrants in general, to learn from each other to maintain or improve their health.

Keywords: eating patterns, food, phenomenological, international students

INTRODUCTION

The international student population in the United States has steadily grown for more than half a century and has increased more than 25 times, with current enrollment at 764,495 students (1). Throughout the past decades, many studies have examined international college

---

* Correspondence: Cecilia S Obeng, PhD, Associate Professor, Indiana University, School of Public Health, 1025 E. 7th Street, SPH 116, Bloomington, IN 47405, United States. E-mail: cobeng@indiana.edu.

students' cultural adjustment issues such as culture shock, confusion about role expectations, lack of social support, social self-efficacy, and language barriers, collectively referred to as acculturative stress (2). Individuals experiencing significant amounts of acculturative stress typically encounter a deterioration of overall health status (3).

The transitional period between adolescence and adulthood is known as a critical time for adopting and developing health behaviors related to prevention and wellness (4).

Living independently in new environments, such as those for undergraduate college students, further make this transition an important time. International college students of all ages may face similar issues related to cultural assimilation and stress of transitional periods (5). International student health, particularly nutritional health, is not well known and warrants exploratory and in-depth study.

One of the numerous health related changes that often occurs with immigration is change in diet. It is well known that undesirable changes in diet can lead to lifestyle-related diseases such as obesity, and obesity-related conditions such as heart disease, diabetes, and certain forms of cancer (6). The nutritional health and wellbeing of international students in institutions of higher education in the US is understudied despite the fact that it supports the goal of academic success.

A study by Pan et al. (7) discovered that changes in eating behaviors identified by Asian students living in the US involved skipping breakfast, increased frequency of consumption of salty and sweet snack items, and decreased frequency of consumption of vegetables. Another study in Belgium examined the change in dietary habits of international students from 60 different countries and concluded that healthier choices were hindered by a perceived unavailability of healthy food products (8).

It is necessary to understand the process by which international students adopt or blend the dietary practices of the US to their everyday lives. Dietary acculturation and nutrition transition are concepts that refer to the process that occurs when individuals of a minority group adopt eating patterns and food choices representative of the host country (9, 10). Dietary acculturation often focuses on large shifts in diet to more energy-dense foods that can impact nutritional outcomes such as increases in body weight (9, 10). However, it is important to note that dietary acculturation can also result in healthful dietary changes.

The exposure of international college students to a new food supply potentially changes the way food is chosen, acquired, stored and prepared. Often the unavailability of what these international college students consider traditional food and ingredients, results in increased intake of host country foods. Researches done on dietary acculturation often report an overall improvement in nutritional health when traditional healthful eating patterns are retained (9, 10).

Given the above literature on dietary issues, this study examined the shifts in dietary patterns and health status of international students living and studying in the US.

METHODS

The study took place at a large mid-western public university in the spring of 2103 and was designed for both undergraduate and graduate international students. The criteria for selection to participate in the study included being an immigrant and a full-time college student.

Twenty-five participants from five continents representing 13 different countries were recruited using a snowballing and purposeful sampling technique (11). Specifically, students known to one of the authors through personal contacts were identified and asked to provide contact information for other students they knew of who met participant eligibility. The Indiana University Institutional Review Board approved the research project. Participants were not given any incentives.

Procedure

Eligible participants were sent a ten-question survey instrument that contained both closed and open-ended questions via e-mail. Survey Monkey was used to format the instrument that was pilot tested to ensure clarity of the questions and intended meaning. The participants in the pilot study consisted of three females and one male. They were from Senegal, Brazil, China, and Saudi Arabia. The open-ended questions were refined after they were collected on-line to make them more understandable. For example, one student in the pilot study stated that she was confused by the wording of a question that asked about first impressions of the food system in the US. This question was later clarified and retested to ensure that it was easier to comprehend and interpret. Closed-ended questions gave demographic information that included age, gender, and year in school, home country, and length of time enrolled in a US school.

Study design

A phenomenological approach was used to explore the experiences of the research participants' encounters with food and diet changes in the US.

Phenomenology is an umbrella term that comprises both a philosophy and a psychology that co-inform each discipline (12). The word phenomenology comes from the Greeks words phainoemn and phenesti meaning appearance or to show forth, and logos, meaning logic or reason. Phenomenologists seek to describe the central meanings individuals ascribe to their personal experiences in hope of capturing human experience, in all of its simplicities and complexities (13). Phenomenology also seeks to find commonalities of shared experiences as "universal essences" among groups (11, 12, 14-16). An important characteristic about phenomenology that made it most suitable for this study was the fact that it focuses on how people make sense of experiences and how they transform such experiences in subjective meanings of consciousness and describe them (17). This qualitative approach was employed to illustrate the meanings of this shared experience from the viewpoints of the participants, while also revealing the differences that may be unique to different cultural groups. The data was closely examined using elements of grounded theory and placed in seven categories which were clustered into 3 overarching themes [changes in types of foods eaten, factors affecting food decisions and eating patterns, and health outcomes] representing participant's utterances (18).

RESULTS

The participants (international students from five continents) revealed common essences of their lived experiences in food and eating in the US. The only characteristic that was similar among students was coming to the US for college from other lands. Participants were comprised of both genders, had been in the US ranging from one year to more than five years, varied in age from 17-39 years, and represented undergraduate, master's level and doctoral level student-type (see detail characteristics of participants in Table 1).

Table 1. Selected characteristics of participants

Characteristic	n	%
Age		
17-24	6	24
25-29	10	40
30-34	6	24
35-45	3	12
Gender		
Male	10	40
Female	15	60
Student Type		
Undergraduate	2	8
Master's	6	24
Doctoral	17	68
Years in US		
<1	6	24
1-2	8	32
2-3	4	16
4-5	1	4
>5	6	24
Home Country		
Africa	3	12
Kenya	1	4
Nigeria	1	4
Senegal	1	4
Asia	15	60
Austria	1	4
China	4	16
India	1	4
Japan	3	12
Jordan	1	4
South Korea	3	12
Turkey	2	8
South America	5	20
Brazil	5	20
Europe	1	4
Italy	1	4
North America	1	4
Puerto Rico	1	4

Survey results yielded three overarching themes namely: 1) changes in types of foods eaten, 2) factors affecting food decisions and eating patterns, and 3) health outcomes.

Changes in types of foods eaten

The first broad theme was described by the participants as specific changes in diet in their current lives as students in the US. Diet was defined as the food and drink that is eaten habitually or usually. Three sub-themes were prevalent in theme-one. The first subtheme was: (a) negative shifts in dietary choices. An example of dietary acculturation can be seen in this Chinese female doctoral student's statement:

> In China I ate lots of fresh vegetables, soups and various foods made from flour such as dumplings, (now) I eat more dairy, meat, sweets snacks and drinks in the US. I barely have Chinese soups anymore."

The second sub-theme was: (b) resistance to change food choices. An example of participants' resistance can be explained through the words of a male doctoral student from Japan who noted:

> Compared to Japanese convenience stores, the counterparts in the US have so fewer variety and selection of food on shelves...well, except the amount of chips. Hot dogs and corn dogs cannot be the substitute for grilled salmon bento, packs of rice balls (onigiri) that I have used in Japan.

The third subtheme was: (c) negotiation of home country and US food choices. A male master's degree student from China warned:

> You may get use to traditional American food very quick; otherwise, learn to cook to satisfy your Chinese stomach.

Another example comes from a female doctoral student from Turkey who stated:

> Fast food (in the US) was a fast and convenient choice for me (when I first came to the US)...I ended up consuming a lot of burger, burrito, and chicken wings. After spending a year here, I have realized that I was gaining weight, so I tried to change my diet by cooking at home. Now I am trying to eat what I was eating in Turkey, as we call (it) "food."

Factors affecting food decisions and eating patterns

This theme was characterized by three dominant subthemes namely:

- Environmental factors of access;
- Availability and cost, and
- Individual factors.

Environmental factors were inherent in each participant's survey. Access and availability for all but specific national foods was predominately described as easy to acquire as illustrated by the common phrase:

> "Shopping is convenient" and
> "There are many food choices so that should not be a problem,"

Price was addressed by the majority of participants (n=15 or 60%). There were few similarities related to price between participants' excerpts. A participant wrote:

> "Fast food is cheap" and
> "Healthier foods are more expensive."

Individual factors that can be interpreted as eating behaviors were less prevalent than environmental factors but warrant mention because of their dominance in health related research. A female undergraduate student from Brazil described individual factors by stating:

> I spend more time studying, and will frequently have lunch while doing something else, which I never did in Brazil."

Another example of this subtheme is captured by a South Korean doctoral student's words:

> I also began cooking most of my meals so I have more control and responsibility over my diet."

Health outcomes

Participants (n=22, 88%) stated that some aspects of their health were impacted (both positively and negatively) by diet. Weight gain was mentioned by 32% of participants and food and environmental safety concerns such as pesticides in industrialized foods were dominant. Social and emotional aspects of health such as cooking to unwind, (cooking) for fun, and as a way to share time and connect with friends and home were also common in the data.

DISCUSSION

The findings in this study offer insight into the similar ways international students from around the globe experience, navigate, and adapt to changes in food and diet.

The data point to resilience against accepting less indigenous foods and a protective negotiation when adopting foreign (US) foods or eating practices. Many participants noted a trial period of more energy dense food, with most explicitly stating a return to traditional eating practices with negotiated inclusion of foods prevalent in the US diet.

Although participants came from large number of countries in this research, the participants were older and had more years of education acquired than the plethora of studies done on the US college campuses that look at the diet changes of the US undergraduate students, especially freshmen.

Although there is the disproportionate number of undergraduate students, their unique experience and culture differ vastly in food and eating practices.

Because these international students did not feel well-adapted to the US food system, learning and passing on information from those who feel they have, in particular, older graduate students to younger students (undergraduates) from similar parts or areas of the world could be an important way to help new international students with their food choices in order to help maintain or improve their health.

REFERENCES

[1] Open doors report on international educational exchange. Institute of International Education, 2012. URL: http://www.iie.org/opendoors.
[2] Constantine M, Okazaki S, Utsey, S. Self-concealment, social self-efficacy, acculturative stress, and depression in African, Asian, and Latino international college students. Am J Orthopsychiatry 2004;74(3):230-41.
[3] Mori S. Addressing the mental health concerns of international students. J Couns Dev 2000;78(2):137-44.
[4] Williams CL, Berry JW. Primary prevention of acculturative stress among refugees: Application of psychological theory and practice. Am Psychol 1991:46(6):632.
[5] Arnett J. Emerging adulthood: A theory of development from the late teens through the twenties. Am Psychol 2000;55(5):469.
[6] Centers for Disease Control and Prevention. Overweight and obesity: Adult obesity facts. URL: http://www.cdc.gov/obesity/data/adult.html.
[7] Pan Y, Dixon Z, Himburg S, Huffman F. Asian students change their eating patterns after living in the United States. J Am Diet Assoc 1999;99(1):54-7.
[8] Perez-Cuerto F, Verbeke W, Lachat C, Remaut-De Winter A. Changes in dietary habits following temporal migration. The case of international students living in Belgium. Appetite 2009;52(1):83-8.
[9] Satia-Abouta J, Patterson R, Neuhouser M, Elder J. Dietary Acculturation: Applications to nutrition research and dietetics. Am Diet Assoc 2002;102(8) 1105-18.
[10] Popkin B. The nutrition transition: An overview of world patterns of change. Nutr Rev 2004;62 (7Pt2):S140–3.
[11] Creswell JW. Qualitative inquiry and research design: Choosing among five approaches, 2nd ed. Thousand Oaks, CA: Sage, 2007.
[12] Morse JM. Qualitative health research: Creating a new discipline. Walnut Creek, CA: Left Coast Press, 2012.
[13] Finlay L. Debating phenomenological research methods. Phenomenology Pract 2009;3(1):6-25.
[14] Moustakas C. Phenomenological research methods. Thousand Oak, CA: Sage, 1994.
[15] Van Manen M. Researching lived experience: Human science for an action sensitive pedagogy. New York: SUNY Press, 1990.
[16] Patton MQ. Qualitative research and evaluation methods, 3rd ed. Thousand Oaks, CA: Sage, 1990.
[17] Wertz F. Phenomenological research methods for counseling psychology. J Couns Psychol 2005:52(2):167.

Submitted: June 06, 2014. *Revised:* July 04,2014. *Accepted:* July 13, 2014.

In: Public Health Yearbook 2015
Editor: Joav Merrick
ISBN: 978-1-63484-514-4
© 2016 Nova Science Publishers, Inc.

Chapter 31

PARENTS' STRATEGIES TO INCREASE PHYSICAL ACTIVITY AMONG ELEMENTARY-AGED CHILDREN IN RURAL INDIANA

Sean M Bowman, MA, and Cecilia S Obeng, PhD*

Department of Applied Health Science, School of Public Health,
Indiana University, Bloomington, Indiana, United States of America

Children living in rural areas have less designated recreational facilities for use and limited neighboring children to play with compared to children living in other areas. Moreover, the level of safety and the physical ability for individual travel among rural area children to areas of play may not be appropriate. A survey was designed to better understand strategies that parents perform to overcome environmental barriers present in rural environments for the promotion of physical activity among area children. Participating parents completed a survey consisting of both closed and open-ended questions. Fourteen rural area parents of elementary-aged children completed the survey. Parents described the lack of neighboring children, distance to nearest recreational areas, and lack of sidewalks/roadway shoulders as barriers for being physically active among rural area children. Strategies identified by parents to counteract these barriers included transporting their child to areas of play, signing up child for sport leagues and clubs, and encouraging outdoor family activities. Due to limited neighboring children and areas of play present in rural environments, the parents' role in the child's physical activity behaviors may heavily rely on their transportation and participation through physical activity role modeling.

Keywords: rural areas, children, physical activity, sidewalks, transportation

---

* Correspondence: Cecilia S Obeng, PhD, Associate Professor, Indiana University, School of Public Health, 1025 E 7th Street, SPH 116, Bloomington, IN 47405, United States. E-mail: cobeng@indiana.edu.

INTRODUCTION

America's increasing trend of obesity among children is not fully explainable based on genetic predisposition (1). Although genetics have been linked with obesity, it is physical inactivity that remains one of the leading explanations for the recent phenomenon of obese children (2-4). Furthermore, evidence suggests that the physical community in which a child resides can directly impact the child's physical activity behaviors (5-7).

Individual environments are complex and dynamic systems, which can be enabling or disabling in the promotion of healthy behaviors, more specifically, physical activity (8, 9). Past findings suggest that youth living in rural areas have higher prevalence of obesity and participate in less physical activity versus youth living in other areas (10, 11). Therefore, the aim of this research project was to explore certain rural environmental factors that may be unsupportive in the promotion physical activity among children living in rural areas as well to identify strategies that parents use to oppose, mitigate, or eliminate these barriers to promote physical activity within their child's life.

METHODS

This research was done after an approval from an institutional review board. Parent participants were recruited through the local health center and YMCA within one Midwest rural community. Participants were approached at the local YMCA and community center and asked to participate in a short survey.

A parent was eligible if their child was currently enrolled in an elementary school within the community's school corporation. Eligible parents completed a short survey containing both closed and open-ended questions. The survey was designed to better understand barriers within rural environments that promote physical inactivity among children, as well as to identify roles and strategies parents perform to encourage play or physical activity within their child's life. The data were coded by the first author.

Data analysis included finding common statements/themes in participants' written responses. Analyses of the data included supporting analytical claims with verbatim language of participants.

RESULTS

There were a total of fourteen parent participants. All parent participants had at least one elementary-aged child. The age range for the children was 6-12 years old.

All parents stated that there was no access to street sidewalks from their home residence. One parent wrote that there are "very few flat and hard surfaces." Another parent noted, "Roads don't have shoulders, so it's hard to ride bikes safely with hills and ravines." Over half of the parents estimated that the nearest recreational facility was 10-20 driving minutes from their home residence in which they transport their child, two or more times per week to engage in physical activity. One parent stated there are "very few activities organized in a small community, the YMCA is the only." Another parent said, "We come to the YMCA once a week for gymnastics." One parent indicated that the "park is great, it has a pool, but we have to drive to get there."

The majority of parent participants agreed that limited neighboring children within rural areas may be a disadvantage to their child's social play. One parent wrote there are "no other neighborhood kids to engage in activity with." Another parent said that kids "can't run next door to play." Some parent participants did express that the larger amounts of land prevalent in rural areas can provide great opportunities for their child to be active. One parent wrote, "There are hills to climb, lots of room to run and play."

There were four themes identified concerning the question on how parents promote physical activity and play within their child's life. Themes included: limiting TV and computer usage, signing up child for sport leagues and clubs, transporting child to areas of play, and encouraging outdoor play and family activities. Parents expressed the importance of role modeling physical activity to help encourage physical activity in their child's life. One parent wrote, "I'm active myself and make time available to play with my children. I limit TV and computer time as well as drive them to the YMCA and school playground."

DISCUSSION

From our data, rural environments pose unique challenges for children. For instance, one prominent aspect of rural environment is the lack of sidewalks in the communities. Sidewalks help facilitate safe, travel for residents to connect to other areas within the community. All parent participants in this research project expressed the concern that they had no access to sidewalks from their home residence making it difficult and/or practically impossible for children in their individual efforts to negotiate from their homes to areas of play or to the homes of neighboring children. Investigators in one study associated insufficient amounts of sidewalks near residential areas with obesity (5). In addition, investigators in another study found that residents living in walker friendly neighborhoods participated in 52 more minutes of moderate physical activity per week compared to residents living in areas that are not as walker friendly (12). Therefore, it seems reasonable to conclude that the lack of sidewalks becomes a tremendous barrier for active living among residents within rural communities (13, 14).

For most rural area children, walking or biking to school is not an option. Unlike more condensed areas, rural area children do not have wide shoulders for safe travel. Therefore, parents may be more apprehensive to allow their child to travel by foot or bike due to safety issues. This is noteworthy due to the fact that increased safety and access to recreational areas have been shown to promote physical activity (15, 16). Moreover, children may feel scared to traverse down country roads by themselves with speeding traffic and winding roads with blind turns. Whether the parent does not permit the child on the roads, or the child is apprehensive, the lack of safe travel areas may heavily discourage the residing children from accessing neighboring children to play with.

Another challenge that a child living within rural area faces is limited recreational areas of play within their residential vicinity. Past evidence suggests that accessibility levels of recreational facilities are lower among children who live in less affluent, rural areas (6). The majority of the parent participants within this study gauged that the nearest designated recreational area of play was 10-20 driving minutes from their home residence. This indicates that their children needed to travel long distances to access playgrounds or recreational facilities. This is relevant due the fact that being overweight increases and physical activity levels decrease when there are inadequate recreational facilities near home residence (9). Without travel assistant to recreational or social areas of play, rural area children may feel isolated and further discouraged to be active.

Transporting a child numerous miles a day can be financially and mentally burdensome to parents, especially for families that do not have extra money or time for the added transportation. Due to higher gas prices and greater distances needed to travel within rural areas to access recreational opportunities; it may decrease a family's ability to transport their child to these recreational areas as much as a child might desire. Therefore it becomes very important for rural area parents, coaches, recreational leagues, and health educators to communicate about issues such as travel. The promotion of carpooling among families living in relatively close areas may help alleviate some of the expenses and time involved with driving and picking-up children from parks and sport leagues.

Lastly, the immediate social play available for children in rural areas is limited. This may leave a child feeling lonely, as well as isolated. Parents within this study said that they signed their child up for sport leagues; however, this might not be completely adequate due to sport leagues being seasonal and not every day. Since there are limited neighboring children (as indicated by parents participants) to play with and it may be cumbersome transporting a child daily to recreational areas daily, parents can become role models of exercise themselves, while participating in play with their child in the yard or accompanying them during monitored walking and biking on trails or roads. Parent participants within this research project expressed the importance of role modeling physical activity themselves to help encourage physical activity within their child's life.

Conclusion

Past findings suggest that youth living in rural areas have higher prevalence of obesity and participate in less physical activity versus youth living in other areas (10-11). Consequently, this research project was designed to assess what those environmental barriers are, as well to gauge what parents are currently doing to promote physical activity and play within their child's life. In doing so, this research project helped identify major themes that suggest that children in rural environments have special needs compared to children living in other areas. Due to the dynamics of rural areas, the study discovered that children residing in rural communities have limited accessibility to recreational areas, groups of children to play with, and safe ways to independently travel, which is why parents in rural areas may be largely responsible for their child's transportation to social play. Limited neighborhood children within rural communities highlight the need for parents to be role models through participating in their child's play and physical activity.

REFERENCES

[1] Ebbeling CB, Pawlak DB, Ludwig, DS. Childhood obesity: public-health crisis, common sense cure. Lancet 2002; 360(9331): 473-82.
[2] Zhao J, Grant SFA. Gentics of Childhood Obesity. J Obesity 2011; Volume 2011:1-9.
[3] Dennison DA, Yin Z, Kibbe D, Burns S, Trowbridge F. Training health care professionals to manage overweight adolescents: experience in rural Georgia communities. J Rural Health 2008;24(1):55-9.
[4] Trost SG, Kerr LM, Ward DS, Pate RR. Physical activity and determinants of physical activity in obese and non-obese children. Int J Obes Relat Metab Disord 2001;25(6):822-9.
[5] Boehmer TK, Hoehner CM, Deshpande AD, Ramirez LKB, Brownson RC. Perceived and observed neighborhood indicators of obesity among urban adults. Int J Obes 2007;31(6):968-77.
[6] Brownson RC, Baker EA, Housemann RA, Brennan LK, Bacak SJ. Environmental and policy determinants of physical activity in the United States. Am J Public Health 2001;91(12):1995-2003.
[7] Giles-Corti B, Donovan RJ. Relative influences of individual, social environmental and physical environmental correlates of walking. Am J Public Health. 2003;93(9):1583-9.
[8] Frank LD, Engelke PO. The built environment and human activity patterns: Exploring the impacts of urban form on public health. J Plan Lit 2001;16(2):202-18.
[9] Gordon-Larsen P, Nelson MC, Page P, Popkin BM. Inequality in the built environment underlies key health disparities in physical activity and obesity. JAMA Pediatr 2006;117(2):417-24.
[10] Yen IH, Kaplan GA. Poverty area residence and changes in physical activity level: evidence from the Alameda County Study. Am J Public Health 1998;88(11):1709-12.
[11] Martin SL, Kirkner GJ, Mayo K, Matthews CE, Durstine JL, Hebert JR. Urban, rural, and regional variations in physical activity. J Rural Health 2005;21(3):239-44.
[12] Saelens BE, Sallis JF, Frank LD. Environmental correlates of walking and cycling: Findings from the transportation, urban design, and planning literatures. Ann Behav Med 2003;25(2):80-91.
[13] Bennett GG, McNeill LH, Wolin KY, Duncan DT, Puleo E, Emmons KM. Safe to walk? Neighborhood safety and physical activity among public housing residents. PLoS Med 2007;4(10):1599-1607.
[14] Lavizzo-Mourey R, McGinnis JM. Making the case for active living communities. Am J Public Health 2003;93(9):1386-8.
[15] Babey SH, Brown ER, Hastert TA. Access to safe parks helps increase physical activity among teenagers. Los Angeles, CA: UCLA Center for Health Policy Research, 2005:1-6.
[16] Sallis JF, Hovell MF, Hofstetter CR, Elder JP, Hackley M, Caspersen CJ, et al. Distance between homes and exercise facilities related to frequency of exercise among San-Diego residents. Public Health Rep 1990;105(2):179-85.

Submitted: August 01, 2014. *Revised:* September 14, 2014. *Accepted:* September 23, 2014.

In: Public Health Yearbook 2015
Editor: Joav Merrick
ISBN: 978-1-63484-514-4
© 2016 Nova Science Publishers, Inc.

Chapter 32

ORAL HEALTH OF IMMIGRANT AFRICAN MALES IN THE UNITED STATES

Charity G Gichina, MSc, and Cecilia S Obeng, PhD*
Department of Applied Health Science, School of Public Health,
Indiana University, Bloomington, Indiana, United States of America

Studies on Black immigrants in the United States have focused primarily on general health. In particular, there is a dearth of research on oral health of immigrant African males in the United States. This study examined the oral health status of 25 African immigrant males and their utilization of dental service. Analysis of the results indicate that participants reported having experienced or are experiencing dental health problems such as swollen and bleeding gum, tooth ache, periodontal disease, teeth cavities, decay, teeth sensitivity, teeth loss, need for teeth extraction, and the need for braces. The majority indicated non-use of preventive dental health services in their native countries. Findings from this study show the crucial interplay of participants' native country's culture, and access to dental health service utilization experience in the United States.

Keywords: African immigrants, male, oral health, culture, public health

INTRODUCTION

Immigrant African men are part of a huge influx of immigrants from diverse backgrounds in the United States (1-5). As pointed out by Allan and Caswell (6) and Cruz et al. (5), the current discussion on presumed determinants of general health differences among diverse populations and minority groups including immigrants in the United States, has focused on differences in socioeconomic characteristics such as education and income levels (5, 6). As a result, there is a lack of evaluation of other factors that influence immigrant's oral health status. Specifically, such factors as indigenous cultural beliefs and acculturation process

---

* Correspondence: Cecilia S Obeng, PhD, Associate Professor, Indiana University, School of Public Health, 1025 E. 7th Street, SPH 116, Bloomington, IN 47405, United States. E-mail: cobeng@indiana.edu.

encountered in their daily-lived experience upon immigration to the United States have not been studied. Accordingly, little is known about immigrant's oral health (5, 7).

Research on oral health by Davis (8), Borrell et al. (9), Newton and Bower (10), Patrick et al. (7), Vargas and Arevalo (11) revealed that most oral diseases are preventable and are relatively easy and inexpensive to address at early stages. Oral health is essential for one's well-being. There much more to it than an individual having healthy teeth. In particular, it relates to and impacts the overall health and wellbeing of individuals and entire populations. Accordingly, the consequences of lack of dental care reach far beyond aesthetics (7, 11). It is paramount to consider that the impact of oral health on the overall health and well-being of individuals or groups of people remain connected for everyone living in the United States.

Like many immigrants, African men encounter complex and diverse cultural and social processes that affect both oral health and access to effective dental health care upon immigration to the United States. Such processes present problems of access to care and quality of care, cultural differences between providers and patients, history of discrimination and persistent severity of poverty (12). According to Allan and Caswell (6), the primary influences of dental health services utilization among Immigrant African men include a combination of factors such as access to dental insurance, social and cultural values, cultural and socioeconomic changes that have strongly affected diet, cultural marginalization at the hands of the dominant American culture, and generally low levels of income that affect all of these factors. Results from several studies (5, 7, 11, 13) indicated that experiences people bring with them when they migrate are fundamental to how they subsequently view dental health and dental health services in United States.

Available studies on African health care services, for example, indicate that in many African settings dental health services are accessed only when there is a specific need which is perceived to be serious or life threatening (1, 5, 14). As a result the philosophy of health promotion and preventive medicine are not well established in most African communities. This could explain immigrant African men's utilization of dental health services while residing in the United States. A preliminary evaluation of the current dental health status and dental service utilization by population groups such as immigrant African men is an essential step toward achieving improved oral health status in United States.

In view of the above problems, it is therefore crucial to examine immigrant African men's utilization of dental health services and the cultural and acculturation basis of their oral health care habits while residing in the United States of America.

METHODS

The study utilized purposeful sampling with targeted snowball sampling (15) to recruit 25 individuals aged 18 to 55 years living in central Indiana which is residence to a significant population of African immigrant men. Study sample also comprised of individuals who had lived in Indiana or had related to the current Indiana residents. All participants were born outside the United States and spoke English.

Potential participants in this study were contacted through email, phone calls, and where possible, in person after the researchers were given approval by Indiana University Institutional Review Board. Potential participants were notified that taking part in this study is voluntary. They could choose not to take part or may discontinue participation at any time and such a discontinuation decision of the study would not affect their then current or future relations with the investigators. Consenting participants took 20 minutes to independently complete the questionnaire at their convenience. Completed questionnaires were hand-delivered to the researcher where possible or sent by email.

The study used survey as a data collection instrument containing a list of precise, 14 relevant and easy to answer questions, purposed to collect information on dental health status, dental insurance access, and utilization of dental care services, and self-perceived oral health and cultural influence on dental service use.

This study also used a, selective sampling an aspect of grounded theory, to identify participants and their settings for inquiry before data collection; sorting and category creation was done (16). Open-ended structured question survey format encouraged the participants to tell their own story on the research topic. Also, the study utilized narrative analysis as a form of discourse analysis that sought to study the textual devices at work in the constructions of process or sequence within data texts. This perspective is used for collecting and analyzing data during a single research study as discussed by Daly (17). Within this Narrative analysis, cultural influence on immigrant African men's lived experience is recognized as an important aspect of the true representation of the participants' accounts regarding their dental health choices. This analytical strategy enjoins us, first, to define culture.

The American Heritage Dictionary 2000 (18) defines culture as "the totality of socially transmitted behavior patterns, arts, belief, institutions, and all other products of human work and thought." (p. 442). Culture is a major factor in the influence of dental health service utilization for immigrant African men. Cultural values, education, prior experience with dentists, perceived value of dental care, financial costs, time, and access issues influence care seeking. Elder (19) pointed out that medical and therapeutic resources available to an individual influence their health beliefs and health behaviors. For immigrant African men, the authors believed that health beliefs and health behaviors are embedded in the culture of origin.

Coding and analysis

Collected data from the questionnaire were coded according to similar identified answers in the questionnaire, which were then grouped together and sorted into three categories by theme. Data from open-ended questions are recorded word-for-word as evidence in support of the study findings. The analysis also involves noticing interesting responses in the data and assigning 'codes' to them, based on theme. Writing and coding was mainly a descriptive summary representation of what the participants have said or done. However, actual participant responses are reported to deliver the message as clearly as participants intended.

RESULTS AND DISCUSSION

The study results are divided into the following sections: sample characteristics, oral health status and professional dental health service utilization, cultural influence on professional dental health service utilization, C culture, diet and time, dental health care cost and community support.

Sample characteristics

Fifteen participants reported their country of origin as Kenya while three were from Ghana, three from Nigeria, two from Guyana and two from Sierra-Leone.

Participants' reported that they had lived in the United States for 2.5-25 years with an average immigrant status of 9.7 years. All participants are voluntary immigrant. It is worth mentioning that participants' formal educational levels were balanced ranging from high school to graduate level masters and doctoral degrees. Tables 1-2 represent participants' ages, and educational level.

The results also indicated that thirteen participants (52%) had had employer provided dental health insurance, while 12 participants (48%) did not have insurance. All participants who had the highest education level (doctoral), had access to employer-provided dental health insurance.

Table 1. Participants' ages

Age of participants in years	Number of participants in each age group	Percentage rate
27-29	3	12%
30-39	12	48%
40-49	7	28%
50-59	3	12%
Participants total	25	100%
Average age	30.6 years	N/A

Table 2. Participant education level

Participants education level	Participants in each level	Education level percentage
Elementary	0	0%
High school	4	16%
Undergraduate	10	40%
Graduate Masters	7	28%
Graduate Doctoral	4	16%
Participant total	25	100%

Oral health status and professional dental health service utilization

Majority of the participants reported having experienced or experiencing dental problems such as swollen inflamed and bleeding gum, tooth ache, periodontal disease, teeth cavities, decay, teeth sensitivity, teeth loss, need for teeth extraction and need for braces (see Table 3).

Table 3. Participants' reported current dental health status

Reported current dental health status	Number of participants	Percentage rate
Excellent	2	8%
Good	13	52%
Fair	5	20%
Poor	5	20%
Don't know	0	0%
Total	25	100%

On dental health service utilization, seven participants representing a rate of (28%) reported use of dental health services in their country of origin with two out of seven being taken to the dentist at the age of 2 years and 9 years old, by parents. Five participants (20%) used dental services in their adulthood before migrating to the United States. Those who utilized dental health services before migrating to the United States did so because they had access to employer provided dental health insurance coverage. Of the 25 participants, 18 (72%) reported not using and/or no use of preventive dental health services in their country of origin.

This remained true for all participants after migrating to the United States. Eleven participants (44%) reported having dental health insurance after migration to the United States as this excerpt from one participant indicates:

> When I visited the dentist in 2007, my oral health was fair and degrading to poor. I had some minor gum disease. This was because I had not visited a dentist for 18 years prior to that visit. I was advised to visit the dentist every 4 months for proper cleaning and floss my teeth daily. After the 3rd visit my oral hygiene had improved dramatically (teeth and gums in good condition) and I now visit the dentist every 6 months.

Fourteen participants (56%) indicated lack of dental insurance upon migration to the United States. Having dental health insurance after immigrating to the United States increased professional dental health service utilization.

Most participants who reported having dental health insurance indicated that their dental insurance was an employer-provided insurance. However, participants who had access to employer-provided dental health insurance reported only using dental services that were covered by insurance due to high cost. Those who did not have access to employer provided dental insurance reported no utilization of dental health services except on need or emergency basis (see Table 4).

Table 4. Dental health service utilization and dental insurance access before and after immigration

Dental Health Utilization	Percent with dental health insurance		Percent with no dental health insurance	
	Participants	% Rate	Participants	% Rate
Before immigration	7	28%	18	72%
After immigration	11	44%	14	56%

Cultural influence on professional dental health service utilization

Participants in this study also reported cultural background as a major determinant of their use of dental health services. In addition, the process of acculturation upon migrating to the United States is reported as influencing the current dental health status of the studied immigrant African men. These determinants as alluded to earlier in the study included diet, cost, lack of dental health insurance, lack of time for dental care and general cultural beliefs such as "dentists cause more damage to teeth than good."

Culture, diet and time

Several respondents had the following to say about Cultural change and diet upon migration. These participants blamed American diet for their dental problems.

> While teeth hygiene is not so much emphasized as it is in the American culture, there were types of food such as sugar cane that would clean the teeth as you eat. Also, there are many sugary foods in the American culture than there were in my Kikuyu African culture. For example, in my culture deserts are not usually part of the meals, they are only taken during occasions such as weddings.
>
> My culture had superior teeth exercise: chewing tough sugar canes; tough mature meat with bones; tough corn; raw carrots; medicinal plants as tooth brushes…It's just phenomenal.
>
> There is a belief that the moment you let the dentist examines and interferes with your teeth that will be the beginning of your dental problems through your lifetime. There is also a belief that dental care is not important and so long as the teeth are not hurting, you do not mess with them.
>
> In my native country, specifically the village I grew up in to have a routine dental check was not heard. To our parents, it was waste of money or resources to have that kind of service. They also believed on herb medication.
>
> The need for routine checkup was not engrained when growing up. In general, most of the immigrant do not see the need to see a dentist unless when in pain.
>
> Too much sugar available in abundance, the main reason is the amount of sugar in many diets. Too many sweets, there are some foods that would mess up the oral hygiene e.g., rice.
>
> I am usually wary of excessively sugary food products in contrast to organic naturally grown foods in my country of origin.
> In every social gathering, there are always plenty of sweet foods usually for refreshments or just normal snacks. This does not help the teeth maintenance.
>
> Working late shifts it is easy to skip the oral hygiene in before going to bed.
> I see a dentist every once in a while, very hectic schedules, time, time, time. Too tired to brush at bedtime. Very, very dangerous.

Dental health care cost

Participants in this category indicated that the greatest influence on their dental health care decisions had been financial and whether they had dental insurance or not. The following are excerpts from participants about dental insurance and healthcare cost:

>I may not visit a dentist if I don't have dental insurance. This is same for most Americans. American culture has had no influence on my dental health care decisions and my overall health decisions in general. Generally, preventive care in America is non-existent and that is same in my native country. What has influenced my dental health care decisions is employer provided dental insurance which makes the cost of dental care affordable.

There is easy access to dental providers and specialists. However the cost of dental services in the US is very expensive and can sometimes hinder seeking care.

>I am more likely to spend money helping out someone who has more severe /serious visible problem than spend money at the dentist's office. This is more so if the service is just a regular checkup and none of my teeth is on the verge of coming out.

>I believe all I need is insurance or the resources needed for the dental health services.

>I do not have Medical insurance and cannot afford by myself.

>I did not have the means to do it. My job did not offer any insurance plans.

>I did not have insurance and hence I postponed all dental concerns, as long as I could eat, I stayed away from the dentist.

>It is very expensive especially because I have had many issues that needed major interventions.

>My parents never took me to the dentist.

>The only time you went to the dentist was when in severe pain. I was blessed and never had to go to a dentist for teeth removal.

>I visit the dentist whenever I have insurance and there is surplus after meeting the basic needs for my immediate and extended families.

Community support

On community support for better utilization of dental health services, some participants had this to say:

>I would appreciate if the community had group insurance rates for the dental insurance since it would be affordable to see a dentist. The community can also arrange information sessions about dental health awareness especially for the people like me who have not had or discovered dental problems.

The community could organize dental clinics that provide basic dental services such as screenings, cleanings etc. at a subsidized cost.

The community can help by holding open door dental clinics regularly to help those who do not have dental insurance. This is because it very difficult to raise the kind of monies needed to pay for those services which can be a challenge to many.

Affordable community based dental services either through a formal volunteer based dental service or dentist who can offer subsidized service to immigrant and especially to the new ones. They can get education and early intervention before major dental related disease crop in.

Like all immigrants, African men bring with them particular behaviors, dietary practices, values, and attitudes that, in conjunction with their exposure to environmental and sociopolitical factors, may influence their dental health service utilization, oral health status and overall health and wellbeing. Immigrant African men, for example, may be less prone to oral diseases partly because they come from a culture with a traditional diet that is healthy for their teeth. On the other hand, dental health problems may be an indicator of the overall impact of oral health care systems in the country of origin. With limited options, both preventive and curative dental care services become unaffordable for most immigrant African men, even those who are insured, due to high out-of-pocket expenses.

The results of this study show that in the case of African immigrant men, acculturation immigration attributes play an independent and perhaps even more important role in their dental health utilization experience. In addition, the difficulties encountered by immigrant African men influence their dental health service uptake. Dental health is only a priority when one is unwell; otherwise issues around immigration, housing, employment, and childcare take precedence. Country of birth largely determines an immigrant's cultural background.

The results of this study also show that immigrant African men's beliefs of receiving substandard dental health services because they are not insured or they do not utilize dental health services regularly, influence their decisions which may encourage individuals to postpone professional dental treatment in the hope that the problem will resolve itself. Such individuals end up seeking professional dental services only when faced with no other options.

Analyses of the results indicate that immigrant African men's level of education alone did not have influence on access to dental health insurance. It was noted that individual educational level influenced profession and dental health insurance access. However, most participants shared the same beliefs and perceptions on utilization of professional dental health services.

Although, the participants in this research were only 25 African immigrant men, findings from this study could help to develop culturally-grounded strategies for increasing access to formal and informal oral/dental health services among the underserved ethnic groups such as immigrant African men, and contribute to the development of policies to address immigrant racial- cum -cultural based barriers to dental care. In addition, study findings on different immigration experiences among immigrant African men's use of dental health services will contribute to understanding the dental health implications of racial/ethnic identity and acculturation strategies.

CONCLUSION

Study results enrich the dearth of information on the association of immigration and acculturation attributes with access to dental care, utilization of dental care services, oral health practices, self-perceived oral health of immigrant African men in United States (20). The findings of this study show the crucial interplay of Immigrant African men's original country of birth culture, acculturation into the dominant US culture, and access to dental insurance their dental health service utilization experience.

REFERENCES

[1] Lucas JW, Daheia J, Barr-Anderson DJ, Raynard S, Kington RS. Health status, health insurance, and health care utilization patterns of immigrant Black men. Am J Public Health 2003;10:1740-7.
[2] Larsen LJ. The foreign-born population in the United States 2003. Washington, DC: US Census Bureau, 2004.
[3] Bornstein MH, Cote LR. "Who is sitting across from me?" Immigrant mothers' knowledge of parenting and children's development. Pediatrics 2004;114 (5):557-64.
[4] Hwang W. Acculturative family distancing: Theory, research, and clinical practice. J Psychother 2006;43:397-409.
[5] Cruz GD, Yu C, Christian RS, Racquel ZL. The association of immigration and acculturation attributes with oral health among immigrant in New York City. Am J Public Health 2009;99(Suppl 2): 474–80.
[6] Allan S; Noonan AS, Caswell AE. The need for diversity in the health professions. J Dent Educ 2003;67(9):1030-3.
[7] Patrick DL, Shuk R, Lee Y, Nucci S, Grembowski D, Jolles CZ, et al. Reducing oral health disparities: A focus on social and cultural determinants, BMC Oral Health 2006; 6(1):1186-1203.
[8] Davis K. The intersection of socioeconomic variables, oral health, and systemic disease: all health care is cultural Compendium Cont Educ Dentistry 2000;66 (Suppl 30):40-8.
[9] Borrell LN, Taylor GW, Borgnakke, WS, Woolfolk MW, Nyquist LV. Perception of general and oral health in White and African American adults: Assessing the effect of neighborhood socioeconomic conditions. Community Dent Oral Epidemiol 2004;32(5):363-73.
[10] Newton JT, Bower EJ, The social determinants of oral health: New approaches to conceptualizing and researching complex causal networks. Community Dent Oral Epidemiol 2005;33(1):25-34.
[11] Vargars CM, Arevalo O. How dental care can preserve and improve oral health. Dent Clin North Am 2009;53(3):399-420.
[12] Tilashalski KR, Gilbert GH, Boykin MJ, Litaker MS. Racial differences in treatment preferences: oral health as an example. J Eval Clin Pract 2007;13:102–8.
[13] Chen M, Anderson RM, Barnes DE, Leclercq MH, Lyttle CS. Comparing oral health care systems. A second international study. Geneva: World Health Organization, 1997.
[14] Burns FM, Imrie J, Nazroo JY, Johnson AM, Fenton KA. Why the(y) wait? Key informant understandings of factors contributing to late presentation and poor utilization of HIV health and social care services by African migrants in Britain. AIDS Care 2007;19(1):102-8.
[15] Patton MQ. Qualitative evaluation and research methods, 2nd ed. Newbury Park, CA: Sage, 1990.
[16] Rutledge SE. Enacting personal HIV polices for sexual situations: HIV-positive gay men's experience. Qual Health Res 2007;17: 1040-59.
[17] Daly KJ. Qualitative methods for family studies and human development. Thousand Oaks, CA: Sage, 2007.
[18] American Heritage Dictionary of the English Language, 4th ed. Boston, MA: Houghton Mifflin, 2000.
[19] Elder JP. Reaching out to Americas immigrants: community health communication. Am J Health Behav 2003;27(3):197-205.

[20] Obeng CS. Culture and dental health among African immigrant school-aged children in the United States. J Health Educ 2007;34:343-7.

Submitted: August 08, 2014. *Revised:* September 16, 2014. *Accepted:* September 27, 2014.

In: Public Health Yearbook 2015
Editor: Joav Merrick

ISBN: 978-1-63484-514-4
© 2016 Nova Science Publishers, Inc.

Chapter 33

THE INFLUENCE OF RELIGIOSITY ON SEXUAL BEHAVIORS: A QUALITATIVE STUDY OF YOUNG ADULTS IN THE MIDWEST

Jessica R Hauser, MS, and Cecilia S Obeng, PhD*

Department of Applied Health Science, School of Public Health,
Indiana University, Bloomington, Indiana, United States of America

In the United States, a majority of the population (80%) self-identifies with some form of religion. The purpose of this study was to examine the influence of religiosity on sexual behaviors of 13 young adults. The findings covered four themes: (a) religious beliefs and religious leaders matter to them, (b) participants' religion influence their sexual behaviors, (c) sex should not be performed outside of marriage, (d) participants' decisions were influenced by parents, peers, religion, and the media. The findings indicate that by using the identified salient referents in conjunction with each other, and by acknowledging and teaching religious beliefs, interventions could be very effective in promoting sexual health and reducing risky sexual behaviors among young adults.

Keywords: religion, phenomenology, qualitative research, sexual behaviors in young adults

INTRODUCTION

Data from the 2008 American Religious Identification Survey found that 80% of American adults identify with a religion, and of those 80% of religious Americans, 76% of them identify as Christians (1). Christian churches and faith-based organizations (FBOs) have a long history of independently and collaboratively hosting health promotion programs (2). When evaluating these interventions that have been implemented, it has been found that FBOs can significantly increase knowledge of disease, improve screening behavior and readiness to change, and reduce the risk associated with disease and disease symptoms (2).

---

* Correspondence: Cecilia S Obeng, PhD, Associate Professor, Indiana University, School of Public Health, 1025 E 7th Street, SPH 116, Bloomington, IN 47405, United States. E-mail: cobeng@indiana.edu.

While there are many ways this can be accomplished, DeHaven and colleagues (2) cited the following: "behavior modification programs, nutritional/eating programs, exercise programs, counseling programs, smoking cessation programs; including church-led educational activities utilizing lay health advisors, food events (preparing and tasting healthy foods), using booklets and bulletins, pastoral sermons/testimonies, teams, support groups, telephone calls, increasing fruits and vegetables, increasing physical activity with aerobic exercise and stretching (to mention but a few examples)" (p. 1030, 1033). With more churches per person than any other country, the integration of public health and FBOs may be one answer or strategy to assist with healthcare. While FBOs are being integrated more and more in public health, there is still a need in sexual health that may not be addressed by the faith community. There is an inconsistency between Christian beliefs and the sexual behaviors of adolescents and young adults that the statistics clearly show.

An estimated 20 million new cases of sexually transmitted infections (STIs) occur each year, according to the numbers collected in 2008 by the Centers for Disease Control and Prevention (CDC) in the United States (3). The total number of infected individuals in the United States is estimated at 110 million (3). According to the CDC, this costs an economic burden of nearly $16 billion in direct medical costs (4). This does not account for any other "costs" to an individual such as social, emotional, or psychological burdens, or the cost of transportation to and from healthcare facilities, time off of work, et cetera. Sexual behavior was the 8th leading actual cause of death in the United States in 2000, which were approximately 20,000 deaths (5). Adolescents and young adults (15-24 year olds) only account for 25% of the United States population, but this age group accounts for over half of all new STI cases (6). These statistics show that there is an obvious problem with the current state of sexual health in the United States, specifically, among adolescents and young adults.

Hull et al. (7) investigated the relationship between sexuality and religiosity and found that religiosity offered a protective effect over sexual health. Specifically, it was found that religiosity can be an important factor in delaying of both coital and non-coital sexual behaviors.

Other studies have found a relationship between religiosity and delayed sexual behavior through an identified subsample of longitudinal studies, which are not always common (8). Researchers have examined the associations between religiosity and STI/HIV preventative behaviors by discovering that greater religiosity serves as a protective factor, specifically to the delay of sexual debut among adolescents and emergent adults (9). The authors describe a pattern of significant associations between religious involvement and a spectrum of risk and preventative behaviors (9). Specifically, McCree and colleagues (2003) found adolescents with a higher level of religiosity were more likely to: "have higher self-efficacy to communicate with a new partner as well as a steady partner about sex; communicate about STIs, HIV, and pregnancy prevention; have higher self-efficacy to refuse an 'unsafe' sexual encounter; have more positive and supportive attitudes toward condom use; be supportive of safer sex; to initiate sex at a later age; and ever used a condom in the past 6 months" (9, p. 6-7). A similar finding in female college students was that a "strong" belief in God and church attendance (level of religiosity) decreases the likelihood of engaging in risky sexual behaviors, including multiple partners, inconsistent condom use, or no condom use, and other behaviors (10). Among individuals living with HIV, religiosity and religious teachings influence sexual behavior by promoting safer sexual activities or abstaining from sexual activities (11).

Several other studies support and confirm these findings of a higher level of religiosity being a protective factor against risky sexual behaviors, including delaying sexual initiation/debut, number of lifetime partners, influence on condom use, and influence on peers and family members to also have less risky sexual behaviors (12-18).

As suggested by Rostosky and colleagues, (8), the current study bridges the gap previously formed (which focused exclusively on sexual intercourse) by including all sexual behaviors (8). There is also a lack of research exploring the norm perceptions of the young adults to get to the core of what their religion says and why they think they should or should not be participating in sexual behaviors. Therefore, the main goal of this study is to examine the influence(s) of religiosity on young adults' sexual behaviors and attitudes, specifically those regarding perceived norms and salient referents.

METHODS

A phenomenological approach was utilized to recruit 13 participants residing in Midwestern United States to fill out open-ended questionnaires. Phenomenology is a process in which the researcher identifies the essence of perceived human experiences about a phenomenon as described by those with experiential knowledge of the phenomenon (19, 20). Also, a phenomenological approach was taken due to the shared experience all the participants had in their affiliation with a faith-based organization. The exploration of the narratives allowed for analyses of potential perceived norms that were elicited from the data. All protocols for research with human subjects were approved by the institutional review board at the authors' university at the time the study was conducted.

Participants and recruitment

Purposeful and snowball sampling were both utilized to recruit participants in order to gather a rich data set. Participants were recruited through written e-mail invitations, targeting a population that had attended or had an affiliation with a church, temple, or faith-based organization. Announcements were made at local church functions and at a local Midwestern university to assist in recruitment. Once a few participants were willing to partake in the study, they would recommend peers, and the snowball recruitment began through word of mouth.

The recruitment area included rural areas in Indiana and Ohio. In order to be eligible for the study, participants had to self-identify as being 18-24 years old, residing in rural Indiana or Ohio, and having some type of affiliation or attendance at a faith-based/religious organization. The first author provided questionnaires to churches and other faith-based organizations where the participants could fill them out and bring them back or they could fill them out while the author was present. Others chose to place them in blank envelopes and bring them back to the author at separate meeting times. The author assured all participants that the information was confidential and reinforced the participants to not put any identifying information on the questionnaire. Participation in the study was completely voluntary and the open-ended questionnaire took the participants approximately 10 – 20 minutes to complete.

Study instruments

An open-ended questionnaire was developed to elicit narratives from the participants. This was chosen, rather than face-to-face interviews, due to the nature of the questions. For example, one question asked what sexual behaviors/activities they are participating in and then a few questions later a question asked about their religious leader and what sexual behaviors/activities they approve of them doing. After discussion between the authors, it was decided that with this age group and content, an anonymous questionnaire could elicit the best data.

The first nine questions assessed demographic information, such as age, sex, location, religious affiliation, and sexual orientation. For clarity purposes and as suggested by previous research, we listed what "sexual behaviors/activities" could include and did not limit the participants, but also included "any other behaviors you might determine as 'sexual.' " The remainder of the questions attempted to: assess the participation in sexual behaviors/activities; who influenced that decision to participate (or not) in sexual behaviors/activities; gather information on where the participants were taught about sexuality education; assess a level of religiosity of the participants; understand the participants' perceptions and norms relating to their religion's teaching regarding sexual behaviors/activities; and identify the salient referents reported by the participants in relation to sexual behaviors/activities.

Data coding and analysis

All answers to the questionnaire were typed verbatim, and double-checked for accuracy. We used the processes of phenomenological reduction, horizontalization, and imaginative variation. Phenomenological reduction consists of returning to the essence of the participants' perceived experience to develop the meaning in and of itself; therefore we focused on the phenomenon to understand its essence. Horizontalization is the process of gathering all of the data and giving each piece of it equal value and weight in the first data analysis phase. In the following phases, data are placed into themes where the repeated statements are taken out. Imaginative variation includes the analysis of data from different perspectives and frames of reference. The final phase was constructing a fusion of the textual and structural descriptions of the phenomenon of religious leaders' teaching experiences (20, 21).

By utilizing these processes, we were able to elicit several themes from the data. Although all of the data was initially given equal value, after reviewing the narratives it appeared some questions did not reveal any significant information. Other questions elicited answers with repeated phrases and similar wording from the participants. We then fused the information to describe the participants' experiences.

As was appropriate, demographic characteristics were completed to generate descriptive statistics. Demographics of the sample are provided below to contextualize participant quotes.

RESULTS

Participants included 13 young adults, aged between 18 and 23. All participants were single, white, and living in either Indiana or Ohio. Four participants identified as male and nine participants identified as female. All participants identified as being Christian and heterosexual with the exception of two participants, one identified as agnostic and one as bisexual. The authors used a phenomenological approach for data analysis and following Polkinghorne's (1989) recommendation for 5-25 participants, it was decided that 13 participants was sufficient for the study design (22).

Themes

Four main themes were elicited from the data collected in this study: Theme 1) religious beliefs matter; Theme 2) religious leaders matter; Theme 3) religious beliefs influence sexual behaviors; Theme 4) sex within marriage only; and Theme 5) salient referents influence sexual behaviors.

Theme 1: Religious beliefs matter

Participants in this group said their religious beliefs matter to them. Ten out of thirteen participants reported attending religious/faith-based services weekly or more than once a week, indicating a high level of religiosity. When asked about their religious beliefs, there was a majority answer of religious beliefs being very important in their lives. Participants expressed feelings such as, "They make me who I am. Everyone sins, but it's how we handle life's pressures and our beliefs that matter most." Other participants were more short and concise, "it is the most important thing to me" and "If it weren't for my faith I would not be alive…"

Participants were asked how their religious beliefs influenced their lives and they expressed these ideas to also be of importance. One participant stated, "My Jesus died for me! To save me from my sin. The least I can do is glorify him! Without him I'm nothing!" Another participant related this to certain behaviors, "I don't drink or party or smoke. I try to be a good influence to my unsaved friends by not doing these things." This participant states, "I want to show the love of Jesus to everyone through my actions, not just my words (walk the walk)." The following participants showed the ideals of the religion, "it instilled me with a set of morals"; "my religion makes me more acceptable to other types of people"; and "you always want to be nice and caring and my religion might have taught me to be more that way."

Theme 2: Religious leaders matter

The majority of participants in this group said their religious leaders matter to them. When asked why the opinion of the religious leaders mattered to participants, these were some of the results we received. Some participants stated that God placed the leaders in their lives and they were honoring that leadership appointment. One participant stated, "Because God has placed them in my life to bring wisdom and encouragement in my life." Another, similar statement, "I believe that God has placed spiritual authority over me and I am to honor that."

Another participant expressed, "God appointed them and I trust God." Other participants reported the benefits of following their leaders. One participant stated, "They want to see me running after God and that's what I want as well. I want my leader's opinion to line up with the word of God! Not the world's view." Another participant expressed the view, "Because they lead by example and it proves to be fruitful and beneficial." One more participant stated, "[The leader] has more knowledge in certain areas."

Participants were asked what they thought their religious leaders would want or expect them to do regarding sexual behaviors. The majority of participants perceived their leaders as wanting them to wait for marriage for all sexual behaviors, except for kissing in some cases. One participant states, "I think they approve of kissing but there is an appropriate time and place and as long as it doesn't lead to anything else. They think any sexual act other than kissing is for after marriage. Period!" Another participant follows suit and even includes sexual thoughts, "They want us to not think sexual thoughts period. Some may be ok with kissing but anything beyond that would be crossing the line." Other participants are shorter with their answers, but give the same point, "abstain completely"; "be married first and stay faithful"; and "my leaders want me to wait until marriage."

Theme 3: Religious beliefs influence sexual behaviors

The majority of participants reported that their religious beliefs influence their sexual behaviors. Participants were asked directly what sexual activities they participated in. Five participants did not participate in sexual behaviors; four participants participated in sexual behaviors, as well as penile-vaginal sex; two participants participated in sexual behaviors, but not penile-vaginal sex; one participant did not participate in any sexual behaviors beyond kissing; and one participant stated, "Before I was a Christian I engaged in sexual behavior, but not sex."

When asked how their religion influenced their sexual behaviors, participants had various answers. Some felt there was not much influence, "I didn't really go do church very much when learning about sex so I believe it had no influence." Others felt that religion influenced their sexual behaviors. A participant noted: "It used to influence me but after having sex once, it's hard to stop no matter how bad I feel about it." Other participants felt very strongly about their religious beliefs and their sexual behaviors, "My body belongs to God until he sends me my husband. I will stay pure for him!" and "It prohibits it right now in my life, but I know someday when I'm married I will be able to enjoy sexual activities in a safe environment." Other participants expressed their beliefs as such, "I want to wait for my husband," and "the Bible teaches to be a virgin when going into marriage and I believe the Bible."

Theme 4: Sex within marriage only

The majority of participants in this group said sex should not be performed outside of marriage. One participant expressed, "I am waiting for marriage to have any kind of intimacy. I see it as something special to share with one person, your spouse. This influences how I interact with the opposite sex." Another participant stated, "Sex should not exist outside of marriage. Any form of gratification is immoral unless it is with an opposite-sex spouse (masturbation, porn, etc.)" A participant reported, "The Bible says sex is a gift from God, specifically to be enjoyed in the marriage relationship. It is wrong in any other situation, but in marriage it is a wonderful thing."

Theme 5: Salient referents influence sexual behaviors

Participants identified four main referents that influence their sexual decisions: parents, peers, religion, and the media. When asked what and/or who influenced their decision to participate or not in sexual behaviors, participants gave various answers, with the four underlying themes. One participant stated, "My parents, based on their beliefs. Scripture/Bible, ultimately influenced me, through my parents and my own study." Another participant reported, "My parents and friends; my faith and my values." Other participants expressed, "Friends, media"; "Friends, environment"; and "My parents taught me not to but I was a fool and ignored them. I believe in Jesus now and will stay pure until marriage."

Although the majority of these young adults report their religious leaders are important to them and have an influence on their sexual decision making, only three participants reported that they received any "formal" sexuality education that was affiliated with a faith-based organization, in these cases, their churches. All other participants stated they received sexuality education and information from school-based programs or in couple cases from their parents.

DISCUSSION

The findings in this study offer insight into the influence religion and religious leaders have on attitudes and decisions regarding sexual behaviors in young adults. The participants indicated that they chose less risky sexual behaviors, and in some cases, no sexual behaviors beyond kissing. These findings are similar to the findings of previous studies, which is that: religiosity is a protective factor over risky sexual behaviors. However, the findings also show that even though the participants reported that they were knowledgeable about their religious beliefs, what their religious leaders would want them to do regarding sexual activities, and they valued that opinion, many of the participants previously or currently participated in some type of sexual activity. The sexual activities were "less risky" but were still occurring and were not congruent with their religious beliefs outside of marriage. Many of the participants stated that they did not listen to their parents and/or religious leaders and made mistakes and were now living a life that was compliant with their beliefs. Others reported that they had "stayed pure" and would continue this until marriage.

The participants identified their religious leaders to be important to them and to value their opinions, as well as their parents, peers, and the media. The participants stated that the religious leaders were placed in their lives to lead, teach, and encourage them and that this had proven to be beneficial. Further research could explore what is being taught by the leaders regarding sexuality and relationships to produce this "protective factor" that has been found in adolescence and young adults from religiosity. When analyzing this data, it appeared to line up with part of Fishbein and Ajzen's (2010) Reasoned Action Approach (23). The salient referents that the participants cite as important to them, as well as complying with the perceived social norms to meet the salient referents' perceived expectations all appear to fit into the Reasoned Action Approach.

Limitations

The findings of this study are based on a small sample of a qualitative investigation with the aim of a depth of understanding an experience rather than generalizing the findings of the study. In addition, the focus of the study was limited to young adults who had some affiliation with a faith-based organization and who resided in rural Indiana or Ohio. The participants, mainly due to the location in which recruitment took place, all self-identified as White. While this fills a gap in the research, this also limits generalizability to other populations and specific racial groups. In addition, the study was limited to majority Protestant Christians. It cannot be assumed that our results are representative of the larger population of all Christians, Protestant and/or Catholic, in the United States or abroad. This study relied on self-reported experiences and perceptions from participants and self-report can reflect potential biases when used in interviews for data collection (19).

CONCLUSION

Using the identified salient referents (parents, religious leaders, peers, and the media) in conjunction with each other and by acknowledging and teaching the religious beliefs, interventions could be very effective in promoting sexual health and reducing risky sexual behaviors that increase the high rate of STIs in this age group. Future studies on the content of what parents and religious leaders are teaching would be of value to the field of public health and of aid in the reduction of STIs and teen pregnancy.

REFERENCES

[1] Kosmin BA, Mayer E, Keysar A. The American Religious Identification Survey (ARIS 2008): Summary report, 2009. Trinity College: Institute for the Study of Secularism in Society and Culture. URL: http://commons.trincoll.edu/aris/publications/2008-2/aris-2008-summary-report/.

[2] DeHaven MJ, Hunter IB, Wilder L, Walton JW, Berry J. Health programs in faith-based organizations: Are they effective? Am J Public Health 2004;94(6):1030-6.

[3] 3. Satterwhite CL, Torrone E, Meites E, Dunne EF, Mahajan R, Ocfemia MCB, et al. Sexually transmitted infections among US women and men: Prevalence and incidence estimates, 2008. J Sex Transm Dis 2013;40(3):187-93.

[4] Owusu-Edusei KJ, Chesson HW, Gift TL, Tao G, Mahajan R, Ocfemia MCB, et al. The estimated direct medical cost of selected sexually transmitted infections in the United States, 2008. J Sex Transm Dis 2013;40(3):197-201.

[5] Mokdad AH, Marks JS, Stroup DF, Gerberding JL. Actual causes of death in the United States, 2000, JAMA. 2004;291(10):1238-45.

[6] Centers for Disease Control and Prevention (CDC). 2010 sexually transmitted diseasessSurveillance. URL: http://www.cdc.gov/std/stats10/trends.htm.

[7] Hull SJ, Hennessy M, Bleakley A, Fishbein M, Jordan A. Identifying the causal pathways from religiosity to delayed adolescent sexual behavior. J Sex Res 2011;48(6):543-53.

[8] Rostosky SS, Wilcox BL, Wright MLC, Randall BA. The impact of religiosity on adolescent sexual behavior: A review of the evidence. J Adolesc Res 2004;19(6):677-97.

[9] McCree DH, Wingood GM, DiClemente R, Davies S, Harrington KF. Religiosity and risky sexual behavior in African American adolescent females. J Adolesc Health 2003;33:2-8.

[10] Poulson RL, Eppler MA, Satterwhite TN, Wuensch KL, Bass LA. Alcohol consumption, strength of religious beliefs, and risky sexual behavior in college students. J Am Coll Health 1998;46(5):227-32.
[11] Galvan FH, Collins RL, Kanouse DE, Pantoja P, Golinelli D. Religiosity, denominational affiliation, and sexual behaviors among people with HIV in the United States. J Sex Res 2007;44(1):49-58.
[12] Adamczyk A, Felson J. Friends' religiosity and first sex. Soc Sci Res 2006;35:924-47.
[13] Haglund KA, Fehring RJ. The association of religiosity, sexual education, and parental factors with risky sexual behaviors among adolescents and young adults. J Relig Health 2010;49:460-72.
[14] Lammers C, Ireland M, Reskick M, Blum R. Influences on adolescents' decision to postpone onset of sexual intercourse: A survival analysis of virginity among youths aged 13 to 18 years. J Adolesc Health 2000;26:42-8.
[15] Landor A, Simons LG, Simons RL, Brody GH, Gibbons FX. The role of religiosity in the relationship between parents, peers, and adolescent risky sexual behavior. J Youth Adolesc 2011;40:296-309.
[16] Manlove JS, Logan C, Moore KA, Ikramulla EN. Pathways from family religiosity to adolescent sexual activity and contraceptive use. Perspect Sex Reprod Health 2008;40(2):105-17.
[17] Manlove JS, Terry-Humen E, Ikramullah EN, Moore KA. The role of parent religiosity in teens' transitions to sex and contraception. J Adolesc Health 2006;39:578-87.
[18] Nonnemaker JM, McNeely CA, Blum RW. Public and private domains of religiosity and adolescent health risk behaviors: Evidence from the National Longitudinal Study of Adolescent Health, Soc Sci Med 2003;57:2049-54.
[19] Creswell JW. Research design: Qualitative, quantitative, and mixed methods approaches, 3rd ed. Thousand Oaks, CA: Sage, 2009.
[20] Merriam SB. Qualitative research in practice: examples for discussion and analysis. San Francisco, CA: Jossey-Bass, 2002.
[21] Moustakas CE. Phenomenological research methods. Thousand Oaks, CA: Sage, 1994.
[22] Polkinghorne DE. Phenomenological research methods. In: Valle RS, Halling S, eds. Existential-phenomenological perspectives in psychology: Exploring the breadth of human experience. New York: Plenum Press, 1989:41-60.
[23] Fishbein M. Ajzen I. Predicting and changing behavior: A reasoned action approach. New York: Psychology Press, 2010.

Received: August 25, 2014. *Revised:* September 27, 2014. *Accepted:*October 01, 2014.

In: Public Health Yearbook 2015
Editor: Joav Merrick

ISBN: 978-1-63484-514-4
© 2016 Nova Science Publishers, Inc.

Chapter 34

REFLECTIONS OF TWO-SCREEN USERS: HOW PEOPLE USE INFORMATION TECHNOLOGY WHILE WATCHING SPORTS

Ryan P Vooris, MA, Chase ML Smith, MA, and Cecilia S Obeng*, PhD

School of Public Health, Indiana University, Bloomington, Indiana, United States of America

Scholarship on sport fans indicate that they frequently use more than one platform of information technology when they are watching sports. Three focus groups with a total of 20 participants were utilized to find out how people use the internet and information technology at the same time while they watch sports. Nearly all participants noted that they liked to use information technology such as mobile phones and laptops to keep informed about sports statistics. Two-screen users also talked about the ability of technology to keep them informed about what else is going on in the sports world. Participants indicated that they are fans of multiple teams and therefore use technology to keep abreast of other teams and games while they are watching one team on television. Statements from the participants suggest that the easy access to mobile technologies, made it possible to watch sports on television and keep abreast with other teams.

Keywords: technology, sports, social media

INTRODUCTION

Sport fans frequently use more than one platform of information technology when they are watching sports (1). It is estimated that as many as 85% of people use another device while watching television (2). The spread of technology, combined with a reduction in its size, has made it possible for people to use technology while engaging in other activities. For example,

---

* Correspondence: Cecilia S Obeng, PhD, Associate Professor, Indiana University, School of Public Health, 1025 E 7th Street, SPH 116, Bloomington, IN 47405, United States. E-mail: cobeng@indiana.edu.

the size of smart phones and tablets have made it easier for people to be online, while at a sporting event or watching one on television. People who use information technology while consuming other forms of entertainment are often referred to as two-screen users (3). They can also be said to be engaging in the second-screen experience (4). The use of multiple digital devices at once is an area within multitasking research that has seen a recent rise in interest. This interest is primarily rooted in the belief that the rapid spread of digital devices has created an information technology environment for today's young people, which is drastically different from previous generations (5). The second-screen experience can manifest in a number of different ways. Apps for smart phones and tablets can use audio from a television to sync with a television program. These apps then offer content related to the television program one is watching (4). The popular ABC show Grey's Anatomy offers an app that provides show watchers with an interactive experience while watching the show. As a viewer watches the show, content related to the show and its subject matter are displayed on the app (6). Popular apps such as GetGlue, IntoNow, and Viggle offer similar experiences for people. These apps also offer rewards for "checking-into" a show via the audio recognition software included on most smart phones (4). More importantly, two-screen users represent another way for broadcaster partners to generate revenue. Forbes estimated that CBS's online streaming of Super Bowl XLVII to second-screen users could generate between $10 and $12 million in extra revenue for the network. This online steam of the game contained extra features not available during the network broadcast of the 2013 Ravens versus 49ers Super Bowl. These features included additional camera angles and a user-designed Twitter feed that could appear along with the game broadcast (7).

The two-screen experience also presents itself in the use of social media during sporting events. Social networks such as Twitter and Facebook help to facilitate conversations among fans as they watch a live sporting event (8). Social networks also allow this conversation to be unconstrained by geography and encompass many different voices. The broadcasts of many live sporting events incorporate various elements of social media. These include such things as designating a Twitter hashtag for the event and informing viewers that they can visit the network's official Facebook page for more information about the event (1).

Nielsen, the firm that records and reports on television ratings, reported that in the second quarter of 2013, people tweeted about television 263 million times. This was a rise of 38% from one year before (9). People are tweeting about their television entertainment as they consume it and doing so in ever increasing numbers. For example, the series-finale of the popular show Breaking Bad generated 1.24 million tweets from 601,000 Twitter users during the show's airing. Nielsen estimates that these tweets reached an audience of 9.3 million people (9). The year 2013 marked the first year for which Nielsen tracked the social traffic and social rank of television broadcasts. Of importance for this research is that Nielsen's 2013: Year in Sports Media Report (10) reported that almost half of all tweets which were about television last year, referenced sports—49.7% to be exact. This is despite that the fact that sports accounts for only about 1.2% of all television programming. Nielsen also reported that in September 2013, 61.7 million people used their smartphone to access sport content, an increase of more than 21% from the prior year. This rise in mobile traffic is in contrast to a decrease in computer traffic to sport websites, which Nielsen reports decreased by 9.5% in September 2013 when compared to the previous year. According to Nielsen, people now spend almost as much time accessing sport content on their phones as they do accessing sport content on their computers (10).

The Wall Street Journal reported the findings of research firm, eMarketer, in late 2013, found that 15 to 17% of television viewers utilize social media while watching TV. According to this report, the most used social network while watching television is Facebook, followed by Twitter. The most commonly used device used to access social media while watching television is the laptop, with the smartphone, tablets, and gaming devices being used to engage with the content (11).

In view of the above literature, this study examines how people use technology, while watching sporting events, and how mobile technology, such as tablets and smartphones have made it easier for people to be online, while at a sporting event on television. In particular, we plan on examining what people are doing online via their smartphone, tablet, and/or computer while they consume sporting events and why they supplement that consumption with those technologies. In order to accomplish this goal, focus groups were used with people who self-identified as users of information technology while they consume sports.

METHODS

Focus groups were utilized in order to ascertain a better idea of how people might be using the internet and information technology while they watch sports. Three focus groups were held over the span of ten days in April 2014. In total there were 20 participants (16 males and 4 females). Each participant self-reported as being a user of technology while they watch sports. Participants were undergraduates at a large Midwestern university who were recruited from classes within a sport management undergraduate program. Each focus group featured a trained moderator and lasted between thirty and forty minutes. Each of the three focus groups was recorded and an observer recorded notes on the meetings.

The goal of the focus groups was to gain a better understanding of how prevalent technology is used while they watch sports. With this aim in mind, questions centered on what technology people used while watching sports, what they were doing with that technology, how long they had been a user of that technology and how important they viewed that technology as part of their enjoyment of watching sports. Broader questions which dealt with issues such as how technology fit into other aspects of their lives and how they might feel if that technology was removed from their lives were also asked. The benefits they saw from accessing Internet content while watching a sporting event were also asked.

RESULTS

The audio recordings of the three focus groups were analyzed for common themes which could shed light on the research questions. These results are now explained with relevant quotes from the three focus groups.

Nearly all the two-screen users expressed the opinion that they liked to use information technology such as mobile phones and laptops to keep them informed about sports statistics. Mobile apps such as ESPN Scorecenter, Yahoo! Sports, and The Score were mentioned as places to go to find out the statistics about a game a user is watching. As a few users mentioned, these apps update their game and player stats in real-time. As a result, users are able to supplement their viewing experience with statistics related to the game they are watching on television. Users mentioned that television broadcasts do not always provide player and game stats frequently enough. In turn, a quick reference to an app or a web search can bring up information about a player, a team, or a game.

Two-screen users also talked about the ability of technology to keep them informed about what else is going on in the sports world. Many users discussed the fact that they are fans of multiple teams and therefore use technology to keep abreast of other teams and games while they are watching one team on television. In addition, users talked about the need to know what is going on in other games because the outcome of those games affects their team. One user articulated both of these ideas in the following statement:

> If there are other games on, I'll be on Twitter and the ESPN app to look at other games to keep updated. Playoffs are starting soon, so you want to see the standings update. I'm a Knick fan so we're hoping the Hawks lose, while I'm watching the Knick game. I looking into other sports as well. So if I'm watching basketball, I'm still checking hockey updates, football updates, all other sports that are on. You can't watch everything.

Another motivation for using technology while watching sporting events appeared to be the desire of viewers to be plugged into their social networks. Popular social networking sites such as Facebook and Twitter appear to give fans an opportunity to know about other exciting games or events as they are happening. This in turn also helps them to know if and when they might want to change the channel to watch a different game. Users explained that their social networks help keep them updated about games they are not watching. One user explained the experience as follows:

> I'm just constantly on Twitter because I follow a lot of things where they give you interesting stats about a game you are watching and then also then if I see someone tweet something like 'This Warriors/Mavericks game is getting really tense,' then I'll flip the channel. Because I would have no idea if that is going on unless I was looking at my phone.

As a follow-up to this trend of turning the channel when users see people talking about an exciting event on social media, we asked for specific examples to help explain this social-media prompted-channel-change. One user put it this way:

> I forget when it was, but it was when Steph Curry went off in Madison Square Garden. I saw that it was happening on Twitter and I just put it on right away. Because it sounded exciting.

Another participant said:

> During baseball season, if someone says 'a person has a perfect game going through six inning and we'll broadcast his pitching innings on ESPN,' I'll go to ESPN and see if he can do it or not.

Another participant noted this when talking about the NCAA Division 1 Men's Basketball Tournament, commonly known as March Madness:

> I think recently with the whole March Madness, with the first round there's so many games going on at the same time that Twitter keeps you updated. I was watching the Duke/Mercer game and then I saw on Twitter, that another game is real close with 30 seconds left, I'll flip real quick, see what happens—buzzer beater--and then flip back. It's crazy.

When asked to discuss what social networks they prefer to use when watching sporting events, users expressed that Twitter is there go-to network. The reasons for this varied. Some users discussed how Twitter allows them to stay connected to other games they cannot or are not watching. Others mentioned how they like to read Twitter updates about the game they are watching. One user put it this way:

> I like to use Twitter a lot because I can say I how feel about a game and also see what my peers think and I follow some experts too and I like to see how they feel about it.

Another user built off this response by adding:

> I also like looking at what friends, celebrities, insiders, and other athletes are saying about the game that I'm watching along with their reaction as well.

Twitter was frequently mentioned as the impetus for users changing the channel to watch another game. The reverse also appeared true. When a user is watching an exciting game they want to express that feeling on Twitter or see how others are reacting to the exciting events they are watching. One female user put the feeling this way:

> If a big play happens I like to go on Twitter and see people's reactions and what they are saying about it. Or if a game I'm watching is boring and ESPN is tweeting about how another game is exciting I'll switch to that.

A nineteen year-old male from Maryland had this to say:

> I go on just to see what other people are saying and what the analysts are saying. Especially if a big play happens, like the James Young dunk. I like seeing what everyone is saying on Twitter and how crazy that is.

Users also discussed how news can come to them faster on Twitter than from only watching TV. For example, a research participant noted:

> If someone get hurts, someone on Twitter it will say what happens to them first, before TV.

Users frequently mentioned how Twitter helps them keep up-to-date about games they cannot watch. By reading a constant stream of updates posted by friends, analysts, journalists, official team accounts, and media partners, they are able to follow the events of a game even if they are unable to watch a sporting event. Some users mentioned how this helps them follow along with their favorite international teams. Soccer fans in particular mentioned how Twitter allows them to follow along with their favorite English Premiere League teams, even if they cannot watch the game. By following the right combination of fans, journalists, and official accounts they are able to experience the game on Twitter, even though they are unable to watch it on television. A few users also expressed how they enjoyed reading the humorous takes that parody accounts can have on an event.

Users were clear; they liked to have more information than what is coming from the broadcast. This can come by way of looking at player statistics, game statistics and player biographies for the game they are watching on television. It can also come from reflections on the game which other viewers post to their social media accounts.

In addition to statistics and social media, users discussed how they liked to use information technology to check up on the performance of their fantasy sports teams. Fantasy sports allow people to draft and operate a sports teams in which points are awarded based on how real players perform in real games. Fans then compete against each other to see who can create the best fantasy team. It has been estimated that 32 million Americans play fantasy sports and that the industry generates around $15 billion dollars per year (12). One focus group participant talked about his experience:

> During football season, I check my phone for fantasy football. I'm always going on my apps to see how my players are doing and people around my league are doing, while I'm watching just one game.

Of those who participated in the focus groups and played fantasy sports, all but one user admitted to regularly checking the Internet to see how their teams were doing while they were watching other games.

When asked how often they supplemented their sport-viewing experience with information technology such as mobile phones, tablets, and laptops, users expressed very similar answers. Most users approximated their use of information technology while watching sports at between 90% and 100%. One user put it this way:

> It's basically, unless I'm watching it live, I've got my phone in my hand.

Most users explained that the technology they use while watching sports is usually their smart phone or laptop. Users explained that an important distinction about what technology they use is where they are located. If they are in their room or house, they are much more likely to use their laptop to supplement their sports-watching experience. If they are at a friend's house or out at a bar or restaurant they are going to use their mobile phone. The same is true if they are watching alone or with a group. If they are watching alone, users explained that they are more likely to use their laptop, while if they are watching sports with a group of friends, they will instead have their mobile smartphone in their hand. Three users discussed how they frequently watch one game on television and another on their laptop. These users explained that this often happens during times of the year when there are multiple sports taking place at once.

We next asked users to try to identify how long they have been two-screen users and if they could recall how they got into that habit. Answers varied on this, but one common theme was the purchase of a smartphone. For many of this study's participants, that event occurred during the sophomore or junior year of high school. Participants remarked how the smartphone made checking stats, scores, and social media easier and more convenient for them. Many users talked about how the smartphone allowed them to stay in the know when talking about sports with more people. For example:

> I didn't become attached to information right away. It was more when I found out everyone else was doing it, I felt behind. I felt like to should know more, I should be finding out more stats.

And:

> After living with guys who are more like that, more into having their phone with them all the time, I picked up on that. I used to hate that people looked at their phones during games, it bothered me. But now I find myself doing it. It's a little awkward.

One user articulated how he cut back on his usage of their phone while watching sporting events, because he felt like it took away from the experience.

> I noticed that I was on my phone almost as much as I was watching the game and that got really annoying. I would miss a dunk or something because I was looking at Twitter or something. I want to watch it in real time now.

A two-screen user from New Jersey explained how he got his smartphone, adapted to using Twitter, and how that kept him informed about sports as he watched television:

> I got my smartphone in the middle of high school and once I got it, I immediately got the Twitter put on the phone and started following people to see what people are saying about different sports and stuff like that. I don't like to tweet things, but I like to follow along with what people are saying. If I'm watching one thing, I can look at Twitter and follow along with a completely different game or know about something that happened somewhere else that I wouldn't know from just watching this game.

DISCUSSION

There are a number of important theoretical and practical implications which can be derived from the reflections of these two-screen users. As the statistics stated in the beginning of this manuscript demonstrate, more and more people are using information technology while they watch sports. This is a growing trend that requires examination. It appears clear that the thirst for information is growing among young people. This manifests itself in a number of different ways.

The desire to have more information than what is included in the broadcast of televised sporting events was a common theme echoed by many focus group participants. Focus group members were nearly unanimous in stating that they use mobile apps and the internet to access information which compliments their viewing experience. This can come in the form of checking the statistics for a player they are watching on television or keeping themselves updated about overall statistics in a particular game. This desire for more information is one that mobile app makers need to be aware of. It presents the opportunity for them to create and market mobile apps which present players and game statistics in an easy to find method.

Users articulated how they enjoyed checking their social media networks during games to see how other people are reacting to the same events they are watching. This desire to be connected to each other is similar to the findings in some uses and gratifications research that has examined Twitter (13). The desire of sports fans to do more than just watch the sports is a theme expressed by Gantz and Lewis (1) in their work on why sports fans use new media. In their words, television represents only the "tip of the iceberg's worth of activity associated with following sports" (p. 24). Statements from the participants of these focus groups suggest that easy access to mobile technologies, such as smartphones and laptops, makes it incredibly easy for them to engage in other activities while watching sports on television and that they are doing so at very high rate.

Future study will look at the discourse used by the two-screen users and how this influences their social health and the health of those around them (family members, classmates and friends).

REFERENCES

[1] Gantz W, Lewis N. Fanship differences between traditional and newer media. In: Billings AC, Hardin M, eds. Routledge handbook of sport and new media. London: Routledge, 2014:19-31.
[2] Dredge S. Social TV and second-screen viewing: The stats in 2012. Guardian 2012 Oct 29. URL: http://www.theguardian.com/technology/appsblog/2012/oct/29/social-tv-second-screen-research.
[3] Yenigun S. TV broadcasters amp up the 'second screen' experience. URL: http://www.npr.org/blogs/alltechconsidered/2012/12/28/168163835/tv-broadcasters-amp-up-the-second-screen-experience.
[4] Warren C. When did the 'second screen' become a thing? URL: http://mashable.com/2013/05/02/second-screen/.
[5] Spink A, Cole C, Waller M. Multitasking behavior. Ann Rev Inform Sci Technol 2008; 42(0): 93-118.
[6] Warren C. "Grey's anatomy" fans to get an interactive viewing experience on ipad. URL: http://mashable.com/2011/02/01/greys-anatomy-ipad-app/.
[7] Ozanian M. CBS could earn $12 million from super bowl's "second screen" experience. Forbes 2013 Febr 02. URL: http://www.forbes.com/sites/mikeozanian/2013/02/02/cbs-could-earn-12-million-from-super-bowls-second-screen-experience/.
[8] Gregory S. Why sports ratings are surging on TV. Time 2010 Aug 14. URL: http://content.time.com/time/business/article/0,8599,2010746,00.html.
[9] Friedman W. TV tweets raise 38%, cross-promotion expands Twitter TV audience. URL: http://www.mediapost.com/publications/article/211135/cross-promotion-38-rise-in-tv-tweets.html#axzz2iEF4w5r9>.
[10] Year in Sports Media Report: 2013. Nielsen Company. Report number: 2014.
[11] Marr M. How big is the second screen? Wall Street J 2013 Oct 10. URL: http://blogs.wsj.com/corporate-intelligence/2013/10/10/how-big-is-the-second-screen/.
[12] Goff B. The $70 billion fantasy football market. Forbes 2013 Aug 20. URL: http://www.forbes.com/sites/briangoff/2013/08/20/the-70-billion-fantasy-football-market/.
[13] Chen GM. Tweet this: A uses and gratifications perspective on how active Twitter use gratifies a need to connect with others. Comput Hum Behav 2011;27(2):755-62.

Received: September 01, 2014. *Revised:* September 27, 2014. *Accepted:* October 04, 2014.

In: Public Health Yearbook 2015
Editor: Joav Merrick

ISBN: 978-1-63484-514-4
© 2016 Nova Science Publishers, Inc.

Chapter 35

TURKISH IMMIGRANTS' PRACTICES AND PERCEPTIONS OF VOLUNTARY HIV TESTING AND COUNSELING IN THE UNITED STATES

Alper Kilic, MSc, and Cecilia S Obeng, PhD*

Department of Applied Health Science, School of Public Health,
Indiana University, Bloomington, Indiana, United States of America

ABSTRACT

This study was conducted in order to have an insight into HIV testing perceptions and practices of 15 Turkish migrants living in the United States. Turkish refugees were recruited through emails and a social website (Facebook). The web-based survey used in the study consisted of open-ended questions, and closed–ended questions (for demographic information only). Most participants reported that taking HIV testing once a year was acceptable to them, although they did not consider themselves at risk of having HIV. Two older participants did not report of taking any HIV test in their lifetime. Married couples, as well as single and divorced participants, revealed that they were more likely to get HIV testing, if they were requested to get testing by their partners. Participants did not consider medical failures or tattoos as a potential HIV transmission medium. They indicated that availability of free HIV testing and home test kits might increase the proportion of white-collar Turkish immigrants getting HIV testing regularly.

Keywords: Turkish immigrants, HIV testing, counseling, voluntary testing

INTRODUCTION

Today, the number of people living with HIV/AIDS (human immunodeficiency virus/acquired immunodeficiency syndrome) exceeds 35 million worldwide and while there

---

[*] Correspondence: Cecilia S Obeng, PhD, Associate Professor, Indiana University, School of Public Health, 1025 E 7th Street, SPH 116, Bloomington, IN 47405, United States. E-mail: cobeng@indiana.edu

are various developments in response to this pandemic, there is still no cure for it (1). HIV has a unique and direct relationship with socio-political issues and without a consensus on sexual education, gender and migration, programs targeting intervention drug users, and men having sex with men, no prevention program can be properly planned or become successful (2, 3). Note that the HIV epidemic is driven by people's behavior and health disparities within countries might increase HIV risk among certain minorities (4). Therefore, identifying risk groups, determining prevention strategies with behaviors interventions relevant to the epidemic in the each country is necessary (4). As there is still no cure for HIV/AIDS, education on prevention remains the most effective method of tackling the disease until a cure is found (5). There is a consensus on the benefits of testing for HIV and early detection of the infection (6). HIV testing and counseling have constituted important key strategies for preventing further HIV transmission since the virus was identified in the early days of the pandemic.

Concerning information on HIV/AIDS in the Republic of Turkey, in 2005, the number of registered HIV positive cases - was 2,254 (7); however, in 2012, the number of detected HIV positive cases had risen to 5,740 (7). This figure is insignificant when the population of Turkey is taken into consideration. Many researchers believe that lower number of HIV detection is due to the lack of voluntary testing.

Research has shown that the general population in Turkey does not have enough knowledge about STDs and HIV/AIDS (8). In Turkey issues related with sex behaviours are rarely openly discussed in the society. A study which was conducted among female students attending a religious school in Eastern Turkey found that a considerable percentage of the students found talking about sexually transmitted diseases as a taboo and their information about reproductive health was limited (9). Although premarital sex is generally considered as a taboo, research shows that premarital sexual intercourse exists in Turkey among university students (8).

TURKISH MIGRANTS IN THE UNITED STATES

Concerning Turkish Migrants living in the US, the number of economic–opportunity-centered migrants originating from Turkey into the US has been constantly increasing in the last two decades. The exact number of Turkish Americans in the US is hard to accurately determine due to the complicated nature of migration originating from Turkey (10). Earliest recorded Turkish migrants arrived in the US in 1586 after sailors from Ottoman Navy were captured during a sea battle between Spain and the Ottoman Empire and the captured sailors were taken by Spanish ships to the new continent (11). Two hundred of them settled in present day North Carolina. Eventually, 100 of them were returned by the English government to the Ottomans (11). Significant number of immigrants arrived in the US in the mid-nineteenth century. Due to the multi-ethnic composure of the Ottoman Empire, it was not always possible to distinguish the immigrants' ethnic identities, whether they were from Turkish Muslim background with Turkish as native language or they belonged to various ethnic groups. In the nineteenth century, many Ottoman Citizens who migrated to the US were ethnic Arabs, Azeri, Armenian, Greek and Jewish.

Turkish migrants continued to arrive in the US at the beginning of the twenty-first century. During World War One and the Balkan wars, after the establishment of the new Turkish Republic, professional migrants started to arrive in the US. Today there are differences in counting with respect to the number of Turkish migrants in the US and the number varies between 199,000 to 500,000 (12).

Research on the factors related to HIV testing decisions in various groups worldwide has demonstrated that with a few exceptions, accessibility to healthcare services and a recent HIV related risk behavior are the most important factors influencing HIV testing behavior (6). Even in countries with high HIV prevalence such as in South Africa, HIV testing is stigmatized, persons who were not tested for HIV are more likely to have negative opinions about HIV positive people and even people who are receiving tests for HIV (13). In addition, many scholars from around the world have found that higher education and information on the risks associated with HIV, do not necessarily lead to safe sex behaviors (14, 15).

Beliefs concerning causes of illness and being at risk vary considerably across cultures, and gender roles acculturation and education levels tend to play a role.

This qualitative research aimed to identify perceptions, testing preferences and testing attitudes among university affiliated Turkish migrants in the U.S. In addition, we aimed to identify the role of trust of health care providers/governments about confidentiality of test results in taking an HIV testing in the future.

METHODS

Turkish immigrants were recruited through a social website (Facebook) and email with the assistance of personal contacts at the IU Bloomington campus. Participants were sent an anonymous online survey link and asked to forward the link to their colleagues from Turkey and/or their spouses. Snowball sampling method was used for recruitment. Fifteen participants were found eligible to take part in the study with the criteria — being Turkish-born and living in the U.S. for at least a year.

Study design and analysis

This study took place in 2013 after an approval from the Institutional Review Board for the protection of Human Subjects at Indiana University. The web-based survey used in the study consisted of closed ended questions (for demographic information only), and open-ended questions. Participation was voluntary. The words that were considered to be important were grouped during coding and further sorted into themes.

RESULTS

Most of the participants were female (n = 10). Median age for both female and male participants was found to be 40 (one participant did not report his/her age). Among the participants who reported their marital status, the number of married couples was found to be the highest (n = 7), followed by single participants (n = 4) and divorced participants (n = 2).

Only one single male participant reported that he considered himself personally being under HIV risk while three female surveyed participants reported that everyone who is sexually active has a risk of having an HIV infection. All other participants mentioned that they did not consider themselves personally under the risk of acquiring HIV. One participant responded "I do not carry more risk than normal population, because I have a ordinary life and do not work on AIDS." Another response to the same question was "I think I have no risk, I have my husband and we have a trusty relationship. We do not go out much." None of the participants mentioned having a tattoo might have a higher risk factor for acquiring the HIV.

Five participants reported that taking HIV testing once a year was ideal, although they were not considering themselves at risk, they were usually recommending HIV testing to the "people at risk."

Two older participants aged 62 and 65 did not report of taking any HIV test in their life time. Married couples, single, and divorced participants, revealed that they were likely to get HIV testing if they were requested to do so by their sexual partners. However, response to this question varied from:

"I will get the test in order to make my partner feel better and feel safe."
"In my case we don't need such test."
"We were both tested some time ago and we have a monogomous relationship;"
"I wouldn't do it and in addition my partner would not ask me for it."

Participants reported that availability of free HIV testing and home test kits, might increase the likelihood of getting HIV testing regularly.

In most of the responses, perceived risk for acquiring HIV was low and almost all of the participants reported that they do not consider HIV to be a threat in any way to their daily lives. Survey participants did not report of belonging to any particular HIV risk group. They indicated that not belonging to any of the special risk groups associated with HIV naturally decreases their risk of HIV transmission. Moreover, all participants except one reported that people without any HIV risk behavior did not have to test for HIV regularly. Participants did not consider HIV test as necessity and this can be considered as normal as they reported they have unconditional support and confidence in their spouses sexual fidelity. Most participants recommended that HIV test should ideally be taken once a year by those who are in any risk group. Four participants were skeptical about confidentiality of HIV testing results. One of the respondents mentioned "No, I don't think they are announced but people can receive this information whenever they want to, governments have all informations."

Participants identified HIV risk groups correctly although none of them listed having a tattoo as a risk factor. They reported the following as risk groups: "Sex workers, persons who deal with blood tests, everyone who has sex with more than one partner, people having sex out of marriage, homosexual individuals, people having unprotected sex, people sharing needles, people being exposed to HIV virus with open wounds, babies who are born to HIV positive parents as having a higher risk for HIV transmission. Since research participants associated HIV testing with people in a high risk group, and they did not consider themselves in these risk groups, it could be argued that our survey participants were less likely to receive an HIV test.

However, for younger migrants this picture can be different. Especially for the children of Turkish migrants who arrived in the US in an early age. Age at arrival among immigrants was found to be related with higher acculturation and income levels in studies from around the world (16, 17, 19). Assimilation hypothesis indicates that Turkish migrants should become more individualistic with increasing length of stay in the United States (18). Individualism acquired with increased time spent in the US would decrease possible stigmatization attached with HIV testing.

DISCUSSION

Research participants did not report any specific stigmatization attached with HIV testing. However, not having self-perceived risk factor for HIV transmission and not feeling a need for the testing suggests there is a potential for stigmatization attached with HIV testing already (having increased risk for HIV transmission) among the survey participants.

On the other hand, we did not include questions that measured the information level of participants on HIV itself in general in this research. All in all, this finding is found to be similar to research outcomes from Turkey, where the general populations' and students' perceptions of HIV risk were found to be low regardless of their sexual activity characteristics (20). Frequency and attitude towards HIV testing among the general population in Turkey is not well studied. HIV testing is limited and not systematic among high risk groups (21). Low knowledge on the virus suggests that there are different mechanisms that might play a role in preventing the spreading of the virus in Turkey. One of those reasons should be the role of male circumcision and its preventive role against HIV transmission although not all researchers found a conclusive result, studies about the interconnectedness between circumcision and the spread of HIV/AIDS in Africa suggest a curb in the spread of the disease if protective action is taken, especially during male circumcision (22, 23, 24).

In our study, most participants reported that availability of HIV testing kits at home would increase their likelihood of using testing kits at home. Only one participant mentioned potential problems associated with home based kits, such as its lower predictability and lack of onsite psychological support mechanisms in the case of encountering an HIV positive result at home.

Among the limitations of this study, is the fact that we had a small number of respondents. Also, after posting the link of the survey questions, we had no control over how accurately respondents answered the open ended online survey questions. In addition, we did not have a direct control regarding who received the survey link in the end through convenience sampling method, since we requested research participants to forward the survey to their Turkish friends who study or work in the U.S. as academicians and originating from Turkey.

In sum, the general picture regarding perceptions of Turkish migrants in the US on HIV testing appears to be inconclusive. Future research may further look into the possible effects of migrants' education and acculturation levels and their trust in health care providers/government in relation to confidentiality of HIV testing.

REFERENCES

[1] UNAIDS Global Report. UNAIDS report on the global AIDS epidemic 2012. URL: http://www.unaids.org/en/resources/publications/2012/name,76121,en.asp.

[2] Champredon D, Bellan DJ. HIV sexual transmission is predominantly driven by single individuals rather than discordant couples: a model-based approach. PloS One 2013;8(12):e82906.

[3] JH & TB (n.d.). Girl power. The impact of girls education on HIV and sexual behaviour. URL: http://www.actionaid.org.uk/doc_lib/girl_power_2006.pdf.

[4] WHO, UNAIDS, UNICEF global HIV/AIDS response. Epidemic update and health sector progress towards universal access progress report 2011. URL: http://apps.who.int/iris/bitstream/10665/44787/1/9789241502986_eng.pdf?ua=1.

[5] Batchelor WF. AIDS: A public health and psychological emergency. Am Psychol 1984;39 (11): 1279-84.

[6] Irwin KL, Valdiserri RO, Holmberg SD. The acceptability of voluntary HIV antibody testing in the United States: a decade of lessons learned. AIDS (London, England) 1996;10(14):1707–17.

[7] HATAM Hacettepe University HIV/AIDS Treatment and Research Center. URL: http://www.hatam.hacettepe.edu.tr/veriler_Haziran_2013.pdf.

[8] Ergene T, Cok F, Tumer A, Ünal S. A controlled study of preventive effects of peer education and single session lectures on HIV/AIDS knowledge and attitudes among university students in Turkey. AIDS Educ Prev 2005;17(3).

[9] Reis N. Sexual and reproductive health needs of adolescent girls from conservative and low-income families in Erzurum, Turkey. Health 2011;3(6):370–7.

[10] Kaya I. Identity and space: The case of Turkish Americans. Geographical Rev 2010;95(3):425–40.

[11] Abd-Allah UF. Turks, Moors and Moriscos in early America: Sir Francis Drake's liberated galley slaves and the lost colony of Roanoke. Burr Ridge, IL: Nawawi Foundation, 2010:1-43.

[12] Assaker R. Census takes aim to tally 'hard to count' populations. The Washington Diplomat 2012. URL: http://www.washdiplomat.com/index.php?option=com_content&view=article&id=6036:census-takes-aim-to-tallyhard-to-count-populations-&catid=205:april-2010&Itemid=239.

[13] Kalichman SC. HIV testing attitudes, AIDS stigma, and voluntary HIV counselling and testing in a black township in Cape Town, South Africa. Sex Transm Infect 2003;79(6):442–47.

[14] Simoni JM, Pantalone DW. Secrets and safety in the age of AIDS: does HIV disclosure lead to safer sex? Top HIV Med 2004;12(4):109–18.

[15] Fisher JD, Misovich SJ, Kimble DL, Weinstein B. Dynamics of HIV risk behavior in HIV-infected injection drug users. AIDS Behav 1999;3(1): 41–57.

[16] Gonzalez A. The education and wages of immigrant children: the impact of age at arrival. Econ Educ Rev 2003;22(2):203–12.

[17] Kuo BCH, Roysircar G. Predictors of acculturation for Chinese adolescents in Canada: Age of arrival, length of stay, social class, and English reading ability. J Multicultural Couns Dev 2004;32(3):143–54.

[18] Aycicegi-Dinn A, Caldwell-Harris CL. Individualism–collectivism among Americans, Turks and Turkish immigrants to the US. Int J Intercultural Relat 2011;35(1): 9–16.

[19] Heath A, Kilpi-Jakonen E. Immigrant children's age at arrival and assessment results. Paris: OECD, 2012.

[20] Cok F, Ann Gray L, Ersever H. Turkish university students' sexual behaviour, knowledge, attitudes and perceptions of risk related to HIV/AIDS. Culture Health Sex 2001;3(1):81–99.

[21] Ay, P. Is there a "hidden HIV/AIDS epidemic" in Turkey? The gap between the numbers and the facts. Marmara Medical Journal. URL: http://www.marmara medicaljournal.org/pdf/pdf_MMJ_391.pdf.

[22] Siegfried N, Muller M, Volmink J, Deeks J, Egger M, Low Williamson P. Male circumcision for prevention of heterosexual acquisition of HIV in men. Cochrane Database Syst Rev 2003;3: CD003362.

[23] Auvert B, Taljaard D, Lagarde E, Sobngwi-Tambekou J, Sitta R, Puren A. Correction: Randomized, controlled intervention trial of male circumcision for reduction of HIV infection risk: The ANRS 1265 Trial. PLoS Med 2006;3(5):e226.

[24] Bailey RC, Moses S, Parker CB, Agot K, Maclean I, Krieger JN, Ndinya-Achola JO. Male circumcision for HIV prevention in young men in Kisumu, Kenya: a randomised controlled trial. Lancet 2007;369(9562): 643–56.

Received: September 08, 2014. *Revised:* October 01, 2014. *Accepted:* October 09, 2014.

In: Public Health Yearbook 2015
Editor: Joav Merrick

ISBN: 978-1-63484-514-4
© 2016 Nova Science Publishers, Inc.

Chapter 36

SIGNIFICANCE OF RACE IN COLLEGE ATHLETICS: COMPARING MISSION STATEMENTS ACROSS RACIAL BOUNDARIES

Chase ML Smith, MA, Cecilia S Obeng, PhD, and Gary A Sales, PhD*

School of Public Health, Indiana University, Bloomington,
Indiana, United States of America

ABSTRACT

The majority of issues and controversies surrounding commercialism in college athletics today focus around the revenue generating sports of men's basketball and football at the division one level in the National Collegiate Athletic Association (NCAA). The intent behind comparing mission statements of predominately white institutions conferences and black colleges and universities conferences is to get a more in-depth idea of who they are, what they do, and where they are heading. Only 38.8% of the PWIs and conferences as a whole showed diversity to be a priority of 'who they are' through their mission statements. The results showed a clear distinction of HBCUs focusing more on the student-athlete, more on diversity without the need for business-type core values, and less on generating revenue. This arguably leads into research centered on the racial formation within the NCAA as a macro-level social process. Also, there is little attention paid to the health needs in the colleges' brochures and mission statements. It is anticipated that this study will draw attention to the above-stated lacuna and consequently generate interest in the health needs of college athlete.

Keywords: HBCU, PWI, mission statements, college athletics, grounded theory

---

* Correspondence: Cecilia S Obeng, PhD, Indiana University School of Public Health-Bloomington, 1025 E 7th Street, HPER 116, Bloomington, IN 47405 United States. E-mail: cobeng@indina.edu.

INTRODUCTION

The racial classifications used in the process of attaching a meaning to a group of individuals producing group identity can be viewed as the determinants toward the "racial practices of opposition ("we" versus "them") at the economic, political, social, and ideological levels" (1). The United States has historically been a nation encompassed of various ethnic immigrant groups, with the white race establishing dominance in the nation's early history through slavery over phenotypically African individuals. The white hegemony and systemic discrimination of race has been a cornerstone within race relations in the U.S. deeming white Americans stereotypically 'true' Americans and black Americans as inferior (2). According to dominant racial theory, society is able to identify groups and individuals in racial terms to place them in categories (3). Essentially, the white identity has sat atop the racial hierarchy throughout time in the United States and, in turn, its development and growth can be linked to the structure of slavery implemented prior to the civil war (2, 4). Prior to the 1954s Brown v. Board of Education decision that ruled racially segregated schools unconstitutional, black college students in the U.S. attended historically black colleges and universities (HBCU) for their academics and athletics. Nevertheless, as much as the upper-class, white decision makers in predominately white institutions (PWI) were reluctant to embrace the idea of black students attending their universities, they were equally open to the idea of recruiting black athletes to compete on their athletic teams to improve the already commercialized collegiate athletics (2, 5).

Issues and controversies

Money is generated within the National Collegiate Athletic Association (NCAA) from the men's basketball tournament commonly known as March Madness. In 2010, the NCAA agreed to a 14 year $10.8 billion dollar broadcasting agreement to cover the men's basketball tournament consisting of 68 teams playing for a national championship (6, 7). The Bowl Championship Series (BCS), separate from the NCAA, reportedly held a four year deal between the years 2011 and 2014 worth $125 million dollars per year to structure a playoff system for football (8, 9). After existing for 16 years, the BCS shifted to the College Football Playoff (CFP), separate from the NCAA, adding a final four aspect to the college football scene similar to the way the men's basketball playoff champion is decided. The new system still includes contracts with the five high-major conferences similar to the BCS system (ACC, SEC, Big Ten, Big 12, PAC12) with another spot being awarded to one of the mid-major conferences' (American, Mountain West, Mid-American, Sun Belt and Conference USA) highest-ranking team (10). The salaries for college football coaches range from Nick Saben for the University of Alabama at the top of the list receiving a total compensation in 2013 of just over $5.54 million, and Steve Sarkisian for the University of Washington as the #25 highest paid coach in college football receiving just over $2.57 million in total compensation in 2013 (11). The salaries for college basketball coaches in the 2013 men's basketball tournament ranged from Mike Krzyzewski for Duke University at the top of the list receiving a total pay for the 2013-14 season of just over $9.68 million, to Sean Miller for the University of Arizona as the #10 highest paid coach in college basketball receiving just over $2.62

million, and finally to Gregg Marshall for Wichita State University as the #25 highest paid coach receiving just over $1.79 million in total pay (12). The top earning athletic directors of institutions within the NCAA receive salaries of just over $3.23 million, $1.41 million, and $1.23 million for David Williams for Vanderbilt University, Tom Jurich for the University of Louisville, and Jeremy Foley for the University of Florida respectively (13).

The significance of race comes into question when addressing the 2012 Racial and Gender Report Card within college sports reported by The Institute for Diversity and Ethics in Sport. Out of the 120 football bowl subdivision (FBS) PWIs in the NCAA that are eligible to play in a bowl, 108 of the presidents within those PWI were white, while only five were black. From an athletic department focus, out of the 120 institutions, only 15 athletic directors were persons of color and 15 of the head football coaches were African-American (14). Further statistics from the report card show that 100% of the 11 FBS conferences which house these PWI have white men as their commissioners. When including all of the Division-1 Conferences within the NCAA, excluding conferences containing HBCU, records show that 29 of the 30 conference commissioners were white. The football student-athlete (SA) demographics on the 2012 report card at the FBS institutions revealed that 51.6% were African-American and 43.3% were white. Across the entire NCAA the demographic distribution was 46.4% white and 43.2% African-American (14 p4). The numbers for Division-1 men's and women's basketball showed a majority by the African-Americans accounting for 57.2% and 47.9% of the student athletes respectively (14). The aim of this investigation is to determine the significance race has on the disposition of a collegiate athletic conference's mission statement.

Defining race in college athletics

Confusion is prevalent in settings of discussion when terms within race and ethnicity are not defined or explained. This study will take the explanations and definitions given by Jay Coakley (15) to define race, ethnicity, ethnic population, and minority. They are as follows:

> Race refers to a population of people who are believed to be naturally or biologically distinct from other populations… Ethnicity is different from race in that it refers to a cultural heritage that people use to identify a particular population… ethnic population is a category of people regarded as socially distinct because they share a way of life, a collective history, and a sense of themselves as a people… minority is a socially identified population that suffers disadvantages due to systemic discrimination and has a strong sense of social togetherness based on shared experiences of past and current discrimination (15).

The definitions above are not meant to ignore the complexity and debate that surrounds the definition of race. Omi and Winant (3) feel energies must be made to understand race in a way that explains the constant unbalanced compound of social implications being distorted by political struggle. With this train of thought, their definition of race becomes "a concept which signifies and symbolizes social conflicts and interests by referring to different types of human bodies" (3).

While racial ideology seems to be so deeply rooted in the US culture that it is commonly mistaken as a fact of nature (15), the concept of race is not biologically practical (3, 15). The nature of this investigation centers on the acknowledgement that the 'African-American' race and ethnic group throughout history have been assigned meanings due to their skin color and existence of a shared culture within HBCU (15).

Racial identities within college sport

The labeling of groups often clouds the realization that ethnicity and race are not only forced, but according to Cornell and Hartmann (16) "they are also identities that people accept, resist, choose, specify, invent, redefine, reject, actively defend, and so forth" (16). A racial or ethnic identity may be assigned by the dominant group, or asserted by the group itself. It may then have the characteristics of being thick if the identity dominates the social organization and daily life of the individuals and group, or it is thin if it just serves symbolically without much influence on everyday life (16). Within college athletics, the media have had an influence in highlighting the negative aspects of black SAs since their "great migration" into PWI. Consequently, black SAs have received labels and discrimination surrounding these aspects of low graduation rates and retention even though they are highly recruited for their athletic prowess (17). In turn, the experiences of black students and black SAs have been filled with feelings of alienation, racial and social isolation, and racism due to the choice or necessity in asserting their racial identity on campus (2). Institutions that are successful in generating revenue have gone as far as to separate SA living quarters from the rest of the student body so that SA can bond. These actions can further isolate the black SAs causing them to gravitate toward their likeness in terms of race and/or ethnicity (17). Arguably this situation is evidence of racism with the white decision-makers raising their social position by controlling and exploiting these black SAs who have been categorized racially or ethnically on campus (1).

The interest of black athletes in basketball and football to attend a HBCU over a PWI has decreased over the last 40 years due to the amount of television exposure and state of the art facilities athletes receive at PWI (18). It is this attractiveness that gives support for college sports moving even more toward the business model and commercialism. It has generated an intangible product, brand development and recognition, and overall it is raw entertainment bringing in high revenues that accurately labeling college sports as a commercial enterprise (6) much like other business organizations in the United States.

Mission statements

The mechanics of a mission statement for organizations is to use as a communication tool (19) to state who they are and what they do (20, 21). In addition to these two things, it may also signify where the firm plans on heading to next along with their priorities, values, and beliefs that set it apart from other entities (20). In a content and textual analyses investigation on Fortune 1000 companies ranked 1 to 25 and 975 to 1000, Williams (20) found the "higher-performing firms mentioned respect, leadership, diversity, citizenship, and responsibility somewhat more often, and they included teamwork and safety to an even greater degree" (p.113). Furthermore, the objectives mentioned nearly the same in the mission statement of both groups were excellence, integrity, and innovation.

Previous research into mission statements in higher education has revealed that institutions may use them for the purpose of distinguishing the institution's laws and rules. Also, the statements purpose can serve as inspirational or motivational in addition to relaying the institution's position on its values, characteristics, and historical significance (22). Morphew and Hartley (22) investigated the elements of higher education institutions' mission statements by examining the organizational differences, communications within constituents, and if mission statements are used as legitimating tools. They reported significant findings in institutional control, a commitment to diversity, and the idea of 'service' to the students (p462).

Aims

Much of the existing literature revolving around the commercialism of college athletics deals with the SA experience and the controversies involved in the contradiction that the SA are actually athlete-students.. Furthermore, college athletic institutions operate under the belief that these SA are amateur athletes leaving the questions about the SA actually working as an employee under the business model of athletic departments (6). The intent behind comparing mission statements of PWI conferences and HBCU conferences is to get a more in-depth idea of who they are, what they do, and where they are heading (20).

METHODS

Grounded theory was selected as the design for this investigation to better understand the characteristics surrounding college athletic department mission statements since little has been reported on the topic. Grounded Theory has been defined by (23) as a qualitative research design that: "examines a phenomenon as related to theory" (p24). This method is ideal for extracting the intentions and meanings from the data (24, 25, 26). The act of asking theoretical questions with thinking comparatively opens the investigator's mind to a plethora of possibilities giving investigations the ability to show sameness and variation in categories giving relevance to application (25, 26). Grounded Theory also gives the investigator the ability to avoid standard ways of thinking about phenomena, discover properties and dimensions of categories, and force the asking of questions without the giving of provisional answers (26 p. 89). This investigation is the first step to examining the larger questions behind the structure of the NCAA, and its conferences' and institutions' mission statements. The purpose is to develop a theory from existing data that offers an explanation by using constant comparison (27). Strauss and Corbin (26) describe this type of analysis as a precursor to theorizing with the intent of collecting data to reach theoretical saturation.

Data collection

Purposeful sampling was used to collect the data for the eight conferences and 103 institutions in the NCAA. The athletic conference mission statements with HBCUs as the majority of members under analysis were the four left existing today: Central Intercollegiate Athletic Association (formally known as Colored Intercollegiate Athletic Association) (CIAA), Southern Intercollegiate Athletic Conference (SIAC), Southwestern Athletic Conference (SWAC), and the Mid-Eastern Athletic Conference (MEAC). In addition to the 39 HBCU athletic institutions with a mission statement, all four of the HBCU athletic conferences contained a conference mission statement that was also included in the investigation. The athletic conference mission statements with predominately white institutions as members under analysis were the top four revenue generating conferences according to Forbes (28) in ranking order: Big Ten (B10), Pacific 12 (PAC12), Atlantic Coast Conference (ACC), and the Southeastern Conference (SEC).

The CIAA today has 12 membered institutions. Out of the 12 members, 10 of the athletic departments contain a mission statement. The SIAC today has 14 membered institutions. Out of the 14 members, 12 of the athletic departments contain a mission statement. One of the 12 members, Central State University, is a member in the conference only for the sport of football. Due to the significance of the study aimed around the revenue-generating sports of men's basketball and football, their mission statement was included in the results. The SWAC contains 10 members in its conference, and seven of the athletic departments contain a mission statement. Nine of the 13 schools in the MEAC had an athletic mission statement. The Big Ten has 12 members in the conference, and 10 of those institutions were found to have a mission statement available. The PAC12 has 12 members in the conference, and 11 of those institutions were found to have a mission statement available. The ACC had 14 of its 15 members provide an athletic mission statement. It should be noted that the University of Notre Dame was included in this investigation since they are members of the ACC in every sport besides football, and have a considerably high historical significance in the realm of college football (29). The SEC has 14 athletic institutions in its conference, and 11 had mission statements available for investigation. In addition to the 46 PWI athletic institutions with a mission statement, a total of three of the four PWI athletic conference's contain a conference mission statement that were also included in the investigation.

Access to the athletic conferences' mission statements was mainly obtained from their official websites. From there, the institutions' official athletic department websites within each conference were found on the conference's official website accordingly. The mission statement for each institution for PWIs and HBCUs on the institution's official website were mainly under the tab 'inside athletics.' Mission statements not found under a palpable link within the official website were searched out on a general search engine using appropriate terminology. Once all online resources were exhausted, a phone call was made to an administrator (Athletic Directors, Assistant or Associate Athletic Directors, Director of Compliance, Senior Woman Administrator, Sports Information Director, Human Resources, etc...) within the athletic department to find out if a mission statement for the athletic department or conference existed, and if a request could be granted via email. It is worth noting that 81 of the 85 athletic departments in the sample contained official websites separate from the higher education institution of affiliation. Alcorn State University, Mississippi Valley State University, LeMoyne-Owen College, and Morehouse College had official athletic department websites within the construction of their institution's educational website.

The nature of the mission statements was textual in single paragraph form and of concise objectives. Some athletic departments chose to elaborate and lengthen the statement with additional paragraphs of objectives. Other athletic departments chose to complement the mission statement with a set of core values to further support the mission of the athletic department. The common objectives mentioned in the mission statement of both HBCU and PWI groups were competitive excellence and integrity. This aids in the development of the two research questions used in this investigation:

- RQ1: What are the characteristics in the mission statements for NCAA institutions in predominately white athletic conferences?
- RQ2: What are the characteristics in the mission statements for NCAA institutions in historically black athletic conferences?

Data analysis

The investigators used an open coding approach to implement the initial analytic process of categorizing the properties and dimensions discovered in the data (25, 26). A range of potential meanings were found within the mission statements to discover categories along with links to subcategories giving justification for the axial coding (26, 30). "Axial is appropriate for studies employing grounded theory methodology,…Grouping similarly coded data reduces the number of Initial Codes you developed while sorting and re-labeling them into conceptual categories" (30). The data were then transcribed using selective coding to ultimately come to a degree of understanding (26, 31). The five themes derived from the selective coding were; 1) student-athlete focus; 2) institutional control; 3) diversity directive; and 4) brand focus. Properties-also known as characteristics of a category-were recognized for each of these categories to give the investigator the ability to compare and contrast the characteristics in the mission statements to find the four themes listed above (31). Once a category or feature was found to be within the data of a conference or institution's overall mission, it was simply recorded as existing to avoid monotony and redundancy in the results of the investigation.

RESULTS

The properties and dimensions of the mission statements investigated within the NCAA conferences and institutions provided a clearer understanding in the purpose for athletic departments in higher education institutions. The terminology for labeling the mission statements at times varied throughout the process. Instead of the term mission, other labeling was recognized accompanying the term statement to substitute while still giving the impression of a mission, vision, philosophy, or statement of purpose (20). Additionally, one conference and 41 of the athletic departments contained a set of core values to complement their mission statement. While these core values also serve a purpose to relay who the institution is and what they stand for (20), a separate count was tallied for themes contained in the mission statement alone without contributing core values. The terminology for labeling the core values feature included with the mission statements varied and included the terms; principles, goals, objectives, priorities, or criteria for excellence. Additionally, if a distinct segment's format within the page was displayed in an arrangement of being isolated from the mission statement itself, along with a collection of single-word or phrased ethos, then the segment was considered as a core value. The core values showed characteristics and dimensions congruent with the mission statements giving further validity for the four themes created in the investigation.

Student-athlete focus

The higher educational system operates with the initiative to educate its students. At the core of the SA focused theme is the idea consistent with the overall well-being of the SA.

Table 1. Student-Athlete Focus Properties as a Percentage of the Sample

Conference	Development	Learning	Commencement
HBCU			
CIAA	63.6	81.8	27.3
MEAC	80.0	70.0	60.0
SIAC	71.4	78.6	57.1
SWAC	75.0	87.5	75.0
PWI			
ACC	60.0	66.7	53.3
Big10	63.6	63.6	36.4
Pac12	81.8	54.5	36.4
SEC	58.3	33.3	50.0

* Percentages do not include Core Values.

This is supported by the properties of the athletic department striving to improve the personal development of the SA, to adopting the role of a higher education entity, and creating an emphasis with the athletic department aiding their SAs toward graduating. See Table 1 the percentages of HBCU and PWI institutions that included evidence of a student-athlete focus within their mission statement without taking into consideration core values.

The MEAC and the PAC12 showed considerable focus within the personal development of the SAs. All four HBCUs showed evidence of a focus on supplementing the institution's mission for higher learning, and the SWAC put forth a purpose to aid their SAs all the way to graduation.

Serving personal development

A student-athlete focus from an athletic department must be solely directed toward the SA's well-being. This is represented by any statement within the overall mission statement that shows direct intentions by the athletic department toward the SA's experience being bettered without any mention of gains or control by the athletic department or institution within the context of the message. The University of Arizona, a PWI, states "the individual rights, welfare and academic goals of the student athlete should not be compromised by the

University's desire to conduct successful athletic programs." The contradicting dimensions representing gains can be expressed through the words success, excellence, championships, and/or core values. These dimensions are considered to be contradictory to the overall focus on the SA due to the absolute bias the athletic department is declaring in the meanings behind how it defines success, excellence, and core values. The dimension of championships being encouraged shows a focus toward athletics and away from education. Examples of acceptable phrases to support a focus for personal development within a SA are as follows: proper balance between academics and athletics in SA life, dedicated to the development and, interests of our students. Fort Valley State University, a HBCU, contained an understanding for the personal development of the SA by stating:

> We seek to provide diversified and challenging programs to meet educational needs resulting from societal changes and to provide learning and living environments that enable our graduates to become innovative and critical thinkers, problem solvers, and responsible citizens."

Supplement to education

An athletic department's desire to enhance the overall educational experience of the SA shows a strong focus to the teaching the SA, and the learning experience that is received by the SA. Supplementing the existing educational setting is the mentioning of academics or education with direct intentions for the SA's experience being bettered academically absent any focus for gains by the athletic department through success, excellence, championships, or core values. In addition, there is an expressive intent to advance the educational setting of the university. The contradicting dimensions representing control by the athletic department can be represented with the words integrity, sportsmanship, and compliance. For example, a PWI that is the University of Mississippi's athletic "department will prepare SAs to be productive members of society by assisting in their development of academic, athletic, social, and leadership skills within an environment which fosters integrity, sportsmanship, and emotional, physical, and mental well-being." Clear distinctions of a focus by the department to oversee the SAs' development of integrity and sportsmanship represent a property of institutional control influenced by the rules and bylaws of the NCAA, conference, and institution. Examples of acceptable phrases to support the focus for the SA are as follows: dedicated to teaching, research, and service, challenging and/or inspiring SAs, and conduct a service for sovereignty. North Carolina Central University, a HBCU, has a strong mission toward enhancing the educational initiative as well as the physical, mental and social health or well-being by placing:

> The highest priority on the quality academic and athletic experience as part of the overall education of student-athletes. We affirm academic excellence as the cornerstone to the mission of the institution; as well as the physical, mental and social well-being of those admitted. In so doing, we seek to strengthen the integration of the athletic program objectives with academic development objectives. We seek to promote the personal and social development of our student-athletes, coaches and all others associated with the NCCU athletics programs.

Commitment to commencement

The aspects of development for graduating SAs included success such as in Boston College's affirmation regarding "the personal formation and development of students, preparing them for citizenship, service, and leadership." In addition, other mission statements showed a purpose to "lead to the development of a well-rounded, more enlightened individual," "produce young men and women able to become constructive contributing members of society," and "promote the matriculation and retention of students." It is worth noting that four HBCUs included the term multicultural society as the setting transitioned from the university to the workplace for students' post-graduation life.

Overall, the investigations within the mission statements of institutions and conferences considered to be HBCUs, showed more focus on the SA specifically without any other intentions behind servicing their experiences during college. The percentages shown in table 2 provide a clear discrepancy between HBCUs and PWIs toward a student-athlete focus within their mission statements when core values are not taken into consideration.

Table 2. Student-Athlete Focus Properties as a Percentage of the Institution Type

Type	Development	Learning	Commencement
HBCU	72.1	79.1	53.5
PWI	65.3	55.1	44.9

*Percentages do not include Core Values.

Institutional control

The structure of the NCAA is one that requires the membered institutions to operate with institutional control to maintain the amateur status of the SAs that represent their institution's athletic teams (6). Through the property of compliance to the NCAA's rules and by-laws, conferences and institutions strive to implement institutional control. Additionally, the accumulation of other dimensions contributing to institutional control exists within the properties of excellence and success through academic and athletic gains. The most frequently used term to represent institutional control was integrity. This was due to the nature of the dimension carrying the mission to be fair and honest, and signifying the adherence to NCAA rules through the mission statement.

Academic success

The property of academic excellence and success expressed in the athletic mission statements voiced an intent different than the learning property within the SA focus expressed in the missions of athletic departments showing an effort to leverage onto the existing university missions and principles. Athletic departments have required academic standards within the NCAA bylaws in the form of the academic progress rate (APR). The implementation of the APR is the product of NCAA efforts to improve retention and graduation rates for SA (32). The criteria for this property includes the term academics accompanied with subjective terms of achievement such as success, excellence, highest standards, and/or integrity. Benedict College's athletic mission statement states "the administration and staff of the Athletic Department espouses a student-centered philosophy, which ranks academic achievement as the number one priority for its athletes." When comparing the institutions within HBCUs and PWIs, the focus on academic success deemed within the standards of the athletic department are 69.8% and 67.3% respectively. It is worth noting that 80% of the MEAC's institutions and their conference mission statements included a property of academic success, and 81.8% of the PAC12's institutions also contained the property contributing to institutional control. The percentages calculated were all absent core values.

Athletic success

The stance an athletic department may take when the controversy of the terms student-athlete versus athlete-student are being considered to label the individuals that participate in competitive collegiate athletics is one to maximize human potential in the pursuit of comprehensive excellence. This stance combines both athletic and academic excellence as properties for institutional control. However, the primary purpose surrounding collegiate athletics is the ability to compete, and compete to win. The property of athletic success can be expressed by any mention of athletics as a priority, a focus on excellence, sportsmanship, winning championships, or overall competition. Athletic departments operating under the structures implemented by the NCAA are subjected to the influences from post-season competition that decides a winner and a loser. This type of property tends to show priority within the athletic department of athletics over the overall experience included in higher education, thus controlling the experiences of its student-athletes. The institutions and conferences within PWIs showed 83.7% of the mission statements to have a strong academic success focus even without including the core value numbers.

Compliance

Investigating the property of compliance within the NCAA, athletic conferences, and its member institutions is a multi-faceted task. While the Georgia Institute of Technology, a PWI, feels "the integrity of our mission is enhanced by our commitment to adherence to the rules of the Institute, the Atlantic Coast Conference and the National Collegiate Athletic Association," it is the basis for the idea of institutional control to rely on the institutions within the NCAA to operate with integrity in adherence to the rules and bylaws that make up the NCAA constitution. Compliance contains dimensions including the overall essence of abiding by the rules and displaying integrity while participating in amateur athletics with the assumption that conferences, institutions, and SAs will do what is right in the eyes of the NCAA. The University of California, a PWI, is "committed to incorporating our mission, vision and values into the culture of our department in order to achieve our goals." The commitment to compliance and integrity within HBCU mission statements without core values was greater than PWIs by a 69.8% to 53.3% margin.

Diversity directive

The theme of diversity directive did not contain any properties. The selective coding was supported by any evidence of showing focus in the mission statement toward bringing an awareness of gender and minority equalities. Some of the identifying phrases were represented with equitable treatment or opportunities for all, pledges to be steadfast in the encouragement of cultural, supporting ethnic and gender diversity, attention to diverse backgrounds, promoting diversity, and equal access for all. Some institutions included measures of diversity in their mission statement (Mississippi State University, Southern University, Bethune-Cookman University, and North Carolina Agricultural and Technical State University). Washington State University, a PWI, emphasized an awareness for diversity in their mission statement, "The Athletics Department values diversity, including gender and ethnicity, and is committed to providing equitable opportunities for all students and staff." The following tables represent the recorded themes of diversity showing their occurrence in conference and athletic department missions within the NCAA.

Brand focus

Athletic institutions in the NCAA have been known to operate within the business model of commercialism (6). Within this model is the acknowledgement of an existing brand to preserve and prosper within an organization's mission. The properties within the themed brand focus were devotions to generating revenue, portraying an image, and service to the community.

Table 3. Diversity Directive Theme as a Percentage of the Sample

Conference	Core Values With	Core Values Without
HBCU		
CIAA	63.6%	45.5%
MEAC	50.0%	50.0%
SIAC	42.9%	35.7%
SWAC	50.0%	50.0%
PWI		
ACC	60.0%	40.0%
Big10	54.5%	18.2%
Pac12	81.8%	54.5%
SEC	58.3%	41.7%

Table 4. Diversity Directive Theme as a Percentage of the Institution Type

Conference	Core Values With	Core Values Without
HBCU	51.2%	44.2%
PWI	63.3%	38.8%

Table 5. Generating Revenue Properties as a Percentage of the Institution Type

Conference	Core Values	
	With	Without
HBCU	18.6%	14.0%
PWI	49.0%	26.5%

Devotions to generating revenue

The mission statements for a number of the PWIs in the SEC showed a purpose for generating revenue. Two-thirds of the PWIs within the SEC that contained mission statements or a core values section included a fiscal responsibility within the athletic department. Other identifying dimensions to the property of devoting a purpose to generating revenue included mentioning a championship experience, elevating the brand, providing direct financial support, impressing alumni, and Benedict College, a HBCU expresses efforts to "contributing significantly to the successful marketing of the college." The focus of the PWIs compared to the HBCUs proves worthy of mentioning, especially when taking into consideration the core values of PWIs. Table 5 illustrates this comparison.

Portraying an image

The concerns and efforts for portraying a positive, respectable image was consistent between the two institutional types. The majority of HBCU athletic mission statements contained the initiative for a strong public image. Without the use of core values, which specifically focuses on image with terms of ethos, 62.8% of all the HBCU mission statements focused on image. If the data with core values is included, the total percentage increases to 72.1%. PWIs seemed to rely heavily on the core value supplement to their statement. Without the core values, only 46.9% of the PWIs contained an image property for focusing on their brand. When the core values were identified, the number of PWIs containing an image property increased to 65.3%. The core values of passion, integrity, excellence, respect, innovation, teamwork, personal development, leadership, and accountability are all terms used to provide a positive brand image. In addition, there were efforts of supporting the property of image through the themed brand focus in the following phrases: a model university, promotion of core values, reflecting the interests of more than one entity (students, faculty, conference, NCAA, and community), recruiting SAs with expectations of excellence, professionalism, success, integrity, and becoming positive contributors to society. The University of Nebraska's athletic department, a PWI, went as far as to extend their image to everyone involved with the program by "Maintaining LOYALTY to student-athletes, co-workers, fans and the University." Albany State University, a HBCU, showed multiple purposes behind their statement:

> The Department strives to recruit, enroll and retain academically sound student-athletes who are capable of academic success and who have the desire and motivation to graduate and to become responsible citizens that positively contribute to society.

Service to the community

The property supporting this theme touches on the public relations of the athletic department and the institution as a whole. The dimensions of selflessness in identifying a service to the community involved direct intentions by the athletic department to the community being bettered absent any focus for gains by the athletic department or institution through success, excellence, championships, or core values. Exempting phrases include success through community involvement and promote community involvement of our student-athletes, coaches and staff as necessary for our program's success. These two examples give reason to believe there are alternative motives to the service to the community. The University of Southern California displayed a very selfless dimension to the property of service to the community by stating, "The principal means by which that mission (statement) is accomplished consists of teaching, research, artistic creation, professional practice and selected forms of public service." Even with the inclusion of core values, only 37.2% of HBCU athletic institutions and 40.8% of PWI's athletic departments contained a service to the community property within their Brand's Focus.

DISCUSSION

The components of critical race theory (CRT) applied to the institutionalization of college athletics' supports the stereotypes of African-American athletes as poverty stricken individuals being exploited on the premise of their athletic abilities by the National Collegiate Athletic Association (NCAA) and its membered PWI through commercialism (2, 17, 33). The significant percentages within the results without the presence of core values surrounding the promotion and focus on diversity within the mission statements for PWIs seems to support the institutionalization of college athletics' exploiting African-American athletes. Just 18.2% of the B10 conference and institutions' mission statements within the results supplied a voice for diversity, and only 38.8% of the PWIs and conferences as a whole showed diversity to be a priority of 'who they are' through their mission statements (20, 21). This intent by PWI seems inconsistent with the heavy focus on revenue-generating sports of men's basketball and football considering the participation of the African-American athlete is dominant for both sports (14). The unrecognized statistic of the low HBCU percentages for a diversity directive within their mission statements and core values is due to the idea that "Black institutional racism" or "reverse institutional racism" does not exist (34, 35). This stems from the history of White supremacy in American society and sport with perceived or real absence of any occurrences of people of color having the same privileges, rights, and seats off power within society.

Limitations

The concept of institutional isomorphism must be considered for the entire sample due to the association every conference and institution has being members of the NCAA. DiMaggio and Powell (36) concluded that "the greater the dependence of an organization on another organization, the more similar it will become to that organization in structure, climate, and behavioral focus" (36). The concept behind the need for institutional control within the NCAA as a whole gives a reciprocal dependency between the association and the conferences and institutions. This position of dependency has the ability to influence the missions throughout the entire association. Continued limitations within institutional isomorphism is that "the more uncertain the relationship between means and ends the greater the extent to which an organization will model itself after organizations it perceives to be successful" (36). It can be argued that the PWIs are deemed success due to the large amount of revenue generated leaving reason to believe the HBCUs will model their mission after these prospering institutions. This essentially limits the fields of creativity and innovation within the mission of HBCUs or other PWIs who were deemed not successful enough in terms of generating revenue, and were excluded from the purposeful sample.

Conclusion and future research

The majority of issues and controversies surrounding commercialism in college athletics today focus around the revenue generating sports of men's basketball and football at the division one level in the NCAA. The higher education institutions with athletics in this group run their operations like a business. Coakley (15) feels "all amateur sport organizations share an interest in two things: 1) Controlling the athletes in their sports and 2) Controlling the money generated from sponsorships and competitive events" (15). The percentages within the results centered on the generating revenue property of the brand focus show nearly half of the PWIs display purpose behind operating a business with the NCAA influencing big-business core values. Omi and Winant (3) might argue for future research due to the percentages in tables 2, 4, and 5 showing a clear distinction of HBCUs focusing more on the student-athlete, more on diversity without the need for business-type core values, and less on generating revenue. These results show encouragement for research centered on the racial formation as a macro-level social process. There seems to be evidence in the percentages supporting a political spectrum within the NCAA that includes radical projects. Analysis of racial projects may be able to take place not only at the NCAA level for policy-making, conference level, and institutional level, but also at the core of student-life for minorities at PWIs and HBCUs alike (3). While it is argued within this piece that "Black institutional racism" or "reverse institutional racism" does not exist, there still remains a possibility for investigations in HBCUs encompassing interpersonal racism since it "takes place on the ground level and has to do with attitudes and habitual actions" (34).

In sum, it goes without saying that college athletics, besides revenue generation and emphasis on specific academic and social values, does impact the social, mental and emotional health of the student athletes. There is however, little attention paid to the above-mentioned facets of health in the colleges' brochures and mission statements. Furthermore, there is a dearth of scholarship on the interconnectedness between colleges' mission statements and the actual effort made at ensuring that their clientele, the student athletes, stay healthy to help them achieve the objectives stated in their mission statements. It is anticipated that this study will draw attention to the above-stated lacuna and consequently generate interest in the health needs of college athletes with the view to ensuring that colleges document these in their mission statements and follow through with assisting student athletes.

REFERENCES

[1] Bonilla-Silva E. Rethinking racism: Toward a structural interpretation. Am Sociol Rev 1997;62(3):465-80.
[2] Francique A, Singer J. Representation, participation, and the experiences of racial minorities in college sport. In: Sailes G, ed. Sports in higher education: Issues and controversies in college athletics, 1st ed. San Diego, CA: Cognella, 2013:111-36.
[3] Omi M, Winant H. Racial formation in the United States, 1st ed. New York: Routledge; 1994.
[4] Harris CI. Whiteness as property. Harvard Law Rev 1993;106(8):1707-91.
[5] Sage G. Introduction. In: Brooks D, Althouse R, eds. Diversity and social justice in college sports: Sport management and the student-athlete, 1st ed. Morgantown, WV: Fitness Information Technology, 2007:1-17.
[6] Gilde C, Malec M, Sailes G. Commercialism in college sports. In: Sailes G, ed. Sports in higher education: Issues and controversies in college athletics, 1st ed. San Diego, CA: Cognella, 2007:53-85.
[7] NCAA.com. CBS Sports, Turner Broadcasting, NCAA reach 14-Year agreement, URL: http://www.ncaa.com/news/basketball-men/2010-04-21/cbs-sports-turner-broadcasting-ncaa-reach-14-year-agreement.
[8] Staurowsky E, Abney R. Intercollegiate athletics. In: Pedersen P, Parks J, Quarterman J, Thibault L, eds. Contemporary sport management, 4th ed. Champaign, IL: Human Kinetics, 2011:142-63.
[9] Frommer F. Game-changing call to college football: Playoff. URL: http://abclocal.go.com/wpvi/story?section=news/sports&id=6791526.
[10] Barnhart T. Before BCS ends, the whens, wheres, whys of College Football Playoff. URL: http://www.cbssports.com/collegefootball/writer/tony-barnhart/24400200/before-bcs-ends-the-whens-wheres-and-whys-of-college-football-playoff.
[11] Gaines C. The 25 highest-paid coaches in college football. Business Insider, 2013. URL: http://www.businessinsider.com/the-25-highest-paid-coaches-in-college-football-2013-11?op=1.
[12] Berkowitz S, Upton J, Schnaars C, Dougherty S. USA Today 2014. URL: http://www.usatoday.com/sports/college/salaries/ncaab/coach/
[13] Berkowitz S, Upton J, Dougherty S, Durkin E. USA Today 2014. URL: http://www.usatoday.com/sports/college/salaries/all/director/.
[14] Lapchick R, Agusta R, Kinkopf N, McPhee F. The 2012 racial and gender report card: College Sport Orlando: TIDES 2013. URL: http://www.tidesport.org/RGRC/2012/2012_College_RGRC.pdf.
[15] Coakley J. Sports in society, 10th ed. New York: McGraw-Hill, 2009.
[16] Cornell S, Hartmann D. Ethnicity and race, 2nd ed. Thousand Oaks, CA: Pine Forge Press, 2007.
[17] Hawkins B. The new planation: The internal colonization of black student athletes, 1st ed. Winterville, GA: Sadiki Press; 2000.
[18] Despite great strides, HBCUs and NCAA recognized athletic conferences face challenges. Diverse 2013. URL: http://diverseeducation.com/article/50844/
[19] Bartkus B, Glassman M, Bruce McAfee R. Mission statements: are they smoke and mirrors? Business Horizons 2000;43(6):23-8.
[20] Williams L. The mission statement A corporate reporting tool with a past, present, and future. J Business Commun 2008;45(2):94-119.
[21] Falsey T. Corporate philosophies and mission statements, 1st ed. New York: Quorum Books, 1989.
[22] Morphew C, Hartley M. Mission statements: A thematic analysis of rhetoric across institutional type. J Higher Educ 2006;77(3):456-71.
[23] McMillan J, Schumacher S. Research in education, 7th ed. Upper Saddle River, NJ: Pearson, 2010.
[24] Dickson G, Flynn L. Nurses clinical reasoning processes and practices of medication safety. Qual Health Res 2012;22(1):3-16.
[25] Corbin J, Strauss A, Strauss A. Basics of qualitative research, 3rd ed. Los Angeles, CA: Sage, 2008.
[26] Strauss A, Corbin J. Basics of qualitative research, 2nd ed. Thousand Oaks, CA: Sage, 1998.
[27] Glaser B, Strauss A. The discovery of grounded theory, 1st ed. Chicago, IL: Aldine. 1967.

[28] CBSSports.com. Forbes: Big ten most valuable college conference. SEC fourth 2013. URL: http://www.cbssports.com/collegefootball/story/21563564/forbes-big-ten-most-valuable-college-conference-sec-fourth.

[29] Bruening J, MinYong L, others. The University of Notre Dame: an examination of the impact and evaluation of brand equity in NCAA Division IA football. Sport Marketing Quart 2007;16(1):38-48.

[30] Saldana J. The coding manual for qualitative researchers, 1st ed. London: Sage, 2009.

[31] Komives S, Owen J, Longerbeam S, Mainella F, Osteen L. Developing a leadership identity: A grounded theory. J Coll Stud Dev 2005;46(6):593-611.

[32] Hamilton K. Putting the "student" back into the student-athlete: In an effort to improve retention and graduation rates, the NCAA rolls out new rules and regulations. Black Issues Higher Educ 2005;22(4):28.

[33] Hawkins B. The new plantation: Black athletes, college sports, and predominately white NCAA institutions, 1st ed. New York: Palgrave Macmillian, 2010.

[34] Desmond M, Emirbayer M. What is racial domination? Du Bois Rev 2009;6(02):335-55.

[35] Valelly R. White-washing race: The myth of a color-blind society by Michael K Brown, Martin Carnoy, Elliot Currie, Troy Duster, David B Oppenheimer, and Marjorie M Shult. Political Sci Quart 2004;119(4):699-700.

[36] DiMaggio P, Powell W. The iron cage revisited: Institutional isomorphism and collective rationality in organizational fields. Am Sociol Rev 1983;48(2):147-60.

Received: September 09, 2014. *Revised:* October 02, 2014. *Accepted:* October 11, 2014

In: Public Health Yearbook 2015
Editor: Joav Merrick
ISBN: 978-1-63484-514-4
© 2016 Nova Science Publishers, Inc.

Chapter 37

ENCOURAGING ARAB WOMEN TO BEAT THE CANCER EPIDEMIC: AN INVESTIGATION INTO POSITIVE ATTRIBUTES THAT ENCOURAGE ARAB WOMEN TO PRACTICE PREVENTION METHODS FOR CANCER

*Sara A Suhaibani, MPH, and Cecilia S Obeng, PhD**

Department of Applied Health Science, School of Public Health,
Indiana University, Bloomington, Indiana, United States of America

ABSTRACT

Breast cancer in Arab countries tends to occur at younger age, with almost half under the age of 50 years. This study investigates 25 Arab women living in the United States and their knowledge about breast cancer prevention methods. Findings indicate that participants reported lack of knowledge on how to practice breast self-exam. Majority of participants indicated they never attended any community program on breast cancer prevention or go for mammogram examinations. Participants noted that knowing how to do breast exam and being reminded at the clinics would help them practice breast self-exam. Given that research indicates that breast self-exam and mammograms help save lives, it is recommended that health professionals and family members remind women, especially Arab women, about breast cancer prevention methods.

Keywords: breast cancer, Arab women, mammogram, breast self-exam

INTRODUCTION

Worldwide, cancer is a leading cause of death among men and women. In the year 2004, approximately 7.4 million deaths were from cancer alone. Amongst women, breast cancer is

---

* Correspondence: Cecilia S Obeng, PhD, Associate Professor, Indiana University, School of Public Health, 1025 E 7th Street, SPH 116, Bloomington, IN 47405, United States. E-mail: cobeng@indiana.edu.

one of the main types of cancer leading to "overall cancer mortality" (1, 2). In the United States, among women, breast cancer is the foremost diagnosis of new cancers and the second leading cause of death after lung cancer (3). An epidemiological surveillance indicates that during the year 2005, the age-adjusted mortality rates of breast cancer was 24.8 per 100,000 among U.S. female population (4). According to the World Health Organization, cancer is the fourth ranked cause of death in the Arab world after cardiovascular diseases, infectious/parasitic diseases, and injuries (5). In the next two decades, cancer is predicted to increase 100-180% in the Eastern Mediterranean Region (5). In the Arab world, including the Kingdom of Saudi Arabia, breast cancer is increasingly occurring among young pre-menopausal women as opposed to what happens in western countries, where breast cancer is common among women at menopausal age. More disturbingly, most cases of breast cancer in the Arab world are detected at advanced stages (1, 6, 7).

The published facts and statistics about breast cancer are indicators of a serious problem that needs to be addressed. The lack of knowledge and awareness about breast cancer, primary and secondary prevention, and how to detect breast cancer in its early stages are causing preventable fatalities among women in this part of the world.

WHY THIS TOPIC?

The topic of breast cancer is chosen due to the situation in the Arab world in general. Breast cancer is increasing tremendously in the Middle Eastern countries. Many young females are losing their lives due to being diagnosed with breast cancer in advanced stages (5). In the Kingdom of Saudi Arabia (KSA), women are diagnosed with breast cancer between the ages 20-50 years, reflecting a diagnostic that starts at younger age for that specific type of cancer. These facts are raising concerns about the lack of knowledge about breast cancer and attitudes regarding primary and secondary prevention, especially about breast self-exam and other early detections methods.

OVERVIEW OF BREAST CANCER

The American Cancer Society's most recent estimates for breast cancer in the United States indicate that the chance of a woman having invasive breast cancer some time during her life is a little less than 1 in 8. The chance of dying from breast cancer is about 1 in 35. In addition, during the year 2010, it was estimated that there was approximately 207,090 new cases of invasive breast cancer in women, about 54,010 new cases of non-invasive carcinoma, and around 39,840 deaths from breast cancer in the U.S. female population alone (3). Breast cancer is the most common cancer among women in the United States, other than skin cancer. It is the second leading cause of cancer death in women, after lung cancer (3). In the American population, breast cancer death rates have been going down as a result of increased awareness about breast cancer prevention and early detection, as well as the improvement of treatment techniques. Today, with primary and secondary prevention and the advancement in treatments methods, there are more than 2.5 million breast cancer survivors in the United States (3).

ON DEFINING BREAST CANCER

To help the reader understand the issue at hand, a short background on what constitutes breast cancer is presented. "Breast cancer is cancer that forms in the cells of the breasts" (10). The American Cancer Society defines breast cancer as a "malignant tumor that starts from cells of the breast." A malignant tumor is a "group of cancer cells that may grow into or invade surrounding tissues or spread to distant areas of the body" (3). According to the Mayo Clinic, breast cancer occurs among men and women, but mostly in women (10). Early menarche: women who started their period before age 12 years, late parity: women who had their first child after the age of 30 years, women with nulliparity

TYPES OF BREAST CANCER

According to the National Breast Cancer Foundation, "Breast cancer is categorized by whether it begins in the ducts or lobules, which are the organs responsible for breast milk production" (11). Types of breast cancer include:

Ductal carcinoma in-situ (DCIS)

This type of breast cancer is one of the earliest stages where the tumor is still in place and has not yet spread out. The tumor is found inside the ductal system (11).

Infiltrating ductal carcinoma (IDC)

IDC makes up 78% of breast cancer diagnoses in the United States, which makes it the most common type among other types of breast cancer (11). On the mammogram, IDC shows in one of two shapes: either star-like shape or rounded shape; the star-like shape is more aggressive (11).

Medullary carcinoma (MC)

MC represents 15% of all types of breast cancers and has a good prognosis. It is called medullary, because it looks like the gray matter of the brain, which is called the medulla (11)

Infiltrating lobular carcinoma (ILC)

Representing 5% of all diagnosis, ILC forms in the upper outer quadrant of the breast. ILC tumors give positive results when conducting estrogen and progesterone receptors tests and response well to hormone therapy (11).

Tubular carcinoma (TC)

TC appears like a tubular shape under the microscope. This type of breast cancer is common among women aged 50 and over. TC represents 2% of the diagnosis and has a good prognosis (11).

Mucinous carcinoma (Colloid)

This type of breast cancer makes up 1-2% of all breast cancers. Mucinous carcinoma is different from other types of breast cancer, because it sets off mucus production inside the breast (11).

Inflammatory breast cancer (IBC)

IBC is rare but invasive, it accounts for 1% to 5% of all breast cancer cases in the United States. IBC is called "inflammatory" because the breast is inflamed. The breast appears swollen and red because the cancer cells block the lymph vessels in the breast skin which lead to very aggressive consequences (11).

BREAST CANCER STAGES

According to the National Cancer Institute, "staging is the process of determining whether a cancer has spread within the breast or to other parts of the body" (12). According to the Mayo Clinic, "Breast cancer stages range from 0 to IV, with 0 indicating cancer that is very small and noninvasive. Stage IV breast cancer, also called metastatic breast cancer, indicates cancer that has spread to other areas of the body" (10). Each of the stages is briefly explicated below:

Stage 0

This is the first stage of cancer where the tumor is still in situ and non-invasive; for example, Ductal carcinoma in situ is a stage 0 type of cancer. The tumor is local (10).

Stage I

This is the first stage of an invasive breast cancer. In this early stage the tumor has certain characteristics in measures and location. The size of the tumor is 2 centimeters (3/4 inch) or less and the cancer has not spread to the lymph nodes or to other organs (10).

Stage II

This stage describes invasive breast cancer in which one of the following is true: the tumor measures less than 2 cm (3/4 inch), but has spread to the lymph nodes under the arm; or no tumor is found in the breast, but breast cancer cells are found in the lymph nodes under the arm, or if the size of tumor is between 2 and 5 cm (about 3/4 to 2 inches) and may or may not have spread to the lymph nodes under the arm, finally a stage II may show the T larger than 5 cm (2 inches) but has not spread to any lymph nodes (10).

Stage III

Stage III is an advanced stage of breast cancer where tumors start to invade surrounding tissues. This stage is subdivided into three categories IIIA, IIIB, and IIIC based on a number of criteria including: (size of the tumor, location of the tumor in surrounding tissues By definition, stage III cancer has extended to the immediate region but has not spread to distant sites (the tumor is regional) (10).

Stage IV

Stage IV is an advanced stage cancer and is considered to be invasive because the cancer has spread to other organs of the body (the tumor is distant) usually the lungs, liver, bone, or brain (10).

SYMPTOMS

According to the Centers for Disease Control and Prevention (CDC), when breast cancer formulates no visible signs and symptoms appear until the tumor grows. The symptoms start to be evident due to changes in how the breast looks or feels. These symptoms include: a new lump in the breast; lump that has changed; change in the size or shape of the breast; pain in the breast or nipple that does not go away; flaky, red, or swollen skin anywhere on the breast; and a nipple that is very tender or that suddenly turns inward" (13).

RISK FACTORS

Several factors may affect an individual's risk of developing breast cancer. These risk factors include unchangeable and modifiable risk factors. Unchangeable risk factors include: "gender, age, genetic risk factors, family history of breast cancer, personal history of breast cancer, race and ethnicity, dense breast tissue, previous chest radiation, starting first menstrual period at an early age, and beginning menopause at a late age" (3, 13). Modifiable risk factors, typically related to a person's lifestyle including: "Not having children, or having your first child later in life, and lack of breast feeding." In addition, lack of physical activity, being overweight "particularly after menopause," using hormone replacement therapy for a long time, and using oral contraceptives can increase risk factors of cause breast cancer (3, 13).

BREAST CANCER PREVENTION

Avoiding risk factors for breast cancer aids in the prevention of disease development. The National Cancer Institute recommends several steps to minimize the chances of developing breast cancer. One of the most important, precautious procedures is to become familiar with your breasts through breast self-exam.

Cancer prevention strategies include avoiding or limiting hormone therapy, especially after menopause, eating a healthy diet that is low in fat and high in fruits and vegetables, maintaining a healthy weight, and making physical activity part of the daily routine (12). In addition, other preventable practices to lower the chance of developing breast cancer are: avoiding smoking and avoiding exposure to environmental pollution, limiting alcohol intake, and avoiding the use of oral contraceptive pills. Moreover, becoming pregnant at early age and breast-feeding prevent the onset of breast cancer (12).

EARLY DETECTION AND DIAGNOSIS

Anderson et al. (3) define early detection as "the identification of breast cancer at a point in its natural history when it can be treated with techniques that have the least physical impact and the greatest chance of producing a cure" (14).

Early detection and screening for breast cancer help in finding a tumor, if it exists, well before any symptoms develop and in a stage where the cancer is controllable. Going through early detection tests and exams lead to early diagnosis, a situation that potentially increases the likelihood of a successful treatment and better prognosis. There are many instruments and tools used to detect breast cancer including:

Mammogram. This X-ray instrument is the most common screening method used for detecting breast cancer. It is recommended for women to do their mammogram yearly, as long as no breast cancer symptoms are showing, at age 40 years old (2).

Breast ultrasound. "Breast Ultrasound are waves to produce images of structure deep within the body." This diagnostic method is used to determine if the breast malformation is a cyst filled with fluid (3).

Breast magnetic resonance imaging (MRI). MRI is a machine that formulates images of the inner section of the breast by using magnetic and radio waves to formulate image of the interior of one's breast. Before implementing this method the patient is given a dye injection (2).

Breast biopsy. A breast biopsy is removing a sample of breast cells for testing. To determine whether a patient has breast cancer or not, the doctor will have a biopsy by removing a sample of any abnormal breast cells. The sample is sent to a laboratory for testing. In addition, biopsy sample helps in determining the type of cells involved in the breast cancer and the aggressiveness (stage) of the cancer (3).

TREATMENT OPTIONS FOR BREAST CANCER

When diagnosed with breast cancer, a doctor determines treatment options based on the type of breast cancer, it's stage, whether the cancer cells are sensitive to hormones, the overall health of the patient, and an individual's own preferences for treatment. Most women prefer surgical treatment for breast cancer; however, the surgical treatment usually comes along with additional treatment, such as chemotherapy, hormone therapy, or radiation. Breast cancer treatments include:

Surgical treatment

This treatment involves removing only the breast cancer (lumpectomy) or removing one or several lymph nodes (sentinel node biopsy) or removing the entire breast (mastectomy) (10).

Hormone therapy

Hormone therapy is usually used to treat breast cancers that are sensitive to hormones. These cancers are referred to as "estrogen and progesterone receptor positive cancers" (10).

Targeted drug

"Targeted drug treatments attack specific abnormalities within the cancer cell" (10).

Chemotherapy

Chemotherapy is a common treatment for cancer in which drugs are used to destroy cancer cells, but it usually causes many side effects such as loss of hair, weight loss, and nausea (10).

CLINICAL TRIAL

Clinical trials are unproven treatments that may or may not be better than the other treatment options, but a doctor may give the patient this treatment option depending on the condition of the illness (10).

DOCUMENTATION OF BREAST CANCER IN THE ARAB WORLD

Worldwide, it is estimated that around 11 million people developed cancer in 2002. Of these, 53.7% were in developing countries and 46.5% were in developed countries. Among women in Saudi Arabia, breast cancer is the most common form of cancer followed by colon-rectal cancer (15). Cancer is an increasing problem in the Arab world. According to the World Health Organization (5), cancer is a leading cause of death in this part of the world and is estimated to kill 272,000 individuals annually. The Arab world (also called the Eastern Mediterranean Region or Middle East) refers to the Arabic-speaking countries extending from Lebanon and Syria in the north, Morocco in the west, Yemen in the south and Iraq in the east. The population of the Arab countries is over 300 million spreading along North Africa and Western Asia (5). Arab countries share common demographic problems and embrace the same culture and beliefs but different socio economic status (7).

Cancer is considered to be a "taboo" in most of the Arab world, and people call it "that other disease" and fear to mention it by name due to lack of knowledge and awareness (16). Breast cancer is the most frequent type of cancer among females in the Arab world. Patients with breast cancer in Arab countries tend to be young and almost half of the patients are under age 50 years; the median age of 49-52 years of Arab women with breast cancer is a decade lower when compared to the age 60 years of women developing breast cancer in Western developed countries (1, 7, 17). In many Arab countries "political instability, military conflicts, and poor planning have hindered the development of medical advances for breast cancer detection and treatments (17)." In addition, political and economic issues slow down research on cancer-related issues leaving the responsibilities of investigation and advancement under "individuals' and institutional motivation" (16). Salim et al. (7) stated that the risk factors for breast cancer in the Arab world are the same as those in developed countries. Further, some risk factors appear to be more significant in some Arab countries than others. According to Salim et al. (7) some risk factors like late age at last full-term pregnancy and long term use of oral contraceptive were significant predictors for breast cancer among females in Egypt, while in Jordan, increased numbers of pregnancies and obesity among postmenopausal women were significant predictors for breast cancer (7). In Kuwait, significant risk factors for breast cancer included "high Body Mass Index, lack of physical activity, early age at menarche, late age at first pregnancy hormonal therapy, and frequent consumption of carbohydrates, sweets, animal fat, and vegetable oil (margarine) with low intake of fresh vegetables and olive oil" (7).

On the other hand, significant risk factors for breast cancer among Iraqi females were tied with having a family history of breast cancer and oral contraceptives use, whereas high-risk human papilloma virus infections showed a significant predictor for breast cancer among women in Syria (7). In many Arab countries the age-adjusted incidence rates for breast cancer are increasing tremendously (1, 7).

For example, in Lebanon, the breast cancer incidence rate grew from 20 per 100,000 women in 1996 to 46.7 per 100.000 in 1998. In Jordan the incidence rate for breast cancer increased from 7.6 per 100,000 women in 1982 to 32.8 per 100,000 in 1997 (16). Although the incidence of cancer is lower than developed countries, it is expected to reach the highest increased incidence among all World Health Organization's regions in the coming years (5). Unfortunately, although the increase in breast cancer incidence is noted worldwide, there is still a lack of national and regional cancer registries in some Arab countries. Also, there is inadequate mortality and disease specific mortality rates recorded in almost all Arab countries (16).

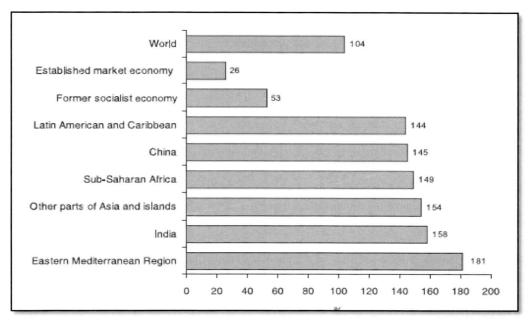

Source: WHO, 2009.

Figure 1. Increases in death from cancer (%).

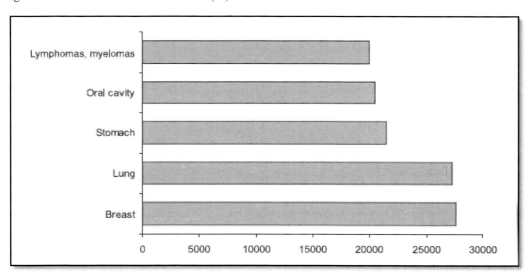

Source: WHO, 2009.

Figure 2. Top 5 cancer causes of death in Eastern Mediterranean Region.

PRIMARY AND SECONDARY PREVENTION AWARENESS OF BREAST CANCER

According to the American Cancer Society (3), the risk of developing breast cancer can be reduced by primary and secondary prevention. The best prevention practice is to avoid risk factors that increase the likelihood of developing breast cancer and adopt a healthy lifestyle including eating healthy, maintaining physical activity, and taking the breast cancer screening when one reaches the appropriate age or as a doctor recommends (18). In addition, early detection for breast cancer plays a significant role in finding tumors at an early stage which subsequently increases the survival rate to as high as 93% if found in the first stage (stage 0) and if the appropriate treatment is implemented (3). Therefore, following early detection practices can reduce the impact of breast cancer and allow for a greater range of treatment options.

Unfortunately, there is a rapid increase in obesity in Arab countries due to embracing an unhealthy lifestyle of unhealthy food consumption and lack of physical activity, primarily among children, adolescents, and young adults (3, 18, 19). Adopting Western cuisine and increasing the production of processed food and fast food restaurants have affected health in the Eastern Mediterranean Region, and has contributed to the rising numbers of cancer cases (5, 20). Low intake of fruits and vegetables among Arab countries has increased the prevalence of breast cancers. At the same time, changes in lifestyle and rapid urbanization have led to less physical activity (20, 21). In addition to the important role of dietary factors at play in the etiology of cancer, it is documented that obesity, consumption of a specific food like high consumptions of food that are high in fat or processed ingredients, and tobacco use are all linked to the development of breast cancer (19). Note, however, that the tobacco epidemic is less advanced in developing countries. Tobacco use is responsible for about 30% of the cancer burden in some industrialized countries, but much lower in developing countries since the tobacco epidemic is in its early stage (3, 18). Moreover, environmental factors are associated with cancer, yet studies have shown that pollution contributes to less than 2% of cancer risk factors in developed countries and is not expected to be higher in developing countries (3, 18).

Conversely, attitudes and beliefs regarding health in Arab countries differ from those in Western countries. Many Arabs would only go to the doctor when they noticed severe symptoms. They do not believe in taking precautions or going to the doctor for screening or early detections (22). Most cancers present at an advanced stage in Arab countries when a cure is improbable, even with the best treatments. In a study conducted by El Saghir et al. (16) large numbers of women in Arab countries presented with locally advanced and metastatic breast cancer because of poor health education, fear of finding out they have cancer, shyness, and difficult access to healthcare facilities. The primary reason behind improved survival rates for breast cancer in the U.S. and Europe has been shown to be finding the tumor in earlier stages of disease. Cautious attitudes regarding breast cancer and implementing early detection among women in Western countries were achieved through public education and increasing awareness of breast cancer prevention. It is important to note that data have shown that knowledge and attitudes regarding breast cancer prevention and early detection are absent in Arab countries. There is an urgent need for a public health plan to increase the knowledge and attitudes regarding breast cancer prevention. Increasing knowledge about breast cancer is the most effective approach of reducing cancer mortality in the Eastern Mediterranean Region (3).

BREAST CANCER MANAGEMENT AND PROFESSIONAL IMPLICATIONS IN THE ARAB WORLD

It is estimated that more than 50% of the cancers in the world are attributable to three factors: tobacco, infection, and unhealthy lifestyle (diet, obesity, and lack of physical activity). Early detection and appropriate treatment for breast cancer increase the ability to control the disease and lead to a better survival rate. However, Arab countries lack proper health education and advanced treatment options for breast cancer. The public knows very little about breast cancer risk factors and prevention methods and when an individual develops a cancer he/she cannot find many treatment options (1). Even knowledge about secondary prevention methods such as breast self-exam and early detection are limited. In addition, most Arab countries lack national programs for screening unless a motivated institution or private corporation sponsors the screening program (23). However, few motivated women would undergo the screening due to poor knowledge about the importance of screening and because it is too expensive for the majority of people since governmental and private insurers do not usually cover the expenses of screening. Further, when a female is diagnosed with breast cancer, treatment options are limited in most Arab countries. Medical development in the Arab world is far behind the developed countries. For example, if an individual has radiotherapy services as a treatment for breast cancer, one would find it far below international standards in Arab countries. When comparing Arab countries and the U.S., in terms of available radiation therapy centers, all Arab countries combined have 84 radiation therapy centers, while the U.S. has 1,875. Furthermore, whereas all the Arab countries have 256 radiation oncologists, the U.S. alone has 3,068, which reveal an enormous resource shortage of facilities and health personnel in the Arab world (16).

BREAST CANCER IN THE SAUDI FEMALE POPULATION

The Kingdom of Saudi Arabia KSA(KSA) has witnessed an enormous increase in breast cancer in the last several years (1, 6, 7, 17, 24). The latest released data from KSA National Cancer Registry shows breast cancer as the leading cancer among women in KSAin 2005, accounting for 22.4% of all newly diagnosed female cancers with the median age of 46 years at diagnosis (15, 25). The data revealed an increase in the incidence rate of breast cancer within a year from 2004 to 2005 (see Figures 4 and 5). The data confirm a growth in the age-standardized incidence rate from 15.4 per 100,000 in 2004 to 24.4 in 2005 (24). The five regions with the highest breast cancer incidence were in the Eastern region at 30.0 per 100,000 the Makkah region at 20.9 per 100,000, the Riyadh region at 18.6 per100,000, the Jouf region at 16.9 per 100,000 and the Tabuk region at 12.5 per 100,000 (24). The majority of cases are identified in advanced stages; for example, 44% of breast cancer cases are found in advanced stages (regional) (see Figure 6). Further, a higher frequency of breast cancer patients are among younger pre-menopausal women who do not seek help until the cancer reaches an advanced stage (26). A comparison of the referral patterns from the different regions of KSA shows that while there is an increase in numbers of cancer cases in all regions of KSA, it is most striking in the Eastern, Southern and Northern regions. The age distribution and menopausal status are similar in the different regions (8, 26). In a study conducted on the stages of breast cancer among female patients who came to King Faisal Hospital and Research Centre, it was found that 36% of the cases were early stage breast cancer (stages I, II), while 64% of the cases were at advanced stages (stages III, IV) (24).

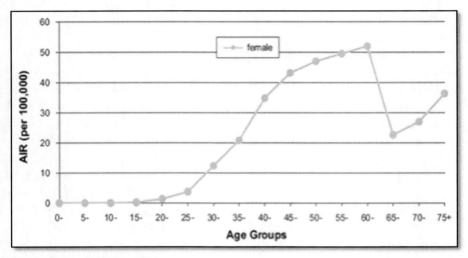

Source: Saudi Cancer Registry, 2004.

Figure 3. Incidence rate for female breast cancer in the year 2004, Saudi Arabia.

In another study conducted by Ezzat et al. (24) most women who came at King Faisal Specialist Hospital seeking breast cancer treatment were premenopausal women at median age of 46 years and the cancer was found in stage III (24). However, there is a lack of accuracy regarding the number of cases of breast cancer in these two studies. The number of breast cancer cases is estimated to be more than what was mentioned but they were not recorded due to malfunctioning of the hospital staff (28).

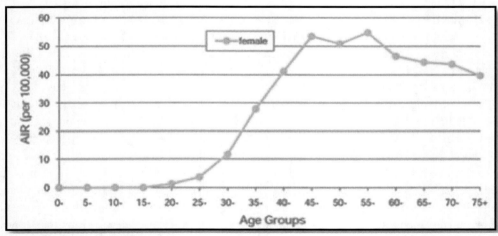

Source: Saudi Cancer Registry, 2005.

Figure 4. Incidence rate for female breast cancer in the year 2005, Saudi Arabia.

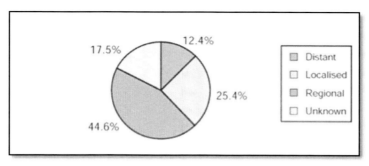

Source: Saudi Cancer Registry, 2005.

Figure 5. Distribution of female breast cancer in Saudi Arabia.

Risk factors for breast cancer among Saudi females are similar to the risk factors in the U.S., yet some of the emphasized risk factors include "estrogen use, hormone replacement, oral contraceptive pills, early menarche: women who started their period before age 12 years, late parity: women who had their first child after the age of 30 years, women with nulliparity, women who did not have any children or who did not report any pregnancies" are at high risk of breast cancer (27) (see Figures 3, 4, and 5).

KNOWLEDGE AND PREVENTION OF BREAST CANCER AMONG SAUDI FEMALES

Promoting health education and breast cancer preventable behavior is essential to decrease the odds of developing breast cancer and to improve the quality of life for the population (20, 27). In Saudi Arabia, breast cancer is increasing among younger females in all different regions (8, 15, 26). The increased prevalence of breast cancer among Saudi women at a younger age is tied with a lack of awareness about primary and secondary prevention implications (6, 17, 29). Many women have no access to mammograms due to "racial, environmental, financial/insurance barriers; lack of education; and, most importantly, lack of encouragement by a physician" (9). Social and demographic factors play an important role regarding the level of knowledge of breast cancer leading to an unfavorable outcome of breast cancer in KSA (27). However, even individuals who are knowledgeable about breast cancer prevention methods will not necessarily use the information to avoid risk factors of breast cancer (6, 27). In a study by Amin et al. (27) trying to assess the "level of knowledge about risk factors and utilization of screening methods used for breast cancer among Saudi women, the results show that knowledge about breast cancer risk factors and early detection methods were low and dependent upon educational and occupational status." In addition, early screening is underutilized among participants due to several perceived barriers. Moreover, the study showed early detection methods were employed by less than 5% and mammography by only 3% of cases (27).

Dandash and Al-Mohaimeed (6) discovered that most of the 90% of respondents (women) in the Al-Qaseem region who participated in their study showed lack in basic knowledge regarding breast cancer prevention. The study also revealed that persons with higher socioeconomic lifestyle had higher knowledge about breast cancer prevention, but even then people did not practice early detection (6). Also Milaat (29) assessed the level of awareness regarding breast cancer prevention and breast self-examination among students in Jeddah city, and discovered a very low knowledge level among the students. Specifically, over 80% of the participants showed lack of knowledge about breast cancer (29). Additionally, students who demonstrated better knowledge of breast cancer were among older students, married, or having a child, and students who experienced breast problems personally or in the family (29).

The presented data point to the urgent need for educational programs and national campaigns to promote awareness about breast cancer, since it has been estimated that there will be a 350% increase of breast cancer in KSA by the year 2025. The only way to stop these appalling predictors is to spread knowledge in the community and to educate individuals to avoid risk factors of breast cancer and implement early detection methods (20, 30). Breast cancer programs should be structured and implemented on a wide scale and tailored to fit individual communities (6). These statistical disparities in the Arab world in general and KSA in particular, imply the importance to establish community based promotion programs to enhance the knowledge about breast cancer, expand access to breast cancer screening, diagnostic services, and treatment. This approach can be achieved by focused efforts and collaboration between governments and healthcare system.

STRATEGIC PLAN TO PROMOTE BREAST CANCER PREVENTION AND EARLY DETECTION

It is estimated that 40% of cancers can be prevented by risk factors modifications. Therefore, prevention offers the greatest public health potential and the most cost effective long-term approach for cancer control (3). Since breast cancer is commonly diagnosed at late stages in Arab countries, efforts should be directed to increasing knowledge about prevention and promoting awareness regarding early detection of breast cancer. Such a focused plan can lead to diagnosis at earlier stages, potentially improving the odds of survival and successful treatment of breast cancer, and enabling simpler and more cost effective treatments. Reducing the impact of breast cancer in the Arab world will require modifications and improvements to the healthcare system and public education. Strategic health communication campaigns for breast cancer prevention that use multiple channels of communication can be used to effectively disseminate relevant information regarding breast health risks to vulnerable populations and encourage adoption of health-promoting behaviors (31, 32). Such recommendations can be broadened to be used in the Arab world in general or in one specific country like Saudi Arabia.

The focus of our strategic plan is promoting primary and secondary awareness regarding breast cancer. A proposed approach once implemented effectively would serve the purpose of breast cancer prevention through promoting awareness regarding risk factors about breast cancer and the importance of early detection. This approach is a culturally sensitive health communication program, in which cultural traditions, norms, and settings are taken into consideration while conducting the program in order to meet the health consumer preferences and draw a large population to the program (33). An example of such an approach is the Cancer Care Mission Program in Pune, India. In this program health professionals addressed the targeted population by categorizing them according to their religion, language, literacy and education, financial status, villagers and city residents (33). In addition, the team in this program made additional efforts to address the multiple languages, cultures, and religions through appropriate research and knowledge of the different cultures. In communicating the targeted knowledge about breast cancer, the project members addressed each individual according to their level of education and literacy, so for highly educated people the team presented statistics and scientific information, and for the illiterate, basic knowledge and visuals like posters and PowerPoint presentations in their local languages, needs, and beliefs were utilized Also, cultural sensitivity is crucial for such programs to succeed. Health professionals in this project integrated images and pictures from the local heritage in presenting sensitive images like breasts and other women body parts. Overall the issue of cultural and religious sensitivity and how they are being treated in any initiative, whether a health promotion program or an awareness campaign, is of a high priority in Arab countries and specifically in KSA where such aspects of life are considered more important that any given health issue (see Figures 6 and 7).

Type of Barrier	Examples
Taboos	"Putting aside" a family member diagnosed with breast cancer; "placing a curse" on individuals with breast cancer; "silencing" individuals with breast cancer
Myths	Having no pain means no breast cancer; believing breast cancer is a disease of "the old"
Religion	Religious leaders bless "traditional healers" over "western or modern" medicine; believing "It is God's will"
Communication	Graphics or pictorial representations of breasts may not be culturally appropriate; assuming print is the best medium in countries with high literacy rates
Decision-makers	Not identifying tribal and clan leaders who allow programs to happen; not identifying key family member(s) who make decisions for women related to their health
Awareness and educational materials, programs, and outreach activities	Importing and using inappropriate materials; assuming everyone knows English; assuming that what works "back home" will be successful here
Defining what constitutes knowledge	Discounting "local" knowledge for the most part as useless; defining the only reliable and valid knowledge as evidence-based
Complex changes	No understanding that complex change is a process that takes time and not an event; believing all changes that are being promoted are the best for the individuals being served
Funding agencies and organizations	Presuming that those receiving the funds will do "their bidding"; assuming funding from countries with high levels of resources is always wanted and welcomed
Local ways of learning	Overlooking local ways of learning (for example, singing, drama, story telling); judging local ways of learning as inappropriate in breast cancer education
Power	Knowing "for sure" who wields the power to ensure their programs will be successful; using power through a participatory process for the "common good" is sound practice
Countries and regions at war and/or in turbulent times	Obtaining funding sources is very difficult; perceiving breast cancer as a major problem is not likely

Source: Yip et al. 2008.

Figure 6. Barriers to awareness, education, and outreach programs and activities for early detection programs for breast cancer.

Level of resources	Patient and Family Education	Human Resource Capacity Building	Patient Navigation
Basic	General education regarding primary prevention of cancer, early detection and self examination Development of culturally adapted patient and family education services	Primary care provider education re breast cancer detection, diagnosis and treatment Nursing education re cancer patient management and emotional support Pathology technician education re tissue handling and specimen preparation Trained community worker	Field nurse, midwife or healthcare provider triages patients to central facility for diagnosis and treatment
Limited	Group or one-on-one counselling involving family and peer support Education regarding nutrition and complementary therapies	Nursing education re breast cancer diagnosis, treatment and patient management Imaging technician education re imaging technique and quality control Volunteer recruitment corp to support care	On site patient navigator (staff member or nurse) facilitates patient triage through diagnosis and treatment
Enhanced	Education regarding survivorship Lymphedema education Education regarding home care	Organization of national volunteer network Specialized nursing oncology training Home care nursing Physiotherapist & lymphedema therapist On-site cytopathologist	Patient navigation team from each discipline supports patient "handoff" during key transitions from specialist to specialist to ensure completion of therapy
Maximal		Organization of national medical breast health groups	

Source: Anderson et al., 2007.

Figure 7. Breast care programs: human resource allocation table.

FUTURE TRENDS

The trend has been attributed to several factors including emphasis on early detection and education of professionals and public yet these trends are going slowly and need to be emphasized. In addition, in the Arab world in general and in KSA specifically, there is a need to improve the healthcare system as a whole in order to promote the health outcomes among the population. Many taboos need to be overcome and replaced with knowledge and valid facts. Breast cancer is one side of the story and for just that issue one will find that there is a lot to do to reduce breast cancer morbidity and mortality. To fix the problem we need to start from zero and renovate the health system. Primary healthcare workers are rarely provided with sufficient education about the early signs of cancer or where to refer suspected cases. This could be remedied by short training courses like continuing education programs, brochures or posters, and by establishing links between those who deliver primary healthcare and referral centers (5). Authorities in the Arab countries and KSA should embrace the concept of training sufficient numbers of nurse practitioners and physician assistants to promote health knowledge about breast cancer (17). Also, access to multi-disciplinary tumor boards and clinics will improve breast cancer care. Development of centralized, specialized cancer centers may be a cost effective way to deliver breast cancer care to some women. Panelists of the Global Summit Consensus Conference noted that measures to educate the public and healthcare providers about breast health and breast cancer detection, diagnosis, and treatment are considered more important than screening in countries with limited resources to deliver such care to women nationwide (16). Also, awareness campaigns and screening should be applied according to resources. Awareness campaigns should also be directed to the whole family and to husbands instead to encourage their daughters and wives to enroll in early detection programs. Radiation therapy facilities and manpower remain very limited and deserve better planning and investment, and to be more widely available and distributed in major cities and distant regions (16, 31). Health promotion is a new concept in the Arab world but with strategic planning and resourcing, hopefully the health status will improve among all Arab communities and cancer will no longer be an epidemic concern.

In view of the above literature in the Arab world, this study examines Arab immigrant women in the United States and their perspectives on breast cancer. The purpose of this study was to investigate the reasons behind an increasing number of breast cancer cases in their advanced stage among Arab women in general and among women in Saudi Arabia, and find the solutions to promote prevention against breast cancer.

METHODS

Twenty-five Arab females aged 18 to 54 years were recruited for this research. Purposeful sampling (34) was used to recruit the participants. Participants came from different backgrounds, specifically KSA, Egypt, Syria, Sudan, Jordan. However, more than half of participants came from KSA. During this study, all participants resided in the United States for academic purposes. Majority of participants were married 60% with a bachelor degree or beyond.

The authors used a phenomenological approach for data analysis (35). The questionnaire was distributed to participants by hand as well as via email. The data collection instrument contained a list of eight questions. The questionnaires were composed of open-ended and closed-ended questions.

After approval by Indiana University's Institutional Review Board, potential participants for the study were contacted through email, phone calls, and, where possible, in person by one of the authors. Potential participants were notified that taking part in this study was voluntary. It took 25 minutes for each participant to complete the questionnaire. Completed questionnaires were hand delivered where possible, or sent by email.

Data from open-ended questions were used for this research. Because this study used a phenomenological approach, it allowed the researchers to code according to similarity in the identified answers. Commonalities in participants' personal experiences were also grouped together and sorted into categories by theme (34-37).

RESULTS

Research findings indicated that participants lack knowledge regarding how to practice breast self-exam. Participants cited several reasons, such as not knowing how to do the breast self-exam. A participant stated: "I do not know how." There was also lack of time to do the exam as expressed by a participant: "I don't have an opportunity to do it." Some participants noted that influences from family members and medical practitioners also impacted their choice of not going to a clinic. A participant noted: "because no one in my family has, the doctor said I do not need it."

Additionally, the majority of participants (64%) indicated they never attended any program in their community to gain knowledge regarding breast cancer prevention. However, we also noticed that the group of participants who positively reported doing the exam also reported attending an educational program on breast cancer and prevention.

Furthermore, the majority of participants (80%) reported not ever getting a mammogram. We had hoped to explore such practices within the specific age (40 years and above), however we could not do so due to lack of participants in this age range. Some participants attested that if healthcare professionals would help them learn about breast cancer prevention methods and remind them at the clinics, it would go a long way to help them practice breast self-exam.

DISCUSSION

Findings from the study confirm the existing literature emphasis on the lack of knowledge and awareness among Arab women about breast cancer awareness and prevention measures (6, 27, 29). Knowledge among individuals in the Arab community concerning breast cancer and its prevention including breast self-examination and having a mammogram is insufficient. Inadequate personal knowledge on the issue of breast cancer seems to be a big factor in allowing this life threatening disease to continue in the Arab world. As participants reported, educating the public about prevention measures would be a good start in addressing the problem. However, as time problems were also reported, such educational efforts should reinvent themselves in manners that accommodate the public needs and correct any false ideas. Collaborative efforts from public service offices, health officials, and interested groups might consider creating educational materials that take into the consideration people's culture and the sensitivity of the subject and reach out to the public in a variety of ways.

The taboo nature of the issue could also be providing misinformed grounds for the disease to flourish. As women rarely talk about it or only talk to very close family members and relatives (16), misinformation could be the only source for deciding on what to be done about preventing the disease. This conundrum amplifies the role of physicians and their responsibility in informing their patients and explaining measures available to them.

Given that research indicates that primary and secondary prevention, especially breast self-exam and mammogram help save lives, it is highly recommended that health educators, nurses, physicians, and family members routinely remind female members about breast cancer prevention methods.

Proper knowledge about the issue should facilitate the development of better informed citizens who are able to navigate through misinformed arguments. The lack of time obstacle was particularly interesting as breast self-examination takes little time and could be done while in the shower.

From this study we conclude how crucial it is to make available proper awareness and practices about breast cancer as our observations showed a positive correlation between attending an educational program about breast cancer prevention and taking proper measures in preventing breast cancer.

REFERENCES

[1] Najjar H, Easson A. Age at diagnosis of breast cancer in Arab nations. Int J Surg. 2010;8(6):448-52.
[2] World Health Organization. The World Health Organization's cancer fact sheet 297, 2009. URL: http://www.who.int/mediacentre/factsheets/fs297/en/print.html.
[3] American Cancer Society. Cancer facts and figures 2010. URL: http://www.cancer.org/acs/groups/content/@epidemiologysurveilance/documents/document/acspc-026238.pdf.
[4] National Cancer Institute. Surveillance Epidemiological End Results Program: State cancer profiles: Death rates, 2009. URL: http://statecancerprofiles.cancer.gov/cgi-bin/deathrates/deathrates.
[5] World Health Organization, Regional Office for the Eastern Mediterranean. Strategy for cancer prevention and control in the Eastern Mediterranean region. Cairo, Egypt: WHO/EM/NCD/060/, 2009.
[6] Dandash K, Al-Mohaimeed A. Knowledge, attitudes, and practices surrounding breast cancer and screening in female teachers of Buraidah, Saudi Arabia. Int J Health Sci 2007;1(1):L61-71.
[7] Salim E, Moore M, Al-Lawati J, Al-Sayyad J, Bazawir A, Bener A, et al. Cancer epidemiology and control in the Arab world: Past, present and future. Asian Pacif J Cancer Prev 2009;10:3-16.
[8] Ezzat A, Raja M, Rostom A, Zwaan F, Akthar M, Bazarbashi S, et al. An overview of breast cancer. Ann Saudi Med 1997;17(1):10-5.
[9] Abulkhair O, Al Tahan F, Young S, Musaad S, Jazieh A. The first national public breast cancer screening program in Saudi Arabia. Annals of Saudi Med 2010;30(5):350-357.
[10] Mayo Clinic. Definition. Breast cancer. URL: http://www.mayoclinic.com/health/breast-cancer/DS00328.
[11] National Breast Cancer Foundation. - Breast cancer types. Accessed 2010. URL: http://www.nationalbreastcancer.org/types-of-breast-cancer.
[12] National Cancer Institute. Breast cancer treatment. URL: http://www.cancer.gov/cancertopics/pdq/treatment/breast/patient/allpages/print.

[13] Centers for Disease Control and Prevention. Breast cancer and you: what you need to know. URL: http://www.cdc.gov//cancer/breast/pdf/BreastCancerFS_2010.pdf.
[14] Anderson B, Braun S, Lim S, Smith R, Taplin S, Thomas D. Early detection of breast cancer in countries with limited resources. Breast J 2003;9(2):51-59.
[15] Ministry of Health, Saudi Cancer Registry Cancer incidence report. URL: http://www.scr.org.sa/reports /SCR2005.pdf.
[16] El Saghir N, Khalil M, Eid T, El Kinge A, Charafeddine M, Geara F, et al. Trends in epidemiology and management of breast cancer in developing Arab countries: a literature and registry analysis. Int J Surgery 2007;5(4): 225-33.
[17] Ibrahim E, Zeeneldin A, Sadiq B, Ezzat A. The present and the future of breast cancer burden in the Kingdom of Saudi Arabia. Med Oncol 2008;25(4):387-93.
[18] Vogel, V. Breast cancer prevention: a review of current evidence. CA Cancer J Clin 2000;50(3):156-70.
[19] Holmes M, Willett W. Does diet affect breast cancer risk? Breast Cancer Res 2004;6(4):170-8.
[20] Al-Amri A. Prevention of breast cancer. J Fam Commun Med 2005;12(2):71-74.
[21] Khatib O. Noncommunicable diseases: risk factors and regional strategies for prevention and care. East Mediterranean Health J 2004;10(vi): 778-88.
[22] Lipson J, Meleis A. Issues in health care of Middle Eastern patients. West J Med 1983;139(6): 854-61.
[23] Hanna T, Kangolle A. Cancer control in developing countries: using health data and health services research to measure and improve access, quality and efficiency. BMC Int Health Hum Rights 2010;10:24.
[24] Ezzat A, Ibrahim E, Raja M, Al-Sobhi S, Rostom A, Stuart R. Locally advanced breast cancer in Saudi Arabia: high frequency of stage III in a young population. Med Oncol 1999;16(2):95-103.
[25] Ministry of Health, Saudi Cancer Registry. Cancer incidence report 2005. URL: http://www.emro.who.int/ncd/pdf/saa_cancer_registry_2005.
[26] Khan A R Hussain NK Al-Saigh A Malatani T, Sheikha AA. Pattern of cancer at Asir Central Hospital, Abha, Saudi Arabia." Ann Saudi Med 1991;11(3):285-8.
[27] Amin T, Al Mulhim A, Al Meqihwi A. Breast cancer knowledge, risk factors and screening among adult Saudi women in a primary health care setting. Asian Pacific J Cancer Prev 2009;10(1):133-8.
[28] Al-Zahrani A, Baomer A, Al-Hamdam N, Mohamed G. Completeness and validity of cancer registration in a major public referral hospital in Saudi Arabia. Ann Saudi Med 2003;23(1-2):6-9.
[29] Milaat W. Knowledge of secondary-school female students on breast cancer and breast self-examination in Jeddah, Saudi Arabia. East Mediterranean Health J 2000;6(2/3):338-44.
[30] Alam A. Knowledge of breast cancer and its risk and protective factors among women in Riyadh. Ann Saudi Med 2006;26(4):272-7.
[31] Anderson B, Yip C, Smith R, Shyyan R, Sener S, Eniu A, et al. Guideline implementation for breast healthcare in low-income and middle-income countries: overview of the Breast Health Global Initiative Global Summit. Cancer 2008;113(8):2221-43.
[32] Yip C, Smith R, Anderson B, Miller A, Thomas D, Ang E, et al. Guideline implementation for breast healthcare in low- and middle-income countries: early detection resource allocation. Cancer 2008;113(8):2244-56.
[33] Kreps G, Sivaram R. Strategic health communication across the continuum of breast cancer care in limited-resource countries. Cancer 2008;113(8):2331-7. doi:10.1002/cncr.23832.
[34] Patton MQ. Qualitative evaluation and research methods, 2nd ed. Newbury Park, CA: Sage, 1990.
[35] Moustakas C. Phenomenological research methods. Thousand Oaks, CA: Sage, 1994.
[36] Smith JA, Osborn M. Interpretative phenomenological analysis. In: Smith JA, ed. Qualitative psychology: A practical guide to research methods. Thousand Oaks, CA: Sage, 2007:53-80.
[37] Van Manen M. Researching lived experience. Ontario, Canada: Althouse Press, 1990.

Received: September 12, 2014. *Revised:* October 06, 2014. *Accepted:* October 15, 2014

In: Public Health Yearbook 2015
Editor: Joav Merrick

ISBN: 978-1-63484-514-4
© 2016 Nova Science Publishers, Inc.

Chapter 38

CULTURE, HEALTH, AND THE USE OF HOUSEHOLD CLEANING PRODUCTS BY AFRICAN WOMEN

Nesrin Omer, MSc, and Cecilia S Obeng, PhD*

School of Public Health, Indiana University, Bloomington,
Indiana, United States of America

ABSTRACT

This study focuses on African women's use of cleaning products and their awareness of the health and environmental effects of these products. There were 15 participants in the study. Analyses of the findings indicate that participants' culture has an influence on the way most of the women view and respond to harmful cleaning products. Some participants noted that they did not practice safety measures to protect their health, although all of them believed there was some risk from using cleaning products. Others indicated that they did not mix cleaning products according to the instructions on the product and some were unfamiliar with the effects of such mixing, or did not see the need for following the instructions. Environmental and health campaigns should develop accessible and effective methods to increase the awareness of African women about the health hazards associated with the use of cleaning products, and the importance of practicing or adopting safety and protective measures when using such products. Also, information should be provided to these women as to where alternative affordable and effective non-toxic products may be purchased, and the real long-term costs of using chemical products.

Keywords: African immigrants, of cleaning products, environmental health, culture

---

[*] Correspondence: Cecilia S Obeng, PhD, Associate Professor, Indiana University, School of Public Health, 1025 E 7th Street, SPH 116, Bloomington, IN 47405, United States. E-mail: cobeng@indiana.edu.

INTRODUCTION

Scholarship on women's health have focused mainly on their reproductive health (1), while factors like environmental effects on women's health have received little or no attention especially on African women's health (2, 3). In Africa as in many developing countries, issues such as AIDS, poverty, teen aged pregnancy and Ebola have got some attention. In general, concerning women's health related to dangerous domestic and environmental factors few studies have considered evaluating them (4).

Scholarship on women's health indicates that women in developed and developing countries have the main responsibility for household activities (5), For African women, the fact that they usually do the -household chores and farm work make their situation particularly difficult (6). In some parts of the world, particularly, in Sub Saharan Africa men have to do less domestic chores than women (7).

Women in work-places (especially where commercial chemicals is used), can encounter considerable health risks from minor to life-threatening. For example, epidemiological scholarship indicates that daily used of chemically-based cleaning products, with organochlorines content is connected to breast cancer (8, 9).

Note that studies on cleaning products focused mainly on the health of Caucasian, Hispanic, African Americans, among others (10-12). Unfortunately, African immigrant women's knowledge on cleaning products and how their culture influences the use of these products has not been sufficiently investigated.

In addition, the literature on the use and impact of chemicals on the health of Africans has focused on - chemical poisoning in the household in general and on other toxic chemicals such as Dichloro-Diphenyl-Trichloroethane (DDT), which is not used since 1972 in the USA (United Nations Environment Program, 2008. There has also been a study in Zimbabwe on chemical poisoning that indicated that some chemical poisoning admissions at the hospitals are due to the outcome of exposure to kerosene (13).

In view of the above literature, this study addresses the effects of cleaning products on the health of African women, including their utilization and storage, and their children's use and access to these products. Consumer behavioral factors that expose them and their families to health risks are also addressed.

METHODS

This study uses phenomenology in data collection and analysis. In a phenomenological study, participants should not located at a single place rather they must be persons who have experienced the phenomenon (topic) being investigated (14). All involved in this study are African women who use household cleaning products. Most of the fifteen participants live in Bloomington, Indiana and the rest reside in Michigan, Ohio, Virginia, and Maryland. They come from nine African countries: Egypt, Ethiopia, Libya, Mali, Morocco, Senegal, Sudan, Swaziland, and Tanzania, and have different backgrounds, briefly described below. They range in age from their early 20s to mid-50s, and most have children. All were very willing to participate in this study, and we excluded potential candidates who were not especially interested in participating, as well as two who travelled back to Africa before we had a chance to validate their answers. For the sake of anonymity, we named the participants using the alphabets A, B and C, and so forth. For list of participants see Table 1.

Table 1. List of Participants

Participant	Age	Marital Status	# of Children	Education/Occupation	Date of Arrival to USA	Residency
A	50	M	2	Accounts Receivable Manager	1982	Bloomington, Indiana
B	31	M	2	Bachelor in Media	2009	Bloomington, Indiana
C	Mid-30s	S	None	Environmental analyst	1990	Maryland
D	Mid-20s	M	None	Bachelor in English Language	2010	Bloomington, Indiana
E	22	M	1	Clinical Laboratory Science	2008	Bloomington, Indiana
F	Mid-30s	M	2	Assistant Professor	Mid-90s	Michigan
H	30	S	1	PhD student in Linguistics	2007	Bloomington, Indiana
G	39	M	2	Master in Physical Therapy	1999	Michigan
I	Mid-50s	M	3	High school	2001	Ohio
J	Mid-40s	M	None	Master in Mathematics	2001	Michigan
K	30	M	3	High School	2009	Virginia
L	50	D	3	PhD in Linguistics	2001	Bloomington, Indiana
M	Mid-40s	M	4	Associate degree in Computer Science	2005	Bloomington, Indiana
N	Mid-30s	M	3	Seamstress	2001	Bloomington, Indiana
O	Mid-30s	M	1	Master student in Second Language Studies	2006	Bloomington, Indiana

Procedure

This study was carried out in accordance with the ethical standards stated by the Human Research Protection Program (HRPP) at Indiana University so as to protect the rights and welfare of human research participants.

The questionnaires for this study were sent to the participants via email; thus, this study collected data via long interviews of approximately 60-90 minutes featuring open-ended questions. It followed a procedure as described by Seidman (14), where three detailed interviews should be done when doing phenomenological inquiry. The first interview should focused on the participants past experiences, followed by participants present experiences and the third joined the two together to describe participants individual's experiences with the phenomenon. Prior to conducting these interviews, we wrote a full description of one of the authors' own experiences with household cleaning products in order to bracket off her experience from those of the participants. In addition to the open-ended questions, we sometimes used phone, email, and face-to-face interviews to check information with participants and to validate their narratives. For data analysis, Moustakas (15) suggested two phenomenological analysis, the Van Kaam Method and the Stevick-Colaizzi-Keen method. We chose to analyze our study data using Moustakas's modified van Kaam method because it focuses on the validation of data.

For example, we often returned to the participants to make sure that they understood the questions from their point of view. Moustakas (15) provided example of data validation borrowed from Humphrey's (1991) study that focused on the concept of "searching for life's meaning." Humphrey's approach was to send his participants copies of his descriptions of participant's answers for them to examine. Before analysis their answers were read back to them several times and we asked them what they thought of their answers in order to enable them to make corrections and additions accordingly. Due to this approach, the two participants who traveled back to Africa, with whom we lost contact before we could validate their information, were excluded from this study. In this case, we did not want to wait for their responses to finish the study syntheses, a potential delay that posed the risk of losing contact with the rest of the participants.

RESULTS AND DISCUSSION

From our data it appears that culture has an influence on the way most of these women viewed and responded to health practices or concerns about protecting themselves from harmful chemicals. The effect of culture was evident regarding the protection of their privacy; some participants were Muslim women and took measures to prevent outsiders from viewing them or their private spaces. These participants indicated that they generally do not open the curtains when using cleaning products, but in upper rooms that cannot be seen by passersby, some of these women chose to open their windows while cleaning. Our data also shows that a great volume and variety of powerful cleaning products were used on a regular basis since participants indicated that it was very important for them to have clean homes. The effectiveness of cleaning products was more important for the women than the products' effect on their health, and the environment. None of the participants used cleaning products categorized as "green," although they were aware of these products.

Household cleaning and safety practices

According to our data, most of the participants did not lock their cleaning products in their African homes, and continued this practice in the United States. The same can be said for practicing safety measures when cleaning. Most of the women did not wear gloves or mask in Africa while cleaning, and did the same when moved to United States. Most used very simple cleaning products in their African homes, such as liquid and bar soap, which do not require wearing gloves or mask. But upon coming to the United States, they adopted the practice of using the commercial chemical products, most of which can have adverse effects on their health. It appears that most of the participants did not practice safety measures to protect their health, although all of the participants believed there was some risk from using cleaning products, and all with the exception of one had experienced adverse health effect, as well as some members of their families.

Choice and use of cleaning products

Eleven of the fifteen participants used chemical cleaning products daily and indicated that they were responsible for carrying out all their household cleaning activities. This means the majority of the African women who participated in this study were exposed daily to health risks from using cleaning products, because they did not practice safety measures to reduce their exposure as mentioned by the participants. Some participants did not read the cautionary labels. Others indicated that they did not mix cleaning products according to the instructions on the product and some were unfamiliarity with the effects of such mixing, or do not see the need for following the instructions.

Involvement of children in cleaning

Regarding the involvement of children in cleaning, all participants, except for two, seemed to be very protective of their children, and did not allow them to use cleaning products but in some cases helped with other chores. Although in Africa they did allow their children to use cleaning products, most of these products are mild liquid and bar soap. A few participants had their children help in cleaning where they also used these products, where adverse effects are noted by many of the women, and in one case, the use of the product had to be discontinued. One of the two participants, who had their children use cleaning products in the United States, stated that 'due to the practices in her home country, daughters must be trained from early age to participate in household work.'

Getting information on product safety and cleaning effectiveness

Almost half of the participants did not know where to get information on cleaning products, and half got information from the labels on the products and from online, or both. In addition, none of the participants knew about the Soap and Detergent Association (SDA), a non-profit trade association that has an online resource containing information on the safety and effectiveness of household cleaning products.

IMPLICATION ON FUTURE RESEARCH

The results of this study point out and highlight the importance of incorporating culture as a key factor in future research that deals with African women's health and the use of household cleaning products. This study also demonstrates the need for research dealing with African women's behavioral use and storage of cleaning products and the impact on their families' health. Other important issues that arose from this study, was that as some participants allowed their children to use cleaning products to train them for household work as a cultural practice, there is the need for research/surveys to determine the percentage of African women who allow their children to use cleaning products, and the impact of this practice on their children's health. Moreover, environmental and health campaigns should develop accessible and effective methods to increase the awareness of African women of the health hazards associated with the use of cleaning products, and the importance of practicing or adopting safety and protective measures when using cleaning products. Given the prevalence of using unsafe cleaning products among the participants, information should be provided to these women as to where alternative affordable and effective non-toxic products may be purchased. Also information on real long-term costs of using chemical products should be communicated to African women.

REFERENCES

[1] Lewis N, Kieffer EC. The health of women: Beyond maternal and child health. In: Verhasselt V, Philips D, eds. Health and development. London: Routledge, 1998.
[2] Brems S, Griffiths M. Health women's way: Learning to listen. In: Koblinsky M, Timyan J, Gay J, eds. The health of women: A global perspective. Oxford, OH: Westview Press, 1993.
[3] Lewis N. Safe womanhood: A discussion paper. Toronto, ON: Intern Federation of Instit for Advanced Study, 1994.
[4] Ardayfio-Schandorf E. Women's health status in Africa: Environmental perspectives from rural communities. Health Care Women Int 1993;14(4):375-86.
[5] MacCormack C. Planning and evaluating women's participation in primary health care. Soc Sci Med 1992); 35(6):831-7.
[6] Ilahi N, Grimard F. Public infrastructure and private costs: Water supply and time allocation of women in rural Pakistan. Econ Dev Cultural Change 2000;49(I):45-75.
[7] World Bank. Engendering development: Through gender equality in rights, resources, and voice. World Bank Policy Res Report. Washington, DC: World Bank, 2001.
[8] Calle EE, Frumkin H, Henley S J, Savitz D A, Thun M J. Organochlorines and breast cancer risk. Can Cancer J 2002;52:301-9.
[9] Zota AR, Aschengrau A, Rudel RA, Brody G. Self-reported chemicals exposure, beliefs about disease causation, and risk of breast cancer in the Cape Cod breast cancer and environment study: A case-control study. Environ Health 2010;9:40.
[10] Hondagneu-Sotelo P. Domestica: Immigrant workers cleaning and caring in the shadow of affluence. Berkeley, CA: University of California Press, 2001.
[11] Mulvaney C, Kendrick D. Engagement in safety practices to prevent home injuries in preschool children among white and non-white ethnic minority families. Inj Prev 2004;10(6):375-8.
[12] Bello A, Quinn MM, Perry MJ, Milton DM. Characterization of occupational exposures to cleaning products used for common cleaning tasks-a pilot study of hospital cleaners. Environ Health 2009;8:11.
[13] Nhachi CF, Kasilo OM. Household chemicals poisoning admissions in Zimbabwe's main urban centres. Hum Exp Toxicol 1994;13(2):69-72.
[14] Creswell JW. Qualitative inquiry and research design: Choosing among five traditions. London: Sage, 1998.
[15] Moustakas C. Phenomenological research methods. Thousand Oaks, CA: Sage, 1994.

Received: September 14, 2014. *Revised:* October 06, 2014. *Accepted:* October 16, 2014

SECTION FIVE - ACKNOWLEDGMENTS

In: Public Health Yearbook 2015
Editor: Joav Merrick

ISBN: 978-1-63484-514-4
© 2016 Nova Science Publishers, Inc.

Chapter 39

ABOUT THE EDITOR

Joav Merrick, MD, MMedSci, DMSc, born and educated in Denmark is professor of pediatrics, child health and human development, Division of Pediatrics, Hadassah Hebrew University Medical Center, Mt Scopus Campus, Jerusalem, Israel and Kentucky Children's Hospital, University of Kentucky, Lexington, Kentucky United States and professor of public health at the Center for Healthy Development, School of Public Health, Georgia State University, Atlanta, United States, the medical director of the Health Services, Division for Intellectual and Developmental Disabilities, Ministry of Social Affairs and Social Services, Jerusalem, the founder and director of the National Institute of Child Health and Human Development in Israel. Numerous publications in the field of pediatrics, child health and human development, rehabilitation, intellectual disability, disability, health, welfare, abuse, advocacy, quality of life and prevention. Received the Peter Sabroe Child Award for outstanding work on behalf of Danish Children in 1985 and the International LEGO-Prize ("The Children's Nobel Prize") for an extraordinary contribution towards improvement in child welfare and well-being in 1987. E-mail: jmerrick@zahav.net.il.

In: Public Health Yearbook 2015
Editor: Joav Merrick
ISBN: 978-1-63484-514-4
© 2016 Nova Science Publishers, Inc.

Chapter 40

ABOUT THE NATIONAL INSTITUTE OF CHILD HEALTH AND HUMAN DEVELOPMENT IN ISRAEL

The National Institute of Child Health and Human Development (NICHD) in Israel was established in 1998 as a virtual institute under the auspices of the Medical Director, Ministry of Social Affairs and Social Services in order to function as the research arm for the Office of the Medical Director. In 1998 the National Council for Child Health and Pediatrics, Ministry of Health and in 1999 the Director General and Deputy Director General of the Ministry of Health endorsed the establishment of the NICHD.

MISSION

The mission of a National Institute for Child Health and Human Development in Israel is to provide an academic focal point for the scholarly interdisciplinary study of child life, health, public health, welfare, disability, rehabilitation, intellectual disability and related aspects of human development. This mission includes research, teaching, clinical work, information and public service activities in the field of child health and human development.

SERVICE AND ACADEMIC ACTIVITIES

Over the years many activities became focused in the south of Israel due to collaboration with various professionals at the Faculty of Health Sciences (FOHS) at the Ben Gurion University of the Negev (BGU). Since 2000 an affiliation with the Zusman Child Development Center at the Pediatric Division of Soroka University Medical Center has resulted in collaboration around the establishment of the Down Syndrome Clinic at that center. In 2002 a full course on "Disability" was established at the Recanati School for Allied Professions in the Community, FOHS, BGU and in 2005 collaboration was started with the Primary Care Unit of the faculty and disability became part of the master of public health course on "Children and society." In the academic year 2005-2006 a one semester course on "Aging with disability" was started as part of the master of science program in gerontology in our collaboration with the Center for Multidisciplinary Research in Aging. In 2010 collaborations with the Division of Pediatrics, Hadassah Hebrew University Medical Center, Jerusalem, Israel around the National Down Syndrome Center and teaching students and residents about intellectual and developmental disabilities as part of their training at this campus.

RESEARCH ACTIVITIES

The affiliated staff have over the years published work from projects and research activities in this national and international collaboration. In the year 2000 the International Journal of Adolescent Medicine and Health and in 2005 the International Journal on Disability and Human Development of De Gruyter Publishing House (Berlin and New York) were affiliated with the National Institute of Child Health and Human Development. From 2008 also the International Journal of Child Health and Human Development (Nova Science, New York), the International Journal of Child and Adolescent Health (Nova Science) and the Journal of Pain Management (Nova Science) affiliated and from 2009 the International Public Health Journal (Nova Science) and Journal of Alternative Medicine Research (Nova Science). All peer-reviewed international journals.

NATIONAL COLLABORATIONS

Nationally the NICHD works in collaboration with the Faculty of Health Sciences, Ben Gurion University of the Negev; Department of Physical Therapy, Sackler School of Medicine, Tel Aviv University; Autism Center, Assaf HaRofeh Medical Center; National Rett and PKU Centers at Chaim Sheba Medical Center, Tel HaShomer; Department of Physiotherapy, Haifa University; Department of Education, Bar Ilan University, Ramat Gan, Faculty of Social Sciences and Health Sciences; College of Judea and Samaria in Ariel and in 2011 affiliation with Center for Pediatric Chronic Diseases and National Center for Down Syndrome, Department of Pediatrics, Hadassah Hebrew University Medical Center, Mount Scopus Campus, Jerusalem.

INTERNATIONAL COLLABORATIONS

Internationally with the Department of Disability and Human Development, College of Applied Health Sciences, University of Illinois at Chicago; Strong Center for Developmental Disabilities, Golisano Children's Hospital at Strong, University of Rochester School of Medicine and Dentistry, New York; Centre on Intellectual Disabilities, University of Albany, New York; Centre for Chronic Disease Prevention and Control, Health Canada, Ottawa; Chandler Medical Center and Children's Hospital, Kentucky Children's Hospital, Section of Adolescent Medicine, University of Kentucky, Lexington; Chronic Disease Prevention and Control Research Center, Baylor College of Medicine, Houston, Texas; Division of Neuroscience, Department of Psychiatry, Columbia University, New York; Institute for the Study of Disadvantage and Disability, Atlanta; Center for Autism and Related Disorders, Department Psychiatry, Children's Hospital Boston, Boston; Department of Pediatric and

Adolescent Medicine, Western Michigan University Homer Stryker MD School of Medicine, Kalamazoo, Michigan, United States; Department of Paediatrics, Child Health and Adolescent Medicine, Children's Hospital at Westmead, Westmead, Australia; International Centre for the Study of Occupational and Mental Health, Düsseldorf, Germany; Centre for Advanced Studies in Nursing, Department of General Practice and Primary Care, University of Aberdeen, Aberdeen, United Kingdom; Quality of Life Research Center, Copenhagen, Denmark; Nordic School of Public Health, Gottenburg, Sweden, Scandinavian Institute of Quality of Working Life, Oslo, Norway; The Department of Applied Social Sciences (APSS) of The Hong Kong Polytechnic University Hong Kong.

TARGETS

Our focus is on research, international collaborations, clinical work, teaching and policy in health, disability and human development and to establish the NICHD as a permanent institute at one of the residential care centers for persons with intellectual disability in Israel in order to conduct model research and together with the four university schools of public health/medicine in Israel establish a national master and doctoral program in disability and human development at the institute to secure the next generation of professionals working in this often non-prestigious/low-status field of work.

Contact

Joav Merrick, MD, MMedSci, DMSc
Professor of Pediatrics and Public Health
Medical Director, Health Services,
Division for Intellectual and Developmental Disabilities,
Ministry of Social Affairs and Social Services, POB 1260, IL-91012
Jerusalem, Israel.
E-mail: jmerrick@zahav.net.il

SECTION SIX - INDEX

INDEX

A

acquired immunodeficiency syndrome (AIDS), xix, 71, 90, 102, 135, 136, 138, 140, 142, 148, 149, 150, 151, 189, 201, 262, 339, 342, 378, 379, 441, 461, 462, 464, 465, 466, 508
adolescence, 206, 217, 219, 221, 240, 241, 257, 277, 281, 347, 375, 412, 420, 449
adolescents, 13, 33, 34, 35, 57, 63, 64, 65, 69, 70, 71, 142, 150, 181, 182, 183, 184, 186, 187, 188, 205, 206, 207, 208, 209, 211, 212, 213, 214, 215, 216, 217, 218, 219, 221, 222, 223, 224, 225, 226, 228, 230, 233, 235, 236, 237, 238, 239, 240, 241, 249, 253, 255, 256, 261, 271, 272, 273, 274, 277, 278, 279, 288, 289, 334, 379, 431, 444, 451, 466, 496
African immigrants, 333, 334, 433, 507
alcohol, 17, 40, 41, 42, 54, 93, 94, 95, 102, 103, 189, 193, 207, 208, 209, 212, 213, 214, 215, 217, 218, 221, 222, 223, 224, 225, 226, 227, 228, 229, 231, 232, 233, 240, 241, 243, 244, 245, 246, 247, 248, 249, 250, 251, 253, 254, 255, 261, 270, 273, 277, 278, 279, 280, 281, 289, 290, 291, 323, 324, 325, 326, 327, 328, 329, 330, 331, 352, 362, 378, 379, 451, 492
alcoholism, 102, 323, 324, 329, 330
American physicians, 411, 413, 414, 415, 416
Arab women, xiv, 487, 494, 503, 504
Arsenic, 173
assessment, 17, 23, 24, 30, 36, 51, 56, 57, 58, 70, 78, 79, 82, 91, 103, 106, 107, 118, 136, 160, 162, 163, 165, 166, 170, 171, 178, 197, 201, 205, 207, 214, 216, 217, 218, 244, 255, 279, 289, 295, 311, 314, 318, 321, 466

B

biosphere reserves, 105, 106, 108, 118
Black faith community, 136, 137, 138, 140, 141, 143, 147, 148
blood donors, 381, 382, 383, 384, 389
breast cancer, 264, 487, 488, 489, 490, 491, 492, 493, 494, 496, 497, 498, 499, 500, 501, 503, 504, 505, 506, 508, 512
breast self-exam, 487, 488, 492, 497, 500, 504, 505, 506
breastfeeding, 281, 282, 283, 286, 287, 288, 289, 291, 343, 344, 345, 346, 347, 348
bridging organizations, 105, 106, 107, 109, 111, 115, 117, 118

C

capacity building, 89, 91, 92, 96, 97, 98, 99, 100, 101, 108, 164, 171, 201
cardiovascular disease, 16, 40, 51, 54, 57, 60, 264, 327, 328, 329, 330, 333, 488
cardiovascular risk, 40, 41, 42, 46, 47, 48, 49, 50, 51, 53, 56, 57, 58, 60
Chicago, 73
childhood obesity, 3, 4, 5, 6, 7, 8, 9, 11, 12, 13, 40, 51, 54, 60, 431
children, xv, xviii, 3, 4, 5, 6, 7, 9, 12, 13, 17, 20, 21, 31, 39, 40, 41, 42, 43, 44, 46, 47, 48, 50, 51, 53, 54, 55, 56, 57, 58, 61, 112, 122, 123, 124, 125, 126, 127, 128, 129, 130, 133, 134, 135, 176, 179, 188, 196, 206, 207, 208, 209, 210, 211, 212, 213, 214, 215, 216, 217, 218, 225, 231, 233, 236, 237, 238, 240, 241, 252, 256, 263, 268, 270, 271, 279, 282, 324, 334, 335, 341, 344, 345, 346, 347, 352, 356, 357, 382, 389, 390, 392, 393, 394, 396, 397, 399, 400, 401, 402, 403, 405, 406, 414, 416, 427,

428, 429, 430, 431, 441, 442, 465, 466, 491, 496, 499, 508, 509, 511, 512, 515, 517, 518
chimpanzees, xvi
chronic disease, 11, 17, 57, 156, 196, 295, 298, 303, 306, 310, 518
cigarette smoking, 241, 247, 251, 282, 359, 360, 365, 367, 373, 374, 375, 376, 377, 378, 379
citizen science, 163, 164, 165, 166, 167, 174, 178, 179, 180
cleaning products, 507, 508, 509, 510, 511, 512
collaboration, 3, 4, 5, 10, 16, 17, 19, 20, 21, 28, 29, 30, 32, 34, 35, 36, 60, 73, 74, 75, 76, 77, 78, 80, 82, 83, 84, 85, 86, 87, 88, 105, 106, 107, 111, 115, 116, 117, 121, 136, 154, 155, 156, 158, 161, 166, 194, 500, 517, 518
college, xv, 15, 16, 18, 21, 24, 34, 39, 43, 49, 53, 56, 63, 65, 73, 87, 88, 135, 153, 191, 192, 194, 195, 200, 243, 244, 245, 246, 247, 248, 249, 250, 251, 252, 253, 254, 255, 268, 275, 278, 295, 303, 305, 312, 313, 314, 318, 341, 349, 351, 367, 375, 377, 378, 382, 385, 388, 389, 390, 393, 395, 399, 411, 412, 413, 415, 416, 417, 419, 420, 422, 425, 444, 450, 451, 469, 470, 471, 472, 473, 474, 478, 479, 481, 482, 483, 484, 485, 518
college athletics, 469, 471, 472, 473, 482, 483, 484
college students, 34, 243, 244, 245, 246, 247, 248, 249, 250, 251, 252, 253, 254, 255, 312, 313, 314, 375, 377, 378, 411, 412, 413, 415, 416, 417, 419, 420, 425, 444, 451, 470
community based participatory research, 17, 89, 90, 102, 134, 164, 179
community centered, 23, 121
community engagement, 16, 21, 23, 25, 119, 149, 167, 183, 186, 192
community-academic partnership, 163, 164, 165, 167, 176, 177, 178
community-engaged research, 181, 182, 185
co-morbidity, 205
concept mapping, 102, 135, 136, 138, 139, 141, 143, 150
contaminated sites, 164, 165, 180
continuing professional education, 73, 74, 75, 76, 86, 88
counseling, 56, 61, 136, 137, 150, 196, 207, 252, 281, 289, 349, 393, 417, 425, 444, 461, 462
critical consciousness theory, 89, 92
cross-sectoral collaboration, 105, 106, 107, 115, 116, 117
culture, xvi, xvii, xviii, 110, 111, 112, 113, 143, 150, 151, 162, 189, 195, 198, 200, 207, 235, 246, 333, 334, 335, 337, 338, 339, 340, 409, 411, 412, 413, 415, 416, 420, 425, 433, 434, 435, 436, 438, 439,

440, 441, 442, 450, 466, 471, 479, 494, 505, 507, 508, 510, 511

D

design, 9, 21, 32, 35, 66, 76, 77, 78, 79, 86, 92, 101, 121, 123, 124, 128, 130, 132, 133, 134, 137, 138, 143, 148, 149, 157, 158, 159, 161, 167, 169, 178, 209, 210, 295, 401, 421, 425, 431, 447, 451, 463, 473, 512
diverse cultures, xv
doping, 257, 258, 260, 261, 262, 266, 269, 270, 271, 272, 274, 275
dual degree program, 15, 16, 17, 19

E

eating patterns, 419, 420, 421, 423, 425
Ebola virus, xvi, xix
education, xix, 6, 8, 9, 10, 12, 15, 17, 18, 19, 24, 29, 30, 31, 33, 34, 39, 40, 41, 43, 47, 48, 49, 50, 51, 53, 54, 55, 56, 58, 59, 60, 61, 63, 66, 69, 71, 73, 74, 75, 76, 78, 79, 80, 81, 86, 87, 88, 108, 113, 121, 122, 123, 124, 125, 126, 127, 133, 멸134, 136, 141, 142, 143, 148, 149, 150, 153, 154, 155, 157, 162, 164, 165, 166, 174, 178, 180, 192, 193, 194, 195, 196, 197, 198, 199, 201, 207, 246, 247, 259, 282, 290, 333, 340, 343, 344, 346, 347, 349, 350, 355, 382, 383, 385, 388, 389, 390, 393, 394, 395, 396, 400, 406, 413, 420, 424, 425, 433, 435, 436, 440, 446, 449, 451, 462, 463, 465, 466, 470, 473, 474, 475, 476, 477, 479, 483, 484, 496, 497, 499, 500, 501, 503, 509, 518
environmental exposure assessment, 164
environmental health, 17, 19, 63, 105, 106, 107, 111, 112, 113, 116, 118, 135, 163, 165, 174, 175, 179, 180, 507
exercise, 4, 40, 41, 42, 44, 46, 48, 57, 59, 88, 111, 153, 157, 159, 187, 263, 267, 270, 272, 274, 275, 333, 334, 335, 336, 337, 338, 339, 340, 341, 352, 378, 430, 431, 438, 444

F

females, 64, 68, 70, 183, 221, 223, 225, 226, 227, 234, 238, 240, 339, 340, 341, 385, 389, 421, 450, 455, 488, 494, 499, 503
filoviridae, xvi
financial, xvii, 23, 29, 39, 40, 41, 42, 43, 44, 45, 47, 48, 49, 50, 51, 53, 54, 55, 56, 57, 58, 59, 60, 90,

99, 110, 121, 179, 184, 186, 193, 200, 216, 333, 404, 435, 439, 481, 499, 501
financial stress, 40, 44, 48, 50, 53, 54, 56, 58, 59, 60
fitness, 8, 9, 271, 273, 275, 333, 337, 339, 484
food, vi, xviii, 4, 5, 8, 9, 39, 40, 41, 42, 44, 46, 48, 49, 56, 63, 64, 92, 106, 111, 112, 113, 115, 123, 126, 127, 128, 132, 171, 173, 175, 197, 199, 200, 237, 254, 259, 261, 267, 323, 330, 334, 339, 346, 347, 348, 419, 420, 421, 422, 423, 424, 425, 438, 444, 496
fruit bats, xvi

G

gardening, 134, 164, 166, 167, 169, 170, 173, 174, 180
Ghana, 336, 337, 342, 343, 344, 346, 347, 436
girls, 63, 64, 65, 70, 125, 221, 222, 223, 224, 225, 226, 227, 228, 229, 232, 233, 234, 235, 236, 238, 239, 240, 241, 261, 263, 391, 466
gorillas, xvi
grounded theory, 342, 421, 435, 469, 473, 475, 484, 485

H

HBCU, 469, 470, 471, 472, 473, 474, 475, 476, 477, 478, 479, 480, 481, 482
health care delivery, 76, 86, 153, 182, 185, 186, 187, 188
health care workers, 343, 344
health promotion, 17, 105, 106, 107, 108, 109, 110, 111, 112, 113, 114, 115, 116, 117, 118, 119, 150, 151, 159, 191, 341, 434, 443, 501, 503
healthcare system, xv, 191, 193, 194, 198, 402, 412, 416, 500, 503
hemorrhagic fever, xvi
HIV, 71, 89, 90, 92, 94, 95, 96, 97, 98, 101, 102, 135, 136, 137, 138, 139, 140, 141, 142, 143, 144, 145, 146, 147, 148, 149, 150, 151, 193, 201, 262, 264, 286, 338, 339, 342, 377, 378, 379, 441, 444, 451, 461, 462, 463, 464, 465, 466, 467
HIV intervention strategies, 136, 137
HIV testing, 461, 462, 463, 464, 465, 466
HIV/HCV prevention, 89, 90
homeless adolescents, 181, 182, 183, 184, 185, 186, 187, 188, 189
human immunodeficiency virus, 136, 262, 461
Human papillomavirus, 64, 70, 71

I

IgG sero-prevalence, 382
immigrants, xv, 201, 327, 333, 334, 335, 336, 339, 340, 341, 411, 412, 416, 419, 433, 434, 440, 441, 462, 465
India, 349
infant mortality, 27, 28, 30, 31, 32, 33, 34, 35, 36
international students, 412, 413, 415, 416, 417, 419, 420, 422, 424, 425
interprofessional, 15, 16, 17, 18, 21, 53, 56, 57, 58, 60, 73, 74, 75, 76, 77, 78, 79, 80, 81, 82, 85, 86, 87, 88, 153, 154, 155, 156, 157, 158, 159, 160, 161, 162, 191, 192, 194, 201
interprofessional collaboration, 16, 21, 53, 56, 73, 74, 75, 76, 78, 79, 80, 82, 85, 86, 87, 154, 162, 191
Interprofessional education, 73, 77, 79, 80, 87, 88, 153, 154, 162
ischemic priapism, 349, 351, 352, 355

L

landscape, 11, 28, 111, 112, 113, 118, 121, 122, 123, 124, 128, 130, 132, 134
locus of control, 61, 360, 375, 377
loneliness, 295, 296, 297, 298, 313, 314, 315, 316, 317, 318, 320, 321

M

macaques, xvi
male, 43, 66, 67, 95, 97, 125, 183, 185, 222, 223, 226, 238, 239, 245, 250, 261, 263, 265, 272, 273, 301, 329, 337, 339, 353, 365, 367, 379, 385, 386, 388, 395, 399, 421, 422, 423, 433, 447, 457, 463, 464, 465, 466, 467
mammogram, 487, 489, 492, 504, 505
master of public health, 15, 16, 19, 517
medical education, 15, 16, 17, 18, 23, 24, 25, 88
mission statements, 109, 469, 472, 473, 474, 475, 478, 479, 481, 482, 483, 484
monkeys, xvi, 283
Moscow, 323
MSW, 89, 181

O

obesity prevention, 3, 6, 7, 8, 9, 12, 13, 334
Oklahoma, 181

oral health, 17, 416, 433, 434, 435, 436, 437, 440, 441

P

partnership, 8, 15, 17, 27, 29, 30, 31, 32, 33, 34, 35, 36, 37, 56, 58, 60, 65, 69, 75, 108, 112, 113, 116, 122, 135, 137, 139, 141, 149, 160, 164, 165, 166, 167, 175, 176, 179, 180, 192, 194, 197, 201, 202, 395, 396, 403
peer teen educators, 64, 65, 69
phenomenological, 320, 336, 343, 344, 411, 414, 417, 419, 421, 425, 445, 446, 447, 451, 504, 506, 508, 509, 512
phenomenology, 217, 335, 342, 421, 425, 443, 445, 508
physical activity, 5, 6, 7, 8, 9, 12, 13, 61, 111, 115, 121, 134, 334, 336, 340, 341, 342, 427, 428, 429, 430, 431, 444, 491, 492, 494, 496, 497
pregnancy, 27, 28, 31, 33, 34, 35, 36, 202, 226, 227, 229, 230, 231, 236, 238, 240, 241, 277, 278, 279, 280, 281, 282, 283, 284, 286, 287, 288, 289, 290, 291, 360, 377, 382, 383, 391, 444, 450, 494, 508
prevalence, 4, 5, 7, 12, 13, 54, 58, 64, 70, 71, 137, 193, 205, 216, 217, 226, 228, 243, 245, 246, 253, 254, 255, 261, 271, 272, 321, 329, 330, 342, 349, 350, 352, 356, 381, 382, 383, 389, 390, 392, 394, 405, 428, 430, 450, 463, 496, 499, 512
priapism, 349, 350, 351, 352, 353, 354, 355, 356, 357
problem-based learning, 73, 74, 76, 88
psychiatry, 18, 103, 202, 205, 206, 216, 217, 218, 219, 221, 241, 243, 255, 256, 272, 290, 321, 330, 352, 405, 518
public health, xv, xvi, xix, 3, 4, 5, 6, 7, 8, 10, 11, 12, 13, 15, 16, 17, 18, 19, 20, 21, 22, 23, 24, 27, 28, 29, 30, 32, 33, 34, 35, 36, 37, 53, 54, 58, 60, 61, 63, 64, 71, 73, 74, 75, 78, 86, 87, 88, 89, 102, 105, 106, 107, 110, 111, 112, 113, 114, 116, 117, 137, 143, 148, 150, 151, 167, 180, 191, 192, 194, 195, 200, 202, 240, 241, 244, 245, 247, 248, 253, 254, 272, 273, 274, 293, 321, 323, 326, 330, 331, 333, 334, 341, 342, 343, 348, 356, 359, 360, 363, 367, 368, 372, 373, 376, 379, 381, 382, 391, 393, 394, 401, 402, 403, 404, 405, 407, 411, 419, 427, 431, 433, 441, 443, 444, 450, 453, 461, 466, 469, 487, 496, 500, 507, 515, 517, 518, 519
public participation in scientific research, 163, 164, 178, 179
PWI, 469, 470, 471, 472, 473, 474, 475, 476, 477, 478, 479, 480, 481, 482

Q

qualitative research, 88, 118, 181, 186, 188, 189, 335, 336, 342, 425, 443, 451, 463, 473, 484, 485

R

rare disease, 295, 296, 297, 315, 318, 319, 320
refugees, 191, 192, 193, 194, 195, 196, 197, 198, 199, 200, 201, 202, 334, 336, 425, 461
religion, 95, 150, 151, 192, 337, 338, 341, 378, 443, 445, 446, 447, 448, 449, 501
reoffending, 89, 90, 92, 94, 98, 101
risk communication, 163, 164, 165, 166, 171, 177, 178, 179, 401
rubella, 381, 382, 383, 384, 385, 386, 388, 389, 390, 391, 392, 405, 407
rural areas, xvii, 121, 122, 129, 132, 326, 349, 352, 385, 427, 428, 429, 430, 445
rural India, 349, 427, 445, 450
rural schools, 121
Russia, xiii, 323, 326, 327, 328, 329, 330, 331

S

sexual behaviors in young adults, 443, 449
sickle cell disease, 349, 350, 351, 352, 353, 355, 356, 357
sidewalks, 427, 428, 429
Sinai, 243
social isolation, 295, 296, 297, 298, 300, 302, 313, 315, 316, 317, 318, 319, 320, 321, 366, 370, 472
social media, 59, 63, 65, 66, 68, 69, 453, 454, 455, 456, 458, 460
sports, 113, 124, 126, 127, 134, 257, 258, 259, 260, 261, 262, 263, 264, 266, 267, 268, 269, 270, 271, 272, 273, 274, 275, 338, 341, 453, 454, 455, 456, 458, 459, 460, 469, 471, 472, 474, 482, 483, 484, 485
Spring, 295
stress, 40, 44, 50, 51, 53, 54, 58, 59, 60, 61, 188, 193, 206, 217, 225, 230, 232, 234, 248, 282, 308, 324, 325, 326, 330, 412, 416, 420, 425
students, 4, 7, 8, 13, 15, 16, 17, 18, 19, 20, 21, 22, 23, 27, 29, 30, 31, 32, 33, 34, 36, 56, 58, 71, 74, 80, 87, 121, 122, 123, 124, 125, 126, 127, 128, 129, 130, 132, 133, 140, 153, 154, 155, 156, 157, 158, 159, 160, 161, 162, 192, 194, 195, 196, 197, 198, 199, 201, 226, 227, 240, 243, 244, 245, 246, 247, 248, 249, 250, 251, 252, 253, 254, 255, 272, 288, 303, 308, 324, 335, 336, 375, 383, 411, 412, 413, 414, 415, 416, 419, 420, 421, 422, 423, 425,

462, 465, 466, 470, 472, 473, 476, 477, 478, 480, 481, 500, 506, 518
stuttering, 349, 351, 352, 353, 355
substance abuse, 17, 37, 89, 90, 92, 93, 100, 101, 102, 182, 203, 205, 207, 216, 217, 218, 221, 222, 223, 224, 225, 226, 227, 228, 229, 230, 232, 233, 234, 235, 236, 237, 238, 239, 240, 241, 243, 244, 248, 250, 252, 253, 255, 257, 273, 277, 278, 279, 282, 286, 289, 290, 378, 379
substance abuse treatment, 37, 89, 90, 100, 235, 236, 237, 239
sustainability, 9, 23, 30, 48, 105, 106, 107, 109, 111, 112, 113, 114, 115, 116, 121, 148, 179, 189, 200, 201
sustainable development, 105, 106, 107, 108, 109, 110, 112, 113, 114, 115, 116, 117, 118

T

task force, 3, 4, 5, 6, 7, 9, 10, 11, 12, 20
technology, xiv, 19, 166, 265, 270, 330, 414, 453, 455, 456, 458, 459, 460, 479, 484
teenage pregnancy, 240, 277, 278
tobacco regulation, 360
translational research, 27
transportation, 6, 8, 10, 17, 112, 127, 129, 199, 200, 335, 339, 383, 427, 430, 431, 444
Turkish immigrants, xiv, 461, 463, 466

U

Uganda, xvi, 121, 122, 123, 124, 126, 128, 129, 133, 134, 336, 337

United States (USA), xv, 3, 15, 27, 39, 53, 63, 73, 89, 121, 135, 153, 163, 181, 191, 205, 221, 243, 257, 277, 295, 333, 343, 393, 411, 419, 427, 433, 443, 453, 461, 469, 487, 507

V

voluntary testing, 461, 462
vulnerable population, 92, 154, 155, 156, 157, 159, 161, 162, 205, 379, 412, 500

W

Washington, 393
WHO, 381
Wisconsin, 63
women, xviii, 28, 31, 33, 35, 36, 39, 40, 41, 43, 44, 47, 48, 49, 50, 51, 53, 54, 55, 56, 57, 58, 59, 60, 64, 71, 97, 99, 102, 103, 142, 193, 199, 202, 221, 231, 232, 233, 234, 235, 236, 237, 238, 240, 241, 244, 245, 264, 277, 278, 280, 282, 284, 286, 288, 289, 290, 291, 305, 324, 333, 334, 337, 338, 339, 341, 342, 347, 348, 356, 374, 378, 381, 382, 389, 390, 391, 450, 471, 478, 487, 488, 489, 490, 492, 493, 494, 496, 497, 498, 499, 501, 503, 505, 506, 507, 508, 510, 511, 512
workforce training, 73, 74, 86

Z

Zambia, 381, 382, 383, 384, 389, 390, 391